Modified-Release
Drug Delivery Technology

DRUGS AND THE PHARMACEUTICAL SCIENCES
A Series of Textbooks and Monographs

Executive Editor
James Swarbrick
PharmaceuTech, Inc.
Pinehurst, North Carolina

Advisory Board

Modified-Release Drug Delivery Technology

Second Edition

Volume 2

edited by

Michael J. Rathbone
InterAg
Hamilton, New Zealand

Jonathan Hadgraft
University of London
London, UK

Michael S. Roberts
University of Queensland
Brisbane, Australia

Majella E. Lane
University of London
London, UK

informa
healthcare

New York   London

Informa Healthcare USA, Inc.
52 Vanderbilt Avenue
New York, NY 10017

International Standard Book Number-10: 1-4200-4435-4 (v. 1: Hardcover)
International Standard Book Number-13: 978-1-4200-4435-5 (v. 1: Hardcover)
International Standard Book Number-10: 1-4200-5355-8 (v. 2: Hardcover)
International Standard Book Number-13: 978-1-4200-5355-5 (v. 2: Hardcover)

Library of Congress Cataloging-in-Publication Data

Modified-release drug delivery technology/edited by
Michael J. Rathbone . . . [et al.]. - - 2nd ed.
    v. < 1- > ; cm. - - (Drugs and the pharmaceutical sciences ; v. 183, etc.)
    Includes bibliographical references and index.
    ISBN-13: 978-1-4200-5355-5 (hb : alk. paper)
    ISBN-10: 1-4200-5355-8 (hb : alk. paper) 1. Controlled release technology. 2. Controlled
release preparations. I. Rathbone, Michael J., 1957- II. Series.
    [DNLM: 1. Delayed-Action Preparations. 2. Drug Delivery Systems. 3. Technology,
Pharmaceutical. W1 DR893B v. 183 2008 / QV 785 M692 2008]
    RS201. C64M63 2008
    615′.6–dc22   2007047360

For Corporate Sales and Reprint Permissions call 212-520-2700 or write to:
Sales Department, 52 Vanderbilt Avenue, 16th floor, New York, NY 10017.

Visit the Informa web site at
www.informa.com

and the Informa Healthcare Web site at
www.informahealthcare.com

To my son Benjamin

—Michael J. Rathbone

Preface

Over the last few decades, rapid developments have occurred in the area of modified-release drug delivery technology, and significant research and development has occurred in all routes of drug delivery. This is an ever-expanding area of pharmaceutical research, and so we decided to update and expand *Modified-Release Drug Delivery Technology* to achieve a more comprehensive compilation of information.

To this end, the Second Edition is divided into two volumes. Volume 1 addresses modified-release drug delivery technologies developed for the oral mucosal and gastrointestinal routes. Volume 2 addresses modified-release drug delivery technologies for the parenteral, dermal, pulmonary, nasal, vaginal, and ocular routes. Both volumes assume that the reader is already familiar with fundamental controlled-release theories. The volumes are divided into discrete parts, each of which is defined by the route for drug delivery. Individual parts begin with an overview, written by the leaders in the respective fields. They cover the anatomical, physiological, and pharmaceutical challenges inherent in formulating a modified-release drug delivery technology for a particular route of drug delivery. Each overview is followed by chapters that provide specific examples of the different approaches that have been taken to design and develop an innovative modified-release drug delivery system for those routes (written by experts in that specific technology).

Modified-Release Drug Delivery Technology, Second Edition, aims to describe as many examples of modified-release drug delivery technologies as possible. Ultimately, however, inclusion of a given technology in this book was based on author availability, rather than the desire to include a particular technology or to select or reject a particular technology based on its relative merits. We hope that the selection is representative of each field.

The first part of Volume 2, edited by Stephen Perrett and Michael J. Rathbone, contains chapters that provide an overview of the modified drug release landscape as observed from the commercial (Perrett) and academic (Siepmann) viewpoints. An evaluation of the role of modified-release formulations to address patient and doctors' needs (Anelli), and a viewpoint on investors' requirements (Walton) are also discussed in this part. These chapters provide an interesting insight into how these different disciples view this area of research. In Part II, Robert Gurny and colleagues provide an overview of currently available and emerging modified-release ophthalmic drug delivery systems. Most of these systems are in the developmental stage, but several technologies that have reached commercialization are described in depth. Part III addresses implant and injection technologies. In their introduction section leaders Majella Lane, Franklin Okumu, and Palani Balausubramanian offer a comprehensive overview of this evolving and challenging area of drug delivery. They complement their overview with chapters that cover a diverse range of implant and injection technologies. Section leaders for Part IV, Jonathan Hadgraft, Majella Lane, and Adam Watkinson, have written a thorough overview of the dermal and transdermal area and have organized a series of chapters that cover a wide range of diverse technologies, from wound dressings, through nail delivery, to propulsion of solid drug particles into the skin by means of a high-speed gas flow. Patches that deliver drugs via diffusion, iontophoresis, sonophoresis, or microprojections are also covered.

The nasal route is covered in Part V. Section leader Ashim Mitra offers an instructive overview into this interesting route of drug delivery that highlights how difficult drug delivery can be for this route of administration. David Woolfson (Part VI leader, vaginal route) presents a comprehensive account of the biological and pharmaceutical challenges to the vaginal route of drug delivery, which is restricted to 50 percent of the population and is limited by cultural and societal constraints. The chapters associated with this section provide an insight into the different approaches that can be employed to deliver drugs via the vaginal mucosa. In the final section of this book (Part VII) section leader Paul Myrdal provides an informative overview of the unique challenges associated with delivering drugs via the pulmonary tract. The chapters in Part VII describe the various systems, devices, formulations, and methods of drug delivery to the lung. The focus of pulmonary drug delivery systems tends not to be on the control of medicament release from the formulations in which they are presented, but rather on inhalation systems that deliver drugs practically instantaneously to the target organ (which is the "release" part for therapeutic activity for many of the currently approved products for inhalation). Numerous different technological approaches are described in the chapters associated with this section, each of which provides descriptive comments on the complexity of this route of drug delivery.

We would like to express our thanks to each of the section leaders, who spent a great deal of time identifying technologies, writing informative overviews, and editing the chapters associated with the routes of drug delivery in which they are expert. We would also like to thank all of the authors who contributed chapters to this book, whose individual innovative research activities have contributed so much to the current modified-release drug delivery technology portfolio that exists today. We thank them for taking the time to share their experiences and work.

Michael J. Rathbone
Jonathan Hadgraft
Michael S. Roberts
Majella E. Lane

Contents

PART III: INJECTION AND IMPLANT TECHNOLOGIES

PART IV: DERMAL AND TRANSDERMAL TECHNOLOGIES

Contributors

Marco M. Anelli   Research and Development, Keypharma, Milan, Italy

B. Steven Angersbach   College of Pharmacy, University of Arizona, Tucson, Arizona, U.S.A.

Ian C. Ashurst   GlaxoSmithKline Research and Development, Ware, Hertfordshire, U.K.

Jay Audett   ALZA Corporation, Mountain View, California, U.S.A.

Mimoun Ayoub   Genzyme Pharmaceuticals, Liestal, Switzerland

Palani Balausubramanian   DURECT Corporation, Cupertino, California, U.S.A.

Leila Bossy   Department of Pharmaceutics and Biopharmaceutics, School of Pharmaceutical Sciences, University of Geneva, University of Lausanne, Geneva, Switzerland

Keith R. Brain   An-eX Analytical Services Ltd., Cardiff, U.K.

Gregor Cevc   IDEA AG, Munich, Germany

Hak-Kim Chan   Faculty of Pharmacy, University of Sydney, Australia

Guohua Chen   ALZA Corporation, Mountain View, California, U.S.A.

David C. Cipolla   Aradigm Corporation, Hayward, California, U.S.A.

Andrew R. Clark   Nektar Therapeutics, San Carlos, California, U.S.A.

Michel Cormier   ALZA Corporation, Mountain View, California, U.S.A.

Peter Crocker   Imprint Pharmaceuticals Ltd., OCFI, Oxford, U.K.

John Culwell   DURECT Corporation, Cupertino, California, U.S.A.

Peter E. Daddona   Zosano Pharma, Fremont, California, U.S.A.

Eric J. Dadey   QLT USA, Inc., Fort Collins, Colorado, U.S.A.

Florence Delie   Department of Pharmaceutics and Biopharmaceutics, School of Pharmaceutical Sciences, University of Geneva, University of Lausanne, Geneva, Switzerland

John Denyer   Respironics Respiratory Drug Delivery (UK) Ltd., Chichester, U.K.

Signe Erickson   SurModics, Inc., Irvine, California, U.S.A.

Olivia Felt   Department of Pharmaceutics and Biopharmaceutics, School of Pharmaceutical Sciences, University of Geneva, University of Lausanne, Geneva, Switzerland

Warren Finlay   Department of Mechanical Engineering, University of Alberta, Edmonton, Alberta, Canada

Kirk D. Fowers   Protherics Plc, West Valley City, Utah, U.S.A.

Pascal Furrer   Department of Pharmaceutics and Biopharmaceutics, School of Pharmaceutical Sciences, University of Geneva, University of Lausanne, Geneva, Switzerland

Ripal Gaudana   University of Missouri-Kansas City, Kansas City, Missouri, U.S.A.

Harvinder S. Gill   The Wallace H. Coulter Department of Biomedical Engineering at Georgia Tech and Emory University, Georgia Institute of Technology, Atlanta, Georgia, U.S.A.

Marc Giroux   Kurve Technology, Inc., Bothell, Washington, D.C., U.S.A.

Marshall Grant   Formulation Development, MannKind Corporation, Danbury, Connecticut, U.S.A.

Darren M. Green   An-eX Analytical Services Ltd., Cardiff, U.K.

Jennifer Gudeman   KV Pharmaceutical Company, St. Louis, Missouri, U.S.A.

Robert Gurny   Department of Pharmaceutics and Biopharmaceutics, School of Pharmaceutical Sciences, University of Geneva, University of Lausanne, Geneva, Switzerland

J. Richard Gyory   Transform Pharmaceuticals, Lexington, Massachusetts, U.S.A.

Jonathan Hadgraft   School of Pharmacy, University of London, London, U.K.

Janet A. Halliday   Controlled Therapeutics (Scotland) Limited, East Kilbride, Lanarkshire, U.K.

Anthony J. Hickey   School of Pharmacy, Division of Molecular Pharmaceutics, University of North Carolina-Chapel Hill, Kerr Hall-Dispersed Systems Laboratory, Chapel Hill, North Carolina, U.S.A.

Peter Hwang   Stanford Sinus Center, Stanford University School of Medicine, Stanford, California, U.S.A.

Rajni Jani   Pharmaceutical Research and Development, Alcon Research Ltd., Fort Worth, Texas, U.S.A.

Eric Johansson   Aradigm Corporation, Hayward, California, U.S.A.

Gunjan Junnarkar   ALZA Corporation, Mountain View, California, U.S.A.

Pradeep K. Karla   University of Missouri-Kansas City, Kansas City, Missouri, U.S.A.

Troels Keldmann   DirectHaler A/S, Copenhagen, Denmark

Patrick F. Kiser   Department of Bioengineering, University of Utah, Salt Lake City, Utah, U.S.A.

Martin Knoch   PARI Pharma GmbH, Starnberg, Germany

Joseph Kost   Department of Chemical Engineering, Ben Gurion University of the Negev, Beer-Sheva, Israel

Deep Kwatra   University of Missouri-Kansas City, Kansas City, Missouri, U.S.A.

William J. Lambert   Pacira Pharmaceuticals, Inc., San Diego, California, U.S.A.

Majella E. Lane   School of Pharmacy, University of London, London, U.K.

Mathew Leigh   PHARES Drug Delivery AG, Muttenz, Switzerland

Andrea Leone-Bay   Pharmaceutical Development, MannKind Corporation, Danbury, Connecticut, U.S.A.

R. Saul Levinson   KV Pharmaceutical Company, St. Louis, Missouri, U.S.A.

Kathy Los   Pacira Pharmaceuticals, Inc., San Diego, California, U.S.A.

Tamar Lotan   NanoCyte Inc., Jordan Valley, Israel

R. Karl Malcolm   School of Pharmacy, Queen's University Belfast, Medical Biology Centre, Belfast, Northern Ireland, U.K.

Heidi M. Mansour   School of Pharmacy, Division of Molecular Pharmaceutics, University of North Carolina-Chapel Hill, Kerr Hall-Dispersed Systems Laboratory, Chapel Hill, North Carolina, U.S.A.

Juan A. Mantelle   Noven Pharmaceuticals, Inc., Miami, Florida, U.S.A.

Francis J. Martin   Eclipse Nanomedical, Inc., San Francisco, California, U.S.A.

Kevin Maynard   Imprint Pharmaceuticals Ltd., OCFI, Oxford, U.K.

Ashim K. Mitra   University of Missouri-Kansas City, Kansas City, Missouri, U.S.A.

Samir Mitragotri   Department of Chemical Engineering, University of California, Santa Barbara, California, U.S.A.

Achim Moser   Boehringer Ingelheim MicroParts GmbH, Dortmund, Germany

Rainer H. Müller   Department of Pharmacy, Free University of Berlin, Berlin, Germany

Paul B. Myrdal   College of Pharmacy, University of Arizona, Tucson, Arizona, U.S.A.

Kurt Nikander   Respironics, Inc., Respiratory Drug Delivery, Parsippany, New Jersey, U.S.A.

Franklin W. Okumu   DURECT Corporation, Cupertino, California, U.S.A.

Rama Padmanabhan   ALZA Corporation, Mountain View, California, U.S.A.

Jung-Hwan Park   Kyungwon University, Seoul, Korea

Steven Percival   ConvaTec Wound Therapeutics™, Global Development Centre, Deeside, Flintshire, U.K.

Stephen Perrett   Eurand, Vandalia, Ohio, U.S.A.

Rolf D. Petersen   Department of Pharmacy, Free University of Berlin, Berlin, Germany

J. Bradley Phipps   ALZA Corporation, Mountain View, California, U.S.A.

Bernard Plazonnet   Chamalières, France

Ajay Prasad   University of Delaware, Newark, Delaware, U.S.A.

Mark R. Prausnitz   School of Chemical and Biomolecular Engineering, Georgia Institute of Technology, Atlanta, Georgia, U.S.A.

Lakshmi Raghavan   Vyteris, Inc., Fair Lawn, New Jersey, U.S.A.

Ramesh C. Rathi   Protherics Plc, West Valley City, Utah, U.S.A.

Erin Rhone   Pharmaceutical Research and Development, Alcon Research Ltd., Fort Worth, Texas, U.S.A.

Steve Robertson   Controlled Therapeutics (Scotland) Limited, East Kilbride, Lanarkshire, U.K.

Ashutosh Sharma   Vyteris, Inc., Fair Lawn, New Jersey, U.S.A.

Florence Siepmann   College of Pharmacy, University of Lille, Lille, France

Juergen Siepmann   College of Pharmacy, University of Lille, Lille, France

Alan Smith   Altea Therapeutics Corporation, Atlanta, Georgia, U.S.A.

Eliana B. Souto   Health Sciences Department, Fernando Pessoa University, Porto, Portugal

Janet Tamada   ALZA Corporation, Mountain View, California, U.S.A.

Daniel J. Thompson   KV Pharmaceutical Company, St. Louis, Missouri, U.S.A.

Eric Tomlinson   Altea Therapeutics Corporation, Atlanta, Georgia, U.S.A.

A. Neil Verity   DURECT Corporation, Cupertino, California, U.S.A.

Herbert Wachtel   Boehringer Ingelheim Pharma GmbH & Co. KG, Ingelheim, Germany

Michael Walker   ConvaTec Wound Therapeutics™, Global Development Centre, Deeside, Flintshire, U.K.

Kenneth A. Walters   An-eX Analytical Services Ltd., Cardiff, U.K.

Fintan Walton   Pharma Ventures Ltd., Oxford, U.K.

Adam C. Watkinson   Acrux Ltd., Melbourne, Australia

Christina Wedemeyer   Genzyme Pharmaceuticals, Liestal, Switzerland

Jeffry G. Weers   Nektar Therapeutics, San Carlos, California, U.S.A.

Torsten Wöhr   Genzyme Pharmaceuticals, Liestal, Switzerland

A. David Woolfson   School of Pharmacy, Queen's University Belfast, Medical Biology Centre, Belfast, Northern Ireland, U.K.

Jeremy C. Wright   DURECT Corporation, Cupertino, California, U.S.A.

*Part I: Using Modified-Release Formulations
to Maintain and Develop Markets*

1

The Modified-Release Drug
Delivery Landscape

The Commercial Perspective

Stephen Perrett
Eurand, Vandalia, Ohio, U.S.A.

The life cycle management of pharmaceutical products through reformulation is an established practice in the industry and, historically, many commentators have recognized the opportunity that reformulation can represent for specialist companies and technology-focused innovators. The 1990s saw an increasing number of companies being created that based business models on the development of established therapeutic compounds as this offered pharmaceutical product development which was faster, cost less, and had a large part of the therapeutic risk removed. The estimated size of market represented by reformulation varies between commentators and relies upon the definition of drug delivery, but figures from Datamonitor estimate it to be currently worth in the region of $114 billion. If one also considers that on average between 2002 and 2005, 39% of all new product launches by the top 50 manufacturers were reformulations of existing drugs (MIDAS prescribing insights: IMS Health March 2006) and that IMS placed the global Pharmaceutical Market in 2006 at $643 billion, then the monetary value of reformulation is clearly significant.

COMMERCIAL DRIVERS OF REFORMULATION

The goal and driver for product reformulation is the generation of a positive return on the investment made to develop and launch a reformulated product and both innovators and companies specializing in reformulation must carefully consider the financial implications in deciding whether or not to adopt this strategy for a given compound as although reformulating a product may improve it, it may not ultimately be worth it. Reformulation strategies generally seek to expand the market for a compound, to defend the market of a compound or to create a new market for a compound. There is inevitably some crossover in the strategies used and the approach taken is also a function of the competitiveness of the compound as it is and the actions of competitors.

In seeking to expand a market innovators are looking to take a compound into new areas through label expansion, this generally involves new clinical studies, it may also involve the concurrent production of dosage forms that are more friendly to a particular patient group—such as orally disintegrating tablets (ODTs) or suspension formulations.

In defending their markets, innovators are seeking to make their products more competitive by, e.g., launching once a day formulations into a therapeutic area where competing products are dosed multiple times per day. The most common form of market defense, however, is defense against generic launch and innovators seek to extend the life cycle of the brand by making it non-substitutable by a generic product, this means that for-mulation changes need not necessarily improve product performance, although this would be a desired outcome.

The final reformulation approach is to seek to create a new market for an already generic compound and, when they are not partnered with innovators, this is where specialist reformulation companies operate. This is not just the preserve of specialist companies and innovators will also play in this space if they see an opportunity. The strategic driver of reformulation depends on the position of a compound in the life cycle of a brand. The weights that are given to differentiation, in the sense of just being different, and true therapeutic differentiation vary greatly at different points in the life cycle. As discussed below, differentiation for generic defense need only mean that the product is different from the product used in an abbreviated new drug application (ANDA) filing, whereas a reformulation launched into an already generic market must represent a significant therapeutic improve-ment over the now commoditized product.

GENERIC DEFENSE

Differentiation from Generic Products

The goal of reformulation as a means of generic defense is clear: to prevent the substitution of the branded product by generics on patent expiry. To do this it is sufficient to alter the branded product only to the extent that it is no longer the same as the product that the generic companies are using as the reference for their registrations. This prevents pharmacies substituting generic product for the reformulated branded product which will not have been used as a reference formulation. It is essential that the brand holder switch their patients to the new formulation prior to generic launch and the timing of the launch of the new formulation is crucial. If it is launched too soon then the generics will simply use the new formulation as the reference, if it is launched too late then the market for the brand will have already been lost to the generics.

One of the clearest and most successful instances of this has been the successive reformulations of fenofibrate by Fournier (now Solvay), who have succeeded in defending Tricor® (Abbott) through changing the dosage strength or the form of the product. The first product iteration was a 300-mg capsule containing particulate drug; the second, a capsule containing 200 mg of finely milled drug; the third a 160-mg tablet containing finely milled drug and surfactant; the fourth a 145-mg tablet containing nano-particulate drug—all of these formulations are bioequivalent to one another. Progressive size reduction resulted in more than a two-fold increase in bioavailability, but all were bioequivalent to one another and essentially directly substitutable formulations from a medical perspective: however, they are not directly substitutable from a regulatory perspective. This means that scrips written for Tricor® cannot be substituted in the pharmacy and this is true even if the dosage from is changed from a capsule to a tablet. That said, the final nanoparticulate formulation did enable Abbot to remove the food requirement for dosing from the label.

It is debatable whether any of these changes represented anything other than a repackaging of the same ingredient; however, through the use of successive periods of market exclusivity associated with the new dosages the brand has been able to avoid substitution by generics, thus preserving its value through three successive expirations of market exclusivity, as the innovator was able to switch patients to the new formulation prior to this. The great advantage to this approach was that it was a relatively inexpensive series of progressions from the perspective of the clinical registration requirement in that no efficacy studies were required for formulations that aimed only at bioequivalence.

That it is the brand that drives value is further illustrated in the case of this drug by Scieles nanoparticulate product of fenofibrate licensed from Skyepharma, which is a low-dose small-particle formulation. The Sciele product was largely similar to Tricor® and had a similar label, including the lack of a food requirement, yet it was reported by Sciele to have only 1.8% of total prescriptions at the end of the first quarter 2007. That sales are a tiny fraction of those of the Tricor® brand may seem predictable, but it is perhaps salutary to those who might think that the pharmaceutical market differs substantially from any other.

While the market considerations driving Tricor® seem to have been paramount, there are other reformulation examples that more readily retain a link between product improvement and market defense. Pfizer's Procardia XL®, which used the Alza [now Johnson & Johnson; (J&J)] Oros® sustained release tablet technology, changed the dosage form from a capsule to a tablet, changed the divided dosage form to a once daily dosage form which also provided for a zero-order drug release. Despite the fact that pharmacokinetic profile of this formulation was eventually duplicated, the proprietary nature of the formulation and its differentiated release characteristics were enough to prevent direct generic substitution of the brand for over 10 years.

Timing of Reformulation

As mentioned above, timing is of crucial in optimizing the commercial returns from a compound through its product life cycle and innovators must launch at the right time, to launch too soon is to squander the 3 years of market exclusivity offered by the FDA on the basis of new clinical studies, to launch too late is not only to have missed this, but to launch into a market in which reference pricing will have seriously eroded.

As an illustration, GlaxoSmithKline's (GSK's) Paxil CR®, a reformulation of GSK's paroxetine obtained U.S. marketing approval for the controlled-release form based on SkyePharma's Geomatrix® technology in February 1999; however, the product was not launched until three years later in 2002. This allowed Paxil® to progress further in its life cycle as no generic entry was anticipated prior to 2003, thereby allowing GSK to switch patients to the new dosage form at an appropriate time and not prematurely. Generic attack of the CR form will now only began in June 2007 when Mylan's ANDA filing for a controlled release dosage form received approval on the expiry of pediatric exclusivity related to a patent covering the crystalline form of the active pharmaceutical ingredient (API). This also illustrates an interesting point regarding reformulation; the new formulation uses a proprietary technology with patent coverage until 2012, yet it is not this that has prevented a generic from entering the market. This is worth mentioning because, although formulation patents provide a significant barrier, does not have the same defensive power as patents covering the compound itself.

It is also worth recalling at this point that Paxil was a compound that was dosed once-a-day; the CR form did not change that. In circumstances where the brand was not available or where the market was already generic reformulation in this way would not have been a viable option. The therapeutic benefits of the reformulation are arguably minimal, as we saw previously with Tricor, but the submission of new clinical studies qualifies the product for 3 years regulatory exclusivity and renders it nonsubstitutable by generic Paxil.

The D2/D3 agonists ropinirole (Requip®) from GSK and pramipexole (Mirapex®) and their use in the treatment of Parkinson's disease are also illustrative of timing as a driver for the development launch of reformulated products. GSK have again chosen to defend this brand against generic attack and to extend its life cycle with an extended-release formulation using the Geomatrix® technology—Requip CR®. In this case, however, there is the bonus of a less frequent dosing schedule, which is welcome for this patient group. GSK originally filed for approval with the FDA in April 2006 in anticipation of patent term expiry in May 2008; however, administrative problems with the submission meant that the FDA only finally accepted the filing in April 2007. This means that GSK will struggle to switch their Parkinson's patients to the new formulation, before generic appearance in the United States should they receive approval before May 2008, if they receive approval after this date then they may be entering a reduced value generic market. It is therefore fortunate that there is a clearly defined difference between the two products.

Mirapex (pramipexole) has an estimated patent constraint date of 2011, although Barr now has final approval for a generic version, Pfizer hold patents to an extended-release dosage form, but as yet there are no reports on the development of such a formulation, despite the fact that this would be a better dosage form. To launch, at this stage in the product life cycle would be to waste 3 years of regulatory exclusivity. That the development of Requip CR® has not caused Pfizer to move may be due to the fact that the revenue that might be lost to during the 2 to 3 year period that it will exist alongside Mirapex, would be as great as the 2 to 3 years' of revenue that would be lost to generics after 2011, if a CR formulation were brought forward now. Mirapex easily outsold Requip in 2005, $254 as opposed to $159 (IMS data) and one assumes that it is perception as a better drug will to some extent counter the convenience of Requip CR. Certainly of greater importance at this time is the registration of Mirapex for the treatment of restless legs syndrome as this is a new market in which Requip is currently unopposed. Since its approval in this indication in June 2005, U. S. sales have increased from $159 in 2005 to $315 in 2006 (IMS data).

This speculated timing of the launch of a Mirapex CR can be contrasted with Pfizer's reformulation of Detrol® to Detrol LA®. This reformulation occurred early on in the product life cycle in response to the appearance of Ditropan XL®, as the market began its move to once-a-day therapy. At this stage it was not possible to allow the competition to erode the revenue expectation of Detrol over an extended period. In this case, the potential loss over the remaining life span of the product would likely be much greater than would have been recouped through the delay of generic entry for a period of 2 to 3 years.

Defensibility and Value of Reformulation

Extended-release technology for oral drug delivery is a mature technology. Approaches that are able to also build features that go beyond converting multiple dose schedules to once-a-day are likely to fare best.

An interesting modification of the extended release angle was used in Pfizer's Azithromycin Zmax® azithromycin suspension. Azithromycin has a long half-life and dosing of Zithromax® was already once daily. By combining a high dose (2 g) with a sustained release technology, Pfizer was able to establish that a complete course of treatment was possible with a single dose. It is unclear as to whether the high dose or the formulation technology is the more important factor, but by using both, more defensibility can be built into the formulation.

That the dose of the formulation may be the technology is very well illustrated by Merck's alendronate, where the 70-mg dose can now be dosed once per week rather than being taken daily. This truly is a therapeutic benefit to patients and, as a result, it created a very competitive product. This has proven more difficult to defend from a patent viewpoint, but not entirely due to the fact that the dosing schedule is harder to defend per se.

The best technology patents look like new chemical entity (NCE) patents and in some cases they are. The recent launch of GSK's extended release Coreg® was based on Flamel's Micropump® technology: however, this product owes much to the phosphate salt of carvedilol used in the formulation. Carvedilol is poorly soluble at neutral and alkaline pH, meaning that absorption of the immediate release formulation occurs primarily in the upper part of the GI tract. A sustained release formulation would need either to be based on upper GI retention and/or the use of a bioavailability enhancement technology suited to insoluble drugs for the delayed-release portion of the dose. Through consideration of Flamel and GSK's patent application (1) a key mechanistic part of the formulation is linked to the increased solubility of the phosphate salt in combination with acidic excipients in the delayed release fraction of the formulation. The contribution of the Micropump technology is unclear, but should this patent proceed to grant substitution of the formulation becomes much less straightforward, being based more upon the chemistry of salt forms and combinations of chemical species in a particular dosage construct it becomes a more difficult task to duplicate without encroaching on the patents covering the product.

The move to use the phosphate salt and switch to a capsule from a tablet also resets the competitive clock of technology-focused developers, such as Biovail and Egalet, that were developing sustained elease carvedilol formulations. The substitution of the sustained release formulation that GSK had in development may not have been an express aim of their program, but now it is no longer an option. Controlled release formulations for substitution will need to be based on the phosphate form and on a capsule.

If one pursues this theme, the very best of all defense strategies would be new chemical entities, and one can reasonably say that Shire have taken such an approach to the life cycle management of Adderall XR®. The recent settlements between Shire and Barr and Shire and Impax will allow Barr to market generic versions of Adderall XR in the United States on April 1, 2009 and Impax to market generic versions of Adderall XR in the United States 181 days following Barr's launch. Through a $2.3 billion acquisition of New River, Shire have obtained lisdexamphetamine, Vyvanse®, a dex-amphetamine pro-drug, something that can be looked upon as a molecular sustained release technology. Vyvanse is also claimed to have less abuse potential and to be safer that its active moiety, but its biggest commercial advantage is the fact that it is a NCE and consequently entitled to 5 years of NCE exclusivity as well as benefiting from patents covering the compound itself.

We should not leave this area of life cycle management without considering the relatively recent phenomenon of reformulations through the separation of the active isomers from drugs that were previously marketed as the raecemate. This approach has been largely pioneered by the specialty pharmaceutical company Sepracor, who were among the first to recognize this business opportunity. Through the purification and selection of the most active isomer from a previously mixed product, medications with equivalent efficacy can be made using a lower dose of API, thus qualifying for market exclusivity in much the same way as we saw above for Tricor fenofibrate: however, in this case the protection is much more robust. The compound is also an NCE and may be eligible for much longer term patent protection. The weakness of this approach is that medical benefits, if present, are difficult to tease out. Despite this, Astra Zeneca's rebranding of raecemic omeprazole, Prilosec®, to the single isomer esomeprazole Nexium® has been successful—the clinical benefits being generated largely through what is effectively a dose increase.

A second example is Forest/Lundbeck's citalopram (Celexa®), whose franchise has been protected through the registration and launch of escitalopram with patent coverage now extending to March 2012 following a U.S. District Court ruling in July 2006 in Lundbeck/Forest's favor (2).

This launch was not as successful as it might have been as Lexapro is subject to more generic competition than anticipated due to Forest's failure to switch patients quickly enough from Celexa to Lexapro® before generic Celexa entered the U.S. market; with 29% of Forest's depression prescriptions still being written for Celexa on that date.

While there is price pressure from payers where the raecemic generic is available, and the very close similarities between the two products are self-evident, the fact that this strategy works (and that it works to the extent that it does) illustrates once again the power of marketing structures and the brand.

We have considered a series of formulation approaches with varying degrees of complexity and have seen that a simple reformation does not generally buy any more time from generic competition than is offered by the three years of exclusivity for the new dosage form given by the regulatory authorities. In many ways, the more challenging or suboptimal the formulation is in the original product, the greater are the possibilities for the innovator to retain control as improvements are sequentially added.

MARKET EXPANSION

There is a disincentive to add new formulations, such as extended release formulations, at points other than the late phases of the life cycle as this is to forgo the extension of life cycle as a means of generic defense. There is also a second disincentive: the cannibalization of the existing product. This will inevitably occur, making this a questionable move in terms of return on investment. Unless competitive products are gaining market share owing to a better dosing regimen, innovators will not move in this direction until the appropriate point in the life cycle.

At the approximate midpoint of a product life cycle, an appropriate means to grow sales of the product, as it is within any market, is to enter new markets. The expansion into new geographies is part of the normal progression of the product. In addition, the product progresses into new therapeutic areas through the performance of new clinical trials to add new indications to the product label. These can be incremental or moves into unrelated therapeutic areas or even the characterization of new disease states, such as restless legs syndrome, which has become an important market for Requip with sales almost doubling since approval.

Combination Products

The reformulation strategies used around the midpoint or a little beyond are, therefore, designed to add value through expanding the market reach of the compound, in these cases the original formulation will continue to exist with the new. Examples of this type of approach are found in combination products such as Novartis's Exforge®, a fixed dose combination of valsatran and amlodipine, and Lotrel, a fixed dose combination of amlodipine and benazepril. Other examples include Pfizer's Caduet®, a fixed dose combination of atorovastatin and amlodipine and Merck's Vytorin®, a fixed dose combination of simvastatin and ezetimibe. The Caduet® and Vytorin® products are interesting as they are arguably good and bad examples of the combination formulation approach, from a commercial perspective.

Caduet was intended to be the first combination therapy to target both dyslipidemia and hypertension. Although there is a strong correlation between the disease states the cross-risk factors and the titration schemes make the product difficult to use and the message of greater convenience is lost in a cumbersome prescribing regimen that involves 11 different formulations. Conversely, Vytorin®, a combination of two cholesterol-lowering drugs, is available in only 4 dosage combinations. The marketing message—that it is superior to monotherapies in lowering cholesterol—is clear and its prescribing is simple. This joint venture between Schering Plough and Merck has been very effective in extending the life cycle of Zocor® even though generic simvastatin is now readily available.

These reformulation strategies may not make as much use of the formulation scientists' art as controlled release formulations, but there are examples where technically innovative approaches are found in combination product or in products that coexist with the original dosage forms. Abbott's Kaletra®, a fixed dose combination of lopinavir and ritonavir, in which a liquid product requiring refrigeration dosed as a liquid or six soft shells was replaced by four tablets not requiring refrigeration. This was achieved using Abbott's Soliqs® technology and was approved by the FDA in October 2005 and in the European Union (EU) in July 2006.

The now abandoned combination of atorvastatin and torcetrapib, a product aimed to raise HDL levels while lowering LDL, which was under development by Pfizer as part of the management of the life cycle of Lipitor®, also incorporated a solubility enhancement technology to increase the absorption of torcetrapib (3). This added formulation complexity and, of course, enhances defensibility.

One of the most successful combination products has occurred in pulmonary medicine, and although there may be less opportunity for this delivery route, some reformulated products have been strikingly successful. Advair®, in which the combination of two drugs, salmeterol and fluticasone, which were previously separately available and remain so, has enabled GSK to create product with over $6 billion in sales. This was the first fixed dose combination of a bronchodilator and a steroid and accounted for 56% of new scrips after its launch in 2004.

This field has also seen one truly innovative product reach the market through the development of Exubera®, inhaled insulin, which represents a true breakthrough in the delivery of large molecules. Unfortunately, this has not led to commercial success.

Other noteworthy examples in this space are the development of a dry powder inhalation of the antimicrobial tombramycin for the treatment of bacterial lung infections in patients with cystic fibrosis. The present formulation is an air-jet nebulized delivery of a solution with an inhalation time of at least 15 minutes, which is bulky and not portable. The new formulation under development by Nektar and Novartis promises to be rapid and easily portable. In this patient group, who are the subjects of a high pharmaceutical burden, reduction in treatment times or treatment approaches that contribute to an increase in their freedom is very welcome.

New Routes of Administration

The extended release formulations of J&J's risperidone, Risperdal Consta® is an injectable formulation based on the Medisorb® biodegradable microsphere technology of Alkermes, with a single injection providing therapeutic coverage for a two-week period. The oral form, Risperdal® was launched in the United States in 1994 and in the EU in 1997. Consta® was launched in the United States in 2003 and in the EU in 2002. It is the only injected antipsychotic and it could reasonably be said that it has 100% of the market represented by those patients who are unwilling to comply with oral therapy; in 2006 worldwide sales of Risperdal Consta® were $870 M (IMS data). It should be noted that worldwide sales of the tablet form were $3.6 billion (IMS data) and it has been suggested that there would have been more take up of Risperdal Consta if pricing had not been at such variance to the tablet—the difference being approximately five-fold in the United States.

J&J have chosen to manage the life cycle of Risperdal® with an NCE paliperidone, which is an active metabolite of risperidone. Invega® (paliperidone) was launched in the United States in January 2007 using J&J's Oros® sustained release tablet technology. The fact that the product is an NCE is currently providing the only means of U.S. defense for this product as it qualifies for five years NCE exclusivity from the FDA, giving it exclusivity until December 2011. The only Orange Book listed patent, which is specific to the NCE, expires in October 2009. Despite this less than ideal situation, which should be qualified by saying that this type of regulatory exclusivity is watertight, the technology does offer advantages that will help to drive the switching strategy, the Oros formulation of paliperidone is a true once-a-day, which is not always the case with Risperdal. The formulation also removes the need for titration at the onset of therapy; the complement long-acting injectable formulation of paliperidone palmitate has a longer period of action and can be injected less frequently, about six weeks. The injectable form also uses Elan's nanoparticle technology, creating a further entry barrier.

On the negative side, the product does face its stiffest competition from generic risperidone. There may be enough to prevent the product from being seen as purely created for the purposes of patent extension by physicians and payers, but the pricing pressure exerted by a generic product which is essentially therapeutically equivalent will be significant. Although the medical advance offered by this reformulation is more incremental, there is probably enough differentiation in the package for J&J to switch patients to the new forms with appropriate pricing.

The reformulation of products that were always injectables has also provided a successful means to expand markets. They have added the most in terms of the use of biodegradeable polymers to extend the efficacy of LHRH agonists, which has been continued to the point where formulations will provide coverage for several months and even as long as one year if the Viadur® titanium implant from Alza (now J&J) is used. One of the advantages of this type of technology is that duplication is not a simple task. The only real alternative is the Atrigel® implant technology from QLT.

There are also approaches in the injectable arena that employ a technology to sustain therapeutic effect through modifying the molecule itself. Pegylated interferon has largely replaced the nonconjugated parent molecule as a drug product. Frequent injections are both unpleasant and time-consuming and products that alleviate this do well. Other reformulations of injectable products have sought to decrease the toxicity of certain products, most notably paclitaxel. Also, the removal of the surfactant Cremophore® from Taxol® was seen to be desirable for the reduction in premedication that this would bring, as the delivery vehicle itself was pyrogenic and contributed to the dose-limiting toxicity of the medication. This proved considerably more challenging than would-be formulators of next generation Taxol imagined. But the eventual launch of Abraxane®, in which insoluble paclitaxel is absorbed to the surface of albumin particles, promises to be both a safer and more efficacious therapy.

New Dosage Forms

Successful formulation-based approaches aimed at expanding markets need not involve a switch to a different route of administration. The production of more convenient dosage forms or dosage forms suited to a particular type of patient are also used to expand the market reach of products and to enhance the competitive profile of the brand. The production of more convenient dosage forms, such as ODTs and suspension formulations, are popular means of doing this. The development of such formulations may also qualify for extension of patent terms of six months if directed toward pediatrics.

The suspension formulation is particularly suited to pediatrics as it can be easily titrated and is suited to all ages. The ODT is a relatively recent development tablet and early formulations were brought to the market by Cima (now Cephalon), Yamanouchi, Lafon (now Cephalon) and Ethypharm. These early formulations were rather fragile, required special packaging, and were not well-suited to high drug doses of active. Second-generation technologies such as Eurand's Advatab® and Cephalon's Durasolv® have characteristics that are similar to conventional tablets, while still possessing the ability to disintegrate very rapidly in the oral cavity.

The ODT dosage form has proven useful, not only for pediatric and geriatric dosage forms, but also for particular types of patients and disease states. In cases where symptom onset is sudden and unpredictable, such as migraine or acute pain, the ODT is useful as it can be taken immediately by the patient, without the need for water, e.g., Zomig®, and Fentora® (fentanyl). In cases such as psychiatric disease, where the patient may not wish others to be aware that they are taking medication or where they may avoid taking it by holding conventional pills in their cheek or under the tongue, the ODT is useful. Examples of such products in include Risperdal ODT, Remeron® ODT, and Zyprexa® ODT.

A particular problem that has been encountered in formulating tablets that are designed to disintegrate in the oral cavity is that many drugs have an unpleasant taste and an additional technology of taste-masking is required to overcome this. This involves coating the drug particles so that a polymer barrier exists between the drug particle and the tongue. This ideally has to be achieved without delaying the release of the drug. This is particularly relevant to drugs that need to act rapidly, such as those for the relief of acute pain such as migraine and the 3-hour T_{max} of zolmitriptan in ODT form as opposed to the 2-hour T_{max} (Zomig® prescribing information) of the conventional tablet form is clearly a move in the wrong direction for a drug designed to bring rapid pain relief.

Other applications where the ODT dosage form is used are those in which the patient is extremely nauseas and would prefer not to contemplate swallowing water. ODT dosage forms are found in Zofran® (ondansetron), which is used for the prevention of nausea and vomiting during chemotherapy. It is also found in other applications where GI symptoms may also be a concern, such as the Prevacid® ODT form.

It is thus necessary to have both a sophisticated ODT technology and a sophisticated taste-masking technology to create successful products. Companies, such as Eurand, that are able to combine a diversity and experience in particle coating with advanced ODT technology are well positioned to further expand the use of the ODTs as a means to extend the market reach of products.

USING FORMULATION TO CREATE NEW PRODUCTS

The final area where reformulation can represent a commercial opportunity is in the reformulation of drugs whose patent has already expired. In this area, specialist companies need not partner with the innovator and brand owner; brand owners may also be opportunistic and attack markets created by others.

A well-publicized and illustrative example of this is the reformulation of methylphenidate by J&J into a once-a-day formulation using the Oros® technology it acquired from Alza, to both revitalize a market with a superior product and to take this market from the original franchise holder. J&J did not have a methylphendidate franchise prior to their launch of Concerta®, a once-a-day Oros formulation, in 2000. Methylphenidate (Ritalin®), a Novartis compound, had already endured four years of patent expiry and sales had largely stagnated in the attention-deficit/hyperactivity disorder (ADHD) market. The patient group is primarily school children and the drug is a controlled substance. This had meant that the original twice-a-day dosing schedule required that the drug be dispensed under the supervision of a school nurse, making those on medication conspicuous with consequent embarrassment.

The ability to dose methylphenidate once daily for ADHD offers particular advantages, so despite a lack of a methyliphendiate franchise, J&J were able to step in and not only transform the ADHD market, but to take the ADHD market from the original franchisee through possession of a formulation technology and foresight. There were also thought to be additional advantages linked the Oros release kinetic, as ascending dose is thought to be a more effective way for the drug to enter the body. Concerta® soon dominated the market for methylphenidate-based drugs. Following the introduction of Concerta, between 2001 and 2003, the market exhibited a compound annual growth rate of 28% reaching $852 million in 2003. Concerta almost exclusively drove this growth, with 74% of all methylphenidate sales in 2003 (IMS data). In 2006 J&J reported sales growth of 20.2% and sales of approximately $900 million. This product has not been substituted in a now highly genericized market and still retains Orange Book exclusivities until 2008.

J&J were not alone in exploiting the particular advantages offered by once-a-day formulations in this market. Shire's Adderall XR®, a sustained release formulation of mixed amphetamine salts, was approved by the FDA on October 12, 2001. Although it was launched only six months prior to the market entry of Barr's generic, strong patient switching from Adderall to Adderall XR was achieved. In its first quarter on the market, Adderall XR accounted for 21% of total Adderall franchise sales. The momentum of uptake of the new formulation was maintained following the launch of further amphetamine generics from Eon and Ranbaxy in 2002. After three companies had launched generics, the XR reformulation still represented 83% of franchise sales and 68% of total molecule sales. That Shire has been able to regularly increase the price of Adderall XR, is entirely due to the fact that it is such a highly differentiated product.

The effect of both Concerta and Adderall XR has been to transform a generic market with products that have profiles similar to those of new entrants rather than the follow-on profiles of reformulations associated with generic defense that we considered earlier. These two products and their market illustrate well the ability of reformulation to drive growth and alter market structure. Further, the conception of these two approaches also illustrates two distinct drivers for reformulation. In the case of Adderall XR, the defense against generic attack and in the case of Concerta the opportunistic conquest of an existing market with a superior product.

This is worth comparing with the reformulation of Xanax®. After patent expiry by Pfizer (Pharmacia and Upjohn), the extended-release formulation was approved in the United States in January 2003, nine years after patent expiry. This product offered a more convenient dosage scheme, but that was all that it offered. It did not overcome a particular problem in the way that Concerta did and could not claim any particular advantages associated with the technology used or offer any patent protection, and after regulatory exclusivity expired it was rapidly substituted by generics. In the three years before generic substitution occurred, revenues increased by approximately $48 million (Datamonitor), but the combination of clinical and launch costs probably make this a marginal product in terms of return on investment. Xanax XR® was never able to gain the momentum of Concerta, and although this strategy would have worked well for life cycle extension it did not work well as a means to revitalize the market for this compound.

There are a limited number of examples where reformulation has delivered a benefit to therapy to the extent that Concerta and Adderal XR have and these were more associated to the particular problems associated with the disease demographic than any unusual property of the formulation itself.

The reformulation of fentanyl has provided examples where the innovation associated with the formulation has also contributed in a large part to the success of the product. Fentanyl was originally developed by J&J in 1962. It is a highly potent opioid analgesic, with a potency approximately 100-fold that of morphine, and it is an important molecule in the management of severe and chronic pain.

In collaboration with Alza, which J&J subsequently acquired, J&J developed the Duragesic® patch, which has a number of important advantages over the injectable or oral means of delivery that had been used. Patients were exposed to a smooth flow of drug, without the need for infusion, over a long period (up to 72 hours). This was a better and more convenient therapy than those offered by generics allowing Duragesic to easily out-compete alternatives. At its peak, Duragesic represented a $1.6 billion market and worldwide sales have only just begun to decline 15 years post-launch with the appearance of generics in 2005: Duragesic sales reported by J&J for 2006 were $1.295 billion.

The approach that Anesta (now Cephalon) took with fentanyl was to enter a new market with a formulation designed to meet the needs of patients in that market. Actiq® was specifically targeted to break through cancer pain, which is a condition in which cancer sufferers experience acute, unpredictable spikes of severe pain that overcome their pain therapy. Actiq is a lollipop formulation of fentanyl, which patients place into their mouths when they experience an episode of breakthrough pain. The very high potency of fentanyl together with its ability to cross the buccal mucosa means that pain relief is achieved very rapidly without the need for injection, furthermore patients can optimize dosing by removing the lollipop once the pain has abated. From 200 to 2003 U.S. sales of Actiq grew from \$14 to \$245 million in 2003 giving Actiq a 16% of the fentanyl market (Datamonitor). In that time the price of Actiq almost doubled. Sales of Actiq reported by Cephalon for 2006 totaled \$572.1 million, representing a year-on-year growth of 39%. Cephalon has managed the life cycle of this franchise through the launch in October 2006 of Fentora®, an ODT tablet for buccal absorption based on the Oravescent® technology acquired from Cima.

A very recent example of an innovative formulation of an old drug to produce a differentiated product is provided by the launch in June 2006 of Vivitrol®, a sustained release injectable formulation of naltrexone licensed from Alkermes. Following subcutaneous or intramuscular administration a steady release rate of naltrexone release into the bloodstream is sustained for up to 1 month.

Naltrexone is an opioid receptor antagonist and was approved for the treatment of alcohol dependence in 1994 and for opioid dependence a decade prior to that. Naltrexone acts at μ, δ, and κ opioid receptors, each of which is implicated in at least one aspect of alcohol and opiate dependence. The blockade of the μ opioid receptor in particular inhibits the reward received from opioids or alcohol and is linked with diminished dependence. The value of oral naltrexone in the long-term treatment of alcohol or opiate dependence has been greatly undermined by the failure of the substance abusers to adhere to the daily dosing schedule. There is an absence of suitable alternative products in this arena, with only Disulfiram and Acamaprosate available. Disulfuram relies on the severe aversive effect produced by inhibition of acetaldehyde dehydrogenase during the metabolism of ethanol, but the adverse side effects associated with this can be severe and even fatal. Acamprosate is thought to act on γ-aminobutyric acid and glutaminergic receptors, but it is administered orally requiring a total dose of 2 g to be administered in three divided doses.

Market uptake to date has been slow, partly due to the fact that this is a difficult market to define and manage. It will be interesting to see how this product will progress. It has solved an important therapeutic drawback associated with naltrexone and entered an area of unmet therapeutic need. The challenge for this product will be to convince doctors and patients alike that pharmacotherapy is an effective treatment for alcohol dependency. Unlike methylphenidate or fentanyl, naltrexone is not a gold standard for the treatment of the condition which the improved formulation addresses.

CONCLUSION

The great majority of drug reformulations are driven by the life cycle of the product and must occur in the right sequence and at the right time if the value of the product is to be fully realized. With efficient planning, this would be built into the life cycle management plans prior to product launch. Timing is crucial, particularly toward the end of product life cycles, at which time it is very difficult to recover from prior delays. The therapeutic advance offered by a reformulation need not be great and may even be minimal if it is allied to the brand. In this case, it is sufficient that it differentiates the new product from its predecessor only to the extent that it can enjoy an extended period of regulatory exclusivity or patent protection. In addition, a reformulation that improves the competitive profile of a compound only to the extent that it takes sales from the previous formulation would be a pointless exercise.

Reformulations that occur beyond the product life cycle face a much higher bar, the benefits offered by reformulation in this case must be akin to those features possessed by new products: they must offer a clear therapeutic advantage and they must be robustly defensible if their life cycle is to last beyond the three years of exclusivity offered by Waxman Hatch. Only a handful of these more independent products created by formulation have emerged, and these have been successful as they have solved special inconveniences present in their therapeutic area or have allowed the treatment of a previously poorly or untreated condition.

In considering the target of reformulation, during the course of the product life cycle this will be heavily biased to market need. It is only after the completion of life cycle that priority can be given to therapeutic need. This is not to give the impression that brands somehow do not respect therapeutic need, it is the therapeutic compound that is leading the response to this challenge in the earlier parts of the life cycle, priorities shift after this goal has been met and the market is given up to generics.

REFERENCES

1. Castan, C, et al. Carvedilol FreeBase, salts, anhydrous forms or solvate thereof corresponding pharmaceutical compositions, controlled release formulations and treatment or delivery methods. Patent WO2005/051322 A2.
2. Press Release 2006, July 13: www.frx.com
3. Freisen DT, et al. Pharmaceutical compositions of cholesteryl ester transfer protein inhibitors and HMG-Co—A reductase inhibitors. Patent WO 20061129167.
4. Garbutt JC, et al. Efficacy and tolerability of long-acting injectable Naltrexone for alcohol dependence: A randomized controlled trial. JAMA 2005; 293(13): 1617–25.

2

The Modified-Release Drug Delivery Landscape

Academic Viewpoint

Juergen Siepmann and Florence Siepmann
College of Pharmacy, University of Lille, Lille, France

INTRODUCTION

Two types of modified (or controlled) drug delivery systems can be distinguished: (*i*) devices that *de*crease the release rate of the drug compared to conventional dosage forms, often during prolonged periods of time (e.g., several hours, days, or months) (1–3), and (*ii*) systems that *in*crease the release rate compared to conventional dosage forms (e.g., in the case of poorly water-soluble drugs) (4,5). Both types of systems can be very helpful to improve the therapeutic efficacy of many pharmaco-treatments.

   The steadily increasing practical importance of modified drug delivery systems can be attributed to the major advantages they can offer over conventional dosage forms, including:

- The possibility to optimize the resulting drug concentration time profiles at the site of action in the human body over prolonged periods of time (1,2,6). Every drug is characterized by its "minimal effective concentration" (MEC) (below which no therapeutic effect occurs), and its "minimal toxic concentration" (MTC) (above which undesired side effects occur) (Fig. 1, dotted lines). The range in-between the MEC and MTC is called "therapeutic range," or "therapeutic window." Depending on the type of drug, this concentration range can be more or less narrow. If a highly potent

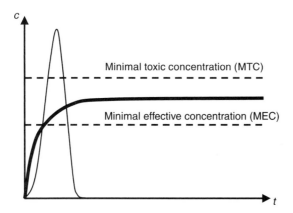

Figure 1 Schematic presentation of the "therapeutic window" of a drug and possible drug concentration time profiles upon administration of oral immediate (*thin curve*) and controlled release dosage forms (*bold curve*). (c) denotes the drug concentration at the site of action in the human body, *t* the time after administration.

drug with narrow therapeutic window (e.g., anticancer drug) is administered using a conventional dosage form, the entire drug dose is generally rapidly released. In the case of oral administration, the drug is subsequently absorbed into the blood stream, distributed throughout the human body and reaches the site of action. Depending on the administered dose and therapeutic range of the drug, the risk can be considerable that toxic concentrations are achieved. In addition, as there is no further drug supply (the entire dose is rapidly released) and as the human body eliminates the drug, its concentration at the site of action decreases again. In many cases, therapeutic drug concentrations are attained only during short periods of time (Fig. 1, thin curve). To overcome this restriction, the first step, the release of the drug out of the dosage form can be time–controlled. For example, a constant drug supply can be provided, compensating the drug elimination out of the human body and, thus, resulting in about constant concentrations within the therapeutic range at the site of action during prolonged periods of time (Fig. 1, bold curve). Consequently, toxic side effects and time periods with sub-therapeutic drug concentrations can be minimized.

■ The possibility to reduce the administration frequency of drugs exhibiting short half-lives in vivo. For example, three times daily oral administration might be replaced by once daily administration only. This is particularly important for elderly patients with multiple drug treatments. Also, required daily injections of drugs (that need to be administered parenterally and are rapidly eliminated out of the human body) might be replaced by injections of depot systems twice a year only. Obviously, this very much facilitated administration schedule allows to significantly improve patient compliance and, thus, the therapeutic efficacy of the treatments.

- The possibility to *enable* new pharmacotherapies. For example, the treatment of brain diseases is particularly difficult due to the blood–brain barrier (BBB), which effectively hinders the transport of most drugs from the blood stream into the central nervous system (CNS). Generally, only small, lipid-soluble molecules and a few nutrients can cross this barrier to a significant extent, either by passive diffusion or using active transport mechanisms (7,8). One possibility to overcome this restriction is to directly inject the drug into the brain tissue (intra-cranial administration). However, due to the generally short half-lives of the drugs within the CNS, frequent administration would be required over long periods of time for the treatment of many brain malignancies. For instance, brain tumors and neurodegenerative diseases (e.g., Alzheimer's and Parkinson's disease's) require therapeutic drug con-centrations at the site of action during several weeks/months/years. As each intracranial administration implies a significant risk to provoke severe CNS infections, this type of treatment method is not feasible. Modified release microparticles or implants can help to overcome this restriction: Ideally, one single injection/implantation is sufficient to provide therapeutic drug concentrations at the site of action during prolonged periods of time.

- The possibility to simulate night time dosing. For the treatment of cer-tain diseases (e.g., asthma) it is important that the drug is available at the site of action in the very early morning. Thus, the patient should take a conventional dosage (e.g., standard tablet) during the night to allow for drug absorption into the blood stream and appearance at the site of action in the very early morning. Alternatively, so-called "pulsatile" drug delivery systems can be administered in the late evening (Fig. 2). During the first couple of hours, no drug is released. Then, after a pre-determined lag time (e.g., 4 hr), the entire drug dose is rapidly released without the need for the patient to wake up. An example for a pulsatile drug delivery system is a polymer coated pellet, with a rupturable coating that is poorly permeable for the drug as long as it is intact (Fig. 2). Upon contact with aqueous body fluids, water penetrates into the pellet and builds up a steadily increasing hydrostatic pressure within the core, which acts against the polymeric film. As soon as a critical threshold value is attained, the coating ruptures and the drug is rapidly released through water-filled pores/channels (Fig. 2).

- The possibility to simulate multiple dosing with one or several drugs. Combining different types of pulsatile drug delivery systems with various lag-times (e.g., different types of polymer coated pellets, filled into hard gelatin capsules or compressed into tablets), several drug doses can be released at pre-determined time points upon one single administration.

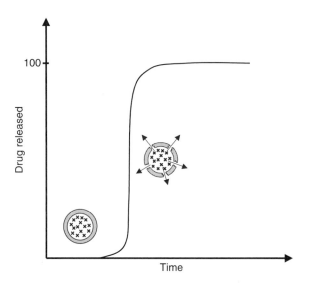

Figure 2 Schematic presentation of a pulsatile drug release profile: negligible release
at early time points, followed by rapid and complete drug release after a predetermined
lag-phase. A polymer-coated pellet is illustrated as an example: The intact macromolecular membrane effectively suppresses drug release until the monotonically increasing hydrostatic pressure within the pellet core reaches a threshold value at which
crack formation within the coating sets on, resulting in rapid drug release through
water-filled pores/channels.

This can substantially facilitate the administration schedule for many
elderly patients.

To be able to control the rate at which a drug leaves its dosage form,
the active agent is generally embedded within a matrix former. Often
polymers are used for this purpose (9–11). For parenteral administration the
polymer should ideally be biodegradable to avoid the necessity to remove
empty remnants after drug exhaust. Depending on the type of drug, type of
polymer, composition and geometry of the device, preparation technique
and release conditions [e.g., contents of the gastrointestinal tract (GIT)
versus muscle tissue], different physico-chemical processes can be involved
in the control of the resulting drug release rate. This might include e.g.,
water diffusion, polymer chain relaxation, glassy to rubbery state transitions, polymer degradation, diffusion of degradation products, drug
dissolution and diffusion, polymer dissolution, creation of acidic micro-
environments, autocatalytic effects, crystallization of degradation products,
re-dissolution of the latter, drug degradation, a decrease or increase in
system size, an increase in polymer chain mobility as well as drug polymer
interactions. If several of these phenomena are simultaneously involved and
of importance for the resulting drug release kinetics, it is generally difficult

to optimize the system, because effects of formulation and processing parameters on the resulting drug release kinetics are not straightforward and device development is often based on series of time-consuming trial and error experiments. However, in some systems only one or two mechanisms are dominant (12–14). If for example, several processes take place in sequence and one of them is significantly slower then the others, this process determines the overall drug release rate. In the following section, the most important drug release rate controlling mechanisms are briefly described.

INVOLVED MASS TRANSPORT PHENOMENA

Diffusion

Diffusional mass transport is occurring in almost all modified drug delivery systems. Different species can be diffusing, including water, drug, soluble polymer chains, drug and polymer degradation products, additional excipients present in the modified release system, as well as substances dissolved within body fluids the device is exposed to. In practice, often the diffusion of the drug through a polymeric network is the rate limiting step for drug release.

Diffusional processes can best be described using Fick's first and second law of diffusion (15,16). Depending on the structure of the device and solubility of the drug within the release rate controlling excipient(s) [generally polymer(s)], different types of diffusion controlled drug delivery systems can be distinguished (Fig. 3):

- *Reservoir devices with a core-shell structure.* The drug is located at the center of the system (e.g., pellet or tablet). The shell consists of the release rate controlling polymer. Generally, drug diffusion through the coating barrier controls the release rate. Depending on the drug solubility within the core upon water penetration and on the drug loading, two types of reservoir systems can be distinguished:
  - Devices with a *non-constant activity source.* In this case, only dissolved drug exists within the system's core upon water penetration (Fig. 3). Thus, drug molecules that diffuse out of the device are not replaced and the drug concentration at the inner membrane's surface decreases with time. If the system does not swell, perfect sink conditions (negligible drug concentrations in the release medium; no hindrance of further drug release by already released drug) are maintained, and if the membrane's properties do not change with time, first order release kinetics (exponentially decreasing release rates) are observed with this type of modified drug delivery system, irrespective of the geometry of the device.
  - Devices with a *constant activity source*: In this case, the initial drug loading is much higher than the amount of drug that is soluble

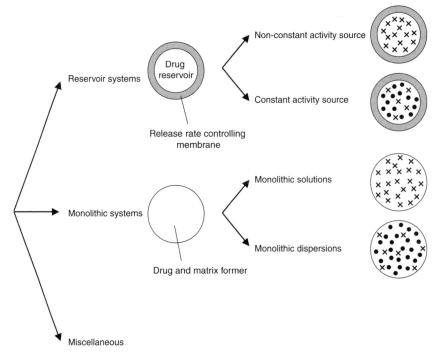

Figure 3 Classification system for primarily diffusion-controlled drug delivery systems.

within the wetted core. Thus, dissolved and non-dissolved drug coexist during major parts of the release period (Fig. 3). Importantly, drug molecules that diffuse through the polymeric barrier out of the device are replaced by the partial dissolution of the excess amount of drug. Consequently, a saturated drug solution is provided at the inner membrane's surface over prolonged periods of time (as long as non-dissolved drug exists). If the system does not swell, perfect sink conditions are maintained and the membrane's properties do not change with time, this leads to constant drug concentration gradients (being the driving forces for diffusion). In this case, the resulting drug release rate is constant as long as drug excess is provided in the system's core, irrespective of the geometry of the device (zero order release kinetics).

- *Monolithic devices*. The drug is distributed (generally homogeneously) throughout the system. This type of devices is also called "mono-bloc" system. Again, depending on the drug solubility within the wetted device and on the drug loading, two types of monolithic systems can be distinguished:

- Monolithic *solutions*, in which the drug is molecularly dispersed within the wetted matrix former (Fig. 3). In case of the simple geometry of thin films that do not swell, dissolve or degrade and under perfect sink conditions, a square root of time relation can be used to describe the first 60 % of drug release (17). This mathematical description should not be confused with the famous square root of time relationship introduced by Takeru Higuchi for thin ointment films with very high initial drug loadings in relation to drug solubility (18). In the case of poorly water-soluble drugs, monolithic solutions can be used to increase the resulting drug release rate in the human body compared to conventional dosage forms. As the drug is molecularly dispersed, no crystals or amorphous aggregates need to be destroyed prior to drug dissolution. In this case, a rapidly hydrating polymer should be chosen as matrix former, and drug release should not significantly be hindered by the macromolecular network. A major challenge during the development of this type of modified drug delivery system can be to provide long-term stability during storage, avoiding, e.g., the formation of thermodynamically more advantageous crystalline structures.
- Monolithic *dispersions*, in which the drug is partially molecularly dispersed and partially non-dissolved within the wetted device (Fig. 3). For the simple geometry of thin films, significant initial drug excess (drug concentration >> drug solubility), perfect sink conditions and a matrix former that does not swell, dissolve or degrade, Takeru Higuchi derived the famous square root of time relationship (18). Unfortunately, it is often misused and applied to drug delivery systems that do not fulfill one or more assumptions the Higuchi equation is based on.

- *Miscellaneous systems.* This can, for instance, be a coated pellet or tablet containing the drug not only in the core, but also in the film coating, or a device that consists of a monolithic drug polymer core and an additional polymer coating, with the core and coating controlling the resulting drug release rate.

Swelling

Depending on the physicochemical properties of the matrix former, polymer swelling can be of major importance (19,20). For example, hydroxypropyl methylcellulose (HPMC)-based matrix tablets can significantly swell (17). The two most important consequences of polymer swelling are:

1. The increase in the length of the diffusion pathways (increase in volume of the systems). This can lead to decreasing drug concentration gradients and, thus, decreasing drug release rates.

2. The increase in the polymer molecular mobility. This can lead to significantly increasing drug mobility within the polymeric network and, thus, increasing drug release rates. For example, in dry tablets, diffusion is generally negligible (the diffusion coefficients approach zero). In contrast, in a fully swollen polymer matrix drug diffusivities can be of the same order of magnitude as in aqueous solutions (17).

Depending on the type of polymer and type of drug, one of these effects can dominate, resulting in decreasing or increasing drug release rates.

Figure 4 schematically illustrates the phenomena which can be involved in the control of drug release from a swellable delivery system. This can for instance be a cross section through half of a matrix tablet which is exposed to an aqueous bulk fluid in radial direction. On the right-hand side, the tablet is still dry and non-swollen, on the left-hand side the bulk fluid is located. Due to concentration gradients, water diffuses into the drug delivery system. With increasing water content, the mobility of the polymer chains and drug molecules increases. At a certain, polymer-specific water concentration, the macromolecular mobility steeply increases ("polymer chain relaxation"). The front at which this phenomenon occurs is called "swelling front," separating the swollen from non-swollen matrix. Importantly, this is not a stationary boundary, but a moving one. If the initial drug concentration in the system is higher than the solubility of the drug in the swollen matrix, dissolved and non-dissolved drug co-exist within

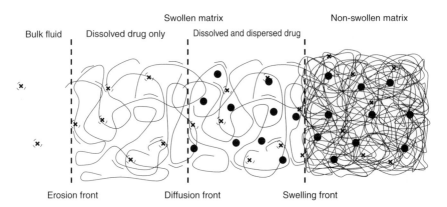

Figure 4 Schematic presentation of a swelling, controlled drug delivery system containing dissolved and dispersed drug (crosses and black circles, respectively), exhibiting the following moving boundaries: (*i*) an "erosion front," separating the bulk fluid from the delivery system; (*ii*) a "diffusion front," separating the swollen matrix containing dissolved drug only and the swollen matrix containing dissolved and dispersed drug; and (*iii*) a "swelling front," separating the swollen and non-swollen matrix.

the matrix directly next to the swelling front. Due to concentration gradients and the significantly increased mobility, dissolved drug molecules diffuse out into the bulk fluid. As long as a non-dissolved excess of drug exists, the concentration of dissolved drug in this part of the matrix is constant (released drug molecules are replaced by the partial dissolution of non-dissolved drug, providing a saturated drug solution). But as soon as all excess drug is dissolved, the drug concentration within the swollen matrix decreases. The front that separates the swollen matrix containing only dissolved drug from the swollen matrix that contains both, dissolved and non-dissolved drug, is called "diffusion front" (Fig. 4) (21,22). Importantly, also this front is not stationary. Furthermore, a third front can be distinguished, which separates the drug delivery system from the bulk fluid: the "erosion front," which is also moving.

Dissolution

Various species can dissolve during drug release and contribute to the overall control of the release rate, including the drug itself, the matrix former and potential further excipients present in the delivery system. To quantify the rate at which a *low* molecular weight substance dissolves, generally the Noyes-Whitney equation can be used (23). To describe the dissolution of a *high* molecular weight material, the so-called "reptation theory" can be applied (24,25). In the case of water-soluble, swellable polymeric matrix formers, the initially dry system consists of highly entangled macromolecules (Fig. 4, right-hand side). Upon water penetration the polymer swells, resulting in decreasing polymer concentrations and increasing macromolecule mobility (as discussed above). On a molecular level, the snake-like motions of the polymer chains ("reptation") permanently change the structure of the network. Entangled chains can either disentangle or modify their entanglement configuration, and disentangled chains can entangle or remain disentangled. At high and moderate polymer concentrations, the resulting macrostructure of the system is approximately time-invariant. However, below a certain polymer concentration, the number of disentangling polymer chains exceeds the number of newly entangled macromolecules, resulting in a destruction of the polymer network. Once the macromolecules are disentangled at the device's surface, they diffuse through the unstirred layer surrounding the system (not shown in Fig. 4), which is characterized by a distinct polymer concentration gradient. Then, convection leads to a homogeneous distribution of the polymer chains within the bulk fluid.

Erosion/Degradation

Unfortunately, different definitions of the terms "erosion" and "degradation" are used in the literature (26). In this chapter, polymer degradation is understood as the chain scission process by which polymer chains are cleaved into oligomers and finally monomers. In contrast, erosion is understood as the process of material loss from the polymer bulk. Such materials can be monomers, oligomers, parts of the polymer backbone or even parts of the polymer bulk.

Two polymer erosion mechanisms can be distinguished: (*i*) surface (= heterogeneous) erosion; and (*ii*) bulk (= homogeneous erosion) (27–29). The basic principles of these two mechanisms are illustrated in Figure 5. In the case of surface eroding drug delivery systems, polymer degradation is much faster than water penetration into the polymer bulk. Thus, degradation occurs primarily in the outermost polymer layers. Consequently, erosion affects only the surface and not the inner parts of the system (heterogeneous process) (Fig. 5A). The inner structure of the systems remains unaltered, but the device shrinks. Drug molecules that are embedded within the polymer matrix are predominantly released by the disappearance of the surrounding macromolecular network. In contrast, polymer chain cleavage is slow compared to water penetration in the case of

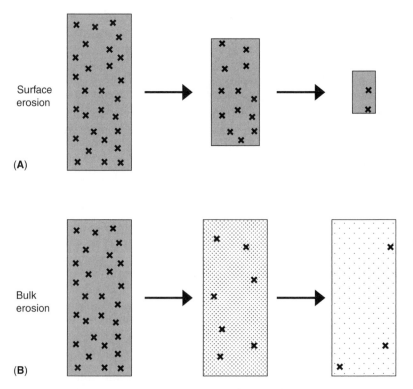

Figure 5 Schematic presentation of: (**A**) Surface eroding drug delivery systems, and (**B**) bulk eroding drug delivery systems. The crosses represent drug molecules.

bulk eroding drug delivery systems (Fig. 5B). In this case, the entire device is rapidly hydrated and the polymer chains are cleaved throughout the system. Consequently, erosion is not restricted to the polymer surface (homogeneous process). The outer dimensions of the drug delivery systems remain unaltered, while the average polymer molecular weight decreases, leading to an increased macromolecular mobility. Due to the release of polymer degradation products into the bulk fluid, the density of the macromolecular network decreases and the porosity increases. Thus, embedded drug molecules become more and more mobile within the device and diffuse out into the release medium.

As a basic rule, polymers that are built from very reactive functional groups tend to degrade fast and to undergo surface erosion, whereas polymers containing less reactive functional groups tend to be bulk eroding. Polyanhydrides are examples for predominantly surface eroding polymers, while poly(lactic acid) and poly(lactic-co-glycolic acid) (PLGA) are examples for predominantly bulk eroding materials. However, it has to be kept in mind that the ratio polymer chain cleavage rate/system wetting rate determines whether the device is surface or bulk eroding, and the system wetting rate also depends on the dimensions of the device (e.g., nanoparticles are much more rapidly completely wetted than large implants). Consequently, drug delivery systems based on the same polymer can be primarily surface or bulk eroding depending on their size. von Burkersroda et al. (30) introduced a critical device dimension ($L_{critical}$). If a drug delivery system is larger than $L_{critical}$, it undergoes surface erosion, while bulk erosion predominates if the device is smaller than this polymer-specific threshold value. For polyanhydrides the $L_{critical}$ value is in the order of 100 μm, for poly(α-hydroxy esters) (e.g., PLGA) it is in the order of 10 cm. However, it has to be pointed out that in the vicinity of the $L_{critical}$ values, both, surface as well as bulk erosion are of importance and the overall erosion behavior of the system shows characteristics of both types of erosion.

Miscellaneous

In practice, a combination of two or more of the above described physico-chemical phenomena might be simultaneously involved in the control of drug release from a specific delivery system (31,32). For example, HPMC-based matrix tablets (being generally the first choice for an oral controlled drug delivery system) are can be governed by a combination of three different phenomena (33–36) (Fig. 6):

1. *Diffusion*: At least three species can be diffusing: water, drug, and disentangled polymer chains. As soon as the tablet comes into contact with aqueous fluids, water molecules (represented as diamonds) diffuse into the system (due to concentration gradients). Then, dissolved drug

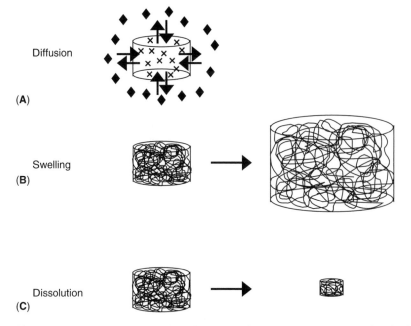

Figure 6 Schematic presentation of the most important physical and chemical phenomena involved in the control of drug release from HPMC-based matrix tablets: (**A**) Diffusion, (**B**) swelling, and (**C**) dissolution. The crosses and diamonds represent drug and water molecules, respectively. *Abbreviation*: HPMC, hydroxypropyl methylcellulose.

    molecules (crosses) diffuse out of the device. Thirdly, polymer chains that have disentangled from the macromolecular network diffuse through the liquid unstirred layer surrounding the tablet (not shown) into the bulk fluid.

2. *Polymer swelling*: The increase in volume of HPMC-based matrix tablets and increase in macromolecular mobility can be considerable. This leads to a drastic increase in the length of the diffusion pathways and mobility of the drug molecules (as discussed above).

3. *Polymer dissolution*: HPMC is water-soluble. Depending on the average polymer molecular weight and degree of substitution, the macromolecules more or less rapidly disentangle from the polymeric network and diffuse into the surrounding bulk fluid.

    If a poorly water-soluble drug is incorporated within the tablets, also drug dissolution can significantly contribute to the overall control of drug release. Due to the complexity of the underlying drug release mechanisms it is not straightforward to mathematically describe the resulting drug release kinetics and to make quantitative predictions of the effects of formulation and processing parameters on the system's properties (17,36).

PLGA-based microparticles are generally the first choice for controlled *parenteral* drug delivery (37,38). Unfortunately, also in these systems generally not only one of the above described physico-chemical phenomena is solely controlling the resulting drug release rate. As water penetration into the microparticles is much faster than the subsequent polymer chain cleavage (ester hydrolysis), the system undergoes bulk erosion. Consequently, shorter chain acids are generated throughout the device (Fig. 7). Due to concentration gradients, monomeric and oligomeric acids diffuse out into the surrounding bulk fluid, where they are neutralized. In addition, bases from the surrounding liquid diffuse into the microparticles and neutralize the generated acids. However, diffusional mass transport is relatively slowly and the rate at which the acids are generated can be higher than the rate at which they are neutralized. Consequently, the micro-environmental pH within the system (in particular at the center of the

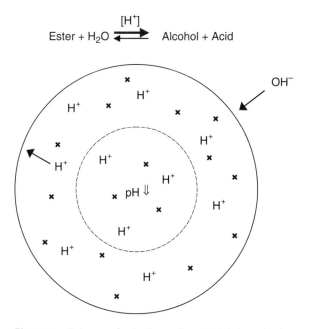

Figure 7 Scheme of a bulk eroding PLGA-based microparticle: Generated shorter chain acids diffuse out of the system, while bases from the surrounding bulk fluid diffuse in. Depending on the relative acid neutralization and acid generation rate, the micro-environmental pH within the system (in particular at the center of the microparticle) can significantly drop and cause drug degradation and autocatalysis: the hydrolytic ester bond cleavage is catalyzed by protons. *Abbreviation*: PLGA, poly(lactic-co-glycolic acid).

microparticles) can drop significantly (39–41). This can lead to drug inactivation (e.g., of protein-based drugs) and accelerated polymer degradation: hydrolytic ester bond cleavage is catalyzed by protons (42). Thus, also drug release can be accelerated (43,44). The two most critical parameters determining the relative importance of such autocatalytic effects are: (*i*) the microparticle size (determining the length of the diffusion pathways), and (*ii*) the microparticle porosity (determining the mobility of the diffusing acids and bases). As in the case of HPMC-based matrix tablets, the complexity of the underlying drug release mechanisms render the optimization of this type of controlled drug delivery systems challenging (45).

FUTURE OUTLOOK

Major challenges in the future development of modified drug delivery systems include (from an academic viewpoint):

1. The development of novel polymeric carrier materials: A serious restriction for the administration of highly promising novel protein-based drugs is the lack of appropriate pharmaceutical dosage forms. Due to the significant advances in biotechnology, numerous proteins can now be made available in sufficient quantities and at relatively low costs. Due to their limited half-lives in the human body, modified drug delivery systems will be required to allow for efficient therapies. Nowadays, proteins are generally administrated parenterally. Unfortunately, the standard parenteral controlled drug delivery system (PLGA-based microparticles) often leads to the loss of bioactivity of encapsulated proteins, due to the creation of acid micro-environments (as discussed earlier). The establishment of novel polymeric materials offering less aggressive environments for protein drugs would represent a major breakthrough for many future therapies. For instance, new dextran-based hydrogels might offer non-acidic, aqueous microclimates and be able to appropriately control the resulting protein release rates (46–48).
2. The possibility to allow for more convenient administration routes for the patient. Nowadays, the necessity to frequently administer drugs parenterally still presents a major practical limitation for many pharmaco-treatments. The use of long term releasing parenteral delivery systems can be of significant help, but obviously the complete circumvention of parenteral administration would be of even greater benefit in the future. Alternative routes might include pulmonary administration (e.g., an inhalable insulin product has recently been commercialized), nasal administration as well as the oral route. Major research efforts are ongoing to allow for oral administration of proteins (49,50). For example, muco-adhesive devices that protect the drug against enzymatic degradation and aggressive pH values within the GIT are under

investigation. The simultaneous release of substances that temporarily enhance drug absorption across the GIT mucosa might be of great practical importance. Obviously, it will be crucial to appropriately control the release of the drug as well as of absorption enhancers from such systems. Thus, modified drug delivery systems can be expected to play a central role in these novel treatment strategies.

3. The possibility to allow for overcoming the BBB in order to effectively treat brain diseases (51–53). Malignancies of the CNS will be of steadily increasing practical importance, especially in the industrial countries. The increasing life expectancy leads to a rising number of patients suffering from Alzheimer's and Parkinson's diseases. The consequences of these disorders (not only for the patients, but also for their family members) will be of fundamental importance in the future. Modified drug delivery systems might significantly contribute to the development of novel CNS treatment strategies (54,55).

4. The development of "intelligent" drug delivery systems: In the very long run, the ideal modified drug delivery system should be able to release the drug(s) "on demand." The device should, thus, be able to precisely detect how much drug is needed and be able to release exactly this amount. As an example, the delivery of insulin should be coupled to the plasma glucose level for the treatment of diabetes. Drugs regulating the blood pressure should be released from delivery systems that are sensitive to this parameter. Novel microchip-based technologies might be very useful to fulfill these advanced tasks (56,57).

REFERENCES

1. Tanquary AC, Lacey RE, eds. Controlled Release of Biologically Active Agents. New York: Plenum Press, 1974.
2. Baker R, ed. Controlled Release of Biologically Active Agents. New York: John Wiley & Sons, 1980.
3. Langer RS, Wise DL, eds. Medical Applications of Controlled Release, Vol. 1: Classes of Systems. Boca Raton, FL: CRC Press, 1984.
4. Broman E, Khoo C, Taylor LS. A comparison of alternative polymer excipients and processing methods for making solid dispersions of a poorly water soluble drug. Int J Pharm 2001; 222(1):139–51.
5. Zahedi P, Lee PI. Solid molecular dispersions of poorly water-soluble drugs in poly(2-hydroxyethyl methacrylate) hydrogels. Eur J Pharm Biopharm 2007; 65(3):320–28.
6. Fan LT, Singh SK, eds. Controlled release. A Quantitative Treatment. Berlin: Springer-Verlag, 1989.
7. Grieg NH. Optimizing drug delivery to brain tumors. Cancer Treat Rev 1987; 14:1–28.
8. Abott NJ, Romero, IA. Transporting therapeutics across the blood–brain barrier. Mol Med Today 1996; 2:106–13.

9. Langer R. Polymeric delivery systems for controlled drug release. Chem Eng Commun 1980; 6:1–48.
10. Langer R, Peppas NA. Chemical and physical structure of polymers as carriers for controlled release of bioactive agents: A review. Rev Macromol Chem Phys 1983; C23:61–126.
11. Rosen HB, Kohn J, Leong K, et al. Bioerodible polymers for controlled release systems. In: Hsieh D, ed. Controlled Release Systems: Fabrication Technology, Vol. 2. Boca Raton, FL: CRC Press, 1988: 83–110.
12. Peppas NA. Mathematical Modeling of diffusion processes in drug delivery polymeric systems. In: Smolen VF, Ball L, eds. Controlled Drug Bioavailability, Vol. 1. New York: John Wiley & Sons, 1984: 203–37.
13. Vergnaud JM, ed. Liquid Transport Processes in Polymeric Materials. Englewood Cliffs, NJ: Prentice-Hall, 1991: 26–9.
14. Vergnaud JM, ed. Controlled Drug Release of Oral Dosage Forms. Chichester: Ellis Horwood, 1993.
15. Crank J, ed. The Mathematics of Diffusion. Oxford: Clarendon Press, 1975.
16. Cussler EL, ed. Diffusion: Mass Transfer in Fluid Systems. New York: Cambridge University Press, 1984.
17. Siepmann J, Peppas NA. Modeling of drug release from delivery systems based on hydroxypropyl methylcellulose (HPMC). Adv Drug Deliv Rev 2001; 48: 139–57.
18. Higuchi T. Rate of release of medicaments from ointment bases containing drugs in suspensions. J Pharm Sci 1961; 50:874–5.
19. Colombo P. Swelling-controlled release in hydrogel matrices for oral route. Adv Drug Deliv Rev 1993; 11:37–57.
20. Doelker E. Water-swollen cellulose derivatives in pharmacy. In: Peppas NA, ed. Hydrogels in Medicine and Pharmacy, Vol. 2. Boca Raton, FL: CRC Press, 1986: 115–60.
21. Colombo P, Bettini R, Peppas NA. Observation of swelling process and diffusion front position during swelling in hydroxypropyl methyl cellulose (HPMC) matrices containing a soluble drug. J Control Release 1999; 61(1–2): 83–91.
22. Colombo P, Bettini R, Santi P et al. Swellable matrices for controlled drug delivery: gel-layer behaviour, mechanisms and optimal performance. Pharm Sci Tech Today 2000; 3(6):198–204.
23. Noyes AA, Whitney WR. Über die Auflösungsgeschwindigkeit von festen Stoffen in ihren eigenen Lösungen. Z Physikal Chem 1897; 23:689–92.
24. Narasimhan B, Peppas NA. Disentanglement and reptation during dissolution of rubbery polymers. J Polym Sci Polym Phys 1996; 34:947–61.
25. Narasimhan B, Peppas NA. On the importance of chain reptation in models of dissolution of glassy polymers. Macromolecules 1996; 29:3283–91.
26. Göpferich A. Polymer degradation and erosion: Mechanisms and applications. Eur J Pharm Biopharm 1996; 42:1–11.
27. Göpferich A, Langer R. Modeling of polymer erosion. Macromolecules 1993; 26:4105–12.
28. Göpferich A. Mechanisms of polymer degradation and erosion. Biomaterials 1996; 17:103–14.

29. Göpferich A. Polymer bulk erosion. Macromolecules 1997; 30:2598–604
30. von Burkersroda F, Schedl L, Göpferich A. Why degradable polymers undergo surface erosion or bulk erosion. Biomaterials 2002; 23:4221–31.
31. Pham AT, Lee PI. Probing the mechanisms of drug release from hydroxy-propylmethyl cellulose matrices. Pharm Res 1994; 11:1379–84.
32. Gao P, Skoug JW, Nixon PR, et al. Swelling of hydroxypropyl methylcellulose matrix tablets. 2. Mechanistic study of the influence of formulation variables on matrix performance and drug release. J Pharm Sci 1996; 85:732–40.
33. Siepmann J, Kranz H, Bodmeier R, et al. HPMC-matrices for controlled drug delivery: A new model combining diffusion, swelling and dissolution mechanisms and predicting the release kinetics. Pharm Res 1999; 16:1748–56.
34. Siepmann J, Kranz H, Peppas NA, et al. Calculation of the required size and shape of hydroxypropyl methylcellulose matrices to achieve desired drug release profiles. Int J Pharm 2000; 201:151–64.
35. Siepmann J, Peppas NA. Hydrophilic matrices for controlled drug delivery: An improved mathematical model to predict the resulting drug release kinetics (the "sequential layer" model). Pharm Res 2000; 17:1290–8.
36. Siepmann J, Streubel A, Peppas NA. Understanding and predicting drug delivery from hydrophilic matrix tablets using the "sequential layer" model. Pharm Res 2002; 19:306–14.
37. Hausberger AG, DeLuca PP. Characterization of biodegradable poly (D,L-lactide-co-glycolide) polymers and microspheres. J Pharmaceut Biomed 1995; 13:747–60.
38. Benita S, ed. Microencapsulation: Methods and Industrial Applications. New York: Marcel Dekker, 1996.
39. Shenderova A, Burke TG, Schwendeman SP. The acidic microclimate in poly (lactide-co-glycolide) microspheres stabilizes camptothecins. Pharm Res 1999; 16:241–8.
40. Brunner A, Mäder K, Göpferich A. pH and osmotic pressure inside bio-degradable microspheres during erosion. Pharm Res 1999; 16:847–53.
41. Li L, Schwendeman SP. Mapping neutral microclimate pH in PLGA micro-spheres. J Control Release 2005; 101:163–173.
42. Lu L, Garcia CA, Mikos AG. In vitro degradation of thin poly(DL-lactic-co-glycolic acid) films. J Biomed Mater Res 1999; 46:236–44.
43. Siepmann J, Elkharraz K, Siepmann F, et al. How autocatalysis accelerates drug release from PLGA-based microparticles: a quantitative treatment. Biomacromolecules 2005; 6:2312–19.
44. Klose D, Siepmann F, Elkharraz K, et al. How porosity and size affect the drug release mechanisms from PLGA-based microparticles. Int J Pharm 2006; 314: 198–206.
45. Siepmann J, Göpferich A. Mathematical modeling of bioerodible, polymeric drug delivery systems. Adv Drug Deliver Rev 2001; 48:229–47.
46. Van Tomme SR, De Geest BG, Braeckmans K, et al. Mobility of model pro-teins in hydrogels composed of oppositely charged dextran microspheres studied by protein release and fluorescence recovery after photobleaching. J Control Release 2005; 110(1):67–78.

47. Vlugt-Wensink KD, Jiang X, Schotman G, et al. In vitro degradation behavior of microspheres based on cross-linked dextran, Biomacromolecules 2006; 7(11): 2983–90.
48. Van Tomme SR, Hennink WE. Biodegradable dextran hydrogels for protein delivery applications. Expert Rev Med Devices 2007; 4(2):147–64.
49. Peppas NA. Devices based on intelligent biopolymers for oral protein delivery. Int J Pharm 2004; 277(1–2):11–7.
50. Morishita M, Peppas NA. Is the oral route possible for peptide and protein drug delivery? Drug Discov Today 2006; 11(19–20):905–10.
51. Brem H, Walter K, Langer R. Polymers as controlled drug delivery devices for the treatment of malignant brain tumors. Eur J Pharm Biopharm 1993; 27:2–7.
52. Brem H, Piantadosi S, Burger PC, et al. Placebo-controlled trial of safety and efficacy of intraoperative controlled delivery by biodegradable polymers of chemotherapy for recurrent gliomas. The Polymer-brain Tumor Treatment Group. Lancet 1995; 345:1008–12.
53. Brem H, Langer R. Polymer-based drug delivery to the brain. Sci Med 1996; 3: 52–61.
54. Wang PP, Frazier J, Brem H. Local drug delivery to the brain. Adv Drug Deliver Rev 2002; 54:987–1013.
55. Siepmann J, Siepmann F, Florence AT. Local controlled drug delivery to the brain: Mathematical modeling of the underlying mass transport mechanisms. Int J Pharm 2006; 314:101–19.
56. Li Y, Shawgo RS, Tyler B, et al. In vivo release from a drug delivery MEMSs device. J Control Release 2004; 100:211–19.
57. Li Y, Duc HLH, Tyler B, et al. In vivo delivery of BCNU from a MEMS devices to a tumor model. J Control Release 2005; 106:138–45.

3

The Modified-Release Drug Delivery Landscape

Advantages and Issues for Physicians and Patients

Marco M. Anelli

Research and Development, Keypharma, Milan, Italy

INTRODUCTION

The field of modified-release drug delivery (MDD) has recently expanded from the first marketed "depot injections" of several decades ago to include new types of oral delivery systems, transdermal drug systems, intrauterine devices, and implantable pumps to name a few.

As we mentioned, the first MDD formulations to enter clinical practice were probably the so-called depot injections used to deliver antibiotics or central nervous system drugs.

Today, there are at least four major classes of MDD formulations, these include:

1. Enteral (oral) MDD formulations:
   - monolithic forms
   - multiparticulate forms

2. Parenteral MDD formulations:
   - subcutaneous
   - intramuscular
   - intravenous
   - intraperitoneal

3. Implantable MDD formulations:
    ■ diffusion MDD formulations
    ■ externally activated MDD formulations

4. Transdermal MDD formulations:
    ■ membrane moderated formulations
    ■ diffusion controlled formulations
    ■ matrix type formulations
    ■ reservoir formulations

In this chapter we focus mainly on oral MDD formulations, even though the majority of the concepts that are described apply also to the other forms. A detailed description of the development all the types of MDD formulations and of their characteristics can be found in the comprehensive textbook edited by Robinson and Lee (1).

MODIFIED-RELEASE SYSTEMS: WHY?

The main objective to formulate an active pharmaceutical ingredient (API) in an MDD system is related to pharmacokinetics (PK).

In fact, an appropriate formulation can make the absorption, distribution, metabolism, and excretion (ADME) profile of a drug much more favorable. This change of the ADME paradigm to MDD–ADME (Fig. 1) can have a profound impact on many aspects of the clinical use of a drug, from patient compliance and convenience to its very efficacy, tolerability, and safety parameters.

MDD FORMULATIONS: CLINICAL USES

The main areas where oral MDD formulations are involved are:

■ gastroprotection
■ taste masking
■ improvement of PK characteristics
■ targeting
■ chronotherapeutics
■ life extension

Gastroprotection

Many drugs (most proton pump inhibitors, or pancreatic enzymes, just to name two categories) are not stable in an acidic environment and would be rapidly inactivated by the hydrochloric acid in the gastric juice.

Enteric-coated or gastroprotected forms are usually obtained by covering the whole tablet or capsule (or the single "particles" in case of multiparticulate forms) with a layer of polymers such as Eudragit or HP-55,

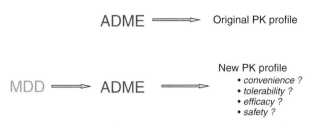

Figure 1 The change of ADME paradigm to MDD-ADME. *Abbreviations*: ADME, absorption, distribution, metabolism, and excretion; MDD, modified-release drug delivery.

which are stable for a very long time at low pH, but dissolve very rapidly once the pH has reached values around 5. The result obtained with this modification is that the drug is isolated from the environment in the stomach and then is rapidly released once the partially digested food is emptied into the duodenum and the contents have been buffered by the bile salts and the pancreatic juice.

Taste Masking

Several APIs have a pungent or unpleasant taste. Ibuprofen—one of the most widely used analgesics—is an example. The problem of unpleasantness is particularly important in pediatric or veterinary formulations, where the oral administration of a bad-tasting medicine could be very difficult or even impossible.

Taste masking is quite relevant also in orally dispersible formulations, also known as fast-melting tablets, which are formulations that can be dissolved in the mouth before swallowing and are usually taken without the need for water.

The masking of the organoleptic characteristics of a compound is usually obtained by covering the whole tablet—or the single particle—with layer or layers of substances, which are stable at the pH of the oral cavity and dissolve rapidly in the stomach. Flavoring agents may also be added. Mixing the right excipients in the right proportions is almost an "art" and also the evaluation of the acceptability of a taste masked formulation is not an exact science and usually involves tasting panels, composed of trained or untrained subjects.

Improvement of PK Characteristics

As we mentioned earlier, an appropriate MDD formulation can change radically the PK profile of a given API. The objectives of these types of formulations are usually to increase the time between two doses as well as to reduce the fluctuation of drug blood levels. The reduction from 3–4 times a day administrations to twice or even once daily, greatly increases patient compliance and reduces the potential for dosing errors, especially in those categories of patients (e.g., the elderly) who routinely assume several preparations. The reduction in the frequency of administration can also have a favorable impact on the cost of care in those situations (long-term care centers, hospitals, etc.) where licensed personnel administered the drugs to the patient.

For the majority of drugs, a constant therapeutic blood level is one of the goals of treatment. Wide fluctuations, in fact, can be the cause of therapeutic failure or of an undesirable toxic effect. This is especially true, for example, in the case of antibiotics, where the blood and tissue levels must be maintained constantly above the minimum inhibiting concentrations of the susceptible germs, in order to avoid the selection of resistant strains.

As shown in Figure 2, the immediate-release formulation of a hypothetical drug (in its native form) could grant 12 hours of coverage at a certain risk of toxicity, since its C_{max} is slightly above the toxicity threshold.

On the other hand, the same drug—administered in a MDD formulation—could eliminate the risk of toxicity and offer longer therapeutic coverage, which may be close to 24 hours.

Targeting

Drug targeting, which is the delivery of a drug only at the site where it is most active and needed, has been the "Holy Grail" of all drug delivery researchers. Despite some remarkable successes, it remains an area that needs to be explored, especially in the field of parenteral administration. A very good description of parenteral drug targeting techniques and issue, with special

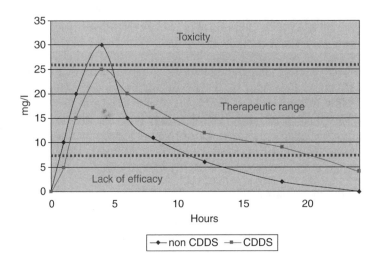

Figure 2 The formulation in a CDDS can reduce the risk of toxicity and extended coverage. *Abbreviation*: CDDS, controlled drug delivery system.

relation to its main field of interest: oncology can be found in the recent textbook edited by Pagé (2). Oral drug targeting may have a less dramatic relevance, but the combination of delayed and prolonged/extended-release techniques allows, just to give an example, to deliver exogenous pancreatic enzymes where they are needed most to promote assimilation of macro and micronutrients (duodenum and upper part of the jejunum). In many cases, such as in cystic fibrosis, where the endogenous pancreatic function is practically nonexistent from birth, this administration is a real life saver.

Another example of successful drug targeting is the administration of 5-aminosalycilic acid directly to the colon, where it is directly active on the lesions of inflammatory bowel disease, avoiding as much as possible its release in the small bowel where it is not needed and, if absorbed, could cause untoward systemic effects.

Chronotherapeutics

Chronotherapeutics can be considered the present frontier of MDD formulations. It is an established fact that many physiological and pathological parameters follow a circadian (that is, "around the day") pattern. For example, the pain and stiffness in arthritic joints are more pronounced in the morning. Similarly, the blood pressure is highest in the early hours of the morning (when the majority of heart attacks and CV accidents occur) and declines during the day. For this reason, it would seem appropriate to deliver an analgesic/antiinflammatory or an antihypertensive when it is needed most. Coverage at the moment of awakening is one of the rationales behind the common practice of prescribing NSAIDs at bedtime on a full stomach, to exploit the intrinsic retardant effect of food.

A recent example of chronotherapy is verapamil controlled onset extended release (COER), a special formulation of verapamil where a prolonged-release formulation of the calcium channel blocker is covered with a polymer layer meant to dissolve—and therefore start the release of the API—a few hours after ingestion.

Even though this approach makes a lot of sense, the clinical advantages of chronotherapeutics have not yet been scientifically proven (or not proven). In fact, controlled onset verapamil investigation of clinical endpoints (CONVINCE): a very large trial on the effect on the administration of verapamil COER versus standard therapy on the number of cardiovascular events in high risk hypertensive patients (3), was stopped for logistical reasons before any statistical significance was reached which may have yielded some scientific evidence. While a final word on the validity of chronotherapeutics might come from smaller studies presently ongoing in the field of endocrinology, the administration of exogenous hormones (cortisol, growth hormone, etc.) in a way that mimics the physiological secretory peaks may allow a more effective treatment of some patient populations.

Life Extension

Finally, a reason why many APIs undergo reformulation in a new MDD formulation is not scientific, but essentially related to marketing and assets protection. When the patent of a successful drug expires, its owner usually faces a significant drop in revenues (in some cases up to 90%) caused by the competition of generic drugs manufacturers. For this reason, the launch of a new formulation of a well-known brand, with some additional claims of improved convenience, safety and/or efficacy, could considerably extend the "commercial life" of a drug, especially if the technology used to produce the MDD formulation is in itself patentable.

WHICH DRUGS ARE SUITABLE FOR MDD FORMULATION?

The extent of fluctuation in drug concentration at steady state is determined by the relative magnitude of the elimination half-life and the dosing interval. For example, if a drug is given at an interval equal to the elimination half-life, then there is a twofold difference between the maximum and minimum concentrations at steady state.

For drugs with short half-lives and with a clear relationship between concentration and response, it will therefore be necessary to dose at regular, frequent intervals in order to maintain the concentration within the therapeutic range. Higher doses at less frequent intervals, in fact, will result in higher peak concentrations, with the possibility of toxicity.

For some drugs with wide margins of safety, this approach may be satisfactory, e.g., amoxicillin has a half-life of approximately 1 hour, but a dosage frequency of 8 hours. This means that very large fluctuations will occur within a dosing interval, but, in view of the low toxicity of this drug, no difficulty with this approach is encountered provided the concentrations are always above the minimum effective concentration during the dosing interval. On the contrary, clinical efficacy may be enhanced by the transiently high bactericidal concentration of some antibiotics e.g., beta-lactams.

Conversely, drugs with long half-lives can be given at less frequent intervals. There is generally no advantage in formulating these drugs as extended-release formulations unless a rapid rate of change of concentration during the absorptive phase is responsible for transient adverse effects, as it may be the case with antihypertensive drugs.

It must be noted, however, that the pharmacological effect of some drugs with short half-lives can be much more prolonged than their PK would suggest. This happens in cases such as the following:

- The drug binds to the tissues, e.g., tissue-bound ACE inhibitors. For these drugs, less frequent dosing is needed even though the drug may have a short half-life.

- The drugs have irreversible effects, e.g., the acetylation of platelet cyclo-oxygenase by aspirin.
- The relationship between response and plasma/blood concentrations is relatively flat or if the given dose results in concentrations which are in the plateau region of the dose–response relationship, e.g., thiazides in hypertension.
- The drug is metabolized to pharmacologically active metabolite(s), which are more slowly cleared than the parent drug, e.g., quinapril, trandolapril, and venlafaxine.

Therefore, even though a good percentage of drugs could benefit from some tweaking of their PK characteristics, not all APIs are suitable for formulation in a MDD formulation.

MONOLITHIC VS. MULTIPARTICULATE FORMS

Whenever the formulation in a MDD approach is involved, a very important distinction to be made is between monolithic and multiparticulate formulations. A tablet obtained by compression is an example of monolithic form, while a capsule filled with drug beads or granules is an example of multiparticulate. There are also hybrid formulations, such as granules compressed into a tablet, or mini- or microtablets (obtained by compression, but only 1–2 mm in size) put into a capsule. Monolithic and multiparticulate forms tend to have slightly different behaviors in vivo.

POTENTIAL ISSUES WITH MDD FORMULATIONS

Unfortunately, even though the potential benefits of an appropriate MDD formulation are many, the development (and the use) of these formulations have to face some hurdles. Sometimes, in fact, a modified, extended or prolonged release form can actually represent a serious disadvantage from the point of view of the patient or of the clinician. The potential issues that need to be taken into consideration when dealing with MDD formulations relate to: GI transit time (TT), regional absorption, first pass, dose dumping, and food effect.

Gastrointestinal Transit Time

The GI/TT is the time an undigested particle takes to travel from the mouth to the anus. According to the various techniques and the diagnostic needs, different—or segmental TTs—may be measured (i.e., gastro-duodenal, gastro-colic, gastro-cecal, etc.). Subject or population variability in TT may affect drug PKs, notably absorption. This is likely to be of limited relevance for immediate-release formulations, which release all their content in a matter of minutes, but may have greater importance for modified-release (delayed-release, sustained-release) formulations and even more for chronotherapeutic agents. In these cases, in fact, a shorter time may result in a more limited exposure to the drug and viceversa. According to published evidence, TT shows variability among different ethnic groups and/or geographic areas and in particular, major difference exists between Indian people and Caucasians. The mechanism of ethnic difference in TT is not yet ascertained, although various causes have been hypothesized. It is a fact, however, that the intestinal TT of Indians, in fact, is shorter, and their stool weight larger than that of Caucasians.

According to published studies, the possible reasons for this are dietary habits—fiber or spice diet content—and/or genetic factors. A greater fiber intake is widely considered as a likely cause for shorter TT in Indian people, compared to Caucasians, but there is not complete agreement on this issue. Even in studies supporting the importance of a greater fiber intake, in fact, the latter does not completely account for the shorter TT observed in Indian people (4–7). Although the involvement of genetic factors in determining the shorter TT reported in Indian people cannot be excluded, no specific data are available in the published literature.

Other ethnic groups, such as the Chinese and peoples of Africa, also have variability in GI TT. The oro-cecal TT of Chinese people, in fact, is longer than that of Caucasians and the cause may lie again in different environmental factors, data is unavailable on this issue (8).

On the other hand, the intestinal TT of some African peoples, is again shorter than that of Caucasians which speculates that environmental factors may be involved, notably the high fiber consumption, even though genetic factors cannot be ruled out (9,10).

Regional Absorption

The absorption pattern of a given drug in the different parts of the GI tract may be very different and examples will be provided to give the reader insight into some of these differences.

This is the case, e.g., of some beta-blockers, such as atenolol, which show a definite absorption window in the upper tract of the small bowel. The variations in the absorption pattern (especially from jejunum, ileum, and colon) can be due to the differences in the epithelium of the three tracts mentioned above and/or in their content (food in different stages of digestion, pH, water percentage, etc.).

For these reasons, the formulation of some drugs in a delayed or even in an extended/prolonged release formulation, could cause a dramatic reduction in the total bioavailability, as it can be seen from Figure 3, where a delay in the release of the drug—formulated to assure an extended release—versus the immediate release formulation results in a marked reduction of both C_{max}

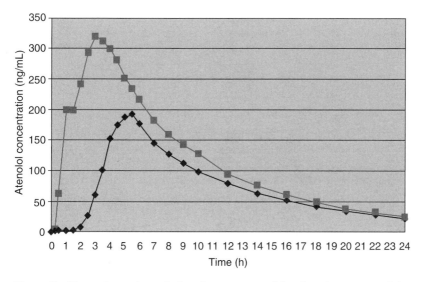

Figure 3 If an absorption window is present, a delay in release can originate a significant reduction in plasma levels.

and AUC, because some of the API is released in a part of the GI tract where the absorption is already reduced. Because of the reduction in bioavailability, reliable information on the differential absorption in the different regions of the digestive tract is rather difficult to obtain. Some data have derived from studying in vitro the permeability and the diffusion through exvivo tissue, but the bulk of the published literature is based on older studies where the GI tract of volunteers was selectively blocked by balloon catheters or on more recent studies using smart capsules, with or without the use of radioactive tracers (Fig. 4).

A smart capsule is a device that can be followed from the outside the body (usually with a scintigraphic camera or an ultrasound machine) and that can be activated with a radio signal when it has reached the desired zone, releasing its content.

First Pass

Another reason why the formulation in an extended/prolonged MDD formulation of a drug may result in reduced bioavailability is the presence of a marked, saturable first pass effect. In some cases, in fact, the relatively quick and elevated peak obtained with an immediate release formulation is capable of saturating the metabolizing capacity of the liver, therefore allowing part of the drug to enter the systemic circulation unchanged. On the contrary, a "smoother" and more gradual release may not be able to saturate the liver metabolism, causing therefore significantly lower systemic levels.

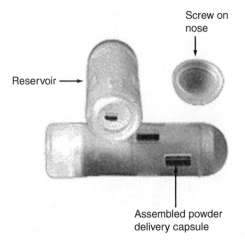

Screw on
nose

Reservoir ⟶

Assembled powder
delivery capsule   **Figure 4**   A smart capsule.

Dose Dumping

One of the biggest concerns when using, or even testing, an extended/
prolonged release formulation is what is technically called dose dumping,
that is, the rapid release of a dose of the drug that was meant to be
administered over several hours. It is easy to imagine that such an event may
have consequences that range from very unpleasant (e.g., in the case of
antihypertensives) to potentially catastrophic (morphine or theophylline).

Another kind of dumping that may occur during everyday clinical use
is when a well-meaning patient (or a caregiver) breaks or even crushes a
monolithic formulation to obtain a half dose or to allow for an easier
administration. The breaking of a monolithic formulation causes in fact, in
the case of MDD formulations based on polymer core erosion, a change in
the surface area and therefore a change in the release characteristics (i.e.,
one half of a 100 mg tablet does not behave like a 50 mg tablet, while the two
halves of the same 100 mg tablet do not behave like a whole one). In the
case of barrier membrane MDD formulations, instead, the breaking of the
tablet turns the system into an immediate release formulation. For this
reason, during the clinical development of a MDD formulation, it is man-
datory that all the necessary steps be taken to evaluate the potential risk of
dumping.

Food Effect

The presence of food in the GI tract can have a profound impact on the PK
characteristics of many APIs. The differences in the environment, gastric

emptying time, transit time, pH, fat content and hydration, in fact, just to name a few, can cause very significant differences in C_{max}, T_{max}, and AUC, differences than can result, in practice, in non-effective or even toxic levels.

In addition to this kind of variability, that we could call intrinsic, since it is related to the physico-chemical characteristics of the API (and is essentially the same for all immediate release formulations), MDD formulations suffer from the additional variability originated by the effect of the food on the different components of the system.

Another important effect of food, which can be neglected for immediate release formulation, is the mechanical stress that the partially digested food, under the influence of peristaltic movements, poses on monolithic formulations. These formulations, in fact, can be broken or crushed during their permanence in the stomach, causing a release of the API potentially very different from what was expected. The MDD formulations that are least affected by this mechanical effect are the osmotic pumps, because of their hard, insoluble shells. The often unpredictable effect of food on drug release is the reason behind the request by all Regulatory Authorities to prove the bioequivalence of two MDD formulations (usually an originator and a lower cost generic) both in the fasted and in the fed state.

In order to determine the effect of food, the Regulatory Authorities suggest a rather heavy and fat-rich English-style breakfast. An example of such a breakfast could be:

High-Fat Content Breakfast (1000 kcal):

- one buttered muffin (fat = 9.2 g),
- one fried egg (fat = 10.0 g),
- 30 g of cheese (fat = 10.2 g),
- one piece of bacon (fat = 4.0 g),
- one serving of boiled potato (fat = 9.6 g),
- 250 mL of whole milk (fat = 8.25 g),
- 180 mL of orange juice.

However, many contract research organizations operating in mostly vegetarian countries, such as India, e.g., use perfectly acceptable meat free alternatives based on local dishes. With the exception of a few countries, however, breakfasts tend to be much lighter than the "standard meal" described above. For this reason—especially since many "once-a-day" MDD formulations are taken at breakfast time—some efforts are being made in order to introduce a lighter meal as a means to evaluate the effect of food on modified release formulations. Even though this approach does have some merits, it seems that a sufficient level of standardization has not yet been reached.

THE BIGGEST ISSUE: INCREASED VARIABILITY

The result of all the potential issues we have examined so far is that the variability in all the PK parameters (and therefore in the in-vivo behavior of a drug) can be much higher whenever MDD formulations are involved. This increased variability has a significant impact, both in clinical practice and in clinical research.

Clinical Practice (Patient Switching)

When a prescriber wishes to transfer a patient from an immediate-release to an extended-release product, generally the equivalent total daily dose should be the same. In some cases, however, an effective response may be achieved with a lower dose of the extended-release product.

In view of the complexity of extended-release products and the potential for greater variability (both inter- and intrasubject) patients should be monitored, at least in the initial phase of the switch, to ensure that the anticipated benefit of switching to such products is actually obtained.

Clinical Research

Whenever in-vivo trials are involved, the result of an increase in variability (i.e., in the dispersion of the data) is always the same. This will increase the sample size if a sufficient power needs to be maintained (11). Since the standard error decreases with the square root of the number of subjects, sometimes the clinical researcher find themselves in situation requiring a prohibitive number of subjects.

REFERENCES

1. Robinson JR, Lee VH, eds. Controlled Drug Delivery: Fundamentals and Applications, 2nd ed. New York: Marcel Dekker Inc., 1987.
2. Pagé M ed. Tumor Targeting in Cancer Therapy. Humana Press, 2002.
3. Black H, et al. Principal results of the controlled onset verapamil investigation of cardiovascular end points (CONVINCE) trial. JAMA 2003; 289(16): 2073–82.
4. Kochlar KP, et al. Gastrointestinal effect of Indian spice mixture. Tropical Gastroenterol 1999; 20:170–4.
5. Jayanthi V, et al. Intestinal transit in healthy Southern Indian subjects and in patients with tropical sprue. Gut 1989; 30:35–8.
6. Tandon RK, et al. Stool weights and transit times in North Indians. J Assoc Physiol India 1976; 24.
7. Shetty PJ, Kurpad AV. Intestinal transit time of South India subjects. Indian J Med Res 1984; December:693–8.
8. Yu LX. An integrated model for determining causes of poor oral drug absorption. Pharm Res 1999; 16(12).

9.   Fakunle YM, et al. Diarrhoea, constipation and intestinal transit time in a Northern Nigerian population. J Tropical Med Hyg 1978; 81(7):137–8.
10. Walker AR. Effect of high crude fiber intake on transit time and the absorption of nutrients in South African Negro schoolchildren. Amer J Clin Nutr 1975; 28 (10):1161–9.
11. Diletti E, et al. Sample size determination for bioequivalence assessment by means of confidence intervals. Int J Clin Pharmacol, Ther Toxicol 1991; 29(1): 1–8.

4

The Modified-Release Drug Delivery Landscape

Drug Delivery Commercialization Strategies

Fintan Walton
Pharma Ventures Ltd., Oxford, U.K.

INTRODUCTION

The drug delivery sector has experienced considerable growth over the past decade as indicated by a variety of measures: the number of pharmaceutical products on the market that incorporate a drug delivery technology, the total sales of such products, the number of drug delivery companies that have been established, and the number and variety of drug delivery technologies upon which these companies are working. This increase in activity is also reflected in the number of drug delivery deals recorded in PharmaDeals® agreements; the number in 2005 was the highest recorded to date (Fig. 1).

In common with many other sectors of the healthcare industry, technological innovation is a major driver in the drug delivery area. To a great extent, but by no means exclusively, such innovation occurs within research-intensive environments. Perhaps only in a minority of cases are highly innovative drug delivery technologies originated within the R&D laboratories of established, vertically integrated drug delivery companies. The foregoing observation is important because it highlights the fact that in the majority of cases, a new drug delivery technology is conceived and initially explored within the context of an organization that is poorly equipped to exploit it. How poorly equipped, however, is in part a function of the form in which such exploitation, or commercialization, is to occur. This chapter focuses on the commercialization options available for a drug

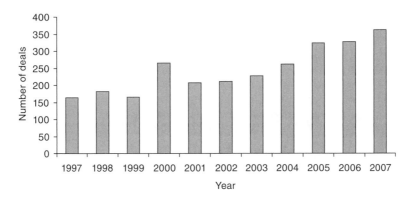

Figure 1 Drug delivery deal activity, 1997–2005. *Source*: Adapted from
©PharmaVentures PharmaDeals® Agreements.

delivery technology, and the criteria that may be used by a drug delivery
innovator to select the appropriate commercialization strategy.

DRUG DELIVERY PRODUCT OFFERINGS

The intended output of the company and its technology is a major factor
that influences strategies and business models, but conversely, a company
may also determine the nature of its product offering in the light of the business model it prefers to adopt. Four potential product offerings may be
defined, as follows:

- Out-licensing either to a service-based company, that will act as direct
  provider of the drug delivery technology to customer/client companies,
  or to pharmaceutical companies for use in-house.
- Sale of devices to pharmaceutical or biotech customer organizations for
  them to market with their pharmaceutical product, or direct to healthcare practitioners and hospitals.
- Service provision, e.g., reformulation of product or processing a product
  to impart defined physico-chemical characteristics.
- New (or enhanced) pharmaceutical product combining the drug delivery
  technology with a specific chemical entity.

EXPLOITATION STRATEGIES

There are six broad strategies that are generally available for the exploitation of an innovation. In increasing order of the degree of involvement of
the innovator in commercialization, and hence in the contribution it must
make to the range of complementary resources required, these are:

- divestment (or single exclusive license)
- licensing to multiple companies
- service offering
- strategic alliance
- joint venture
- internal commercialization

The risks, benefits/returns and resource implications that these six strategies entail are compared in Table 1.

Which of these strategies will allow an innovator to appropriate the most return and provide the most acceptable risk/reward ratio depends mainly on:

- the characteristics of the technology
- the extent of protection through patents
- the resources and capabilities of the innovator

Table 1　Strategies for the Exploitation of Innovation

	Risks	Benefits/returns	Resource implications
Divestment	None	No investment needed, little return	None
Licensing	Some legal risks	Low investment required, returns limited (unless patent position very strong)	Few resources must be provided internally
Service offering	Low risk	Control of proprietary systems, low future returns	Resources must be provided internally
Strategic alliance	Informal structure creates risks	Flexibility	Permits pooling of resources and capabilities from more than one firm
Joint venture	Risks shared. Potential for partner disagreement or culture clash	Investment shared	As for strategic alliance, less flexibility to vary inputs
Internal commercialization	High investment requirement with associated risks	Increased control	All resources required must be provided internally

BUSINESS MODELS

Three distinct business models may be adopted in the commercialization of drug delivery technologies: supplier/service company model; collaborative model; and pharmaceutical company model. In terms of the pattern of activities adopted in pursuit of commercial objectives, these three business models imply a divergence at a very basic level and the differences between the three are quite marked. In addition, it is worth noting that:

- supplier and service company models have certain distinct features
- the three strategy types may not be entirely mutually exclusive
- intermediate forms exist, particularly when the two-stage biotech model is adopted
- the same company may use different strategies for different platform technologies if the characteristics of the technologies are distinct
- the fundamental strategy of a platform technology company may change with time, most notably if occurring with a change in risk aversion/acceptance

PRODUCT, STRATEGY, AND BUSINESS MODELS FOR DRUG DELIVERY TECHNOLOGY

For a typical drug delivery technology, the product offerings that have been defined exemplify the six generic strategies available for the commercialization of innovations, and encompass all three basic business models (Table 2).

Out-licensing, or divesting the drug delivery technology to a larger drug delivery company, absolves the innovator of the majority of responsibility for the commercialization of its technology. This may be appropriate for a very small company with a single technology as it can provide a faster route to full commercialization of the technology than the small company can achieve on its own due to its resource constraints. All the resources necessary for the development and production of a commercial product or service and its marketing/sales would be contributed by the licensee.

Out-licensing the technology to multiple companies will typically require that some basic research work and demonstration studies would have to continue in-house. Although no major investments in additional capabilities may be necessary, substantial effort may be required to provide training and transfer of the technology to the licensees. In a situation where there is weak or absent patent protection and the majority of the intellectual property is held as know-how, this would be a risky strategy to pursue. Potential licensees will require substantial disclosure of methods and proof-of-principle studies, probably in their own laboratories before agreeing significant license terms.

If the product of a company is to be a device, this implies a strategy of internal commercialization and a supplier business model. The device will

Table 2   Generic Strategies for Commercialization

Product offering	Strategy type	Business model implied
Out-licensing (divestment) to larger drug delivery company	Divestment	N/A—essentially all responsibility passed to licensee
Out-licensing to pharmaceutical companies	Licensing	Supplier (of technology)
Device	Internal commercialization	Supplier/service
Fee for service	Service offering	Supplier/service
Pharmaceutical products developed in collaboration with partner companies	Strategic alliance or joint venture	Collaborative
Pharmaceutical products developed through in-house application	Internal commercialization	Pharmaceutical company, or pharmaceutical company followed by collaborative

ideally be applicable to the delivery of multiple different drugs with minimal or no customization required. Interaction with pharmaceutical customers would be much less formalized than in the collaborative model and, rather than develop drug and device in tandem, the device would be customized to the needs of a drug formulation that has been developed independently.

By providing a service offering charged on a fee-for-service basis, the innovator would be able to maintain tight control of its know-how and receive early cash flow. Milestone payments could also be receivable based on technical milestones.

Two very different strategies and business models are compatible with the concept of the drug delivery company's product being a new pharmaceutical product. Both can permit the drug delivery company to appropriate a greater proportion of the overall return to the technology than it could do through the other product offerings, but both will require substantial investment in resources and capabilities by the drug delivery company. A product offering, based on collaborations with partner companies, clearly illustrates a collaborative business model and can be viewed as comprising a strategic alliance strategy. Depending on the degree to which the technology originator is willing to accept risk, the potential returns could be moderate or quite substantial.

An extreme form of the collaborative model would be an exclusive, long-term joint venture with a major pharmaceutical company. This may limit the resource contribution required from the technology innovator, thus reducing the risks involved, although the returns would be reduced accordingly. However, pharmaceutical companies are unlikely to pay a significant premium for exclusive access to an early stage technology that may only be applicable to some of their molecules, and it is generally not the best strategy for drug delivery companies to tie their technology to a single partner in this way. Granting exclusivity for certain therapeutic areas to different partners can be an attractive version of the alliance model, if the partner companies are willing to pay a sufficient premium for exclusivity.

The alternative route to involvement in a new pharmaceutical product is to adopt a strategy of internal commercialization. The drug delivery company would adopt a pharmaceutical company model with the intention of developing potentially enhanced therapeutic products, probably for eventual out-licensing for late-stage development and marketing. The range of resources that would have to be assembled by the drug delivery technology company would be significant, entailing a high level of risk. However, the proportion of the potential returns on the innovation that could be appropriated by it would be increased substantially.

It is worth noting that for certain product offerings, the drug delivery technology innovator has a choice as to the level of direct involvement it needs to have in the product's commercialization. For example, if the company elects to concentrate wholly or partly on the in-house application of its technology to the development of potential improved drugs, there will always be an option to out-license such improved drugs at a relatively early stage of development (thus restricting the scope of the pharmaceutical company model required). By the same token, if it emerges that the production and sale of a device is the preferred commercialization route, the innovator could in principle out-license these rights to a company already established in this market, thus reducing the capital investment and risk-taking required.

APPLICABILITY TO SEGMENTS OF THE PHARMACEUTICAL PRODUCT LIFE CYCLE

The three key phases of a pharmaceutical product's life cycle define three broad market segments to which drug delivery technologies may be applied:

- NCEs—Application to problem NCEs to enable their development or to produce an enhanced product with better market potential than the NCE alone would have;
- Life cycle management—Creation of line extensions, enhanced versions of an existing product and extension of patent life by or for the owner of the original drug;
- Generic plus—Creation of improved versions of off-patent drugs.

ASSESSMENT OF ATTRACTIVENESS OF EACH OPTION

In assessing the attractiveness of the various product offerings and market segments, the valuation of the product or technology on a per-deal basis is certainly relevant, although other factors should also be considered, for example:

- number of deals possible (related to market size and expected penetration);
- competitive structure of the market or market segment;
- investment required;
- risk;
- presence or absence of mutual exclusivity between certain product offerings.

The attractiveness of these offerings will be defined by several inter-related factors, including (but not confined to):

- experience of the drug delivery company in preclinical development, management of clinical trials or device manufacture and sales;
- risk versus reward attitude of management and majority shareholders;
- requirement for near term revenue;
- the need for the commercial leverage offered by a larger partner;
- market conditions.

COMPATIBILITY OF PRODUCT OFFERINGS

The various product offerings, strategies and business models discussed above are not all mutually exclusive. Certain combinations are compatible even if this means that the drug delivery company adopts more than one business model in parallel.

As Table 3 shows, the in-house application of the technology (F) is at least in principle compatible with any other product offering. It is quite normal for a licensor company to retain rights to use a technology on its own account when entering into a licensing arrangement. In contrast, divestment to a service-based company (A) precludes any other possibilities. However, it may be possible to pursue this in combination with the in-house application of the technology for drug development by granting a semi-exclusive license with retention of rights for in-house use. The simultaneous pursuit of device sales (C) together with most other product offerings would imply a degree of competition between the two. Some scope, therefore, exists for drug delivery companies to pursue more than one product offering, providing it avoids combinations that are inherently mutually exclusive.

Table 3 Compatibility of Product Offerings

Product	A	B	C	D	E	F
A		x	x	x	x	(✓)
B			(✓)	✓	✓	✓
C				✓	✓	✓
D					(✓)	✓
E						(✓)
F						

✓ Compatible (✓) Poorly compatible   x Incompatible   Shaded, N/A

Key
A Divestment
B Out-licensing to pharmaceutical companies
C Device sales
D Service provision
E Collaborative drug development
F In-house drug development

CONCLUSION

Drug delivery companies can adopt a variety of different product offerings, strategies and business models when seeking to commercialize their technology. Four potential product offerings have been identified as the output that a drug delivery company may seek to sell:

- licenses to a drug delivery technology
- devices, reagents or equipment
- service provision
- new (or enhanced) pharmaceutical products

    The exploitation strategies that can be adopted are:

- divestment (or single exclusive license)
- licensing to multiple companies
- service offering
- strategic alliance
- joint venture
- internal commercialization

Three generic business models are adopted:

- supplier/service company model
- collaborative model
- pharmaceutical company model

Each management team will adopt a number of criteria when determining what it is feasible to do with their particular technology. These will include: the nature of the technology itself, the demand for it and the form of the competition, the time and resources needed and the amounts available, how complementary resources can be accessed, and the acceptability, suitability and feasibility of the option in the specific context of the company. Furthermore, more than one strategy and business model can co-exist within the same company if chosen and handled carefully.

Part II: Ocular Technologies

5

Ophthalmic Drug Delivery

Pascal Furrer and Florence Delie
Department of Pharmaceutics and Biopharmaceutics, School of Pharmaceutical Sciences, University of Geneva, University of Lausanne, Geneva, Switzerland

Bernard Plazonnet
Chamalières, France

INTRODUCTION

Ocular drug delivery is an extremely important topic, especially with the recent development of new drugs for the treatment of age-related macular degeneration (AMD) (1). Drug delivery to the eye can vary in difficulty and complexity from simple topical eye drops to more sophisticated systems like ocular implants.

The eye (Fig. 1) is a sensory organ that converts light to an electric signal that is treated and interpreted by the brain. Briefly, the eye ball is covered by three layers: an outer fibrous protective layer (sclera and cornea), a middle vascular layer (choroid), and an inner nervous layer (retina) (2–4). The cornea is a clear, transparent, thin (0.5 mm) avascular tissue that is composed of five layers: epithelium, Bowman's layer, stroma, Descemet's membrane, and endothelium (5). The stroma is the only hydrophilic layer. The eye is generally divided into two parts: the anterior and the posterior segments. The anterior includes the cornea, sclera, ciliary body, and the lens; these structures delimit a cavity: the anterior chamber filled with aqueous humor. The posterior segment includes all the structures between the lens and the optic nerve that delimit a cavity: the vitreous filled with an aqueous gel (the vitreous humor).

The eye possesses efficient protective mechanisms like reflex blinking, lachrymation, and drainage, while lid closure protects the eye from external aggression. Tears, the production of which is increased in case of external

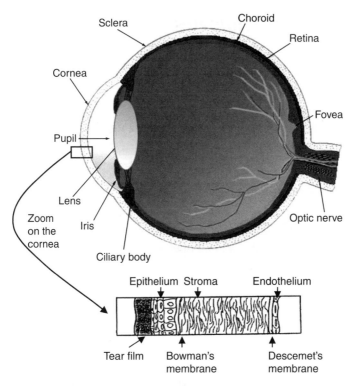

Figure 1 Sagittal view of the human eye with its main anatomic elements and schematic representation of the cross section of the cornea.

aggression, permanently wash the surface of the eye and exert an anti-infectious activity through the lysozyme and immunoglobulins they contain. Finally, the lachrymal fluid is drained down the nasolacrimal pathways, then to the pharynx and esophagus where it is either swallowed or expectorated (Fig. 2). All these protective mechanisms are responsible for the rapid and extensive precorneal loss of topically applied ophthalmic drugs. As a consequence, the ocular residence time of these drugs is limited to a few minutes. Furthermore, their ocular absorption is limited by the highly selective corneal–epithelial barrier, by drug binding to tear proteins and to conjunctival mucin, as well as by overflow of the instilled eye drop (25–60 µl of volume) out of the patient's cul-de-sac which can accommodate only approximately 30 µl of added fluid (6). As a consequence, only 1–10% of the instilled drug is absorbed (7). Moreover, the elderly have difficulty with dosing eye drops to the eye.

Thus, there is a need for innovative drug delivery systems for the ocular route that prolong the contact time between the cornea and the drug.

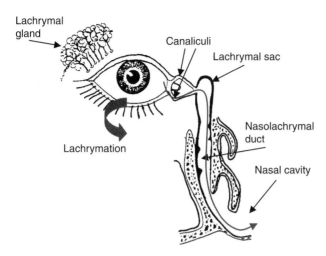

Figure 2 Schematic representation of the lachrymation and the nasolachrymal drainage contributing to the rapid elimination of topically applied ocular drug.

For example, anti-infectious agents would benefit from a longer residence on the surface of the eye and improved compliance and comfort. In addition, greater selectivity (i.e., targeted delivery to specific regions of the eye) would be a plus in order to sustain activity and to decrease the irritation, which is sometimes induced by a bolus dose.

CHALLENGES IN DEVELOPING AN OPHTHALMIC DRUG DELIVERY SYSTEM

Routes of Administration for Ocular Therapeutics

There are several possible routes of ocular drug delivery. The choice depends primarily on the target tissue (8). Traditionally, topical ocular and subconjunctival administrations are used for anterior targets and intra-vitreal or systemic administration for posterior targets.

The topical administration involves two main routes: the transcorneal permeation from the lachrymal fluid into the anterior chamber and the transconjunctival/scleral permeation from the external ocular surface to the anterior uvea–ciliary body and iris. The transcorneal permeation is limited by the corneal barrier. Indeed the tight junctions between the most apical epithelial cells serve as a selective barrier for small molecules, and they completely prevent the diffusion of macromolecules via the paracellular route (9). Moreover, the permeability of lipophilic drugs is higher than hydrophilic drugs (10). On the contrary, the transconjunctival pathway is fairly permeable to hydrophilic and large molecules (11), as the conjunctiva is more a leaky epithelium than the cornea and its surface area is about 20 times greater. Thus the transconjunctival route has recently gained increasing attention for the delivery of large molecules such as proteins and peptides. Topical administration is used to treat pathological conditions of the anterior segment, such as inflammation, allergy, infections, corneal ulceration, and keratoconjunctivis sicca. Subconjunctival administration by injection has been historically used to increase the drug level in the uvea. The injected drug penetrates across the sclera, which is more permeable than the cornea especially to large molecules and whose permeability does not depend on drug lipophilicity (12). The intravitreal administration offers a more direct access to the vitreous to treat diseases of the posterior segment such as endophthalmitis, age-related macular degeneration, proliferative vitreoretinopathy, diabetic macular edema, and retinitis (13).

The systemic administration of drugs, mostly anti-infectious and anti-inflammatory drugs, is also possible, though less convenient for the patient than topical application. The main disadvantage of this route is the potential for systemic toxicity and the limited or variable penetration. Two barriers impair the penetration of drugs from the blood stream into the eye. First, the anterior blood–aqueous barrier that is composed of the endothelial cells of the uvea. This barrier prevents access of large plasma albumin molecules and many antibiotics into the aqueous humor. Some molecules can never-theless be secreted into the aqueous humor during its formation by the ciliary epithelium. Inflammation associated with injury, infection or an ocular disease, e.g., uveitis, may disrupt the integrity of the blood–aqueous humor barrier and drugs may enter the aqueous humor and reach the tissues of the anterior segment. The second barrier between the blood stream and the eye is the so-called blood–retina barrier. This barrier prevents diffusion of the drugs in the posterior part of the eye and is formed by the endothelial cells of retinal capillaries (inner–retinal barrier) and the retinal pigment epithelial cells (outer blood–retinal barrier) (14). Thus, the delivery of drugs to the posterior pole and to the retina is extremely difficult.

Ocular Pharmacokinetics

Human ocular pharmacokinetic experimentation is limited to the non-invasive observation of fluorescent or gamma-scintigraphic probes and to the determination of drug concentration in aqueous humor samples from patients undergoing cataract surgery, where the anterior chamber is open. This latter practice is not carried out very frequently and has serious ethical implications. Precorneal disposition can be studied in humans using tear sampling and subsequent measurement of drug levels in the tear. It should be noted, however, that such a procedure can induce excessive blinking and tear production in subjects sensitive to the sampling pipette, and therefore induce a bias in the results. Moreover, when dealing with formulations that do not mix rapidly with tear film, one can sample a small part of the formulation itself leading to an overestimation, thus making the assay results from such a sample meaningless. Plasma level analyses are irrelevant to assess ocular bioavailability of topically administered ophthalmic drugs. However, it may be considered if a systemic absorption that may lead to undesirable effect is suspected.

The albino rabbit is by far the most commonly used animal model in ocular pharmacokinetic studies. This animal model has various advantages including its availability, docile nature, ease of handling, low cost, relative large ocular surface, important background literature on ocular effects of chemicals and lack of pigmentation enabling better observation of possible hyperemia, especially of the iris (7,15–17). Although the rabbit and human eye do exhibit some similarities (very similar cornea and aqueous humor composition in both species), the rabbit eye differs from an anatomical and physiological point of view from the human eye as it displays a nictitating membrane (a third eyelid), and it has no well-defined Bowman's membrane, slower tear turnover (approximately 7% per minute in rabbits, compared to 16% in man), slower blinking rate (a few times per hour whereas man blinks 15–20 times per minute), slower drainage rate (~0.5 μl/min in rabbits and 3 times larger, ~1.5 μl/min in man), more alkaline tear pH, slower regeneration capability of the corneal epithelium, presence of the nictitating membrane (7,18–23). All these differences may explain, at least in part, the discrepancy between results in rabbit and in human.

As discussed above, the absorption after topical administration is weak. The peak concentration of the drug in the anterior chamber after transcorneal permeation is reached within 20–30 minutes (8). From the aqueous humor, the drug can diffuse to the iris and the ciliary body, where it may bind to melamine and form a kind of reservoir. Drug is eliminated from the aqueous humor by two mechanisms: by aqueous turnover through the trabecular meshwork and Schlemm's canal and by the venous blood flow of the anterior uvea across the blood-aqueous barrier. The first elimination mechanism has a rate of 3 μl/min and does not depend on the nature of the drug, whereas the second mechanism depends on the drug's ability to cross the endothelial walls of the vessel and promotes the elimination of lipophilic drugs whose clearance is in the range of 10–30 μl/min (24). Thus, drug half-life in the anterior chamber is typically short, for instance, nearly 1 hour for timolol.

The drug elimination from the vitreous occurs through two main routes: anterior and posterior (25). Indeed, the drug can by eliminated from the vitreous via the posterior chamber and, thereafter, via aqueous turnover and uveal blood flow. Or, it can be eliminated via the posterior blood-retina barrier if the drug is small and lipophilic.

Drug pharmacodynamics are used when pharmacokinetic properties cannot be measured (26). Some biological responses like miosis, mydriasis, intraocular pressure, and bactericidal activity are easy to assess quantitatively, whereas the appreciation of leakage from the retinal vessels is far more difficult.

TOPICAL OPHTHALMIC FORMULATION APPROACHES

Development of ophthalmic preparations must satisfy the Goldmann's criteria of stability, sterility, tolerance, and efficacy simultaneously (Fig. 3). Stability means that during a particular lapse of time, the essential properties of the preparation do not change or change only in acceptable proportions. In other words, no sign of physical or chemical alteration is detected. On the one hand, the stability may be influenced by the pH of the lachrymal film (close to neutrality) or the preparation. For instance, pilocarpine, a natural alkaloid used in the treatment of glaucoma, contains a lactone ring and undergoes pH-dependant hydrolytic degradation leading to the formation of pilocarpic acid. To achieve suitable stability of pilocarpine, a pH range of 4–5 is necessary (27), and the use of a weak acidic buffer may be necessary. However, the buffer capacity of the preparation, especially if the pH is not in the range of the physiological values, should not overcome the buffer capacity of the tears. Otherwise, the restoration of normal pH, which is itself a function of tear turnover, would be delayed (28). The commonly used ophthalmic buffer systems in ophthalmic formulations are acetic, boric and phosphate buffers. On the other hand, the stability may be also influenced by the sterility of the preparation, as microorganisms can degrade some components. Furthermore, microbiological contamination of eye drops may be synonymous with secondary eye infection. Thus, the use of preservatives or special packaging devices maintaining the sterility of multi dose ophthalmic formulation are required by current pharmacopoeias and regulations (29). Ideally, a preservative should provide qualities such as broad antimicrobial activity, chemical/thermal stability, compatibility with the container and other compounds present as well as being innocuous towards ocular tissues (30). Unfortunately no single preservative has all the required qualities so as to be used universally. Furthermore, some preservatives may lead to ocular cytotoxic or allergic effects (31). Sterility can be achieved by different methods including, in decreasing order of preference, autoclaving, aseptic filtration, dry heat (for ointments), gamma irradiation or gas sterilization with ethylene oxide (32). Unfortunately, many polymers used in ophthalmic formulations do not withstand autoclaving or irradiation and their viscosity precludes the use of sterile filtration. Another important issue in the formulation of ophthalmic preparations is the ocular tolerance, i.e., the ability of ocular tissues to bear a given dose of a chemical without showing evidence of irritation, generally inflammatory reactions, or corrosion (33). A preparation that is not well tolerated induces reflex lachrymation, thus elimination of the drug from the ocular surface

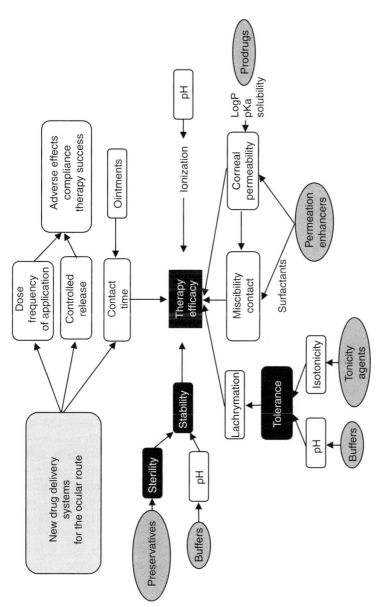

Figure 3 Parameters involved in topical ophthalmic formulations.

accompanied by tissue damage, that in turn impairs the patient's compliance, leading to recurrence of the disease or complications requiring further application of the medicine, a vicious cycle. Ocular tolerance can be assessed in vivo by the Draize test for eye irritation that relies on macroscopic observation and scoring of ocular changes (34) or by alternative methods that are more objective and sensitive (17). Ocular tolerance is influenced by the pH of the preparation and the eye can tolerate small changes in pH, though a large deviation from neutrality cause damage to the ocular surface, leading to ocular discomfort and irritation (35). pH values lower than 2.0 or above 11.5 are considered to be unacceptable (36). Ocular tolerance of aqueous formulation is also influenced by the osmolarity of the solution. Human tears have a mean osmolarity of 310 mOsm/kg and have a tonicity equivalent to that of 0.9% sodium chloride solution (37). Instillation of hypertonic solutions causes lachrymation, a burning sensation and cell desquamation (38–40), whereas a hypotonic solution may cause corneal edema (41). Ophthalmic solutions or suspensions can be made isotonic by the use of tonicity agents such as sodium chloride, buffering salts, dextrose and mannitol, as long as they are compatible with the other ingredients of the formulations. Therapy efficacy is the fourth and most important criterion for ophthalmic preparation. It depends of course on the stability and the tolerance of the preparation, but also on the corneal permeability of the active ingredients. The hydrophilic–lipophilic nature of the cornea clearly indicates that to be well absorbed, active ingredients must exhibit both lipophilic and hydrophilic properties to some extent. For ionizable drugs, the pH of the formulation can be adjusted, within some limits, to favor trans-epithelial permeation of the nonionized form. For instance, pilocarpine has a pKa value of 7.15 (42), which is ideal for transcorneal penetration at physiological pH. The hydrophobicity of chemicals can be represented by the 1-octanol-water partition coefficient logP (43). The use of absorption promoters, also called permeation enhancers, is a way to improve the bioavailability and therapeutic response of topically applied ophthalmic preparations (44,45). These absorption promoters are chemicals that modify transiently the integrity of the corneal epithelium, thus promoting the penetration of drugs through the cornea. The current penetration enhancers include azone, surfactants like polysorbates, surfactants with preservative properties like benzalkonium chloride, or sodium edetate. However, these substances may have adverse effects on the eye, generally inducing irritation and cellular desquamation on the cornea (46). Another approach to improve drug bioavailability at the site of action is to use prodrugs (47,48). These are pharmacologically inactive derivatives of drugs that are chemically (by hydrolysis for instance) or enzymatically (by esterases, ketone reductase or peptidases, enzymes present in the lachrymal film) converted into the active parent drug. Due to the modified solubility or lipophilicity, prodrugs have improved efficacy and stability (49). Dipivefrin, a prodrug of epinephrine, introduced in the late 1970s penetrates the human cornea 17 times better than epinephrine, because its partition coefficient is 100–600 times higher than that of the parent drug (50). Latanoprost (Xalatan®), a prostaglandin $F_{2\alpha}$ prodrug used in the treatment of glaucoma, has a much better tolerance and a 10–30 times improved hypotensive effect than the parent drug (51,52). Finally, a recently developed cyclosporine A prodrug is water-soluble and well tolerated (53). The main limitation of prodrugs is that they are considered as new chemical entities by many Regulatory Agencies, requiring further expensive documented studies. The therapy efficacy also depends on the contact and the miscibility of the active ingredient with the lachrymal film. Surfactants may be added to an ophthalmic preparation to solubilize or disperse the drug effectively (32). Nonionic surfactants like polysorbates are the most commonly used because of the relatively good tolerance (54). However, it should be kept in mind that surfactants may sometimes lower the efficacy of preservatives (55), interact with other polymeric substances present in the preparation (56), and slow down the rate of corneal epithelial healing after injury (57). Another way to improve the water-solubility of sparingly soluble drugs (like sulfonamides inhibiting carbonic anhydrase for the treatment of glaucoma or steroids against inflammation) is to use cyclodextrins (58,59). Cyclodextrins are cylindrical oligosaccharides with a hydrophilic outer surface and a lipophilic inner cavity capable to accommodate lipophilic drugs. Cyclodextrins increase chemical stability, local bioavailability and decrease local irritation (60,61). However, their action might be equivocal, e.g., a cyclodextrin solution of dorzolamide hydrochloride, a topically active sulfonamide, induced intraocular levels lower than the corresponding suspension in rabbits (62). The ophthalmic administration of poorly soluble drugs is also possible as a micronized suspension. Such preparation offers the advantage of prolonged corneal residence, associated with an increased bioavailability. Larger particles theoretically provide a sustained effect due to the increased size of the reservoir. However, these larger particles are associated with irritation, lachrymation, and finally faster elimination from the conjunctival sac (63). Some of the difficulties to formulate suspensions are non-homogeneity of the dosage form, settling, cake formation, aggregation of the suspended particles, and the sterility of the active ingredients (64).

An early attempt to slow down the elimination of the active ingredient drained by the tear flow and to increase the corneal residence time was to formulate ophthalmic ointments (65). These provide the advantage of a prolonged contact time of the drug with the corneal and conjunctival surface (66) and can incorporate low water soluble drugs. Moreover the stability of hydrolyzable drugs, especially of peptidic compounds, is sometimes improved in hydrophobic ointments. However, ophthalmic ointments have some drawbacks including blurred vision (so that their use is restricted to night time application), and inaccurate dosing (67). Indeed, hydrophobic drugs may be entrapped within the ointment base due to a favorable partitioning towards the base, impairing the release of the drug. Another approach to increase the ocular residence time is to enhance the viscosity of the ophthalmic solutions (68).

Viscous Solutions and Hydrogels

Viscous solutions and hydrogels based on the addition of hydrocolloids to mere aqueous solution are the most common formulations. There is no clear-cut delineation between very viscous solutions and gels in terms of biopharmaceutical results (69). However, gels are administered in the same way as an ointment, which is less convenient for the patient than the instillation of a viscous drop. Hydrogels used in ophthalmology are generally classified into two distinct groups: preformed gels and in situ activated gel-forming systems (70). Preformed gels include systems that are administered as viscous preparations on the eye; they are structured before application. The most common polymers in these preformed hydrogels and in viscous solutions are cellulose derivatives, polyvinyl alcohol, polyvinyl pyrolidone, carbomers, polysaccharides, and recently hyaluronic acid (71). The second group refers to polymeric system that are topically applied as solutions or suspensions and that shift from a sol to a gel phase as they are exposed to ocular surface physiological conditions like pH (for pseudolatexes), temperature (for poloxamer hydrogels) or the presence of ions (for gellan gum) (72–75). The main advantage of in situ activated gels over preformed hydrogels is that their administration is easy, since the preparation is conveniently delivered as a drop form and undergoes gelification on the ocular surface (76).

A formulation of timolol based on gellan gum undergoing a sol/gel transition due to the ionic content of the tears, reached the market in 1994 (Timoptic XE™). In situ forming gels have been actively pursued. Products using the gellan gum technology (77) and other polymeric associations like cellulose derivatives and carbomer (78,79) are examples of technologies based on this approach. This field of intricately entangled polymers seems promising since new "patentable" entities might be obtained through in-depth studies of associations of well-established products. The main drawbacks of hydrogels is that they cause a sticky sensation, blurred vision and induce sometimes reflex blinking due to discomfort (80,81).

Bioadhesive Systems

Another strategy developed to increase the bioavailability of ophthalmic drugs is to use mucoadhesive polymers (82). Formulations based on these polymers appear less viscous than those based on traditional viscolyzers. A number of polymers with polar/ionized groups, like carboxymethylcellulose, carbomers, sodium alginate, or acrylic derivatives, have been selected and tested with ophthalmic drugs. In theory, prolonged retention of ophthalmic mucoadhesive formulations is mainly due to electrostatic interactions that occur at the negatively charged corneal surface with the charged groups of the mucoadhesive (83,84). This theory has been explored since the end of the 1980s (85,86). An ophthalmic formulation based on bioadhesive polycarbophil Durasite® is on the market (87). Chitosan is an emerging cationic polymer of great interest for ophthalmic use (88). It has numerous advantages as low toxicity, good biocompatibility and ocular tolerance, bioadhesive properties (89,90). Furthermore, it is endowed with good wetting properties as well as an antibacterial effect that makes it an interesting candidate as a tear substitute (91).

Dispersed Systems

Dispersed systems based on liposomes, micro- or nanoparticles or nanocapsules have been extensively studied for potential ophthalmic use (92,93). The difference between micro- and nanoparticles is based on their size; particles in the micrometer size ($>1\,\mu m$) are called microspheres whereas those smaller than $1\,\mu m$ are known as nanoparticles (94). Liposomes are microscopic vesicles consisting of one or more lipid bilayers separated by an aqueous media. Their diameter typically ranges from 50 nm to 100 μm. They can accommodate both hydrophilic and lipophilic compounds, and due to their structure similar to biological membranes, they come into intimate contact with the corneal/conjunctival surfaces and thus enhance corneal drug absorption (95). Positively charged liposomes were described to have a greater affinity for ocular tissues and their retention in the conjunctival pouch is prolonged (96). They offer the advantage of being completely biodegradable and relatively nontoxic, but are less stable than the other particulate polymeric systems, their sterilization is not easy and their drug loading capacity is limited (97). Ocular dispersed systems are not only used for topical application, but also for systemic administration. Indeed, the use of dispersed systems and in particular liposomes for drug delivery in the retinal space has met undeniable success in the treatment of AMD. Verteporfin (Visudyne®), a photosensitizer used in the photodynamic therapy of AMD, is administered intravenously as a liposomal suspension and is FDA approved since 2000 (98). The drug appears at higher concentrations in the neovessels. A specific laser beam illuminates the neovessel foci and triggers phototoxic effects after activation of the photosensitizer. Such a treatment stops the progression of the disease for periods of several months (99).

For the formulator, the major issues for this type of dispersed systems include the percentage of dispersed phase/entrapment coefficient problem (i.e., how much of the active ingredient will be present in a drop of the final product), stability and shelf life, antimicrobial preservation, tolerance of the used surfactants and last but not least, large scale manufacture of sterile preparations.

Micro-emulsions may be systems of future interest, with the basic caveats concerning sterile manufacturing, long term stability, patient tolerance towards any surfactant, and the difficulty to adequately preserve a biphasic system. Pilocarpine was described to largely benefit from such a formulation, and cyclosporine is a potential candidate for this system (100,101).

Inserts

The earliest official record of a solid insert was described in the *British Pharmacopoeia* in 1948 and was an atropine-containing gelatin wafer, *lamellae*. According to the *European Pharmacopoeia*, ophthalmic inserts are sterile, solid, or semisolid preparations of suitable size and shape, designed to be inserted in the conjunctival sac, to produce an ocular effect. They generally consist of a reservoir of active substances embedded in a matrix or bound by a rate-controlling membrane. These devices are designed to release the drug for a prolonged duration of time, at a constant rate (102). They also promote non-corneal penetration, especially of hydrophilic drugs that are poorly absorbed through the cornea. Despite several advantages such as accurate dosing, absence of preservatives and increased shelf-life, they have one significant disadvantage, which is their solid consistency and are subsequently perceived by patients as a foreign body in the eye (103). Besides the initial discomfort, other potential disadvantages arising from their solid state are possible movement around the eye, occasional inadvertent loss during sleep or while rubbing the eyes, and interference with vision and difficult placement especially for elderly patients. Ophthalmic inserts are generally classified according to their solubility behavior and their possible biodegradability, depending on the polymer(s) used for manufacturing (Fig. 4).

The pilocarpine Ocusert® (Alza Corp.) (Fig. 5) (104) was the first marketed device to achieve zero-order kinetics. The Ocusert® is a soft and flexible elliptical device. The drug is contained in a reservoir with a carrier (alginic acid) enclosed by two release-controlling membranes made of ethylene vinyl acetate copolymer and surrounded by a ring to aid in the positioning and placement (105). The device continuously releases pilocarpine at a steady rate (20 and 40 µg/hr) for 1 week. The product was and is still considered as a technical breakthrough. However, Ocusert® is no longer sold, because of a quite limited market success due to the difficult insertion and removal of the system by elderly patients and to the competition of other more efficient drugs such as beta-blockers and prostaglandins (64). Novel ocular delivery system (NODS) is essentially an "insert with a handle" and will be fully discussed later in a chapter (106).

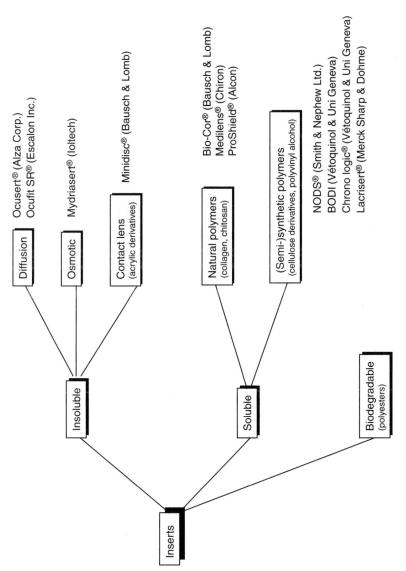

Figure 4 Classification of ophthalmic inserts.

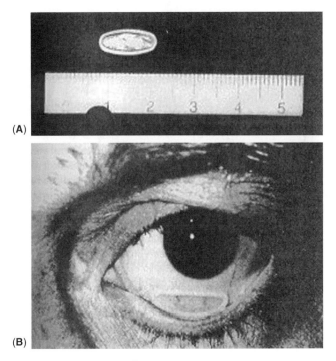

Figure 5 Alza Ocusert® (A) in the conjunctival sac (B).

Although patient complaints have been the major obstacle to the success of ophthalmic inserts, the field of veterinary medicine is still open to these formulations (107). A soluble bioadhesive ophthalmic drug insert (BODI) was recently described and is presently marketed for veterinary use in Europe (see Chapter 7) (108,109).

Implants

Implants are polymeric drug delivery systems designed to be implanted inside the eye through minor surgery (110). They should be sterile and made from a biocompatible, preferably biodegradable, non-inflammatory material (111). The main advantage of ocular implants over traditional drug delivery systems used in ophthalmology is a constant release rate of drug directly to the site of action without systemic side effects or frequent intravitreal injections. The implantation may be subconjunctival for the treatment of anterior segment diseases or intravitreal/suprachoroidal to treat posterior segment diseases. Vitrasert® is an intravitreal reservoir implant approved by the FDA, which can release ganciclovir over a 5–8 month period to treat cytomegalovirus retinitis in patients with acquired immunodeficiency (112). The implant consists of a compressed drug pellet with polyvinyl alcohol that is partially coated with ethylene vinylacetate. After depletion of the active ingredient, the implant may be removed and replaced (113). Surodex, a biodegradable polymer based intraocular insert, is presently developed for post-cataract surgery inflammation (114). Another intraocular implant containing fluocinolone acetonide has been developed for the treatment of chronic non-infectious uveitis affecting the posterior segment of the eye (115). These devices will be thoroughly described in Chapter 6.

RECENT INNOVATIVE OPHTHALMIC DRUG DELIVERY SYSTEMS

There is a real challenge for developing ophthalmic formulations that deliver effective ocular drug concentrations for an extended period (without inducing systemic side effects), which are user-friendly and that do not induce blurring, burning, or foreign body sensation. Many attempts have been made to develop practical approaches to the modified delivery of drugs to the eye as described above. Research is very active in this field and part of the many new technologies will be further described below. Table 1 lists the qualities required for a modified release drug delivery system in ophthalmology.

Gelfoam® is made of absorbable gelatin sponge USP. It can be inserted in the conjunctival pouch in the form of small disks (e.g., 4 mm in diameter and 0.5 mm thick) impregnated with drug solutions. They have been shown to improve the management of pupillary dilation in humans as well as the delivery of pilocarpine (116,117).

Collagen shields have been originally developed as a corneal bandage to promote wound healing (118). They appeared to be useful as a delivery system for anti-infective agents and might possibly be of interest for some other drugs. However, their size and the constraints they impose on vision make them inconvenient for a new drug delivery system. Suspensions of collagen microparticulates (e.g., collasomes or lacrisomes) might be better accepted (119).

Ion exchange resins have been investigated and resulted in the technology used in the product Betoptic S™ to improve bioavailability and to decrease irritation (see the following chapter). The development of this ionic suspension of betaxolol deals with the need to reduce irritability induced by the active ingredient and with the tuning of the sustained release properties. The research and development process resulted in a 0.25% suspension exhibiting the therapeutic activity of a 0.50% solution. Furthermore the suspension is more viscous than the solution, thus prolonging the corneal residence time.

Since the instilled volume of vehicle is a factor of loss and because the use of small instilled volumes/high concentrations of drug is not deemed

Table 1 Qualities of a Modified-Release Ophthalmic Drug Delivery System

A well-designed modified-release ophthalmic drug delivery system must:

Deliver the active ingredient to the right place, i.e., high conjunctival levels are useless when targeting the ciliary body

Improve the ratio of local activity versus systemic effects

Reduce the number of installations per day, once-a-day being considered the optimal goal, although some may consider twice daily to be a better insurance against forgotten administration

Be easy to self-administer

Not induce a foreign body sensation, long lasting blurring or a very bad after taste

Not rely on "exotic" ingredients like New Chemical Entities or difficult to source excipients (unless this is a key element). Preferably, excipients should have a Drug Master File and history of safe use for humans

Be sterilizable at industrial scale by a recognized process

Be compatible with an efficient antimicrobial preservative or packaging in unit doses must be a viable alternative

Preferably be stored without specific conditions

Be covered by a patent, since manufacturers can legitimately expect a return on R&D investment

practical, volatile ophthalmic vehicles have been explored, as well as the concept of dry drops. A dry drop formulation consists of an active ingredient incorporated in a drop of hydrophilic polymer solution (like cellulose derivatives) freeze-dried on the tip of a soft hydrophobic carrier (like polytetrafluoroethylene) (120,121). A dry drop has an improved chemical stability and is declared to be well tolerated as it does not contain preservatives. Ophthalmic rod described at the end of the 1970s is also a "dry" ophthalmic drug delivery system (122). It is made of a nontoxic plastic dipped into a drug solution which after drying forms a thin homogeneous coating and introduced into the conjunctival sac (123,124).

Perfluoro carbon vehicles were patented in the 1990s (125); perfluorodecalin did not induce any ocular irritation in healthy human volunteers, produced an increased ocular retention as well as a good distribution of the vehicle over the cornea (126). This compound was generally well tolerated and the retention of charcoal particulates let the investigators forecast a potential for the perfluorodecalin system for the treatment of periocular diseases.

Sprays are again under consideration although Mitsura®, a pilocarpine spray, was not a success in the mid-1970s (127). Sprays might, however, be useful in pediatric medicine (128).

Iontophoresis is an active drug delivery method utilizing electrical current to transport ionized drugs across and into body tissues. Its application in delivering drugs to the eye was first described more than 50 years ago (129). Iontophoresis has several advantages: it is noninvasive, increases transcleral delivery of many ophthalmic active ingredients (such as anti-virals, steroids, peptides, and nucleotides), and greatly improves their intraocular levels (130,131). However, it does not provide a prolonged drug delivery, it is only applicable with charged molecules and there is a risk of tissue damages inherent to the use of electrical current (132). Recent progress in the technology of the associated hardware has stimulated interest for a renewal of its use in ophthalmology (133).

The use of lectins as mucosal bioadhesins in body cavities, e.g., in the conjunctival pouch, has been advocated (134). The irritancy of lectins from Solanum tuberosum/potato and from Helix pomatia/snail has been studied, and was found to be minimal (135). Further investigations for use in ocular formulations are encouraging (136).

An osmotic micropump has been developed to obtain transcleral delivery of bioactive proteins in pigmented rabbit eyes (137). The anti-intercellular adhesion molecule-1 monoclonal antibody, inhibiting vascular endothelial growth factor, was successfully delivered to the choroid while levels in other eye tissues and plasma were found to be extremely low. This last point has been a recurring concern for all drugs from the ophthalmic formulators viewpoint (138). Osmotic micropumps have also been subconjunctivally implanted by a Purdue University team for continuous ocular treatment in horses (139). Veterinary ophthalmology can certainly benefit from progresses in ocular drug delivery (140).

The posterior segment of the eye is a matter of growing concern due to retinal diseases linked to the increasing elderly population (141). Drug delivery in this part of the eye may be a beneficiary of the recent advances made in biomaterials (142). For instance, the anti-angiogenic agent TNP-470 was conjugated with polyvinyl alcohol and tested in rabbits against experimental choroidal neovascularization (CNV). It was concluded that the targeted delivery of TNP-470-PVA might have potential as a treatment modality of CNV (143).

Identification of the molecular basis for many diseases has led to major advances in the area of gene therapy and ocular diseases are no exception. The eye is particularly suited to gene therapy because of its accessibility and immune privileged status (111,144). Current studies have focused on the use of gene therapy to correct inherited diseases (145). Gene therapy uses viral and non-viral vectors to deliver genes to specific targeted cells. Viral vectors such as adenoviruses, adeno-associated-virus and retro-viruses bear potential risks associated with their immunogenicity and mutagenicity (145,146). On the contrary non-viral approaches such as physical methods or chemical carriers (for instance, liposomes) are relatively non-immunogenic and do not induce inflammatory responses. The use of these vectors holds promise for the future of ocular gene therapy.

CONCLUSIONS

Ocular drug delivery has unique barriers to overcome. Within the last few decades, in response to the advent of potent and versatile therapeutic agents, conventional ophthalmic forms have evolved into a variety of drug delivery systems. Some of the technologies described above are more fully described elsewhere in this section. Such monographs shed light on the different needs for modified-release ophthalmic formulations. The monograph on intraocular implants describes the different drug delivery systems developed to treat specific diseases in the posterior segment. The NODS monograph describes a solution to a basic problem inherent to ocular inserts; the insertion of the device into the patient's eye. It also describes some of the difficulties one can encounter with respect to technology development and regulatory compliance. Finally, the BODI monograph describes a solution to a lesser-known problem, the treatment of ocular infections in animals. The monograph demonstrates that the use of degradable inserts can deliver anti-infectious active ingredients for longer periods than drops, thereby decreasing the need for handling animals.

It is difficult, and probably vain, to forecast the ophthalmic dosage forms of the future but, whatever the future, even when the active ophthalmic ingredients are identified, the development pathway to a marketable ophthalmic product will not be easy. Pharmaceutical research and development provides multiple approaches to achieve this, but it is governed by available technology, innovations in technology and regulatory constraints. Importantly, the cost of the finished product must be bearable by the individuals and/or communities who will use the product, and it has to be economically viable for the manufacturer. As a final thought, it must be kept in mind that the most exquisite modified release technology for an established drug can be made obsolete by the arrival of a new drug; the pilocarpine Ocusert© technology began to decline with the introduction of beta-blocking drugs to ophthalmic medicine.

Nevertheless, the advent of new active ingredients requires a formulation adapted to the ophthalmic use and for this formulation, the four Goldmann's criteria of stability, sterility, tolerance, and efficacy have to be fulfilled.

REFERENCES

1. Ghate D, Edelhauser HF. Ocular drug delivery. Expert Opin Durg Deliv 2006; 3(2):275–87.
2. Arffa RC. Anatomy. In: Arffa RC, ed. Grayson's Diseases of the Cornea. St Louis: Mosby, 1997: 1–22.
3. Hecht G, Roehrs RE, Cooper ER, et al. Design and evaluation of ophtalmic pharmaceutical products. In: Banker GS, Rhodes CT, eds. Drugs and

Pharmaceutical Sciences, Modern Pharmaceutics. New York: Marcel Dekker, 1990: 539–603.

4. McCaa CS. Anatomy, physiology, and toxicology of the eye. In: Hayes AW, ed. Toxicology of the Eye, Ear, and Other Special Senses. New York: Raven Press, 1985: 1–15.

5. Waring GO. Corneal structure and pathophysiology. In: Leibowitz HM, ed. Corneal Disorders, Clinical Diagnosis and Management. Philadelphia: WB Saunders Comp, 1984: 3–25.

6. White WL, Glover AT, Buckner AB. Effect of blinking on tear elimination as evaluated by dacryoscintigraphy. Ophthalmology 1991; 98(3):367–9.

7. Lee VHL, Robinson JR. Review: topical ocular drug delivery: recent developments and future challenges. J Ocul Pharmacol 1986; 2:67–108.

8. Urtti A. Challenges and obstacles of ocular pharmacokinetics and drug delivery. Adv Drug Deliv Rev 2006; 58(11):1131–5.

9. Järvinen K, Järvinen T, Urtti A. Ocular absorption following topical delivery. Adv Drug Deliv Rev 2007; 16:3–19.

10. Huang HS, Schoenwald RD, Lach JL. Corneal penetration behavior of beta-blocking agents II: Assessment of barrier contributions. J Pharm Sci 1983; 72(11):1272–9.

11. Geroski DH, Edelhauser HF. Transscleral drug delivery for posterior segment disease. Adv Drug Deliv Rev 2001; 52(1):37–48.

12. Prausnitz MR, Noonan JS. Permeability of cornea, sclera, and conjunctiva: A literature analysis for drug delivery to the eye. J Pharmaceut Sci 1998; 87 (12):1479–88.

13. Hughes PM, Olejnik O, Chang-Lin JE, et al. Topical and systemic drug delivery to the posterior segments. Adv Drug Deliv Rev 2005; 57(14): 2010–32.

14. Hornof M, Toropainen E, Urtti A. Cell culture models of the ocular barriers. Eur J Pharm Biopharm 2005; 60(2):207–25.

15. Lambert LA, Chambers WA, Green S, et al. The use of low-volume dosing in the eye irritation test. Food Chem Toxicol 1993; 31:99–103.

16. Meyer LA, Nemiroff B, Ubels JL, et al. The role of the nicitating membrane in ocular irritancy testing. J Toxicol Cutaneous Ocul Toxicol 1987; 6:43–56.

17. Daston GP, Freeberg FE. Ocular irritation testing. In: DW Hobson, ed. Dermal an Ocular Toxicology. Fundamentals and Methods. Boca Raton, FL: CRC Press, 1991: 509–39.

18. Saettone MF, Giannaccini B, Barattini F, et al. The validity of rabbits for investigations on ophthalmic vehicles: a comparison for four different vehicles containing tropicamide in humans and rabbits. Pharm Acta Helv 1982; 57: 3–11.

19. Worakul N, Robinson JR. Ocular pharmacokinetics/pharmacodynamics. Eur J Pharm Biopharm 1997; 44:71–83.

20. Prince JH. The rabbit eye related to that of man. In: Prince JH, ed. The rabbit in eye research. Springfield, IL: Charles C Thomas, 1964: ix–xiv.

21. Prince JH, Diesem CD, Eglitis I, et al. The rabbit. Anatomy and Histology of the Eye and Orbit in Domestic Animals. Springfield, IL: Charles C Thomas Publisher, 1960: 260–97.

22. Davies FA. The anatomy and histology of the eye and orbit of the rabbit. Trans Am Ophthalmol Soc 1929; 27:401–41.

23. Mishima S. Some physiological aspects of the precorneal tear film. Arch Ophthalmol 1965; 73:233–41.

24. Schoenwald RD. Ocular Pharmacokinetics/pharmacodynamics. In: Mitra AK, ed. Ophthalmic Drug Delivery Systems. New York: Marcel Dekker, Inc., 1993: 83–110.

25. Maurice DM, Mishima S. Ocular pharmacokinetics. In: Sears ML, ed. Pharmacology of the Eye. Berlin, Heidelberg, New York, Tokyo: Springer-Verlag, 1984: 19–116.

26. Tang-Liu DDS, Acheampong A, Chien DS, et al. Pharmacokinetics and pharmacodynamic correlations of ophthalmic drugs. In: Reddy IK, ed. Ocular Therapeutics and Drug Delivery. A Multiplisciplinary Approach. Lancaster, USA: Technomic Publishing Co, Inc., 1996: 133–47.

27. Pilatti C, Torre MC, Chiale C, et al. Stability of pilocarpine ophthalmic solutions. Drug Dev Ind Pharm 1999; 25(6):801–5.

28. Walz D. Irritation action due to physico-chemical parameters of test solutions. Food Chem Toxicol 1985; 23:299–302.

29. Furrer P, Mayer JM, Gurny R. Ocular tolerance of preservatives and alternatives. Eur J Pharm Biopharm 2002; 53:263–80.

30. Mullen W, Shepherd W, Labovitz J. Ophthalmic preservatives and vehicles. Surv Ophthalmol 1973; 17:469–82.

31. Furrer P, Mayer JM, Plazonnet B, et al. Ocular tolerance of preservatives on the murine cornea. Eur J Pharm Biopharm 1999; 47:105–12.

32. Gangrade NK, Gaddipati NB, Ganesan MG, et al. Topical ophthalmic formulations: basic considerations. In: Reddy IK, ed. Ocular Therapeutics and Drug Delivery. A Multi-disciplinary Approach. Basel: Technomic Publishing Ag, 1996: 3774–403.

33. Chan PK, Hayes AW. Principles and methods for acute toxicity and eye irritancy. In: Hayes AW, ed. Principles and Methods of Toxicology. New York: Raven Press, 1989: 169–220.

34. Draize JH, Woodard G, Calvery HO. Methods for study of irritation and toxicity of substances applied topically to the skin and mucous membranes. J Pharmacol Exp Ther 1944; 82:377–90.

35. Trolle-Lassen C. Investigations into the sensitivity of the human eye to hypo- and hypertonic solutions as well as solutions with unphysiological hydrogen ion concentration. Pharm Weekly 1958; 93:148–55.

36. Hurley PM, Chambers WA, Green S, et al. Screening procedures for eye irritation. Food Chem Toxicol 1993; 31:87–94.

37. Benjamin WJ, Hill RM. Human tears: osmotic characteristics. Invest Ophthalmol Vis Sci 1983; 24:1624–6.

38. Gilbard JP, Carter JB, Sang DN, et al. Morphologic effect of hyperosmolarity on rabbit corneal epithelium. Ophthalmology 1984; 91:1205–12.

39. Motolko M, Breslin CW. The effect of pH and osmolarity on the ability to tolerate artificial tears. Am J Ophthalmol 1981; 91:781–4.

40. Holly FJ, Lamberts DW. Effect of nonisotonic solutions on tear film osmolality. Invest Ophthalmol Vis Sci 1981; 20:236–45.

41. Ludwig A, Van Ooteghem M. The influence of the osmolality on the precorneal retention of ophthalmic solutions. J Pharm Belg 2000; 42:259–66.
42. Pilocarpine (monograph Nr 7505). In: S. Budavari, ed. The Merck Index, 12th ed. Whitehouse Station NJ: Merck & Co, Inc., 2001: 1330.
43. Mitra AK, Mikkelson TJ. Mechanism of transcorneal permeation of pilocarpine. J Pharm Sci 1988; 77:771–5.
44. Liaw J, Robinson JR. Ocular penetration enhancers. In: Mitra AK, ed. Ophthalmic Drug Delivery Systems. New York: Marcel Dekker, 1993; 369–81.
45. Sasaki H, Yamamura K, Mukai T, et al. Enhancement of ocular drug penetration. Crit Rev Ther Drug Carrier Syst 1999; 16(1):85–146.
46. Furrer P, Mayer JM. Ocular tolerance of absorption enhancers in ophthalmic preparations. AAPS Pharm Sci 2002; 4(1):art. 2.
47. Lee VHL, Bundgaard H. Improved ocular drug delivery with prodrugs. In: K.B. Sloan, ed. Prodrugs. Topical and Ocular Drug Delivery. New York: Marcel Dekker, 1992; 221–97.
48. Jarvinen T, Jarvinen K. Prodrugs for improved ocular drug delivery. Adv Drug Deliv Rev 1996; 14:269–79.
49. Tammara VK, Crider MA. Prodrugs: A chemical approach to ocular drug delivery. In: Reddy IK, ed. Ocular Therapeutics and Drug Delivery. Technomic Publishing Co, Inc., 1996; 285–34.
50. Mandel AI, Stentz F, Kitabchi AE. Dipivalyl epinephrine: a new prodrug in the treatment of glaucoma. Ophthalmology 1978; 85:268–75.
51. Bito LZ. Prostaglandins. Old concepts and new perspectives. Arch Ophthalmol 1987; 105(8):1036–9.
52. Cheng-Bennett A, Chan MF, Chen G, et al. Studies on a novel series of acyl ester prodrugs of prostaglandin F2 alpha. Br J Ophthalmol 1994; 78(7):560–7.
53. Lallemand F, Furrer P, Felt-Baeyens O, et al. A novel water-soluble cyclosporine A prodrug: ocular tolerance and in vivo kinetics. Int J Pharm 2005; 295:7–14.
54. Furrer P, Plazonnet B, Mayer JM, et al. Application of in vivo confocal microscopy to the objective evaluation of ocular irritation induced by surfactants. Int J Pharm 2000; 207:89–98.
55. Brown MRW, Norton DA. The preservation of ophthalmic preparations. J Soc Cosmet Chem 1965; 16:369–93.
56. Goddard ED. Polymer/surfactant interaction. J Soc Cosmet Chem 1990; 41: 23–49.
57. Green K, Johnson RE, Chapman JM, et al. Surfactant effects on the rate of rabbit corneal epithelial healing. J Toxicol Cut Ocul Toxicol 1989; 8:253–69.
58. Loftssona T, Järvinen T. Cyclodextrins in ophthalmic drug delivery. Adv Drug Deliv Rev 2000; 36:59–79.
59. Bibby DC, Davies NM, Tucker IG. Mechanisms by which cyclodextrins modify drug release from polymeric drug delivery systems. Int J Pharm 2000; 197(1–2):1–11.
60. Jarho P, Järvinen K, Urtti A, et al. Modified β-cyclodextrin (SBE-β-CyD) with viscous vehicle improves the ocular delivery and tolerability of pilocarpine prodrug in rabbits. J Pharm Pharmacol 1996; 48:263–9.

61. Maestrelli F, Mura P, Casini A, et al. Cyclodextrin complexes of sulfonamide carbonic anhydrase inhibitors as long-lasting topically acting antiglaucoma agents. J Pharm Sci 2002; 91(10):2211–9.
62. Tsien RY. Fluorescent probes of cell signaling. Ann Rev Neurosci 1989; 12: 227–53.
63. Schoenwald RD, Stewart P. Effect of particle size on ophthalmic bioavailability of dexamethasone suspensions in rabbits. J Pharm Sci 1980; 69(4):391–4.
64. Ali Y, Lehmussaari K. Industrial perspective in ocular drug delivery. Adv Drug Deliv Rev 2006; 58(11):1258–68.
65. Kaur IP, Kanwar M. Ocular preparations: the formulation approach. Drug Dev Ind Pharm 2002; 28(5):473–93.
66. Norn MS, Opauszki A. Effects of ophthalmic vehicles on the stability of the precorneal tear film. Acta Ophthalmol 1977; 55:23–34.
67. Bapatla KM, Hecht G. Ophthalmic ointments and suspensions. In: Lieberman HA, Rieger RM, Banker GS, eds. Pharmaceutical dosage forms: Disperse systems. New York: Marcel Dekker, Inc., 1996; 357–97.
68. Ding S. Recent developments in ophtalmic drug delivery. PSTT 1998; 1(8): 328–35.
69. Zignani M, Tabatabay C, Gurny R. Topical semi-solid drug delivery: kinetics and tolerance of ophthalmic hydrogels. Adv Drug Deliv Rev 1995; 16: 51–60.
70. Felt O, Einmahl S, Furrer P, et al. Polymeric system for ophthalmic drug delivery. In: Dumitriu S, ed. Polymeric Biomaterials. New York: Marcel Dekker, 2002; 377–421.
71. Bernatchez S.F, Camber O, Tabatabay C, et al. Use of hyaluronic acid in ocular therapy. In: Edman P, ed. Biopharmaceutics of Ocular Drug Delivery. Boca Raton, FL: CRC Press, 1993; 7:105–20.
72. Gurny R, Ibrahim H., Buri P. The development and use of in situ formed gels, triggered by pH. In: Edman P, ed. Biopharmaceutics of Ocular Drug Delivery. Boca Raton, FL: CRC Press, 1993; (5):81–90.
73. Ruel-Gariepy E, Leroux JC. In situ-forming hydrogels–review of temperature-sensitive systems. Eur J Pharm Biopharm 2004; 58(2):409–26.
74. Miller SC, Donovan MD. Effect of poloxamer 407 gel on the miotic activity of pilocarpine nitrate in rabbits. Int J Pharm 1982; 12:147–52.
75. Rozier A, Mazuel C, Grove J, et al. Gelrite: A novel, ion-activated, in-situ gelling polymer for ophthalmic vehicles. Effect on bioavailability of timolol. Int J Pharm 1989; 57:163–8.
76. Le Bourlais C, Acar L, Zia H, et al. Ophthalmic drug delivery systems—Recent advances. Progr Retinal Eye Res 1997; 17(1):33–58.
77. Alcon laboratories I. US Patent 4,861,760 2007.
78. Kumar S, Himmelstein KJ. Modification of in situ gelling behavior of carbopol solutions by hydroxypropyl methylcellulose. J Pharm Sci 1994; 84(3): 344–8.
79. Kumar S, Haglund BO, Himmelstein KJ. In situ-forming gels for ophthalmic drug delivery. J Ocul Pharmacol 1994; 10:47–56.
80. Dudinski O, Finnin BC, Reed BL. Acceptability of thickened eye drops to human subjects. Curr Ther Res 1983; 33:322–37.

81. Sintzel MB, Bernatchez SF, Tabatabay C, et al. Biomaterials in ophthalmic drug delivery. Eur J Pharm Biopharm 1996; 42(6):358–74.
82. Ludwig A. The use of mucoadhesive polymers in ocular drug delivery. Advanced Drug Delivery Reviews 2005; 57(11):1595–639.
83. Edsman K, Hagerstrom H. Pharmaceutical applications of mucoadhesion for the non-oral routes. J Pharm Pharmacol 2005; 57(1):3–22.
84. Smart JD. The basics and underlying mechanisms of mucoadhesion. Adv Drug Deliv Rev 2005; 57(11):1556–68.
85. Slovin EM, Robinson JR. Bioadhesives in ocular drug delivery. In: Edman P, ed. Biopharmaceutics of Ocular Drug Delivery. Boca Raton, FL: CRC Press, 1993: 145–57.
86. Davies NM, Farr SJ, Hadgraft J, et al. Evaluation of mucoadhesive polymers in ocular drug delivery. I. Viscous solutions. Pharm Res 1991; 8(8): 1039–43.
87. Patel R. US Patent 5,340, 572,23 1994.
88. Alonso MJ, Sanchez A. The potential of chitosan in ocular drug delivery. J Pharm Pharmacol 2003; 55:1451–62.
89. Felt O, Buri P, Gurny R. Chitosan. A unique polysaccharide for drug delivery. Drug Dev Ind Pharm 1998; 24(11):979–93.
90. Felt O, Furrer P, Mayer JM, et al. Topical use of chitosan in ophthalmology: tolerance assessment by confocal microscopy and precorneal retention evaluation by gamma scintigraphy. Proceedings of the 2nd World Meeting APGI/ APV, Paris, 1998; 913–4.
91. Felt O, Carrel A, Baehni P, et al. Chitosan as tear substitute: a wetting agent endowed with antimicrobial efficacy. J Ocul Pharmacol Therapeut 2000; 16(3): 261–70.
92. Gurny R, Boye T, Ibrahim H. Ocular therapy with nanoparticulate systems for controlled drug delivery. J Control Release 1985; 2:353–60.
93. Moshfeghi AA, Peyman GA. Micro- and nanoparticulates. Adv Drug Deliv Rev 2005; 57(14):2047–52.
94. Amrite A, Kompella U. Nanoparticles for ocular drug delivery. In: Gupta R, Kompella U, eds. Nanoparticle Technology for Drug Delivery. New York: Taylor and Francis, 2006; 319–60.
95. Meisner D, Mezei M. Liposome ocular delivery systems. Adv Drug Deliv Rev 1995; 16:75–93.
96. Schaeffer HE, Krohn DL. Liposomes in topical drug delivery. Invest Ophthalmol Vis Sci 1982; 22(2):220–7.
97. Sultana Y, Jain R, Aqil M, et al. Review of ocular drug delivery. Curr Drug Deliv 2006; 3(2):207–17.
98. Ebrahim S, Peyman GA, Lee PJ. Applications of liposomes in ophthalmology. Surv Ophthalmol 2005; 50(2):167–82.
99. Bressler NM, Bressler SB. Photodynamic therapy with verteporfin (Visudyne): impact on ophthalmology and visual sciences. Invest Ophthalmol Vis Sci 2000; 41(3):624–8.
100. Sznitowska M, Zurowska-Pryczkowska K, Janicki S, et al. Miotic effect and irritation potential of pilocarpine prodrug incorporated into a submicron emulsion vehicle. Int J Pharm 1999; 184(1):115–20.

101. Angelov O, Wiese A, Yuan Y, et al. Preclinical safety studies of cyclosporine ophthalmic emulsion. Adv Exp Med Biol 1998; 438:991–5.
102. Bawa S. Ocular inserts. In: Mitra AK, ed. Ophthalmic drug delivery systems. New York: Marcel Dekker, 1993; 223–60.
103. Saettone MF, Salminen L. Ocular inserts for topical delivery. Adv Drug Deliv Rev 1995; 16:95–106.
104. Urquhart J. Development of Ocusert pilocarpine ocular therapeutic systems. In: Robinson JR, ed. Ophthalmic Drug Delivery Systems. Washington, DC: American Pharmaceutical Association, 1980; 105–8.
105. Macoul KL, Pavan-Langston D. Pilocarpine ocusert system for sustained control of ocular hypertension. Arch Ophthalmol 1975; 93:587–90.
106. Diestelhorst M, Krieglstein GK. The ocular tolerability of a new ophthalmic drug delivery system (NODS). Int Ophthalmol 1994; 18(1):1–4.
107. Baeyens V, Percicot C, Zignani M, et al. Ocular drug delivery in veterinary medicine. Adv Drug Deliv Rev 1997; 28:335–61.
108. Gurtler F, Kaltsatos V, Boisramé B, et al. Ocular availability of gentamicin in small animals after topical administration of a conventional eye drop solution and a novel long acting bioadhesive ophthalmic drug insert. Pharm Res 1995; 12(11):1791–5.
109. Baeyens V, Kaltsatos V, Boisramé B, et al. Evaluation of soluble Bioadhesive Ophthalmic Drug Inserts (BODI®) for prolonged release of gentamicin Lachrymal pharmacokinetics and ocular tolerance. J Ocul Pharmacol Ther 1998; 14(3):263–72.
110. Ashton P, Blandford DL, Pearson PA, et al. Review: Implants. J Ocul Pharmacol 1994; 10(4):691–701.
111. Davis JL, Gilger BC, Robinson MR. Novel approaches to ocular drug delivery. Expert Opin Mol Therap 2006; 6(2):195–205.
112. Martin DF, Parks DJ, Mellow SD, et al. Treatment of cytomegalovirus retinitis with an intraocular sustained-release ganciclovir implant. A randomized controlled clinical trial. Arch Ophthalmol 1994; 112(12):1531–9.
113. Ganciclovir intravitreal implant (Vitrasert®). In: Facts and Comparisons®, ed. Ophthalmic Drug Facts. Saint Louis, MO: Wolters Kluwer, 2000; 150–3.
114. Lee SY, Chee SP. Surodex after phacoemulsification. J Cataract Refract Surg 2005; 31(8):1479–80.
115. Lim LL, Smith JR, Rosenbaum JT. Retisert (Bausch & Lomb/Control Delivery Systems). Curr Opin Investig Drugs 2005; 6(11):1159–67.
116. Simamora P, Nadkarni SR, Lee Y-C, et al. Controlled delivery of pilocarpine. 2. In vivo evaluation of Gelfoam device. Int J Pharm 1998; 170:209–14.
117. Negvesky GJ, Butrus SI, Abifarah HA, et al. Ocular Gelfoam® disc-applicator for pupillary dilation in humans. J Ocul Pharmacol Ther 2000; 16:311–5.
118. Hill JM, O'Callaghan RJ, Hobden JA, et al. Corneal collagen shields for ocular delivery. In: Mitra AK, ed. Ophthalmic Drug Delivery Systems. New York: Marcel Dekker, 1993; 261–73.
119. Kaufman HE, Steinemann TL, Lehman E, et al. Collagen-based drug delivery and artificial tears. J Ocul Pharmacol 1994; 10(1):17–27.

120. Diestelhorst M, Grunthal S, Suverkrup R. Dry Drops: a new preservative-free drug delivery system. Graefes Arch Clin Exp Ophthalmol 1999; 237(5): 394–8.
121. Dinslage S, Diestelhorst M, Weichselbaum A, et al. Lyophilisates for drug delivery in ophthalmology: pharmacokinetics of fluorescein in the human anterior segment. Br J Ophthalmol 2002; 86(10):1114–7.
122. Alani DS. The ophthalmic rod–description of a disposable ophthalmic drug delivery device. Acta Pharm Suec 1978; 15(3):237–40.
123. Alani SD, Hammerstein W. The ophthalmic rod–a new drug-delivery system II. Graefes Arch Clin Exp Ophthalmol 1990; 228(4):302–4.
124. Alani SD. The ophthalmic rod: a new ophthalmic drug delivery system I. Graefes Arch Clin Exp Ophthalmol 1990; 228(4):297–301.
125. Meadows D. US Patent 5,173,298. 1992; Dec 1992.
126. Zhu Y, Wilson CG, Meadows D, et al. Dry powder dosing in liquid vehicles: ocular tolerance and scintigraphic evaluation of a perfluorocarbon suspension. Int J Pharm 1999; 191(2):79–85.
127. Doe EA, Campagna JA. Pilocarpine spray: an alternative delivery method. J Ocul Pharmacol Ther 1998; 14(1):1–4.
128. Benvides JO, Satchell ER, Frantz KA. Efficacy of a mydriatic spray in the pediatric population. Optom Vis Sci 1997; 74:160–3.
129. Smith VL. Iontophoresis in ophthalmology. Am J Ophthalmol 1951; 34(5:1): 698–704.
130. Sarraf D, Lee DA. The role of iontophoresis in ocular drug delivery. J Ocul Pharmacol 1994; 10:69–81.
131. Hill JM, O'Callaghan RJ, Hobden JA. Ocular iontophoresis. In: Mitra AK, ed. Ophthalmic Drug Delivery Systems. New York: Marcel Dekker, 1993: 331–54.
132. Lam TT, Fu J, Tso MO. A histopathologic study of retinal lesions inflicted by transscleral iontophoresis. Graefes Arch Clin Exp Ophthalmol 1991; 229(4): 389–94.
133. Halhal M, Renard G, Courtois Y, et al. Iontophoresis: From the lab to the bed side. Exp Eye Res 2004; 78(3):751–7.
134. Clark MA, Hirst BH, Jepson MA. Lectin-mediated mucosal delivery of drugs and microparticles. Adv Drug Deliv Rev 2000; 43(2–3):207–23.
135. Smart JD, Nicholls TJ, Green KL, et al. Lectins in drug delivery: a study of the acute local irritancy of the lectins from Solanum tuberosum and Helix pomatia. Eur J Pharm Sci 1999; 9(1):93–8.
136. Qaddoumi M, Lee VH. Lectins as endocytic ligands: an assessment of lectin binding and uptake to rabbit conjunctival epithelial cells. Pharm Res 2004; 21(7):1160–6.
137. Ambati J, Gragoudas ES, Miller JW, et al. Transscleral delivery of bioactive protein to the choroid and retina. Invest Ophthalmol Vis Sci 2000; 41(5): 1186–91.
138. Urtti A, Salminen L. Minimizing systemic absorption of topically administered ophthalmic drugs. Surv Ophthalmol 1993; 37(6):435–56.
139. Blair MJ, Gionfriddo JR, Polazzi LM, et al. Subconjunctivally implanted micro-osmotic pumps for continuous ocular treatment in horses. Am J Vet Res 1999; 60(9):1102–5.

140. Gurny R, Kaltsatos V, Deshpande AA, et al. Ocular drug delivery in veterinary medicine. Adv Drug Deliv Rev 1997; 28(3):335–61.
141. Geroski DH, Edelhauser HF. Drug delivery for posterior segment eye disease. Invest Ophthalmol Vis Sci 2000; 41(5):961–4.
142. Colthurst MJ, Williams RL, Hiscott PS, et al. Biomaterials used in the posterior segment of the eye. Biomaterials 2000; 21(7):649–65.
143. Yasukawa T, Kimura H, Tabata Y, et al. Targeted delivery of anti-angiogenic agent TNP-470 using water-soluble polymer in the treatment of choroidal neovascularization. Invest Ophthalmol Vis Sci 1999; 40(11):2690–6.
144. Nussenblatt RB, Csaky K. Perspectives on gene therapy in the treatment of ocular inflammation. Eye 1997; 11(Pt 2):217–21.
145. Borras T. Recent developments in ocular gene therapy. Exp Eye Res 2003; 76(6):643–52.
146. Selvam S, Thomas PB, Hamm-Alvarez SF, et al. Current status of gene delivery and gene therapy in lacrimal gland using viral vectors. Adv Drug Deliv Rev 2006; 58(11):1243–57.

6

Intraocular Implants for Controlled Drug Delivery

Leila Bossy

*Department of Pharmaceutics and Biopharmaceutics, School of
Pharmaceutical Sciences, University of Geneva, University of Lausanne,
Geneva, Switzerland*

Signe Erickson

SurModics, Inc., Irvine, California, U.S.A.

Robert Gurny and Florence Delie

*Department of Pharmaceutics and Biopharmaceutics, School of
Pharmaceutical Sciences, University of Geneva, University of Lausanne,
Geneva, Switzerland*

INTRODUCTION

Different pharmaceutical approaches are available to control intraocular pathologies, such as diabetic retinopathy, uveitis, age-related macular degeneration, and cytomegalovirus (CMV) retinitis. Nevertheless, it is still difficult to achieve effective drug levels in the posterior segment tissues of the eye including the retina and vitreous without undesirable side effects. Among these approaches, topical and/or systemic administration of drugs have been widely used due to the advantage of being noninvasive. However, drugs administered orally or topically have limited penetration to ocular tissues such as retina and vitreous and therefore have little therapeutic effect on posterior structures in the eye. Topical applications of drugs at the surface of the eye result in poor intravitreal penetration due to several diffusion barriers preventing the entry of xenobiotics. These barriers are lacrimation, humor turnover, and length of diffusion path (1). Systemically administered drugs penetrate poorly into the eye due to the blood–retinal barrier (2) and require large doses of drug, resulting in potential systemic side effects. Both topical and oral treatments require rigorous patient compliance over an extended period of time to effectively deliver active drugs.

The current standard of care for treating the posterior segment of the eye involves introducing drugs directly into the vitreous chamber by intraocular injection (3,4). Steroids and antibiotics have long been applied clinically by intravitreous injection. However, this route of administration implies repeated applications of large doses to maintain drug concentrations within a therapeutic range for a long period of time because of the eye's natural circulatory processes which rapidly eliminates solution injected into the vitreous (5). These multiple injections are often responsible for severe complications, such as endophthalmitis, glaucoma, vitreous haemorrhage, retinal detachment, and cataract formation (6,7).

Thus, there is a need to find an alternative approach to efficiently treat intraocular pathologies while avoiding repeated intravitreous injections or unwanted side effects due to systemic administration of drugs. Ideally, the drug should be directly delivered in the posterior part of the eye and the drug concentration must be maintained in a therapeutic range over a long period of time. Intraocular drug delivery systems (DDS) offer sustained release of drugs locally for an extended period of time. Among these controlled release systems, intravitreal injection of liposomes (8–10) and microspheres made of biodegradable polymers (11–13) has been considered and may be useful for the treatment of intraocular diseases. However, the injection of small particles presents a major drawback, since particles suspended in the vitreous humor may impair the clarity of the ocular medium. An additional technology for achieving long-lasting and controlled release intraocular drug delivery is the use of solid polymeric implants designed to be inserted in the posterior segment of the eye. This type of device is capable of releasing drug locally into the back of the eye over a long period of time (months or years) while improving patient compliance.

Several studies have demonstrated the use of intraocular implants to be an effective method for achieving therapeutic concentrations of drugs in the posterior segment of the eye and consequently for treating severe chronic eye diseases (14–16). Studies with two such implants (Vitrasert® and Retisert®) have been particularly successful so far, having culminated in their regulatory approval for the treatment of CMV retinitis and uveitis, respectively.

In this chapter we will review the main investigations carried out on solid implants comprised of biodegradable and non-biodegradable polymer matrices. We will see that implants can have several shapes (spiral, rod, plug, pellet, and disc) and are usually implanted in the vitreous through the pars plana (Fig. 1) to treat diseases of the posterior structures of the eye. The drug released from the implant steadily diffuses through the vitreous to the target tissues, the retina, and choroid. Advantages and drawbacks of both biodegradable and non-biodegradable systems will be reviewed. Only solid implants will be covered in this chapter. Injectable systems such as viscous

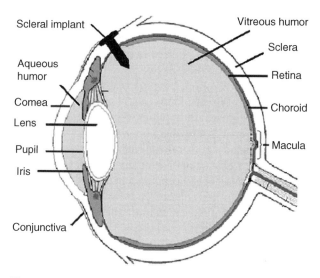

Figure 1 Schematic representation of a human eye with a scleral implant.

polymers (17), microparticles and nanoparticles, as well as liposomes, have intentionally been omitted.

NON-BIODEGRADABLE INTRAOCULAR IMPLANTS

Polyvinyl alcohol (PVA) and ethylene vinyl acetate (EVA) are commonly used together for the preparation of non-biodegradable intraocular implants. PVA is a permeable polymer acting as the scaffold of the implant and controlling the rate of drug passing through the PVA membrane. EVA is an impermeable polymer and is used as a coating polymer. The drug is released out of the system to the surrounding medium by diffusion. The great advantage of implants composed of PVA–EVA is that the release rate of the drug is constant over time (18) and no initial burst is observed. Consequently, the drug is released over a long period of time (months to years) in a controlled manner providing an ideal release pattern. However, implants based on non-biodegradable polymers present a major drawback: they require a surgical procedure for their removal and repeated implantation once the reservoir is empty. Repeated surgery increases the risk of retinal detachment, endophthalmitis, vitreous hemorrhage, and other major complications (19–21). Nevertheless, various intraocular implants based on PVA–EVA have been developed with encouraging results, particularly ganciclovir (GCV) intravitreal implant for the local treatment of CMV retinitis. This implant releases GCV by passive diffusion through a small opening in EVA at the base of the device over a period of 6–8 months (18). Several studies were carried out on animals and in humans (19,22–24), and in 1996 the Food and Drug Administration approved the use of this implant

(Vitrasert) for the treatment of CMV retinitis. The implant requires the creation of a 5-mm scleral incision and is surgically placed in the posterior part of the eye, allowing diffusion of the drug directly to the site of infection. Compared with conventional intravenous injection, Vitrasert can significantly delay progression of CMV retinitis. Apart from the necessity of repeated surgery to remove the empty scaffold, Vitrasert releases GCV only locally. Therefore the concern is raised that patients may develop CMV infections in their unaffected eye and elsewhere in the body. Therefore, treatment with Vitrasert is combined with oral treatment.

A variation of the Vitrasert delivery platform was later developed for the release of fluocinolone acetonide. Encouraging results were obtained with devices releasing the drug at approximately 2 µg/day (25–27). Devices were prepared by compressing pure drug in a 1.5-mm tablet die. Pellets were then coated in a PVA and silicone laminate (rather than EVA) and affixed to a PVA suture strut. Release occurred through a diffusion pore drilled in the coating (26). A clinical study was carried out on patients with severe uveitis (28). The devices were implanted through the pars plana into the vitreous cavity of 7 eyes of the 5 patients and drug was released for at least 2.5 years. Improved visual acuity was observed for all the patients after device implantation. Nevertheless, secondary complications, such as cataract, intraocular high pressure and retinal complications were observed in some patients after implantation of the device (28). After extensive clinical trials, this fluocinolone-releasing implant received Food and Drug Administration approval in 2006 for treatment of uveitis, and is marketed under the name Retisert®.

Other non-biodegradable implants have been developed to treat uveitis or other diseases. Potent anti-inflammatory drugs have been incorporated into sustained-controlled release devices. The efficiency of dexamethasone loaded PVA–EVA implants has been investigated in rabbit eyes and results revealed drug release in the vitreous for more than 3 months with significant reduction of local inflammation (29,30). Another intravitreal PVA–EVA based implant to treat uveitis was developed using cyclosporine A (31,32). Drug was released for at least 6 months inducing significant reduction of inflammation. Implants loaded with two drugs, dexamethasone and cyclosporine were also investigated (33). The device provided sustained release of both drugs for 10 weeks and no significant toxic effects were observed. Studies were also conducted with bethamethasone loaded PVA–EVA (34). The profile of in vitro release from the implant showed an approximately linear pattern, and the drug release could be controlled by changing the concentration of EVA in the solution used for coating the surface of the device (35). The device was implanted in a scleral pocket of pigmented rabbits and concentrations higher than effective levels for suppressing inflammation (0.14–4.00 µg/mL) were reached in the retina-choroid for 28 days.

A triamcinolone acetonide (TA) and 5-fluorouracil intravitreal implant was also tested as sustained-release device and results were very promising for the treatment of experimental proliferative vitreoretinopathy (34).

Other non-biodegradable devices designed for site-specific delivery of drug in the posterior segment of the eye are under investigation, particularly the I-vation™ sustained drug delivery system (SurModics, Inc., MN). The unique helical shape of this implant allows it to be implanted in the pars planar through a 25-gauge needle stick (a 0.5-mm self-sealing incision compared to the 5 mm incision required for Vitrasert implantation) while maximizing the surface area available for drug delivery. The helical drug delivery component of this implant resides fully within the vitreous cavity, while a thin cap resides beneath the conjunctiva and provides sutureless anchoring of the implant to the eye wall (Fig. 2). As such, the implant can be easily located and removed. The 5-mm long implant is comprised of a non-ferrous metal scaffold coated with a polymer matrix containing drug (Fig. 3). Varying the polymer constituents of this matrix confer platform applicability for delivering a wide range of molecules. Diseases such as diabetic macular oedema and age-related macular degeneration could be treated with the I-vation system. The proof of concept has been shown with I-vation TA, developed specifically for sustained release of the steroid TA. Current formulations of the implant contain approximately 1 mg of TA and are designed to release drug in a sustained manner for up to 2 years. Preclinical studies demonstrated that the implant is safe and biocompatible and that it can be easily removed. In a Phase I human clinical trial, 30 patients suffering with diabetic macular oedema were enrolled and early results indicate that the I-vationTA is safe and well tolerated with no sustained elevation of intraocular pressure.

BIODEGRADABLE SOLID IMPLANTS

Altogether intraocular implants have been shown to improve the treatment of intraocular diseases by reducing the unwanted side effects related to systemic administration of drugs and by avoiding repeated injections that can induce severe complications in the eye. Furthermore, non-biodegradable implants have shown a sustained (up to years) and controlled release pattern (no final burst). However, these implants must be removed surgically after release of the drug, producing secondary pathologies. For this reason, implants based on biodegradable polymers have been developed.

Poly(Lactic) Acid and Poly(Lactic-co-Glycolic) Acid

Biodegradable polymers have been the focus of extensive research because of the potential for long-term therapy and site-specific drug administration without the need for device retrieval. Poly(lactic-co-glycolic acid) (PLGA) has

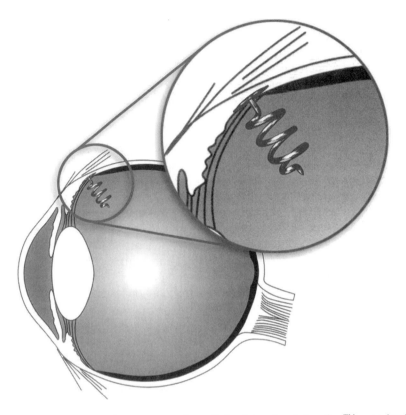

Figure 2 Schematic representation of the intravitreal I-vation™ sustained drug delivery system.

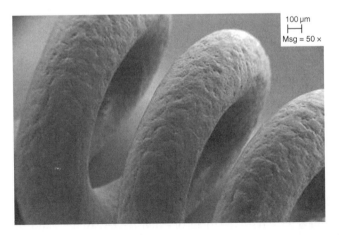

Figure 3 Scanning electron microscope image of the SurModics hybrid protein delivery coating on an intravitreal implant.

been most widely studied because of the long history of its safe clinical use as bioresorbable surgical sutures, implants, scaffolds for tissue-engineered skin and cartilage, and various prosthetic devices (35–38). The polymer undergoes hydrolysis after implantation and resolves into monomers of lactic and glycolic acids. These monomers are metabolized in the body without any adverse reactions.

In general, drug release profiles from biodegradable polymer matrices have a triphasic pattern (39–42): (*i*) an initial burst, (*ii*) a second stage that is derived from diffusional release before erosion and swelling of the polymer begins, and (*iii*) a final sudden burst due to the disintegration of the polymer matrix. The initial burst is most likely due to the rapid release of the drugs deposited on the surface and in the water channels of the matrix. Although this first burst may cause a local adverse effect, the dose of this burst can be reduced by several hours' immersion in a solution before implantation. During the second stage the drug release is controlled by the hydrolysis kinetics of the polymer. Degradation of PLGA is influenced by the ratio of lactide to glycolide as well as the molecular weight: the higher the glycolide content and/or the lower the molecular weight, the faster the degradation rate (43). An increase of the drug loading and/or the total surface area of the device may also increase the release rate. However, an overload of the drug may result in the release of a large amount of drug as an initial burst. The final sudden burst is only barely controllable and thus undesirable. Altogether, the duration and the rate of drug release are affected by the molecular weight and the copolymer ratio of the polymers, the total surface area and volume of the matrices; and the drug loading and physico-chemical properties (43). Several studies have been conducted to improve the release profile of these polymeric implants (44,45), such as using blending ratio of poly(lactic) acid (PLA) to control the release time from several months to one year (46).

One of the first attempts to deliver drug using a biodegradable sustained-controlled device was the use of PLGA rods that were simply placed in the vitreous and thus were free to move in the vitreous cavity with the risk of damaging the retina (47). To anchor the device, implants were designed to be fixed through the pars plana after sclerotomy (Fig. 1) (39,48–50).

Interesting results were obtained with devices composed of PLGA or PLA loaded with GCV for the treatment of CMV retinitis. The in vivo study demonstrated that the drug concentration in the vitreous was maintained in a therapeutic range adequate to treat CMV retinitis for 12 weeks (39,51). However, the second burst in the late phase release profile may induce an overdose of GCV, potentially toxic for ocular tissue and thus a major limitation for the use of these implants. To overcome this undesirable burst, PLGA was replaced by a mixture of different molecular weights of PLA. As a result, the release time could be controlled without a significant burst from several months to 1 year, depending on the blending ratio of PLA (52,53). It has been hypothesised that the low-molecular-weight PLA may avoid gap formation in the matrix made of the high-molecular-weight PLA, which consequently decrease of the adverse final burst of GCV from the implant.

Biodegradable scleral implants made of either PLGA or PLA and loaded with betamethasone phosphate were developed and tested in pigmented rabbit eyes as a long-term intraocular delivery system for the treatment of chronic posterior uveitis. When PLGA was used, the concentration of the drug in the retina and choroid was higher than or within the effective levels required for the suppression of inflammatory processes for more than 1 month (54). In the case of PLA implants, the therapeutic concentration of betamethasone was maintained in the retina-choroid for more than 8 weeks, without showing any toxic effects on the eye (55). As expected, the profile of in vitro betamethasone released from the implant showed a biphasic pattern, with an initial burst and a second phase derived from diffusional release. In contrast to the in vitro release profile, the implant released approximately 8% of the drug during 1 week with no initial burst effect in vivo (55). Thereafter, the implant released the drug faster than in vitro, probably due to the increased drug solubility and to the increased degradation of the polymer in vivo. At the early stage, water absorption by the implant may be less than that found in vitro, limiting the fast release of the drug from the implant. This suggests that the water channels may not be well developed in the matrix. Finally, the drug may be released rapidly after establishment of communication between the inside and outside of the matrix.

Further studies include scleral plugs composed of PLGA containing 1% doxorubicin that were tested in pigmented rabbits. Results demonstrated that the vitreous concentration could be maintained within the therapeutic range for proliferative vitreoretinopathy for four weeks. The long-term results showed no significant toxic reactions to the retina (49).

Implants have also been developed to be placed in the anterior part of the eye such as the Surodex steroid DDS (Oculex Pharmaceuticals, Sunnyvale, CA) (56–58) designed to treat inflammation following cataract surgery. This device made of PLGA is loaded with dexamethasone. It has the shape of a pellet and is placed into the eye at the end of cataract surgery to prevent post-surgical inflammation. Some major disadvantages, such as migration of the device to the anterior chamber and discomfort for the patients have been reported (58). To overcome these drawbacks, a sustained-release implant was combined with an artificial intraocular lens (IOL) (Fig. 4) to be placed in the capsular bag following cataract surgery (59). Therefore, the implant can be immobilized within the capsule. The device is formed of PLGA and contains TA. Different molecular weights of PLGA have been used to study the influence of this parameter on the release profile of the drug. In vitro data showed a tri-phasic release profile (Fig. 5) whereas no initial burst was observed in vivo and the release rate was higher than predicted the in vitro. Both in vivo and in vitro data confirmed that a

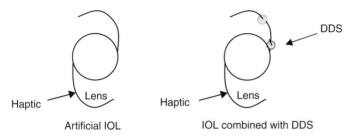

Figure 4 Schematic representation of the IOL combined with the DDS. One or two DDS can be added to the haptic of the IOL. *Abbreviations*: DDS, drug delivery systems; IOL, intraocular lens.

low molecular weight of PLGA results in a higher rate of drug release. The potential for use as a long-term intraocular delivery system to decrease postoperative inflammation was shown on rabbits. Eyes treated with the intraocular device combined with IOL showed a significant reduction of the post-operative inflammatory reaction without any major increase of intraocular pressure. Other drugs could be incorporated in the polymer matrix and up to four discs could be combined with the IOL to increase the amount of drug released. The major advantage of the intraocular drug delivery system is the possibility to combine both the cataract surgery and postoperative treatment in a single procedure.

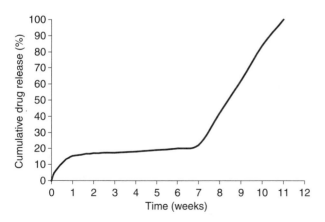

Figure 5 Typical example of a triphasic drug release profile from a polymeric implant made of PLGA. *Abbreviation*: PLGA, poly(lactic-co-glycolic) acid.

Polycaprolactone

Polycaprolactone (PCL) is more hydrophobic and impermeable than PLGA or PLA and does not undergo swelling or bulk diffusion in the body (60). Degradation of PCL by hydrolysis of the ester linkage produces small polymeric fragments that are metabolised after phagocytosis. Drugs loaded in PCL-based implants are released through micropores formed during the drug elution and before degradation of the polymer. The release rate of the drug depends directly on the drug loading: the higher the drug loading, the greater the polymer porosity formed during drug absorption and the higher the rate of drug released. Compared to PLGA and PLA, PCL has a slow degradation kinetic rate and drugs released from the PCL matrix have a linear release pattern without burst effect. Beeley et al. prepared a rod-shaped device loaded with TA using PCL as a polymer matrix (61). Studies carried out on rabbits showed that the subretinal implant was well tolerated by the retina during the one-month follow-up period. Drug levels in different eye compartments demonstrated a posterior eye segment localisation.

PCL has also been used as a polymer matrix for the intraocular implants to deliver 5-FU (62). Results showed that this device allowed slow release of the drug and led to a 100% protection against tractional retinal detachment. Mild vitreous hemorrhage was observed in a few of the treated eyes but no other significant complications were detected.

CONCLUSION

We have seen in this chapter that it is important to develop appropriate devices to treat diseases in the eye that are not properly treated with conventional approaches such as oral/topical administration or intraocular injections of drugs. To improve the treatment of intraocular pathologies, sustained-controlled implants have been developed. These devices are designed to release medications over a long period of time depending on the type and severity of the disease. Biodegradable and non-biodegradable polymers are available as implant matrices. In terms of release profile, devices based on non-biodegradable polymer membranes are more controllable than those based on biodegradable polymers. Furthermore, non-biodegradable devices can release drugs for a longer period (months up to years) than biodegradable devices (weeks up to a few months) and therefore, may be more suitable for chronic intraocular diseases, such as diabetic vitreoretinopathy and age-related macular degeneration. On the other hand, biodegradable implants have the great advantage that they do not need to be removed once the drug has been completely released, whereas in the case of non-biodegradable systems, an additional surgical procedure has to be undertaken to withdraw the implant.

Altogether, there is not a universal device that can be used to treat all the pathologies of the eye. For each pathology a new implant must be accurately developed to release the drug in the appropriate manner. Several parameters must be well studied such as composition, ratio, and molecular weight of the polymers, as well as the shape of the implant and drug concentration.

Overall, intraocular implants have been shown to be efficient in several specific diseases and some of them are clinically used with success. These results are very encouraging and further investigations will surely prove the role of controlled release devices in the treatment of ocular pathologies.

REFERENCES

1. Tojo K, Nakagawa K, Morita Y, Ohtori A. A pharmacokinetic model of invitreal delivery of ganciclovir. Eur J Pharm Biopharm 1999; 47:99–104.
2. Maurice DM, Mishima S. Ocular pharmacokinetics. In: Sears ML, ed. Pharmacology of the Eye. New York: Springer-Verlag, 1984: 19–116.
3. Park CH, Jaffe GJ, Fekrat S. Intravitreal triamcinolone acetonide in eyes with cystoid macular edema associated with central retinal vein occlusion. Am J Ophthalmol 2003; 136:419–25.
4. Bourges JL, Gautier SE, Delie F, et al. Ocular drug delivery targeting the retina and retinal pigment epithelium using polylactide nanoparticles. Invest Ophthalmol Vis Sci 2003; 44:3562–9.
5. Gilger BC, Malok E, Stewart T, et al. Long-term effect on the quine eye of an intravitreal device used for sutained release of cyclosporine. Vet Ophthalmol 2000; 3:105–10.
6. Gillies MC, Simpson JM, Billson FA, et al. Safety of an intravitreal injection of triamcinolone:results from a randomized clinical trial. Arch Ophthalmol 2004; 122:336–40.
7. Jaissle GB, Szurman P, Bartz-Schmidt KU. Ocular side effects and complications of intravitreal triamcinolone acetonide injection. Ophthalmology 2004; 101:121–8.
8. Bochot A, Couvreur P, Fattal E. Intravitreal adminsitration of antisense oligonucleotides: Potential of liposomal delivery. Progr Retin Eye Res 2000; 19: 131–47.
9. Simmons ST, Sherwood MB, Nichols DA. Pharmacokinetics of a 5-fluorouracil liposomal delivery system. Br J Ophthalmol 1988; 72:688–91.
10. Assil KK, Hartzer M, Weinreb RN. Liposome suppression of proliferative vitreoretinopathy. Invest Ophthalmol Vis Sci 1991; 32:2891–7.
11. Ogura Y, Kimura H. Biodegradable polymer microspheres for targeted drug delivery to the retinal pigment epithelium. Surv Ophthalmol 1995; 39:17–24.
12. Moritera T, Ogura Y, Honda Y, Wada R. Microspheres of biodegradable polymers as a drug delivery system in the vitreous. Invest Ophthalmol Vis Sci 1991; 32:1785–90.
13. Moritera T, Ogura Y, Honda Y. Biodegradable microspheres containing adriamycin in the treatment of proliferative vitreoretinopathy. Invest Ophthalmol Vis Sci 1992; 33:3125–30.

14. Geroski DH, Edelhauser HF. Transscleral drug delivery for posterior segment disease. Adv Drug Deliv Rev 2001; 52:37–48.
15. Ambati J, Canakis CS, Miller JW. Diffuion of high molecular weight compounds through slera. Invest Ophthalmol Vis Sci 2000; 41:1181–5.
16. Ambati J, Canakis CS, Miller JW. Transcleral delivery of bioactive protein to the choroid and retina. Invest Ophthalmol Vis Sci 2000; 42:1186–91.
17. Bourges JL, Bloquel C, Thomas A, et al. Intraocular implants for extended drug delivery: Therapeutic applications. Adv Drug Deliv Rev 2006; 58: 1182–202.
18. Smith TJ, Pearson PA, Blandford DL, et al. Intravitreal sustained-release ganciclovir. Arch Ophthalmol 1992; 110:255–8.
19. Martin DF, Parks DJ, Mellow SD, Ferris FL, Walton RC, Remaley NA, Chew EY, et al. Treatment of cytomegalovirus retinitis with an intraocular sustained-release ganciclovir implant. A randomized controlled clinical trial, Arch Ophthalmol 1994; 112:1531–9.
20. Morley MG, Duker JS, Ashton P, Robinson MR. Replacing ganciclovir implants. Ophthalmology 1995; 102:388–92.
21. Martin DF, Ferris FL, Parks DJ, Walton RC, Mellow SD, Gibbs D, Remaley NA, et al. Timong, surgical procedure, and complications. Arch Ophthalmol 1997; 115:1389–94.
22. Anand R, Nightingale SD, Fish RH, Smith T, Ashton P. Control of cytomegalovirus retinitis using sustained release of intraocular ganciclovir. Arch Ophthalmol 1993; 111:223–7.
23. Marx JL, Kapusta MA, Patel SS, LaBree LD, Walonker F, Rao NA, Chong LP. Use of the ganciclovir implatn in the treatment of recurrent cytomegalovirus retinitis. Arch Ophthalmol 1996; 114:815–20.
24. Ashton P, Brown JD, Pearson PA, et al. Intravitreal gancivlovir pharmacokinetics in rabbits and man. J Ocular Pharmacol 1992; 8:343–7.
25. Jaffe GJ, Yang CH, Guo H, Denny JP, Lima C, Ashton P. Safety and pharmacokinetics of an intraocular fluocinolone acetonide sustained delivery device. Invest Ophthalmol Vis Sci, 2000; 41:3569–75.
26. Jaffe GJ, Ben J Nun, Guo H, Dunn JP, Ashton P. Fluocinolone acetonide sustained drug delivery device to treat severe uveitis. Ophthalmology 2000; 107: 2024–33.
27. Jaffe GJ, McCallum RM, Btanchaud B, Skalak C, Butuner Z, Ashton P. Long-term follow-up results of a pilot trial of a fluocinolone acetonide implant to treat posterior uveitis. Ophthalmology 2005; 112:1192–8.
28. Jaffe GJ, Martin D, Callanan D, Pearson PA, Levy B, Comstock T. Fluocinolone acetonide implant (Retisert) for noninfectious posterior uveitis: thirty-four results of a multicenter randomized clinical study. Ophthalmology 2006; 113:1020–7.
29. Hainsworth DP, Pearson PA, Conklin JD, Ashton P. Sustained release intravitreal dexamethasone, J Ocular Pharmacol Ther 1996; 12:57–63.
30. Cheng CH, Berger AS, Pearson PA, Ashton P, Jaffe GJ. Intravitreal sustained-release dexamethasone device in the treatment of experimental uveitis. Invest Ophthalmol Vis Sci 1995; 36:442–53.

31. Jaffe GJ, Yang CS, Wang XC, Cousins SW, Gallemore RP, Ashton P. Intravitreal sustained-release cyclosporine in the treatment of experimental uveitis. Ophthalmology 1998; 105:46–56.
32. Pearson PA, Jaffe GJ, Martin DF, et al. Evaluation of a delivery system providing long-term release of cyclosporine. Arch Ophthalmol 1996; 114: 311–7.
33. Enyedi LB, Pearson PA, Ashton P, Jaffe GJ. An intravitreal device providing sustained release of cyclosporine and dexamethasone. Curr Eye Res 1996; 15: 549–57.
34. Okabe K, Kimura H, Okabe J, Kato A, Kunou N, Ogura Y. Intraocular tissue distribution of betamethasone after intrascleral administration using a non-biodegradable sustained drug delivery device. Invest Ophthalmol Vis Sci 2003; 44:2702–7.
35. Yang C-S, Khawly JA, Hainsworth DP, et al. An intravitreal sustained-release triamcinolone and 5-fluorouracil codrug in the treatment of experimental proliferative vitreoretinopathy. Arch Ophthalmol 1998; 116:69–77.
36. Lingua RW, Parel JM, Assis L. Absorbable copolymer clip: a potential substitute for sutures in strabismus surgery. Binoc Vision 1987; 2:129–36.
37. Lewis DH. Controlled release of bioactive agents from lactide/glycolide polymers. In: Chasin H, Langer R eds, Biodegradable polymers as drug delivery system. New York: Marcel Dekker, 1990, pp. 1-43.
38. Holy CE, Davies JE, Shoichet MS. Bone tissue engineering on biodegradable polymers: preparation of a novel poly(lactide-co-glycolide) foam. In: Peppas NA, Mooney DJ, Mikos AG, Brannon-Peppas L eds, Biometarial, carriers for drug delivery, and scaffolds for tissue engineering. New York: A.I.Ch.E, 1997, pp. 272–4.
39. Kunou N, Ogura Y, Hashizoe M, Honda Y, Hyon S-H, Ikada Y. Controlled intraocular delivery of ganciclovir with use of biodegradable scleral implant in rabbits. J Control Release 1995; 37:143–50.
40. Pitt CG, Gratzl MM, Jeffcoat AR, Zweidinger R, Schindler A. Sustained drug delivery systems. II. Factors affecting release rates from poly(e-caprolactone) and related biodegradable polymers. J Pharm Sci 1979; 68:1534–8.
41. Hora MS, Rana RK, Nunberg HN, G TR, Tice RM, Hudson ME. Release of human serum albumin from poly(lactide-co-glycolide) microspheres. Pharm Res 1990; 7:1190–4.
42. Sanders LM, Kent JS, Mcrae GI, Vickery BH, Tice TR, Lewis DH. Controlled release of a luteinizing hormone-releasing hormone analogue from poly(D,L-lactide-co-glycolide) microspheres. J Pharm Sci 1984; 73:1294–7.
43. Miller RA, Brandy JM, Cutright DE. Degradation rates of oral resorbable implants (polylactate and polyglycolate):rate modification with changes in PLA/PGA copolymer ratio. J Biomed Mater Res 1977; 11:711–9.
44. Yasukawa T, Kimura H, Tabata Y, Ogura Y. Biodegradable scleral plugs for vitreoretinal drug delivery. Adv Drug Deliv Rev 2001; 52:25–36.
45. Yasukawa T, Ogura Y, Sakurai E, Tabata Y, Kimura H. Intraocular sustained drug delivery using implantable polymeric devices. Adv Drug Deliv Rev 2005; 57:2033–46.

46. Kunou N, Ogura Y, Yasukawa T, Kimura H, Miyamoto H, Honda Y, IkadaY. Long-term sustained release of ganciclovir from biodegradable scleral implant for the treatment of cytomegalovirus retinitis. J Control Release 2000; 68: 263–71.

47. Rubsamen PE, Davis PE, Hernandez E, O'Grady GE, Cousins SW. Prevention of experimentla proliferative vitreoretinopathy with biodegradable intravitreal implant for the sustained release of fluorouracil. Arch Ophthalmol 1994; 112: 407–13.

48. Hashizoe M, Ogura Y, Takanashi T, Kunou N, Honda Y, Ikada Y. Implantable bioidegradable polymeric device in the treatment of experimental proliferative vitreoretinopathy. Curr Eye Res 1995; 14:473–7.

49. Hashizoe M, Ogura Y, Kimura H, et al. Scleral plug of biodegradable polymers for controlled drug releas in the vitreous. Arch Ophthalmol 1994; 112: 1380–4.

50. Kimura H, Ogura Y, Hashizoe M, Nishiwaki H, Honda Y, and Ikada Y. A new vitreal drug delivery system with an implantable biodegradabée polymer device. Invest Ophthalmol Vis Sci 1994; 35:2815–9.

51. Hashizoe M, Ogura Y, Takanashi T, Kunou N, Honda Y, Ikada Y. Biodegradable polymeric device for sustained intravitreal release of ganciclovir in rabbits. Curr Eye Res 1997; 16:633–9.

52. Kunou N, Ogura Y, Yasukawa T, et al. Long-term sustained release of ganciclovir from biodegradable scleral implant for the treatment of cytomegalovirus retinitis. J Control Release 2000; 68:263–71.

53. Yasukawa T, Kimura H, Kunou N, et al. Biodegradable scleral implant for intravitreal controlled release of ganciclovir. Graefes Arch Clin Exp Ophthalmol 2000; 238:186–90.

54. Kunou N, Ogura Y, Honda Y, Hyon SH, Ikada Y. Biodegradable scleral implant for controlled intraocular delivery of betamethasone phosphate. J Biomed Mater Res 2000; 51:635–41.

55. Okabe J, Kimura H, Kunou N, Okabe K, Kato A, Ogura Y. Biodegradable intrascleral implant for sustained intraocular delivery of betamethasone phosphate. Invest Ophthalmol Vis Sci 2003; 44:740–4.

56. Wadood AC, Armbrecht AM, Aspinall PA, Dhillon B. Safety and efficacy of a dexamethasone anterior segment drug delivery system in patients after phacoemulsification. J Cataract Refract Surg 2004; 30:761–8.

57. Chang DF, Garcia IH, Hunkeler JD, Minas T. Phase II results of an intraocular steroid delivery system for cataract surgery. Ophthalmology 1999; 106: 1172–7.

58. McColgin AZ and Heier JS. Control of intraocular inflammation associated with cataract surgery. Curr Opin Ophthalmol 2000; 11:3–6.

59. Eperon S, Bossy-Nobs L. Guex-Crosier Y. Petropoulos IK, Gurny R. Cataract and inflammation: a new drug delivery system. Acta Ophtalmol Scandinavica 2006; 84:21.

60. Pitt CG. Poly e caprolactone and its copolymers. In: Chassin M, Langer R, eds, Biodegradable Polymers as Drug Delivery Systems. New York: Marcel Dekker, 1990, pp. 71–119.

61. Beeley NR, Rossi JV, Mello-Filho PA, Mahmoud MI, Fujii GY, de Juan E Jr, Varner SE. Fabrication, implantation, elution, and retrieval of a steroid-loaded polycaprolactone subretinal implant. J Biomed 2005; Mater Res A, 73:437–44.
62. Borhani H, Peyman GA, Rahimy MH, Thompson H. Suppression of experimetnal proliferatvie vitreoretinopathy by sustained intraocular delivery of 5-FU. Int Ophthalmol 1995; 19:43–9.

7

Bioadhesive Ophthalmic Drug Inserts (BODI) for Veterinary Use

Pascal Furrer, Olivia Felt, and Robert Gurny

Department of Pharmaceutics and Biopharmaceutics, School of Pharmaceutical Sciences, University of Geneva, University of Lausanne, Geneva, Switzerland

INTRODUCTION

Most veterinary topical ophthalmic drugs and delivery systems are derived from human ocular formulations (1). However, differences in the eye anatomy and physiology of the animals encountered in veterinary practice and their unique diseases and specific responses to therapeutic agents are sufficient reasons for encouraging and promoting research and development in veterinary medicine. The convenience of medication application by the animal owner is a crucial issue in the selection of the therapeutic system. Indeed, frequent applications are often problematic for the owner and compliance is rather low, in addition to the risk of bite or scratch by the animals. For these reasons, a drug delivery system has been developed with the aim of increasing the residence time of the drug on the ocular surface, sustaining drug release and reducing the number of administrations. This system, the soluble bioadhesive ophthalmic drug insert (BODI), was patented by Gurtler in 1993 and is made of synthetic and semi-synthetic polymers (2).

BODI inserts are primarily composed of a ternary mixture of hydroxypropylcellulose, ethylcellulose, and a cross-linked acrylic polymer, namely carbomer (Table 1). The replacement of natural polymers, such as collagen, used in soluble inserts like collagen shields, by synthetic polymers is undoubtedly advantageous with regard to their safety of use. Indeed, natural biopolymers may be associated with inflammatory responses of the ocular tissues due to the presence of residual proteins. In addition, these

Table 1 Polymeric Composition of BODI

Polymer	HPC (hydroxypropylcellulose)	EC (ethylcellulose)	CP (carbomer)
Characteristic Type	Hydrophilic Klucel® HXF NF	Hydrophobic Ethocel® N50 NF	Bioadhesive Carbopol® 934P
Role	Main vehicle ensuring aqueous solubility	Reduces insert deformation	Reduces risks of expulsion
Concentration (% w/w)	67.0	30.0	3.0

Abbreviations: BODI, bioadhesive ophthalmic drug inserts; HPC, hydroxypropylcellulose; EC, ethylcellulose; CP, carbomer.

days, devices based on collagen may encounter difficulties with approval by regulatory authorities, because of possible prion-infection.

The rationale for developing inserts endowed with bioadhesive properties using Carbopol® (CP) was based on the observation that available ocular inserts did not always allow prolonged release of the incorporated drugs and may be displaced or sometimes expelled by eyeball movements. Despite the fact that the use of non-neutralized CP is controversial due to its acidic nature, which could possibly induce eye irritation (3), Gurtler et al. (4) have demonstrated that it does not cause any damage to the ocular surface at concentrations up to 3%.

DESCRIPTION OF BODI TECHNOLOGY

Size and Shape

BODIs are rod shape inserts obtained by the extrusion of a dried homogeneous powder mixture composed of the polymeric vehicle and the active compound using a specially designed ram extruder. Their final optimal dimensions, customized for placement into the inferior lateral conjunctival cul-de-sac of animals like dogs, are 5.0 mm in length, 2.0 mm in diameter and, 20.5 mg in weight.

Manufacture

In order to ensure a homogeneous distribution of the drug in the matrix, a double extrusion process has been demonstrated to be necessary (4). Briefly, the following manufacturing conditions were applied: a first extrusion at a temperature of 140–160°C with a warming-up time of 2 minutes followed by a second extrusion at a pressure of 200–300 kPa. This extrusion technique offers some advantages such as low cost, rapid development, and good reproducibility.

RESEARCH AND DEVELOPMENT STUDIES

Initial Development Results

The first developed BODIs contained gentamicin sulfate, an aminosidic antibiotic, as the model drug (5,6). However, despite good pharmacokinetic performances when compared with conventional formulations like eye drops, it was demonstrated by Baeyens et al. (7) that due to its high hydrophilicity, gentamicin was almost immediately released from the BODI. This led to a period of efficacy of often lower than 12 hours, similar to ocular inserts based on gelatin (8) or collagen (9–12). Therefore, Baeyens et al. (7) studied different approaches to reduce the solubility of gentamicin using cellulose acetate phthalate (CAP) to obtain either a solid dispersion or a co-precipitate (Fig. 1).

Results showed that CAP was a good release moderator since the duration of efficacy was significantly increased after gentamicin pretreatment. However, it can also be seen from the results in Table 2 that BODI 3 was less effective than BODI 2 in prolonging gentamicin release. On the basis of a modified Draize test, the authors correlated this difference with the bad tolerance score following the deposition of BODI 3 in the

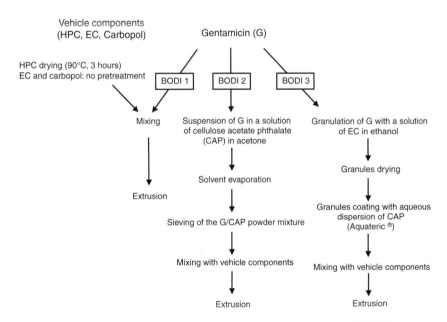

Figure 1 Schematic representation of the fabrication processes of BODIs containing unmodified (BODI 1), or modified gentamicin by the solid dispersion technique (BODI 2) or by the coprecipitate technique (BODI 3). *Abbreviation*: BODI, bioadhesive ophthalmic drug inserts.

Table 2   Half-Life Time of Elimination ($t_{1/2}$) and Time of Efficacy (t_{eff}) of Gentamicin after Deposition on Insert (BODI 1, 2, or 3) in Rabbit Eye

Inserts	Gentamicin state	$t_{1/2}$ (hr)	t_{eff} (hr)
BODI 1	Unmodified	5.11	11.9 ± 0.1
BODI 2	Solid dispersion	21.92	43.8 ± 6.0
BODI 3	Coprecipitate	12.29	23.3 ± 0.3

Source: Adapted from Ref. 7.

inferior cul-de-sac of rabbits (Fig. 2). This is likely related to the presence of surfactants in Aquateric® (CAP), which are well known for their irritating potential.

Further Developmental Studies

From a therapeutic viewpoint, BODIs further evolved by combining a second active compound, namely dexamethasone phosphate, with gentamicin (12,13). The rationale behind co-formulating a corticosteroid with an antibacterial agent into a single ophthalmic drug delivery system was based on the recommendation that, in the case of external infections such as keratitis or conjunctivitis, co-administration of a steroid limits the structural damage related to the inflammatory response (12).

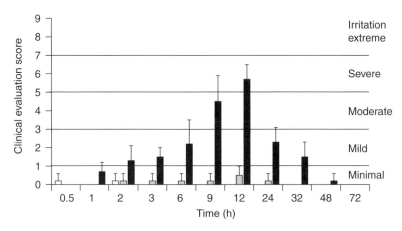

Figure 2   Comparative clinical evaluation of irritation scores after deposition of inserts containing gentamicin without pretreatment (BODI 1) (□), solid dispersion of gentamicin with CAP (BODI 2) (■), and coprecipitate of gentamicin with CAP (BODI 3) (■). *Abbreviations*: BODI, bioadhesive ophthalmic drug inserts; CAP, cellulose acetate phthalate. *Source*: Adapted from Ref. 7.

The main goals of this approach were to avoid the need for a separate administration of dexamethasone and also to limit the side effects associated with repeated installations of dexamethasone, particularly the risk of increased intraocular pressure, which can lead to glaucoma.

In Vitro Studies

These inserts successfully provided a prolonged release of gentamicin above its minimum inhibitory concentration for nearly 50 hours, while also achieving the immediate release of a suitable concentration of dexamethasone in tears for about 12 hours simultaneously (Fig. 3).

Both gentamicin and dexamethasone show a biphasic release profile from a BODI matrix when inserted into the eye. Indeed, the release of drugs from the BODI systems is characterized by two phases: the first one corresponds to the penetration of tear fluid into the insert inducing a high release rate of drug by diffusion and formation of a gel layer around the core of the insert (14). This external gelification then induces the second phase, which corresponds to a slower release rate, controlled by a diffusion

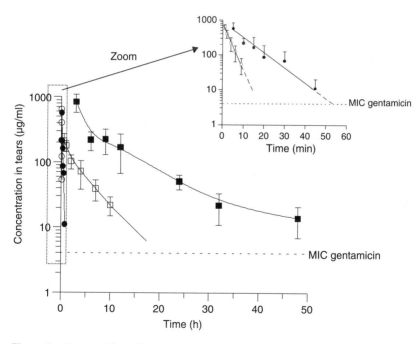

Figure 3   Gentamicin sulfate (■, •) and dexamethasone phosphate (□, ○) pharmacokinetic profiles in tear fluid after deposition of one insert (*squares*) or after administration of 50 µl of a collyrium (*circles*) containing an association of both active ingredients (tested in rabbit, mean ± SEM, $n = 6$). *Source*: Adapted from Refs. 12, 13.

mechanism. This drug release mechanism from a BODI still remains hypothetical since no in vitro tests have been conducted to confirm the mechanism.

In-Vivo Studies

Because previous investigations on BODI successfully demonstrated that the insert was very well tolerated and provided good pharmacokinetic results, the inserts were then studied in clinical randomized trials on 90 Beagle dogs for the treatment of conjunctivitis, superficial corneal ulcers or keratoconjunctivitis and compared with a classical eye drop treatment containing gentamicin and dexamethasone (15). BODI and eye drops provided both similar clinical effects in term of cure rate with no statistical difference. Although both treatments ensured similar clinical recoveries, the insert offered the major advantage of a reduced number of manipulations (one deposition of one insert) when compared with the commercial collyrium therapy (3 applications a day for 7 days). This is particularly crucial in veterinary medicine, as repeated applications can lead to poor compliance.

Evaluating the acceptability of the insert at day 0, the veterinarians reported that more than 80% of dogs did not show a major disturbance during the application of the insert. Only two dogs presented noteworthy disturbance, rubbing the eye to pull out the insert.

Future Developmental Studies

Future studies using the BODI technology may be directed toward the evaluation of other active compounds for ocular therapy. However, it must be noted that the fabrication process limits the choice of therapeutic agents to those that are not heat sensitive.

Another future development of the BODI technology may be to extend its use from its original veterinary applications to human applications. This would involve some design modifications, especially regarding the size and the shape of the inserts.

In order to have data that are more comprehensive on this promising technology, complementary studies may be considered such as: (*i*) evaluation of the effect of the extrusion technique on the stability of the various components of BODI (mainly molecular weight of the polymers), and (*ii*) the effect of a sterilization process on the stability of the formulation components. In the case of the latter, since BODI contains an antibacterial agent and is fabricated at high temperature, it has previously been concluded that inserts were pathogen free. However, it has not been demonstrated using official tests, such as those described in the European Pharmacopoeia, that these two parameters ensure a comparable level of sterility to an actual sterilization process such as gamma-sterilization.

CONCLUSION

BODI are rod shaped soluble inserts made of synthetic and semi-synthetic polymers. The use of synthetic polymers offers advantages with regard to their safety of use. Inclusion of the bioadhesive excipient Carbopol® allows for prolonged release of incorporated drugs and increases residence time of the delivery system in the eye. Furthermore, BODI presents other potential advantages such as accurate dosing, the absence of preservatives that may be noxious to the cornea and good stability due to the absence of water.

BODI inserts are obtained by an extrusion process that offers some manufacturing advantages, but the high extrusion temperatures limit drug candidates to those that are heat resistant.

Several drugs have been incorporated into BODI inserts resulting in release profiles measured in hours to days.

REFERENCES

1. Baeyens V, Percicot C, Zignani M, et al. Ocular drug delivery in veterinary medicine. Adv Drug Deliv Rev 1997; 28:335–61.
2. Gurtler F, Gurny R. Insert ophtalmique bioadhésif. European patent 934 00677-61; 1993.
3. Amin PD, Bhogte CP, Deshpande MA. Studies on gel tears. Drug Dev Ind Pharm 1996; 22:735–9.
4. Gurtler F, Kaltsatos V, Boisrame B, et al. Development of a novel soluble ophthalmic insert: evaluation of ocular tolerance in rabbits. Eur J Pharm Biopharm 1996; 42:393–8.
5. Gurtler F, Kaltsatos V, Boisramé B, et al. Long-acting soluble bioadhesive ophthalmic drug insert (BODI®) containing gentamicin for veterinary use: optimization and clinical investigation. J Control Release 1995; 33:231–6.
6. Gurtler F, Kaltsatos V, Boisramé B, et al. Ocular availability of gentamicin in small animals after topical administration of a conventional eye drop solution and a novel long acting bioadhesive ophthalmic drug insert. Pharm Res 1995; 12:1791–5.
7. Baeyens V, Kaltsatos V, Boisramé B, et al. Evaluation of soluble Bioadhesive Ophthalmic Drug Inserts (BODI®) for prolonged release of gentamicin: Lachrymal pharmacokinetics and ocular tolerance. J Ocul Pharmacol Ther 1998; 14:263–72.
8. Punch PI, Slatter DH, Costa ND, et al. Investigation of gelatin as a possible biodegradable matrix for sustained delivery of gentamicin to the bovine eye. J Vet Pharmacol Ther 1985; 8:335–8.
9. Phinney RB, Schwartz SD, Lee DA, et al. Collagen-shield delivery of gentamicin and vancomycin. Arch Ophthalmol 1988; 106:1599–604.
10. Liang FQ, Viola RS, del Cerro M, et al. Noncross-linked collagen discs and cross-linked collagen shields in the delivery of gentamicin to rabbits eyes. Invest Ophthalmol Vis Sci 1992; 33:2194–8.

11. Bloomfield SE, Miyata T, Dunn MW, et al. Soluble gentamicin ophthalmic inserts as a drug delivery system. Arch Ophthalmol 1978; 96:885–7.
12. Gurny R, Kaltsatos V, Baeyens V, Boisramé B. Therapeutic or hygienic compositions with controlled and prolonged release of the active principles, in particular for ophthalmic use. Patent WO 98/56346; 1998.
13. Baeyens V, Kaltsatos V, Boisramé B, et al. Optimized release of dexamethasone and gentamicin from a soluble ocular insert for the treatment of external ophthalmic infections. J Control Release 1998; 52:215–20.
14. Gurtler F, Gurny R. Patent litterature review of ophthalmic inserts. Drug Dev Ind Pharm 1995; 21:1–18.
15. Baeyens V, Felt-Baeyens O, Rougier S, et al. Clinical evaluation of bioadhesive ophthalmic drug inserts (BODI) for the treatment of external ocular infections in dogs. J Control Release 2002; 82:163–8.

8

Ion Exchange Resin Technology for Ophthalmic Applications

Rajni Jani and Erin Rhone

Pharmaceutical Research and Development, Alcon Research Ltd., Fort Worth, Texas, U.S.A.

INTRODUCTION

Only a few commercially available ophthalmic drug delivery systems have been forthcoming since the introduction of the topical eye drop. However, delivery systems that attempt to increase the residence time in the eye have been extensively studied in the literature. Among these are pre-soaked soft contact lenses (1–7), soluble polymer gels (8,9) and emulsions (10–12), bioerodible ocular inserts (13), diffusional devices or nonerodible inserts (14), and osmotic systems (15). Of these delivery systems, the Ocusert® system (Alza Corporation, Palo Alto, CA), which was introduced in 1975, provided a virtual zero-order release of the drug over a long period of time. Although it was technologically advanced, the Ocusert system was not well accepted by patients.

For a patient with a chronic ocular disease such as glaucoma, efficient drug delivery can make the difference between long-term well being or morbidity of the patient. The conventional method for treating this condition is by the use of eye drops. This approach results in an initial peak dose of drug, which is usually higher than that needed for therapeutic effect, followed by a drop-off in concentration that may fall below therapeutic levels (15). This fluctuating therapeutic course is exacerbated when the patient is reluctant to take the medication because of systemic or localized side effects. The ion exchange resin technology is a means by which this disease can be treated more effectively with the fluctuating drug levels being controlled through formulation.

ION EXCHANGE RESIN TECHNOLOGY

History

The introduction of a topical ophthalmic betaxolol 0.5% solution (Betoptic® Solution 0.5%) in 1985 offered a breakthrough for patients with compromised cardiac and pulmonary function. The beta 1 adrenergic cardioselectivity of betaxolol hydrochloride was proven effective in lowering intraocular pressure with fewer side effects than either timolol maleate or levobunolol. However, the introduction of betaxolol ionic suspension (Betoptic® S) in 1990 provided an even more significant innovation because it provided the same efficacy as betaxolol solution but with a superior safety and tolerance profile.

Product Challenges

The development of topical ophthalmic dosage forms of a nonselective beta-1 and beta-2 adrenergic antagonist provided ophthalmologists with two powerful tools for the treatment of open angle glaucoma and elevated intraocular pressure. However, although beta-blockers are effective in lowering and maintaining normal intraocular pressure, they are also known to have the potential for significant systemic side effects and local irritation.

Systemic Side Effects

Since the majority of glaucoma patients are over 60 years of age and susceptible to age-related body changes (i.e., cardiac and pulmonary function), systemic absorption of any drug following ocular administration must be evaluated carefully to avoid drug toxicity and to avoid exacerbating systemic side effects.

Local Irritation

In addition to systemic side effects, the beta-blockers used in glaucoma topical therapy are known to produce a brief episode of stinging and/or burning upon instillation in some patients. The discomfort associated with topical administration of betaxolol 0.5% solution is due to the high-localized concentration of drug at the cornea nerve endings. Betaxolol is a lipophilic molecule, which resembles a long hydrophobic chain with a small hydrophilic end group. Because of this hydrophobicity, it penetrates the cornea very well. Since the cornea has a network of sensory nerve endings making it very sensitive to external stimuli, exceeding the threshold value causes the nerve ending to fire, resulting in discomfort. Thus to improve comfort (or reduce discomfort) it is necessary to reduce and/or control the penetration of betaxolol into the cornea, thereby reducing the drug concentration below the threshold value at the nerve endings. This hypothetical threshold is shown in Figure 1.

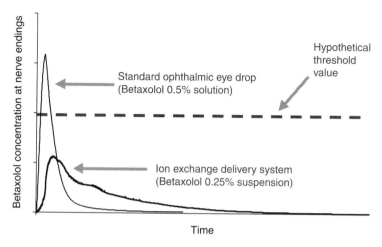

Figure 1 Hypothetical comfort threshold.

Product Requirements

It was this side effect profile that presented pharmaceutical scientists with the challenge of developing a delivery system, which both minimized the ocular discomfort and reduced the systemic absorption that was associated with beta-blockers while maintaining efficacy.

In addition, ideally, the drug delivery system should also provide longer residence time in the precorneal area, and minimize systemic exposure thus providing the same amount (mass) of drug at one half the concentration.

Ion Exchange Resins

The controlled release of a topical ophthalmic beta-blocker at a known release rate was achieved by binding betaxolol to an ion exchange resin.

History and Uses

Interest in the use of ion exchange resins as carriers for drug molecules began in the 1950s. Keating was one of the first to discuss the preparation and evaluation of combinations of carboxylic, sulfonic and phosphoric acid cation exchange resins with a variety of amine drugs (e.g., adrenergics, antihistaminics, antispasmodics, and antitussives) (16).

Ion-exchange resins have been used to modify the release of drug molecules for systemic use for many years. Most major applications of resinate-type dosage forms have been for oral formulation. For example, Burke et al. used ion exchange resins for slow release of propranolol hydrochloride into the gastrointestinal tract (17). Ion exchange resins have also been used as potential phosphate binders for renal failure patients.

The substance to which betaxolol is bound in the formulation is a pharmaceutical grade cationic exchange resin, Amberlite™. Cationic exchange polymers have been used as carriers for cationic drugs in several pharmaceutical preparations, e.g., in numerous tablets (e.g., phentermine maleate), in cough syrups (e.g., Pennkinetic System), and to reduce problems of taste and odor in oral dosage forms. Amberlite ion exchange polymers have also been used in the controlled release of drugs.

Description of Ion Exchange Resins

Ion exchange resins are insoluble ionic materials with acidic or basic groups that are covalently bound in repeating positions on the resin chain. These charged groups associate with other ions of opposite charge. Depending on whether the mobile counter ion is a cation or an anion, it is possible to distinguish between cationic and anionic exchange resins. The matrix in cationic exchangers carries ionic groups such as sulfonic carboxylate and phosphate groups. The matrix in anionic exchangers carries primary, secondary, tertiary, or quaternary ammonium groups. The resin matrix determines its physical properties, its behavior towards biological substances, and to some extent, its capacity.

ION EXCHANGE RESIN TECHNOLOGY FOR OPHTHALMIC APPLICATIONS

The first successful ophthalmic product for topical application using ion exchange resin technology was betaxolol ionic suspension (Betoptic® S, 0.25%) for glaucoma, which was introduced by Alcon Laboratories, Inc. in 1990 (18). Alcon holds worldwide patents directed to sustained release ophthalmic suspensions including Betoptic® S.

The Formulation

Betaxolol ionic suspension contains 0.28% betaxolol hydrochloride equivalent to 0.25% betaxolol bound to Amberlite resin with 0.01% benzalkonium chloride as an antimicrobial preservative. The betaxolol ionic suspension formulation also contains disodium edetate, mannitol, hydrochloric acid or sodium hydroxide to adjust the pH, and purified water as shown in Table 1.

Chemically, betaxolol HCl is (+)-1[p-[2(cyclopropylmethoxy) ethyl] phenoxyl]-3-(isopropylamino)-2-propanol hydrochloride with empirical formula of $C_{18}H_{29}NO_3 \cdot HCl$ and a molecular weight of 343.89. Betaxolol HCl is a white crystalline powder, soluble in water with a melting point of 116°C.

Table 1   Composition of Betoptic S

Ingredient	Concentration
Betaxolol hydrochloride	0.28%[a]
Mannitol	[b]
Disodium edetate	0.01%
Carbomer 934P	[b]
Amberlite[c]	[b]
Benzalkonium chloride	0.01%
Purified water	100.0%

[a]Equivalent to 0.25 % betaxolol base.
[b]Proprietary data.
[c]The cationic exchange polymer is present in the formulation in sufficient quantity to bind 85% or more of the betaxolol present.

Betaxolol base is sparingly soluble in water with a melting point between 70°C –and 72°C. Figure 2 presents the chemical structure of betaxolol HCl.

Chemically, Amberlite resin is a styrene-vinyl copolymer. It is a sulfonic acid exchanger that has a negatively charged (SO_3^-) group that exists on the outer surface of the polymer to which the positively charged betaxolol molecule binds. The resin is the acid form of sodium polystyrene sulfonate, USP. The structure of the functional group is shown in Figure 3.

Manufacture of betaxolol ionic suspension involves dissolution of betaxolol and mannitol in purified water. Milled, acidified sodium polystyrene sulfonate resin is then dispersed into the betaxolol/mannitol solution. The carbomer-suspending agent is dispersed in purified water and added (19). In this ultrafine ophthalmic quality suspension, the ion exchange polymer is milled to a mean diameter, similar in size to steroid particles found in ophthalmic preparations. The particle size of the resin is readily controlled. Controlling and monitoring particle size of the resin employed in betaxolol ionic suspension has allowed for the successful production of this product since 1990 in the United States. The manufacturer has established a stringent specification limit for betaxolol suspension of not less than 99.50% of particles $< 25\,\mu m$; not less than 99.95% of particles $< 50\,\mu m$; and not less than 100% of particles $< 90\,\mu m$.

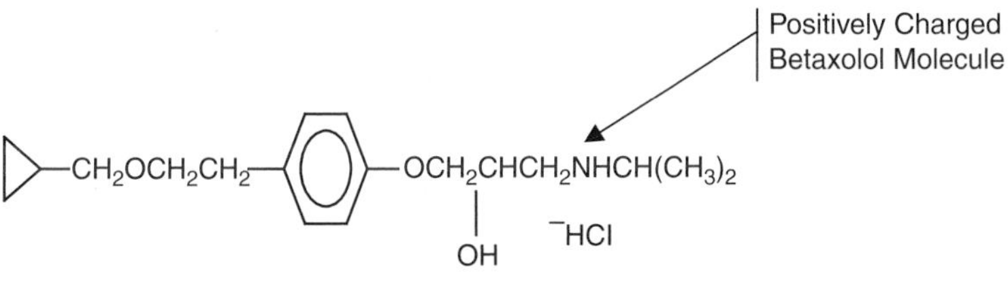

Figure 2   Betaxolol HCl.

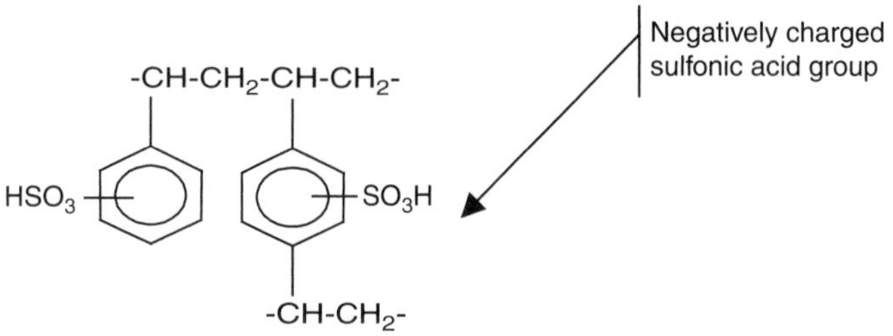

Figure 3   Amberlite resin [poly(styrenedivinylbenzene)sulfonic acid].

Since the formulation contains a carbomer, sodium hydroxide is required to adjust to pH. The pH is targeted to be 7.0 to achieve acceptable bound betaxolol values. This pH value does not alter the comfort of the formulation.

Osmolality of the formulation is a fundamental consideration, which directly relates to ocular comfort. Sodium chloride and other ionic salts, which are frequently employed in formulations to adjust their osmolality, cannot be used in the betaxolol formulation since they would interfere with the betaxolol–resin binding. The non-ionic compound mannitol was selected to render the formulation iso-osmotic since it is very soluble and has no effect on the binding of betaxolol to Amberlite resin (20). The optimum ratio of betaxolol to resin (1:1) remains stable in the finished product.

In this ion exchange delivery system, positively charged betaxolol exists bound to the negatively charged sulfonic acid groups of the Amberlite resin. The extent of betaxolol binding to the resin in the formulation is directly proportional to the resin concentration. The cationic exchange resin of sulfonic acid polymers forms an ion exchange matrix suspended in a structural vehicle containing carbomer polymer. Since betaxolol HCl and the polymer are present in betaxolol ionic suspension in approximately equimolar ratios, conditions in the suspension allow about 85% of the betaxolol to be bound to the cation exchange polymer beads as shown in Figure 4.

Carbopol 934P is added to the formulation to increase its viscosity and therefore increase the residence time of the product in the eye. Carbopol polymer, when hydrated, provides a network of polymer chains forming a structured vehicle in which particles stay suspended for a longer period (21). These attributes are demonstrated by betaxolol ionic suspension's ability to provide uniform dosing of drug for up to four weeks without resuspending the product.

The physical properties of betaxolol ionic suspension distinguish it from other ophthalmic suspensions. Unique among these is the long period of time over which betaxolol ionic suspension remains suspended. To demonstrate this characteristic, eight bottles of betaxolol ionic suspension

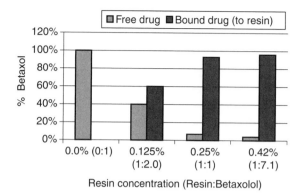

Figure 4 Betaxolol binding to resin.

were resuspended at room temperature at time 0 (Fig. 5) and the betaxolol content was analyzed by high performance liquid chromatography (HPLC) in duplicate samples. The remaining samples were left undisturbed. At weekly intervals, samples from two bottles were dispensed without shaking or resuspension and the betaxolol assayed again by HPLC. As is apparent from Figure 5 the amount of betaxolol, expressed as a percent of label, is constant over the 4-week period. This demonstrated that betaxolol ionic suspension, once suspended, remained suspended over the duration of the study period. A further important characteristic of the suspension technology of betaxolol ionic suspension is that its excellent resuspendibility makes neither vigorous shaking nor shaking for long periods necessary. A few shakes with the wrist are adequate to resuspend betaxolol ionic suspension.

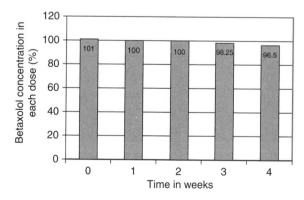

Figure 5 Betaxolol suspension settling time.

Patient Comfort

In the eye, as shown in Figure 6, betaxolol is readily released from the polymer, via exchange with positively charged ions like sodium, potassium, and calcium, which are natural constituents of tears. The net effect of placing one or two drops of betaxolol ionic suspension in the eye is that, as Na^+ is exchanged for betaxolol on the polymer, the beta blocker is released relatively slowly into the lacrimal film. The kinetics of betaxolol release governs the neuronal responses in the eye (particularly those in the cornea) to the molecule. Since betaxolol is released into the lacrimal film more slowly from betaxolol ionic suspension than from betaxolol solution, patient comfort is enhanced.

Time-release profiles for two formulations of betaxolol 0.5% in two ophthalmic dosage forms, solution and suspension, were studied using a controlled release analytical system (CRAS). CRAS is an in vitro technique for measuring time release profiles of ophthalmic dosage forms under conditions closely simulating those prevailing in the precorneal tear fluid (22). The study found that the briefest profile resulted from simple solution. This resulted in rapid dumping, which represented the behavior expected for betaxolol 0.5% solution. Time release for this preparation was essentially complete in 30 minutes. The use of an ion exchange resin in a simple 1:1 drug to resin ratio sustained drug release over a 2-hour period and reduced the maximum drug concentration in the eluent (representing the precorneal tear fluid) to 30% compared to that of the solution.

These data suggested that sustained release formulations should reduce side effects, because the suspension will be retained within the cul-de-sac and drug released from the delivery system continuously (Fig. 7).

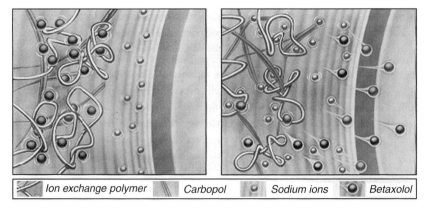

| Ion exchange polymer | Carbopol | Sodium ions | Betaxolol |

Figure 6 Mechanism of action of Betoptic Suspension eye drop.

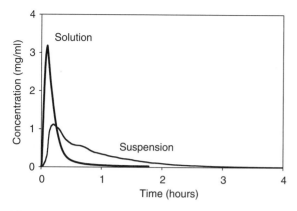

Figure 7 Comparison of time-release profiles from two preparations of betaxolol 0.5%.

Glaucoma is a progressive disease, which puts the patient's visual prognosis at risk. In order to halt the progression of this neuropathological process, treatment should be taken for life. The prolonged daily application of eye-drops demands a high degree of patient compliance. The low potential for adverse events helps to maintain patient compliance. The degree of comfort of any treatment strongly influences patient compliance. To evaluate the degree of patient compliance, the tolerability of betaxolol suspension was studied in a number of clinical trials. In a 3-month double-masked, parallel group clinical study, both betaxolol ionic suspension, 0.25% and betaxolol solution, 0.5% were equally effective in reducing intraocular pressure (23). An equally important conclusion that was drawn from this study was that statistically significantly fewer patients experienced stinging and burning during instillation of betaxolol ionic suspension as shown in Figure 8. The greater ocular comfort of betaxolol ionic suspension

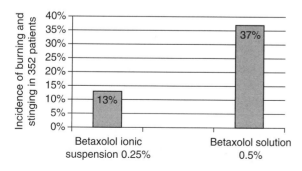

Figure 8 Comfort of Betoptic Suspension as compared to Betoptic Solution.

was attributed to the lower drug concentration and because it was delivered slowly instead of in one bolus.

Finally, in a long-term study, data on the comfort of betaxolol ionic suspension showed that few patients reported stinging or burning on administration of the drops. These numbers were lower than those reported in the 3-month controlled studies. The results indicated that the suspension did not become less comfortable with time (24).

Reduction of Systemic Side Effects

In order to conserve the physiologic integrity of the body, local therapy for glaucoma treatment should not be absorbed into the systemic circulation and should completely be devoid of systemic side effects.

Glaucoma patients frequently present with hepatic and renal changes. This physiologic deterioration affects the tolerability of a drug due to pharmacokinetic changes (including absorption, distribution, metabolism, and drug elimination). To obtain optimal tolerability in these individuals, the ion exchange technology when combined with the beta 1 selectivity of betaxolol resulted in a locally administered betaxolol that exhibited superior systemic tolerability to that of nonselective antiglaucomatous beta-blockers.

Dose Reduction

The ion exchange delivery vehicle that was developed allowed a two-fold reduction in the concentration of topically administered betaxolol without an effect on the drug effectiveness. A study in animals demonstrated the ocular bioequivalence of betaxolol from Betoptic® S and Betoptic® Solution. The same study also showed the superior bioavailability of beta-blocker from betaxolol ionic suspension, compared to that of the 0.5% Betoptic® Solution (Fig. 9).

Comparison with Conventional Ophthalmic Drops

As already discussed, the long period of time over which betaxolol ionic suspension remains suspended, and the ease of resuspendibility of the betaxolol ionic suspension favorably differentiate it from other ophthalmic suspensions.

Betaxolol ionic suspension also differs from conventional suspension products, such as corticosteroid eye drops, in that the delivery system was specifically designed to optimize bioavailability and patient comfort. The suspended exchange resin binds with betaxolol in the formulation and upon instillation, gradually releases it to the eye, thus minimizing ocular discomfort associated with free betaxolol ions.

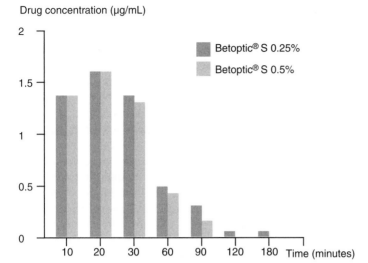

Drug concentration (µg/mL)

Figure 9   Betaxolol concentration in aqueous solutions.

Regulatory Considerations

The original betaxolol ionic suspension was tested in accordance with the USP preservative efficacy test (PET). However, to improve the preservative efficacy of the product beyond its ability to meet USP PET standards, an alternative formulation was developed to meet the more strenuous *European Pharmacopoeia* (EP) PET standards. The new formulation included boric acid and N-lauroylsarcosine.

In addition to the new EP PET standards, a new EP Carbomer Monograph was adopted in 1999. To comply with the EP requirements eliminating benzene in carbomers, Carbopol 974P was substituted for Carbopol 934P. PET testing of betaxolol ionic suspension with boric acid and N-lauroylsarcosine as preservative aids, and Carbopol 974P have shown that the changes in the formulation created a more robust preservative system.

In-Use Experience

Since the introduction of betaxolol solution in 1985, ophthalmologists have used betaxolol for the systemic safety advantages it offers. Although betaxolol ionic suspension was more easily tolerated than betaxolol solution, many ophthalmologists continued to prefer timolol maleate due to its efficacy advantages.

RECENT DEVELOPMENTS

Researchers discovered that by changing the betaxolol molecule, they could make it more effective at lowering intraocular pressure. The result was levobetaxolol 0.5% (BETAXON™). Levobetaxolol is an enantiomer of betaxolol. Animal work has indicated that the "levo" form of betaxolol—the S isomer—possesses greater activity than the dextro form. Betaxolol ionic suspension is composed of both the levo and dextro forms of betaxolol. These have been separated to formulate levobetaxolol ionic suspension, which contains only the levo form.

Since betaxolol and other beta-adrenergic antagonists have been shown to reduce intraocular pressure by a reduction of aqueous production, it is assumed that the mechanism of action of levobetaxolol ionic suspension is similar. Topical administration of levobetaxolol ionic suspension results in systemic exposure to levobetaxolol that is significantly less than that observed with topical dosing with betaxolol 0.5% solution. This suggests a reduced risk of adverse cardiovascular or respiratory events with levobetaxolol ionic suspension. It is thought that the low systemic exposure to levobetaxolol is due to the ion resin exchange suspension that releases the active drug slowly.

CONCLUSIONS

The ion exchange resin technology has been successfully combined with betaxolol and levobetaxolol to optimize the safety and efficacy of topically administered beta-blockers. For the drug betaxolol this drug delivery technology has resulted in a two-fold increase in bioavailability without an associated increase in systemic absorption. In addition the ion exchange resin technology has provided the first viable alternative to eye drops by providing the controlled release of a high performance therapeutic agent that is well tolerated by patients.

ACKNOWLEDGMENTS

We would like to thank our colleagues in the Pharmaceutics, Analytical Chemistry, ADME, Clinical Science, Microbiology and Toxicology Departments of Alcon Research Ltd.

REFERENCES

1. Kaufman HE, Gasset AR. Therapeutic soft bandage lenses. Int Ophthalmol Clin 1970; 10:379–85.
2. Waltman SR, Kaufman HE. Use of hydrophilic conact lenses to increase ocular penetration of topical drugs. Invest Ophthalmol 1970; 9:250–5.

3. Kaufman HE, Uotila MH, Gasset AR. The medical uses of soft contact lenses. Trans Amer Acad Ophthalmol Otolaryngol 1971; 75:361–73.

4. Aquavella JW, Jackson GK, Guy LF. Therapeutic effects of bionite lenses: mechanisms of action. Ann Ophthalmol 1971; 3:1341–5.

5. Maddox YT, Bernstein HN. An evaluation of bionite hydrophilic contact lens for use in a drug delivery system. Ann Ophthalmol 1972; 4:789–90.

6. Podos SM, Becker B, Asseff CF, Harlstein J. Pilocarpine therapy with soft contact lenses. Amer J Ophthalmol 1972; 73:336–41.

7. Assef CF, Weisman RL, Podos SM. Ocular penetration of pilocarpine in Primates. Amer J Ophthalmol 1973; 75:212–5.

8. Leaders FE, Hecht G, VanHoose M, Kellog M. New polymers in drug delivery. Ann Ophthalmol 1973; 5:513–6.

9. Mandell AI, Stewart RM, Kass MA. Multiclinic evaluation of a pilocarpine gel. Invest Ophthalmol Vis Sci 1979; Abstract, Suppl. April.

10. Ticho U, Blumenthal M, Zonis S, Gal A, Blank I, Mazor ZW. A clinical trial with piloplex; a new long-acting pilocarpine compound: preliminary report. Ann Ophthalmol 1979; 11:555–61.

11. Mazor A, Ticho U, Rehany U, Rose L. Piloplex, a new long acting pilocarpine polymer salt. B: comparative study of the visual effects of pilocarpine and piloplex eye drops. Br J Ophthalmol 1979; 63:48–51.

12. Ticho U, Blumenthal M, Zonis S, Gal A, Blank I, Mazor ZW. Piloplex, a new long acting pilocarpine polymer salt. A long term study. Br J Ophthalmol 1979; 63:45–7.

13. Shell JW, Baker RW. Diffusional systems for controlled release of drugs to the eye. Ann Ophthalmol 1974; 6:1037–43.

14. Lerman S, Davis P, Jackson WB. Prolonged release hydrocortisone therapy. Can J Ophthalmol 1973; 8:114–8.

15. Dohlman CH, Pavan-Langston D, Rose J. A new ocular insert device for continuous constant-rate delivery of medication to the eye. Ann Ophthalmol 1972; 4:823–32.

16. Keating JW. Pharmaceutical preparations comprising cation exchange resin absorption compounds and treatment therewith. US patent 2,990,332; 1971.

17. Burke GM, Mendes RW, Jambhekar SS. Investigation of the applicability of ion exchange resins as a sustained release drug delivery system for propranolol hydrochloride. Drug Dev Ind Pharm 1986; 12:713–21.

18. Jani R, Harris R. Sustained release, comfort formulations for glaucoma therapy. US patent 4,911,920; 1990.

19. Jani R, Gan O, Ali Y, et al. Ion Exchange Resins for Ophthalmic Delivery. J Ocular Pharm 1994; 10(1):57–67.

20. Jani R, Gan O, Ali Y, et al. Ion Exchange Resins for Ophthalmic Delivery. J Ocular Pharm 1994; 10(1):57–67.

21. BF Goodrich carbopol polymers product literature.

22. Stevens LE, Missel PJ, Lang JC. Drug release profiles of ophthalmic formulations 1. Instrumentation. Anal Chem 1992; 64:715–23.

23. Weinreb RN, Caldwell DR, Goode SM, et al. A double-masked three-month comparison between 0.25% betaxolol suspension and 0.5% betaxolol ophthalmic solution. Amer J Ophthalmol 1990; 110:189–92.

24. Yarangümeli A, Küral G. Are there any benefits of Betoptic® S (betaxolol Hcl ophthalmic suspension) over other β-blockers in the treatment of glaucoma? Expert Opin Pharmacother 2004; 5(5):1071–81.

Part III: Injection and Implant Technologies

9

Injections and Implants

Majella E. Lane
School of Pharmacy, University of London, London, U.K.

Franklin W. Okumu and Palani Balausubramanian
DURECT Corporation, Cupertino, California, U.S.A.

INTRODUCTION

When considering new options for drug (small molecule, peptide, protein, etc.) delivery, the most direct approach is usually parenteral administration. Because many in vivo preclinical research studies and early clinical trials are performed by direct injection such as intraveneous or subcutaneous administration, the development of injectable dosage forms is more likely to succeed commercially than alternative routes of delivery (oral, topical, pulmonary), assuming that the injectable dosage forms provide the desired pharmacokinetics, efficacy, and safety. Injectable modified release systems are of particular importance due to their ability to alter the pharmacokinetics of the drug. This ability to control the systemic or local residence of a given protein may alter significantly the efficacy or safety of the compound. In the case where the active compound has a short half-life in vivo, a modified release system can extend exposure after a single administration (Table 1). This extended exposure could reduce significantly the number of doses a patient may be required to receive to control their condition. An added benefit of these types of systems is the ability to administer high doses per injection with a fairly low maximum serum concentration (C_{max}). This avoids any undesired side effects or toxicity that may be associated with high C_{max} values observed after direct injection of the drug

Table 1 Injectable and Implantable Modified-Release Systems

Class	Technology	Active agents delivered	Duration (wk)	Ref.
Implant	Osmotic pump, collagen, PLGA	Leuprolide, Ω-INF, rhBMP, rhNGF	12–52	(1–5)
Injectable implant	PLGA, collagen	Leuprolide, GHRP-1, TNF-R, calcium phosphate	1–24	(6–11)
Microsphere	PLGA, POE, PEG-lactide, collagen	Leuprolide, rhGH, GHRP-1, rhNGF, rhVEGF, pegaptanib, risperidone	1–12	(3,12–16)
Nanosphere (liposomes, nanocrystals)	PEG-PLGA, lipids, PLGA, Poly-AA	Lactoferrin insulin, INF-alfa-2b, rhGH, IL-2, doxorubicin, amphotericin B	0.5–1	(17–22)
Injectable gels	PLA, PLGA, PEG-PLGA, SAIB	Leuprolide, rhGH, rhVEGF, BMP-2 deslorelin, bupivacaine	1–24	(23–30)

Abbreviations: PLGA, poly(lactide-co-glycolic acid); POE, poly(ortho ester); PEG, poly(ethylene glycol); PEG-PLGA, poly(ethylene glycol–poly(lactide-co-glycolic acid); PLA, poly(lactic acid); SAIB, sucrose acetate isobutyrate.

compound alone. The focus of this section is modified release systems that are injected or surgically placed in the body where they then deliver the loaded drug. The systems broadly represent four classes of modified release systems: implants, microspheres, injectable gels, and nanospheres (liposomes, nanocrystals). The section covers recent developments in the area of injectable or implantable sustained/controlled release systems including several biodegradable matrices suitable for modified delivery of drugs. In light of the ever-increasing number of products in clinical development which employ polymer conjugation to prolong circulation time in the body a chapter is also included on modification of drug release by chemical modification.

DELIVERY SYSTEMS

Implants

Implants require the use of large gauge needles or surgical procedures for administration. A brief surgical implantation procedure, performed by a trained medical doctor, is required for insertion of most implants and thus the interval between implantation should be sufficiently lengthy (>3 months) to avoid the need for frequent invasive procedures. Because implants contain a fixed dose of drug in a fixed volume (implant size) they are not appropriate for the treatment of diseases requiring drug dosing based on weight (mg/kg) or body surface area (mg/m^2) with the possible exception of a patient population that has a narrow weight or body surface area distribution. The principal advantage associated with implantable devices is that they may operate for long periods of time once implanted and provide a more controlled release than injectable systems. For this reason implants are generally considered when the therapeutic window is sufficient to allow fixed doses, which will yield varying serum levels of the drug depending upon the patient weight, and where chronic administration of the drug is required. The functional lifetime of each implant is controlled by the amount of drug contained in the reservoir (volume < 2.0 ml) and the delivery rate controlled by the implant. The amount of drug implants can deliver is also limited by their size and generally is limited to less than 1.0 g of active drug. The osmotic pump, DUROS® (Durect, Alza), has been approved for treatment of prostate cancer (leuprolide acetate) and is being developed for the management of Hepatitis C Viral infections (4,5) and is reviewed in detail in a separate chapter in this section. For this system a continuous drug dose is delivered over a 3–12 month period providing patient convenience and compliance. This type of implant may be easily removed to stop drug exposure if required.

In contrast to implants that require surgical manipulation, biodegradable implants offer the advantage of a single procedure with no removal of the implant. Several biodegradable implants are either on the market or under development. A good example of this type of system is Zoladex® (AstraZeneca), a poly(lactide-co-glycolic acid) (PLGA) goserelin acetate implant, which is injected into subcutaneous tissue with a 16-gauge needle where it releases goserelin for a period of 28 to 60 days. The choice of matrix used for these biodegradable systems depends on a number of factors, physiochemical properties of the entrapped drug, desired duration of release (<1 day to >3 months), acute (wound healing) or chronic (growth factors, hormones) administration and regulatory status. The U.S. Food and Drug Administration will generally allow clinical investigation of delivery systems based on matrix platforms that have been extensively used for biomedical and pharmaceutical applications (e.g., PLGA, PLA, Collagen, etc.). New materials or materials in use in the food industry can also be used as delivery matrices after sufficient preclinical safety and toxicology studies have been conducted to demonstrate the materials are non-antigenic, non-teratogenic and completely biodegradable. Pilot safety studies of the biodegradable matrix must routinely be performed prior to development of any injectable matrix for parenteral delivery. The injection site reaction to these matrices also requires extensive examination to ensure that they are compatible with the intended injection site.

Microspheres and Injectable Gels

Microspheres and injectable gels offer several advantages, in that they are easy to administer and in many cases can be administered by the patients themselves. As these systems are completely biodegradable, no surgical removal is required. These injectable systems can offer a broad range of delivery profiles ranging from very short (<5 days) to rather long (>3 months) period depending on the desired exposure to the entrapped drug. As these dosage forms are not removed a biodegradable matrix is required such as PLGA (3,12–14). The matrix is fabricated into an easily injectable (small needle size; 20–30 G) form for administration at the desired tissue site (e.g., subcutaneously). The dosage form itself may either be a solid, gel, or liquid. Injectable gels usually consist of a solvent to dissolve the matrix and/or the therapeutic agent and they form an "implant-like" depot upon injection. The amount of drug microspheres can deliver varies depending on the drug loading and the injection volume. Generally these systems are able to deliver up to 0.03 g per injection (1.5 mL total injection volume). Injectable gels are able to deliver higher doses (>0.2 g) due to higher concentrations of drug in the final injection solution.

Both microspheres and injectable gels generally reduce the bioavailability of the entrapped drug when compared to injection of the un-encapsulated drug. This reduction in bioavailability can be attributed to chemical degradation of unreleased drug within the injected matrix or local metabolism of the drug augmented by the presence of the degrading matrix components. Biodegradable microspheres consisting of PLGA have been used as an injectable depot delivery system for small molecule drugs, peptides and proteins (12–14). Examples of injectable gel or in situ forming depot systems include the Alzamer technology, the Atrigel system, the ReGel depot, the PLAD system and the SABRE platform which are reviewed in separate chapters in this book.

Biodegradable Nanoparticles and Liposomes

Biodegradable nanoparticles and liposomes can be administered directly to the blood stream by intravenous infusion (31,32). This class of system may be administered by injection with a conventional needle and syringe. These systems modify the release of entrapped drug as they circulate through the body or accumulate at a specific targeted site of action (e.g., tumor, organ, blood, etc.). This accumulation can be exploited if delivery to specific regions of the body (e.g., solid tumor) that are not accessible or not possible to inject into, but local, high drug levels are desired. Unlike localized injectable systems additional safety studies must be conducted with nanosphere systems to ensure the entrapped drug and delivery matrix are compatible with organ systems where accumulation may occur (lung, liver, lymphatic system, etc.).

Nanospheres and liposomal system offer several advantages over conventional therapy of the same drug because they are able to increase the delivery of drug to the desired location (e.g., tumor, organ, blood, etc.). This increase in concentration at the desired site can lead to increased efficacy and possibly reduced toxicity with lower doses. For example, the accumulation of liposome containing doxorubicin occurs in solid tumors providing a high local drug concentration and minimizing systemic exposure as detailed in a separate chapter in this section on pegylated liposomal technology. The circulation time of nanoparticles will be dependent upon their recognition by the body and their size; particles that have a surface that binds serum proteins (opsinisation) and/or are larger than 100 nm are cleared rapidly through phagocytic pathways. Liposomes containing poly (ethylene glycol) lipids are protected from serum protein binding and phagocytic recognition yielding a longer circulating half-life than conventional liposomes as outlined in more detail elsewhere in this section. The total dose administered is usually limited by the maximum tolerated dose of the entrapped drug. The application of liposomes in parenteral drug delivery with reference to SkyePharma's Depofoam technology is also detailed in a separate chapter. A new particulate long acting rhGH formulation based on polyelectrolye coated crystals is being developed by Altus Inc (33). This system takes advantage of the slower dissolution kinetics of the crystalline protein after subcutaneous injection, a concept that has been used for many years with long acting insulin formulations (34).

MANUFACTURING AND STERILIZATION

Manufacturing drug containing non-biodegradable and biodegradable implants can be challenging and if the drug is a protein this is further complicated by the sensitivity of most proteins to heat and terminal sterilization processes. In general, even if a protein is physically stable to the heat generated during processing or terminal sterilization a loss in activity will be observed due to irreversible chemical modification (35). This intrinsic property necessitates aseptic processing of protein containing implants or validation of alternative sterilization methods (36). Most non-biodegradable implants are filled and sealed by proprietary manufacturing processes that allow for precise control of fill volume and ensure container closure for the drug compartment. Commercial manufacturing of non-biodegradable implants can often be rather complex and costly and should be taken into consideration when a delivery system is selected for clinical investigation. More standardized methods are available for production of biodegradable implants however in most cases the protein or peptide will need to be dehydrated prior to incorporation into the dry polymer blend. This is typically accomplished by dehydrating the protein (air, freeze, or spray drying) in the presence of various stabilizers (37,38). The polymer protein blend is then processed (heat, super critical fluid, or pressure) to yield an implantable device with the desired shape and mechanical characteristics (39,40).

Commercial manufacturing of microparticulate delivery systems can often be rather complex and costly and should be taken into consideration when a delivery system is selected for clinical investigation. Injectable gels are simpler to manufacture and could offer significant cost advantages over other delivery technologies (10,23). The manufacturing process used to produce nanosparticles and liposomes can also be complex and costly due to multiple processing steps and low encapsulation yields. The physical stability of these systems can also be a concern if they are stored as suspensions. For this reason nanoparticle and liposome systems are frequently stored dehydrated and reconstituted at the point of use.

ADMINISTRATION AND DRUG RELEASE

The administration route of implantable or injectable drug delivery systems represents a significant hurdle to market penetration. In general most care providers and patients prefer quick, pain free administration of any parenteral medication. However as noted already, the benefit of a long acting system can outweigh these concerns and lead to acceptance of implants that require surgical implantation after application of a local anesthetic. The goal for most long acting drug formulations is to increase care provider and patient compliance within the prescribed treatment protocol. This is best accomplished if the long acting system can be administered with the same equipment currently in use for administration of short acting formulations. In general fine needles along with low injection volumes are preferred by care providers and patients. Several proprietary kits have been developed to facilitate preparation and administration of long acting drug delivery systems (41–43). Finally since conventional needles and syringes are designed for delivery of Newtonian, non-particulate systems a chapter on novel injection technology (DepotOne) with the potential to delivery higher doses of microparticulate formulations than has previously been achieved completes this section.

CONCLUSION

Formulation scientists have an array of options for modified release drug delivery of therapeutic agents. Appropriate selection of a modified release dosage form will be dependent on the physicochemical properties of the drug, the drug pharmacology and pharmacokinetics, and the disease indications. Modified release delivery systems are generally developed after the bolus injection form (not controlled release) of the drug has been assessed in clinical trials. The increasing number of potent therapeutics such as growth factors and kinase inhibitors will stimulate further research and may require modified release formulation development prior to clinical trial evaluation. The major advantages of such modified release systems are the reduced dose frequency and improved safety profile.

REFERENCES

1. Higaki M, et al. Collagen minipellet as a controlled release delivery system for tetanus and diphtheria toxoid. Vaccine 2001; 19(23–24): 3091–6.
2. Itoh S, et al. The biocompatibility and osteoconductive activity of a novel hydroxyapatite/collagen composite biomaterial, and its function as a carrier of rhBMP-2. J Biomed Mater Res 2001; 54(3):445–53.
3. Saltzman WM, et al. Intracranial delivery of recombinant nerve growth factor: release kinetics and protein distribution for three delivery systems. Pharm Res 1999; 16(2):232–40.
4. Marks LS. Luteinizing hormone-releasing hormone agonists in the treatment of men with prostate cancer: timing, alternatives, and the 1-year implant. Urology 2003; 62(6Suppl. 1):36–42.
5. Gorbakov V. Interim results from a Phase 2 study of Omega Interferon in HCV. In: Proceedings of the 56th Annual meeting of the American Association for the Study of Liver Diseases, San Francisco, CA, 2005.
6. Eliaz RE, Wallach D, Kost J, Delivery of soluble tumor necrosis factor receptor from in-situ forming PLGA implants: in-vivo. Pharm Res 2000; 22(6):563–70.
7. Lee CH, Singla A, Lee Y. Biomedical applications of collagen. Int J Pharm 2001; 221(1–2):1–22.
8. Looss P, et al. A new injectable bone substitute combining poly(-caprolactone) microparticles with biphasic calcium phosphate granules. Biomaterials 2001; 22 (20):2785–94.
9. Ravivarapu HB, Moyer KL, Dunn RL. Parameters affecting the efficacy of a sustained release polymeric implant of leuprolide. Int J Pharm 2000; 194(2): 181–91.
10. Ravivarapu HB, Moyer KL, Dunn RL Sustained activity and release of leuprolide acetate from an in situ forming polymeric implant. AAPS Pharm Sci Tech 2000; 1(1):E1.
11. Ravivarapu HB, Moyer KL, Dunn RL. Sustained suppression of pituitary-gonadal axis with an injectable, in situ forming implant of leuprolide acetate. J Pharm Sci 2000; 89(6):732–41.
12. Cleland JL, et al. Recombinant human growth hormone poly(lactic-co-glycolic acid) microsphere formulation development. Adv Drug Delivery Rev 1997; 28(1):71–84.
13. Yang TH, et al. Effect of zinc binding and precipitation on structures of recombinant human growth hormone and nerve growth factor. J Pharmaceut Sci 2000; 89(11):1480–5.

14. Cleland JL, et al. Development of poly-(d,l-lactideco-glycolide) microsphere formulations containing recombinant human vascular endothelial growth factor to promote local angiogenesis. J Controlled Release 2001; 72(1–3):13–24.

15. Ng EWM, et al. Pegaptanib, a targeted anti-VEGF aptamer for ocular vascular disease. Nature Rev Drug Discovery 2006; 5:123–32.

16. Janssen, Risperdal Consta prescribing information.

17. Trif M, et al. Liposomes as possible carriers for lactoferrin in the local treatment of inflammatory diseases. Exp Biol Med 2001; 226(6): 559–64.

18. Park JW, et al. Tumor targeting using anti-her2 immunoliposomes. J Controlled Release 2001; 74(1–3):95–113.

19. Trepo C. Novel sustained release formulation of INF-alfa-2b-XL, improves tolerability and demonstrates potent viral load reduction in a phase I/IIHCV clinical trial. In Proceedings of the International Symposium on Viral Hepatitis and Liver Disease. Lyon, France, 2005.

20. Oudard S, et al. Novel sustained release formulation of IL-2 improves pharmacokinetics performance and demonstrates potent activation of immunological cell line. In Proceedings of the American Society of Clinical Oncology. Atlanta, GA, 2006.

21. Gabizon AA. Selective tumor localization and improved theraputic index of anthracyclines encapsulated in long-circulating liposomes. Cancer Res 1992; 52:891–6.

22. Richardson M. AmBisome today: Expanding the prospectives on liposomal amphotericin B. ACTA Biomed 2006(2): 3, 4.

23. Okumu FW, et al. Sustained delivery of human growth hormone from a novel gel system: SABER Biomaterials 2002; 23(22):4353–8.

24. Brodbeck KJ, DesNoyer JR, McHugh AJ. Phase inversion dynamics of PLGA solutions related to drug delivery—Part II. The role of solution thermodynamics and bath-side mass transfer. J Controlled Release 1999; 62(3):333–44.

25. Brodbeck KJ, Pushpala S, McHugh AJ. Sustained release of human growth hormone from PLGA solution depots. Pharmaceut Res 1999; 16(12):1825–9.

26. Gutowska A, Jeong B, Jasionowski M. Injectable gels for tissue engineering. Anatom Record 2001; 263(4):342–9.

27. Zentner GM, et al. Biodegradable block copolymers for delivery of proteins and water-insoluble drugs. J Controlled Release 2001; 72:203–15.

28. Kraeling RR, et al. Luteinizing hormone response to controlled-release deslorelin in estradiol benzoate primed ovariectomized gilts. Theriogenology 2000; 40(8):1681–9.

29. Keskin DS, et al. Collagen-chondroitin sulfate-based PLLA-SAIB-coated rhBMP-2 delivery system for bone repair. Biomaterials 2005; 26(18):4023–34.

30. Halladay S. et al. Pharmacokinetic evaluation of subcutaneously administered SABER-bupivacaine (Posidur) following open inguinal hernia repair. In Proceedings of the 33rd Annual Meeting and Exposition of the Controlled Release Society. Vienna, Austria, 2006.

31. Cheng J, et al. Formulation of functionalized PLGA-PEG nanoparticles for in vivo targeted drug delivery. Biomaterials 2007; 28(5):869–76.

32. Swenson S, et al. Intravenous liposomal delivery of the snake venom disintegrin contortrostatin limits breast cancer progression. Mol Cancer Ther 2004; 3(4): 499–511.

33. Govardhan C, et al. Novel long-acting crystal formulation of human growth hormone. Pharm Res 2005; 22(9):1461–70.
34. Basu SK, et al. Protein crystals for the delivery of biopharmaceuticals. Expert Opin Biol Ther 2004; 4(3):301–17.
35. Yaman A. Alternative methods of terminal sterilization for biologically active macromolecules. Curr Opin Drug Discov Dev 2001; 4(6):760–3.
36. White A, Burns D, Christensen TW. Effective terminal sterilization using supercritical carbon dioxide. J Biotechnol 2006; 123(4):504–15.
37. Engstrom JD, et al. Stable high surface area lactate dehydrogenase particles produced by spray freezing into liquid nitrogen. Eur J Pharm Biopharm 2006; 65(2):163–74.
38. Engstrom JD, et al. Morphology of protein particles produced by spray freezing of concentrated solutions. Eur J Pharm Biopharm 2006; 65(2):149–62.
39. Rothen-Weinhold A, et al. Stability studies of a somatostatin analogue in biodegradable implants. Int J Pharm 1999; 178(2):213–21.
40. Rothen-Weinhold A, et al. Injection-molding versus extrusion as manufacturing technique for the preparation of biodegradable implants. Eur J Pharm Biopharm 1999; 48(2):113–21.
41. Bayer, Viadur Leuprolide Acetate Implant prescribing information.
42. Polson AM, et al. Apparatus for forming a biodegradable implant precursor. In: www.uspto.gov. Atrix Laboratories, Inc., USA, 1997.
43. AstraZenica, Zoladex Goserelin Acetate Implant prescribing information.

10

Long-Acting Protein Formulation—PLAD Technology

Franklin W. Okumu

DURECT Corporation, Cupertino, California, U.S.A.

INTRODUCTION

Many polymer based in situ forming implants are currently under development (1,2). The majority of these systems are based on combinations of polymers with hydrophobic or hydrophilic solvents. These solvents either stay associated with or leave the system after injection depending on the aqueous solubility of the solvent. Polylactic acid (PLA) Depot (PLAD) is a novel biodegradable sustained release system based on the combination of PLA with both hydrophilic and hydrophobic solvents. A unique characteristic of the system is its ability to solvate protein powders resulting in a low-viscosity solution that upon injection forms a soft depot that slowly releases the dissolved protein. The presence of hydrophilic solvents facilitates protein dissolution while the hydrophobic solvent solvate the non-water soluble PLA. The main advantages of the PLAD system are ease of preparation and the ability to administer high drug doses in a volume less than 1 mL.

DESCRIPTION OF THE TECHNOLOGY AND MANUFACTURING PROCESS

The PLAD manufacturing process is summarized in Figure 1. The first two steps involve preparation of the PLAD solution as a diluent and formation

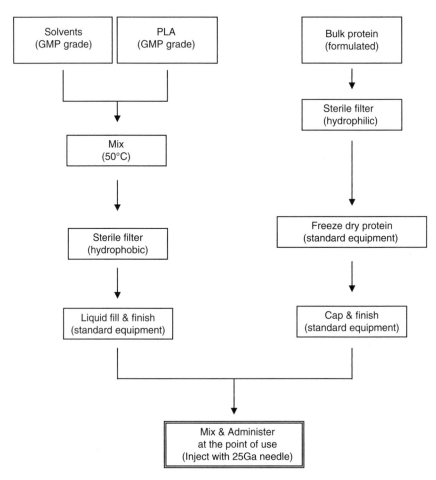

Figure 1 PLAD manufacturing process. *Abbreviation*: PLAD, polylactic acid depot.

of the protein powder that will be mixed with the PLAD solution at the time of use. Both of these processes are standardized and frequently used to aseptically produce marketed pharmaceutical products.

RESEARCH AND DEVELOPMENT—CASE STUDIES

Human Growth Hormone

Human growth hormone (hGH) is a 191-amino acid, single chain endogenous protein hormone that is synthesized, stored, and secreted by the pituitary gland. When secreted hGH stimulates growth and cell reproduction in humans (3). Recombinant hGH (rhGH) has been used since 1985 for hormone replacement therapy in children with growth hormone deficiency that leads to growth failure (4). Several formulations are currently available, yet all require daily injections to maintain growth velocity in growth hormone deficient (GHD) children. The only commercial long acting formulation (Nutropin Depot®) was taken off the market due to high manufacturing costs associated with the production of the microsphere formulation (5). Several improved long-acting formulations are currently under development for treatment of GHD in adults and children (6–8). The objective of this study was to examine the feasibility of using PLAD for sustained delivery of rhGH. The following factors were examined: protein formulation, in vitro initial release, and in vivo pharmacokinetics (PK).

In Vitro Results

Powders produced by spray drying zinc complexed rhGH maintained high monomeric content and produced clear solutions when dissolved in release buffer (Table 1). Formulations A and B contained 60% and 50% rhGH by weight, respectively, the decrease in protein content observed with formulation B is likely due to increased sucrose:protein ratio. Less than 5% of the total dissolved rhGH was released from both formulations in 24 hours (Table 2). Higher protein loading (100 mg/mL) reduced the initial burst (percentage of the total) even though the same total mass of protein was released (0.6 mg). Loss of rhGH monomer was observed after 24 hours incubation of PLAD rhGH formulations at 37°C (Table 3). This loss of monomer may be due to prolonged exposure of dilute rhGH to high-solvent concentrations at elevated temperatures in the aqueous release buffer. Formulations containing less sucrose released more native monomer than the formulations containing higher sucrose. It should be noted that the small amount of protein released in the first 24-hour period might not be representative of the unreleased protein quality. Additionally, it is assumed that these solvents would diffuse away from the injection site in vivo, thus reducing the duration of this exposure to high solvent concentrations.

Table 1 Growth Hormone Formulation Composition and Quality

Formulation	Protein concentration[a] (mg/mL)	Sucrose concentration (mg/mL)	Polysorbate 20 concentration (w/v)	Percent monomer	Moisture content (%)	Composition (w/w)
A	20	2	0.05	99.0 ± 0.1	4.7	60.0
B	20	5	0.05	99.0 ± 0.1	4.5	50.0

[a]Formulated in 25 mM sodium bicarbonate, pH 7.4.

Table 2 PLAD Formulation Composition (w/w)

PLAD formulation number	PLA (%w/w)	Benzyl benzoate (%w/w)	Benzyl alcohol (%w/w)
I	20	79	1.0
II	20	75	5.0

Abbreviations: PLAD, polylactic acid depot; PLA, polylactic acid.

In Vivo Results

After subcutaneous (SC) administration of PLAD II with 50 mg/mL rhGH (A) a rapid rise in serum rhGH level was observed followed by a gradual decline to a plateau (9 ng/mL) after 4 days (Fig. 2). In contrast, after administration of PLAD II with 100 mg/mL rhGH (B) a rapid rise in serum rhGH level was followed by a rapid decline to a plateau (20 ng/mL) after 24 hours. These results indicate a higher sucrose:protein ratio increased the initial release but may not influence the sustained-release phase. Dose ranging data indicate a fairly linear relationship between dose and serum rhGH levels (Fig. 3). These results suggest that injection volume (60–600 µL) should not significantly affect the PK profile of PLAD depots. Histology of injection sites indicate a localized cavitated inflammatory process was associated with rhGH PLAD depots after SC injection in Sprange Dawley® (SD) rats. Walls of cavitated lesions are composed of immature fibrovascular reaction (granulation tissue) admixed with lymphocytes, plasma cells and histiocytes (9). Cellular and formulation debris were present but were not associated with any apparent increase in inflammation or necrosis.

Vascular Endothelial Growth Factor

Vascular endothelial growth factor (VEGF) is an endogenous heparin-binding, endothelial, cell-specific mitogen. Numerous studies have suggested that VEGF is a local regulator of naturally occurring physiologic

Table 3 24 Hour In Vitro Release of rhGH from PLAD

PLAD formulation number	Protein formulation	Burst (% rel in 24 hr)	Monomer (%)
II	50 mg/mL A	3.8	99.6
II	50 mg/mL B	1.4	73.0
II	100 mg/mL B	0.6	85.5

Abbreviation: PLAD, polylactic acid depot.

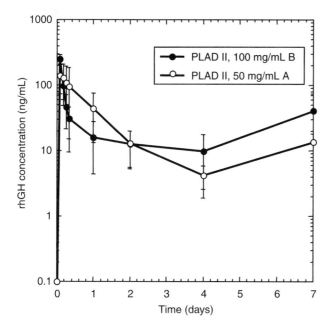

Figure 2 Serum rhGH levels after SC administration of PLAD depots to SD rats (dose 15 mg/kg, *n* = 5). *Abbreviations*: rhGH, recombinant hGH; PLAD, polylactic acid depot.

and pathologic angiogenesis (10,11). In this study PLAD was evaluated as an injectable delivery system for local delivery of recombinant human VEGH (rhVEGF). This local VEGF delivery system could be used for therapeutic revascularization of local tissues of the heart or limbs (12–14).

In Vitro Results

VEGF powders produced by spray freeze-drying rhVEGF maintained high monomeric content and produced clear solutions when dissolved in release buffer (15). Less than 50% of the total dissolved rhVEGF was released from both formulations in 24 hours. Higher PLA content (30% w/w) and a lower amount of BA (1%) resulted in a significantly lower initial burst.

In Vivo Results

After intramuscular (IM) administration of a PLAD formulation with 12 mg/mL rhVEGF B, a rapid rise in plasma rhVEGF concentrations was observed followed by a rapid decline to a plateau (400 pg/mL) after 24 hours (Fig. 4). The plasma concentration versus time profiles indicate that the PLAD rhVEGF formulation indicate rhVEGF is delivered with an initial burst followed by a plateau over the 7-day period examined. These results

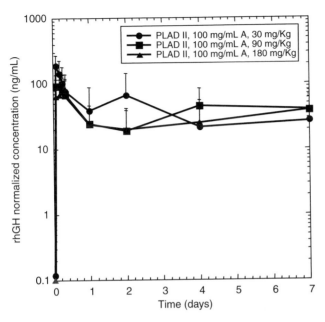

Figure 3 Serum rhGH levels in SD rats after SC administration of PLAD depots (data are dose normalized to 15 mg/kg, *n* = 5). *Abbreviations*: rhGH, recombinant hGH; PLAD, polylactic acid depot.

show the PLAD system may be capable of delivering therapeutic levels of rhVEGF for a period of seven or more days after IM injection through a 25–28 Ga needle. The PLAD liquid system could have several advantages over conventional microsphere systems due to ease of use and simple administration with a conventional syringe and needle.

The PLAD system is capable of delivering therapeutic levels of two important endogenous proteins (rhGH and rhVEGF) for a period of 15 or more days after SC or IM injection through fine needles (25–28 Ga). The PLAD liquid system will have significant advantages over particulate and suspension systems due to ease of use and simple administration with a conventional syringe and needle.

REGULATORY STATUS

The PLAD system utilizes materials and processes that are commonly used in approved parenteral products and registered aseptic manufacturing plants. However, based on current U.S. FDA excipient safety and toxicology guidance documents, any injectable product developed in the future would be required to submit an excipient safety package that contained

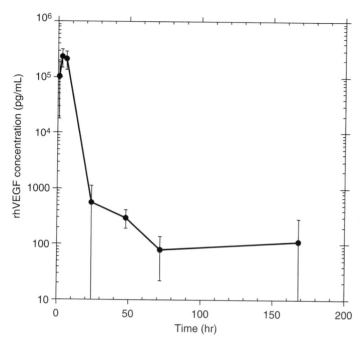

Figure 4 Plasma rhVEGF levels after intramuscular administration to SD rats (3.6 mg/kg, $n = 4$). *Abbreviation*: rhVEGF, recombinant human vascular endothelial growth factor.

sufficient information on the to-be-marketed product delivered by the intended route of administration (16).

COMPETITIVE ADVANTAGES

The PLAD system offers several advantages in comparison to conventional biodegradable polymeric controlled release systems. The administration of PLAD formulations is likely to be less invasive and less painful when compared to implants. This decrease in discomfort and ease of use should improve patient compliance. In addition as mentioned above the manufacture of PLAD based systems is less complex and could significantly lower the investment in manufacturing equipment and plants. The ideal PLAD-based product would possess several of the following key features:

- low viscosity (leading to injection through fine needles)
- high drug loading with simple mixing steps
- biodegradable and biocompatible excipients
- reproducible pharmacokinetic profile after administration
- low initial burst (leading to efficient utilization of loaded drug)

FUTURE DIRECTIONS

With the recent approval of the first biogeneric product and upcoming expiration of key product patents, it is clear that the biotechnology industry is maturing and thus there is increased need for innovative differentiated products. One area where there is clearly a need for improvement is the dosing frequency of most approved protein and peptide drugs. Long acting products based on the PLAD system would clearly provide significant advantages to patients over existing daily injections or multiple daily injections. It is this author's view that the biotechnology industry will move in this direction to maintain competitiveness and maintain market share.

REFERENCES

1. Eliaz RE, Wallach D, Kost J. Delivery of soluble tumor necrosis factor receptor from in-situ forming PLGA implants: in-vivo. Pharm Res 2000; 22(6):563–70.
2. Brodbeck KJ, DesNoyer JR, McHugh AJ. Phase inversion dynamics of PLGA solutions related to drug delivery—Part II. The role of solution thermodynamics and bath-side mass transfer. J Control Release 1999; 62(3):333–44.
3. Li CH, Papkoff H. Preparation and properties of growth hormone from human and monkey pituitary glands. Science 1956; 124(3235):1293–4.
4. Frindik JP, Kemp SF, Sy JP. Effects of recombinant human growth hormone on height and skeletal maturation in growth hormone-deficient children with and without severe pretreatment bone age delay. Horm Res 1999; 51(1):15–19.
5. Johnson F, et al. A month-long effect from a single injection of microencapsulated human growth hormone. Nature Med 1996; 2(7):795–9.
6. Govardhan C, et al. Novel long-acting crystal formulation of human growth hormone. Pharm Res 2005; 22(9):1461–70.
7. Brodbeck KJ, Pushpala S, McHugh AJ. Sustained release of human growth hormone from PLGA solution depots. Pharma Res 1999; 16(12):1825–9.
8. Okumu FW, et al. Sustained delivery of human growth hormone from a novel gel system: SABER. Biomaterials 2002; 23(22):4353–8.
9. Okumu FW, et al. Sustained delivery of growth hormone from a novel injectable liquid, PLAD. In Proceedings of International Symposium on Controlled Release of Bioactive Materials. San Diego, CA: Controlled Release Society, 2001.
10. Ferrara N, et al. Heterozygous embryonic lethality induced by targeted inactivation of the VEGF gene. Nature 1996; 380(6573):439–42.
11. Ferrara N, Henzel WJ. Pituitary follicular cells secrete a novel heparin-binding growth factor specific for vascular endothelial cells. Biochem Biophys Res Commun 1989; 161(2):851–8.
12. Eppler SM, et al. A target-mediated model to describe the pharmacokinetics and hemodynamic effects of recombinant human vascular endothelial growth factor in humans. Clin Pharmacol Ther 2002; 72(1):20–32.
13. Ferrara N. Role of vascular endothelial growth factor in physiologic and pathologic angiogenesis: therapeutic implications. Semin Oncol 2002; 29(6Suppl. 16): 10–14.

14. Street J, et al. Vascular endothelial growth factor stimulates bone repair by promoting angiogenesis and bone turnover. Proc Natl Acad Sci USA 2002; 99 (15):9656–61.
15. Cleland JL, Duenas ET, Okumu FW. Sustained delivery of rhVEGF from a novel injectable liquid, PLAD. In Proceedings of International Symposium on Controlled Release of Bioactive Materials. San Diego, CA: Controlled Release Society, 2001.
16. Guidance for industry non-clinical studies for the safety evaluation of pharmaceutical excipients. US FDA CDER and CBER, 2005.

11

Long-Term Controlled Delivery of Therapeutic Agents by the Osmotically Driven DUROS® Implant

Jeremy C. Wright and John Culwell

DURECT Corporation, Cupertino, California, U.S.A.

INTRODUCTION

Implantable drug delivery systems provide a useful alternative to several current therapies for long-term treatment of chronic conditions. Such systems can free the patient from repeated treatment or hospitalization and can improve patient compliance and quality of life. In addition, implantable systems offer the potential for significantly reducing the cost of care.

The DUROS® implant is a sterile, nonerodible, drug-dedicated system that operates like a miniature syringe, driven by osmosis and releasing minute quantities of drug (Fig. 1). It has been developed to provide long-term, controlled drug delivery for 1–12 months or longer (1). Because of its precise delivery kinetics, DUROS technology is well suited for delivery of potent drugs that require long-term, controlled, parenteral administration, including those that have a narrow therapeutic window or a short half-life. The first regulatory approval of a DUROS product was granted by the U.S. Food and Drug Administration in 2000 for ALZA Corporation's Viadur® (leuprolide acetate implant). While the Viadur implant provides zero-order delivery, DUROS technology can produce additional patterns of drug delivery.

DESCRIPTION OF THE TECHNOLOGY

A schematic of the DUROS system is shown in Figure 1. The system consists of an outer cylindrical titanium alloy reservoir. At one end of the

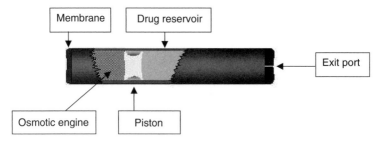

Figure 1   Cross section of the DUROS System. *Source*: From Ref. 3.

system is the rate-controlling membrane, constructed from a specially designed semipermeable polyurethane polymer. Next to the membrane is the osmotic engine, containing primarily NaCl combined with other pharmaceutical excipients. An elastomeric piston separates the osmotic engine from the drug formulation in the drug reservoir. At the far end of the system is the exit port. Exit ports can range from simple, straight channels to more complicated designs based on a number of considerations including rheology (pressure), back diffusion, thermal expansion and drug pharmacodynamics (1,2). The system is designed for subcutaneous implantation. Dimensions can range from 10 mm OD × 44 mm L to 4 mm OD × 44 mm L or smaller.

DUROS drug formulations can be both aqueous and non-aqueous and may be either a solution or a suspension. DUROS formulations should exhibit stability for extended periods of time at body temperature (37°C). Because the DUROS system dispenses formulations at low rates, vehicles containing organic solvents (e.g., benzyl alcohol or DMSO) can be delivered without concerns for adverse effects. Solvents useful for drug formulations for the DUROS system have been described previously (3). Stable formulations have been developed for a number of drugs, including peptides and proteins (4).

The materials in the DUROS system are chosen for their biocompatibility and compatibility with the drug and formulation excipients. Radiation sterilization (γ) can be used to sterilize the final drug product or a DUROS subassembly can be sterilized before aseptically filling the drug formulation.

For a number of applications, the inner aspect of the upper arm is the preferred site for subcutaneous implantation, which is easily accomplished as an outpatient procedure. Once implanted, a constant osmotic pressure gradient is established between body water and the osmotic engine. The osmotic engine expands at a rate controlled by the permeability of the membrane, resulting in controlled displacement of the piston and pumping of the drug formulation. In vivo studies have shown that the rate of osmotic imbibitions into the system is constant, demonstrating that the membrane is not fouled in vivo (5).

The pumping rate of the system can be varied by altering the properties of the polyurethane copolymer in the rate controlling membrane. For a fixed membrane composition, drug delivery rates can be varied by adjusting the drug concentration and a range of dosage strengths of fixed duration can be produced. Mathematics describing the operation of the DUROS system have been presented previously (3,6).

DUROS reservoir volumes up to 1 cc (overall system dimensions of 10 mm OD × 44 mm L) have been investigated. Size can be perceived as a constraint on acceptance of an implantable system, but pumps of much greater dimensions than the 1 cc reservoir system are implanted for treatment of chronic conditions (7). Additional parameters of DUROS system design have been described previously (3).

Osmotic systems generally yield good in vivo/in vitro correlation. For the DUROS Viadur system, in vitro release was within 5% of in vivo release (5). Additionally, an initial clinical study with the DUROS CHRONOGESIC® sufentanil system indicated agreement between in vitro and in vivo delivery rates, with a preliminary bioavailability estimate not different than 100% (8).

RESEARCH AND DEVELOPMENT RESULTS

Viadur (Leuprolide Acetate Implant)

The Viadur DUROS system delivers the GnRH analog leuprolide for 365 days for the palliative treatment of prostate cancer and has been extensively described previously (5,9–11).

CHRONOGESIC® (Sufentanil) Pain Therapy System

For patients with chronic pain, DUROS technology has been applied to the delivery of the opioid drug sufentanil by DURECT Corporation. The resulting CHRONOGESIC sufentanil system delivers the drug in specified doses for 3 months. Sufentanil is 500 times more potent than morphine, allowing for a small 4 × 44 mm implant with a 155-µl reservoir. Figure 2 presents the in vitro release for several dosage strengths of the CHRONOGESIC delivery system.

An initial Phase I clinical trial, a Phase II clinical trial, a pilot Phase III clinical trial and a pharmacokinetic trial have been completed for the CHRONOGESIC delivery system. In the Phase II trial 60% of patients indicated a preference for the CHRONOGESIC delivery system over their pre-study medication. The CHRONOGESIC delivery system also demonstrated improvements in select side effects (12,13).

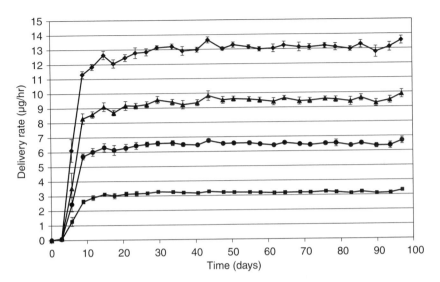

Figure 2 In vitro release rate of sufentanil from four dosage strengths of the CHRONOGESIC® System (phosphate buffered saline, 37°C; standard deviation indicated by error bars). *Source*: From Ref. 3.

Omega DUROS® (Omega Interferon)

Intarcia Therapeutics, Inc. is developing the Omega DUROS system for delivery of the protein omega interferon for treatment of hepatitis C viral infection. The system delivers omega interferon for 3 months utilizing a non-aqueous formulation. Potential advantages of Omega DUROS include eliminating the need for weekly injections, improved patient compliance, reduced side effects and reduced viral breakthrough (14).

Site-Specific Drug Delivery Using DUROS Technology

For site directed drug delivery, a miniaturized catheter can be attached to the DUROS system to direct the flow of drug to the target organ or tissue. Site-specific delivery enables a therapeutic concentration of a drug to be present at the target location without exposing the entire body to a similar dose.

DUROS Intrathecal Opioid Delivery System

Intrathecal delivery of opioids is indicated for a number of chronic pain conditions. By directly delivering into the intrathecal space, much smaller doses of opioids can elicit pain relief.

The DUROS Intrathecal Opioid system under development by DURECT Corporation is designed to be implanted subcutaneously near the target-site of drug administration. A miniature catheter is attached to the

DUROS system and tunneled under the skin to the intrathecal space. The DUROS Intrathecal Opioid system can deliver the drug for 3 months at rates of 10–100 µg/hr (3).

DUROS Delivery into the Brainstem

Experimental and clinical studies have demonstrated improvements in survival associated with local therapy for brain tumors (15). Because the brainstem monitors many basic functions, targeted chemotherapy into this area of the brain should be approached cautiously. DUROS delivery into the brainstem was investigated by insertion of a catheter into the pons of cynomologous monkeys (16,17).

In this study, a catheter with a 30-cm silicone-tubing proximal section and a 2–3 cm nickel titanium alloy distal section was attached to a DUROS system (1 cc reservoir, 10 µL/day pumping rate). The study demonstrated that the pons of monkeys could be safely accessed via catheter and that saline could be safely infused for 90 days (16). Analysis of cerebrospinal fluid and plasma carboplatin levels demonstrated a local CNS pharmacokinetic advantage with intra-pons delivery (17). Local neurotoxicity was dose dependent. The DUROS catheter system thus offers opportunities for advancing antitumor therapy targeted to the brain and brainstem.

DISCUSSION AND FUTURE DIRECTIONS

The DUROS system provides precise zero-order delivery capabilities usually found only in electro-mechanical infusion pumps that are larger and more complicated. The small size makes the system highly suitable for the delivery of potent drugs, including biomolecules, which required precise control of the rate of delivery. Commercialized applications and applications in development include the Viadur, CHRONOGESIC, and Omega DUROS delivery systems.

Site directed delivery offers the potential of utilizing smaller doses of drugs with better selectivity of action and substantially reduced side effects. Miniaturized catheter systems have been developed for the DUROS implant and their utility demonstrated in animals, including delivery to the brainstem. These systems enable the DUROS technology to be applied for local delivery of potent agents that require precise rate control. Applications of DUROS site directed delivery in diverse fields (such as pain management, heart disease and cancer chemotherapy) are anticipated.

ACKNOWLEDGMENTS

The authors wish to acknowledge the contributions of their colleagues on the DUROS project teams and would also like to thank Kirstin C. Nichols for assistance with editing this chapter.

REFERENCES

1. Peery JR, Dionne KE, Eckenhoff JB, et al. Inventors. ALZA Corporation, assignee. Sustained delivery of an active agent using an implantable system. US Patent 5,985,305. 1999.
2. Johnson, RM, Theeuwes, F, Gillis EM, et al. Inventors. DURECT Corporation, assignee. Implantable devices and methods for treatment of pain by delivery of fentanyl and fentanyl congeners, US Patent 6,835,194; 2004.
3. Wright JC, Johnson RM, Yum SI. DUROS® osmotic pharmaceutical systems for parenteral and site-directed therapy. Drug Delivery Technol 2003; 3(1): 3–11.
4. Dehnad H, Berry S, Fereira P, et al. Functionality of osmotically driven, implantable therapeutic systems (DUROS® implants): Effects of osmotic pressure and delivery of suspension formulations of peptides and proteins. Proc Intern Symp Control Rel Bioact Mater 2000; 27:1016–7.
5. Wright JC, Leonard ST, Stevenson CL, et al. An in vivo/in vitro comparison with a leuprolide osmotic implant for the treatment of prostate cancer. J Control Release 2001; 75:1–10.
6. Stevenson CL, Theeuwes F, Wright JC. Osmotic implantable delivery systems. In: Wise D, ed. Handbook of Pharmaceutical Controlled Release Technology. New York: Marcel Dekker, 2000 :225–53.
7. Krames ES. Intraspinal opioid therapy for chronic nonmalignant pain: Current practice and clinical guidelines. J Pain Symptom Manage 1996; 11(6): 333–52.
8. Fisher DM, Kellett N, Lenhardt, R. Pharmacokinetics of an implanted osmotic pump delivering sufentanil for the treatment of chronic pain. Anesthesiology 2003; 99(4):929–37.
9. Wright JC, Chester AE, Skowronski RJ, et al. Long-term controlled delivery of therapeutic agents via an implantable osmotically driven system: The DUROS implant. In: Rathbone RJ, Hadgraft J, Roberts MS, eds. Modified-Release Drug Delivery Technology. New York: Marcel Dekker, Inc., 2002: 657–69.
10. Fowler JE, Flanagan M, Gleason DM, et al. Evaluation of an implant that delivers leuprolide for 1 year for the palliative treatment of prostate cancer. Urology 2000; 55(5):639–42.
11. Fowler JE, Viadur Study Group. Patient-reported experience with the Viadur 12-month leuprolide implant for prostate cancer. Urology 2001; 58(3): 430–4.
12. http://www.durect.com/wt/durect/page_name/chronogesic (accessed December 2006)
13. Fisher DM. Implantable osmotic pump providing continuous subcutaneous delivery of sufentanil for chronic pain. In: Proceedings of the 2nd World Congress of World Institute of Pain, Istanbul, Turkey, June 27–30, 2001.
14. http://www.intarcia.com/products.html (accessed December 2006).
15. Weingaart JD, Rhines LD, Brem H. Intratumoral chemotherapy. In: Bernstein M, Berger, MS, eds. Neuro-Oncology: The Essentials. New York: Thieme Medical Publishers, Inc., 2000: 240–8.

16. Storm PB, Clatterbuck RE, Liu YJ, et al. A surgical technique for safely placing a drug delivery catheter into the pons of primates: Preliminary results of carboplatin infusion. Neurosurgery 2003; 52(5):1169–77.

17. Strege RJ, Liu YJ, Kiely A, et al. Toxicity and cerebrospinal fluid levels of carboplatin chronically infused into the brainstem of a primate. J Neurooncol 2004; 67:327–34.

12

The SABER™ Delivery System for Parenteral Administration

Jeremy C. Wright, A. Neil Verity, and Franklin W. Okumu

DURECT Corporation, Cupertino, California, U.S.A.

INTRODUCTION

The SABER™ delivery system is a biodegradable, in situ forming depot for the controlled delivery of small molecules, peptides, and large biomolecules via parenteral administration. The sucrose acetate isobutyrate extended-release (SABER) system consists of a high viscosity, nonpolymeric liquid carrier material with one or more pharmaceutically acceptable solvents and other excipients (1,2). The system provides controlled delivery for several days to several months.

The primary high viscosity liquid carrier material utilized in the SABER system is sucrose acetate isobutyrate (SAIB), a fully esterified sucrose derivative with a nominal ratio of six isobutyrates to two acetates (Fig. 1). The material is a mixed ester with high hydrophobicity, and as such, does not crystallize but exists as a viscous liquid. As a pharmaceutical excipient, SAIB is currently not a component of any approved drugs but is a direct food additive approved in over 40 countries (3). In a simple SABER delivery system, SAIB is mixed with a pharmaceutically acceptable solvent and the drug to be delivered is dissolved or dispersed in the SAIB/solvent solution for subsequent injection. If a water-soluble solvent such as ethanol is chosen, the solvent will quickly diffuse out of the injected volume leaving a viscous, in situ forming depot of SAIB and drug. The drug will be released in a sustained fashion via diffusion from the depot.

In more complex SABER systems, the concentration of the active pharmaceutical ingredient (API) may exceed the solubility of the API in the

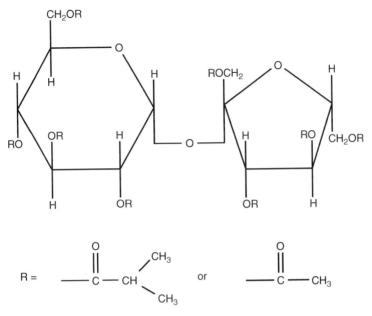

Figure 1 Chemical structure of SAIB. *Abbreviation*: SAIB, sucrose acetate isobutyrate.

SABER matrix, resulting in a dispersed suspension formulation. Drug loadings as high as 30–40% have been achieved in SABER formulations for parenteral delivery. To date, there appear to be no unusual technical obstacles or restrictions on what type or class of drug may benefit from sustained, parenteral delivery utilizing the SABER system, accepting the limitation that the drug must be sufficiently potent to permit a therapeutic dosage to be deliverable in a dosage volume acceptable to the patient. The SABER system can be utilized for systemic therapy (e.g., by injection as a subcutaneous or intramuscular depot) or the system can be utilized for local delivery via administration to the desired site of action.

Drug delivery from depot systems has been characterized by several mathematical treatments (4,5). Based on these mathematical treatments the release of drug from the SABER system depends on the diffusivity of the drug in the SABER matrix, the drug loading and the solubility of the drug in the SABER matrix (i.e., drug release rate increases with increasing diffusivity, solubility and loading in a predictable fashion) (6). The diffusivity and the solubility of the drug can be manipulated by the choice of solvent. Generally, water soluble solvents (such as ethanol, benzyl alcohol, N-methyl-2-pyrrolidone NMP, dimethyl sulfoxicl DMSO) diffuse from the SABER depot, resulting in lower drug diffusivities and drug solubilities in the SABER depot and slower drug release. Conversely, a solvent with negligible water solubility (such as benzyl benzoate) tends to be retained in the SABER matrix, resulting in higher drug diffusivities and drug solubilities in the SABER depot and higher drug release. Drug release can also be adjusted by the inclusion of selected excipients in the SABER matrix. For example, additives such as the bioerodible poly(lactic-co-glycolic) acid polymers have been investigated to adjust drug diffusivity and solubility in the SABER matrix, with polylactic acid being extensively investigated for applications in protein delivery (7). Systematic variation of the above parameters allows the delivery rate of the SABER formulation to be controlled into the target range for a given therapeutic application. Delivery of steroids, antineoplastic agents, peptides and proteins via the SABER system have been previously reported (2,7–10).

Advantages of the SABER Delivery System

The SABER delivery system offers a number of advantages

- flexible, tunable, sustained delivery of a wide range of drugs
- potential for minimal drug "burst" upon injection
- capacity for high drug loadings
- applicable to both systemic and local drug delivery
- inherently drug stabilizing due to the hydrophobic nature of the SABER matrix
- potential for room temperature storage/stability
- injection through standard syringes fitted with fine needles (21–28 Ga)
- reduced volume of administration compared to microspheres
- easily administered to the patient (or easily self-administered)
- potential for less pain upon injection
- ease of manufacture
- low cost of goods
- biodegradable

RESEARCH AND DEVELOPMENT RESULTS

Extended Three-Month Delivery from the SABER Delivery System

A proprietary hydrophobic drug was formulated in a SABER delivery system and administered to rabbits. Plasma concentrations of the drug are shown in Figure 2. Sustained release of the drug was observed over the 3-month testing period.

Application of the SABER Delivery System for Protein Delivery

The SABER delivery system has been used to facilitate local and systemic sustained delivery of several therapeutic proteins and peptides for periods of 1–4 weeks including rhGH (recombinant human vascular endothelial growth

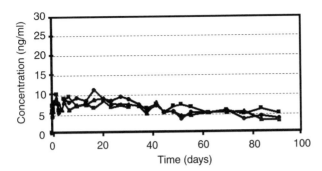

Figure 2 Time versus rabbit plasma concentration curve of a proprietary hydrophobic small molecule released from a single injection of a SABER delivery system.
Sustained plasma levels of drug were detected for 90 days with similar results seen
in each rabbit individually graphed ($n = 3$). *Abbreviation*: SABER, sucrose acetate
isobutyrate extended release.

factor), rhVEGF, deslorelin acetate, and additional undisclosed SABER protein product candidates that are in early development (7,11–13). For example,
recombinant human Growth Hormone (rhGH) was administered to athymic rats as a single subcutaneous injection of a SABER formulation
(15 mg/kg). The rhGH serum levels peaked at approximately 65 ng/mL
within the first 2 hours followed by a decline to plateau levels between 1
and 5 ng/mL by day 5 with maintenance at these levels for >28 days
(Fig. 3). This and other non-clinical studies (data not shown) demonstrate
the utility of the SABER delivery system as a sustained release delivery platform for local or systemic delivery of therapeutic proteins and peptides.

Utility of the SABER Delivery System for CNS Delivery

To evaluate the SABER delivery system for local chemotherapy of brain
tumors, systems were injected into the cerebral cortex of adult and neonatal
(12–24 hr old) rats. Adult rats showed no signs of distress; neonatal rats
showed no reduction in survival. There was a mild to moderate transitory
inflammatory response with the SABER delivery systems considered biocompatible in both adult and neonatal rats. The study concluded that the
SABER delivery system might be a useful pharmaceutical system for local
central nervous system drug delivery (14).

Clinical Experience with the SABER Delivery System

The clinical utility of a SABER delivery system is currently under investigation in multiple Phase 2 clinical studies evaluating the safety and activity of
POSIDUR™, a SABER™ bupivacaine formulation. POSIDUR is currently
under development by DURECT Corp. (Cupertino, CA) and Nycomed

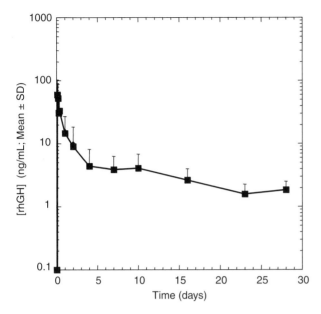

Figure 3 Serum rhGH levels after a single subcutaneous injection of a 1-month SABER rhGH formulation (athymic rat n = 5; 15 mg/kg dose, 25 Ga needle). *Abbreviations*: rhGH, recombinant human growth hormone; SABER, sucrose acetate isobutyrate extended release.

(Denmark). The product is designed to treat and control local, postoperative pain by providing continuous 48–72 hour local delivery of bupivacaine (long acting amide local anesthetic/analgesic) upon instillation within a surgical site. Potential advantages of the POSIDUR formulation over current standard practices of pain control may include overall greater pain relief, reduction in opioid usage and associated opioid side effects, reduced hospital staff burden, and shorter hospital stays. The POSIDUR formulation is an injectable, clear solution of SAIB/benzyl alcohol containing bupivacaine base. To date over 200 patients have been exposed to 1.25–7.5 mL of the POSIDUR formulation or placebo vehicle (SAIB/BA). Subcutaneous injections and wound instillations (subfascial and subcutaneous in wound placement) have been well tolerated and easily administered. As shown in Figure 4, subcutaneous administration of the POSIDUR formulation demonstrates dose linear pharmacokinetics with a rapid onset of delivery and sustained plasma levels for 48–72 hour. Of note, is the absence of any "drug dumping" or "drug burst" upon administration. Bupivacaine bioavailability was estimated to be ~100% (data not shown). The utility of the POSIDUR formulation as a long acting local analgesic is currently under clinical investigation in a variety of surgical procedures.

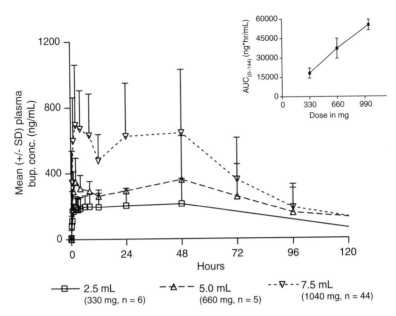

Figure 4 Pharmacokinetics of subcutaneous administered POSIDUR™ formulation. Patients undergoing inguinal hernia repair received paired, s.c. trailing injections on either side of ~5 cm surgical incision. Dose was administered equally on each side of the incision: 2.5 ($n = 6$), 5.0 ($n = 5$), or 7.5 ml ($n = 44$) of POSIDUR (330, 660, and 990 mg buvicaine, respectively). *Note*: The 7.5-ml POSIDUR dose was co-administered with 50 mg of commercial Bupivacaine–HCl (total bupiavacaine dose = 1040 mg). *Insert*: Plasma buvicaine concentrations demonstrated dose-linear kinetics (AUC_{0-144}).

REGULATORY

SAIB is a well-known GRAS food additive (3) approved in over 40 countries for use as an alternative to brominated vegetable oil in soft drinks, where it stabilizes emulsions, primarily by acting as a densifier for citrus oil flavorings. SAIB has an extensive safety profile including carcinogenicity, mutagenicity, and teratology studies. DURECT has conducted additional safety studies to support the use of SAIB in delivery systems for parenteral applications and oral applications (DURECT's ORADUR™ oral delivery platform). DURECT currently holds a drug master file DMF supporting the use of SAIB as a pharmaceutical excipient.

FUTURE DIRECTIONS

The SABER delivery system has shown wide utility in the delivery of active pharmaceutical agents, with durations of several days to 3 months. Ongoing preclinical and clinical studies continue to support the application of SABER delivery systems to parenteral delivery of small molecule, peptide, and protein therapeutic agents. For many therapeutics, localized drug delivery offers the potential to decrease systemic toxicity, increase efficacy, and modify biodistribution. DURECT is developing advanced SABER delivery systems for local drug delivery to meet these objectives.

ACKNOWLEDGMENTS

The authors would like to acknowledge the contributions of their SABER team colleagues, especially John Gibson, and would like to thank Kirstin Nichols for editorial assistance.

REFERENCES

1. Tipton AJ, Holl RJ. High viscosity liquid controlled delivery system. US Patent 5,747,058; 1998.
2. Tipton, AJ. Sucrose acetate isobutyrate (SAIB) for parental delivery. In: Rathbone MJ, Hadgraft J, Roberts MS, eds. Modified-Release Drug Delivery Technology. New York: Marcel Dekker, Inc., 2002: 679–87.
3. Reynolds RC, Chappel CI. Sucrose acetate isobutyrate (SAIB): historic aspects of its use in beverages and a review of toxicity studies prior to 1988. Food Chem Toxicol 1998; 36:81–93.
4. Hirano K, Ichihashi T, Yamada H. Studies on the absorption of practically water-insoluble drugs following injection. I. Intramuscular absorption from water-immiscible oil solutions in rats. Chem Pharm Bull 1981; 29(2):519–31.
5. Higuchi T. Mechanism of sustained-action medication: Theoretical analysis of rate of release of solid drugs dispersed in solid matrices. J Pharm Sci 1963; 52(12):1145–9.
6. Wright JC. In Situ Gelling Technologies for Drug Delivery, Releasing Technologies Workshop, 31st Annual Meeting and Exposition of the Controlled Release Society, June 12–16, Honolulu, Hawaii, 2004.
7. Okumu FW, Dao LN, Fielder, PJ, et al. Sustained delivery of human growth hormone from a novel gel system: SABER^{TM}. Biomaterials 2002; 23:4453–8.
8. Sullivan SA, Gibson JW, Burns PJ, et al. Sustained release of progesterone and estradiol from the SABER^{TM} delivery system: In vitro and in vivo release rates. Proc Int Symp Control Rel Bioact Mater 1998; 25:653–4.
9. Sullivan SA, Gilley RM, Gibson JW, et al. Delivery of Taxol® and other antineoplastic agents from a novel system based on Sucrose Acetate Isobutyrate. Pharm Res 1997; 14:291.
10. Fleury J, Squires EL, Betschart R, et al. Evaluation of the SABER^{TM} delivery system for the controlled release of deslorelin for advancing ovulation in the mare: Effects of formulation and dose. Proc Int Symp Control Rel Bioact Mater 1998; 25:657–8.
11. Pechenov S, Shenoy, B, Yang MX, et al. Injectable controlled release formulations incorporating protein crystals. J Control Release 2004; 96(1):149–58.

12. Kraeling RR, Barb CR, Rampacek GB. Luteinizing hormone response to controlled-release desorelin in estradiol benzoate primed ovariectomized gilts. Theriogenology 2000; 53(9):1681–9.

13. Keskin DS, Tezcaner A, Korkusuz P, et al. Collagen-chondroitin sulfate-based PLLA-SAIB-coated rhBMP-2 delivery system for bone repair. Biomaterials 2005; 26(18):4023–34.

14. Lee, J, Jallo, GI, Penno MB, et al. Intracranial drug-delivery scaffolds: Biocompatibility evaluation of sucrose acetate isobutyrate gels. Toxicol ApplPharmacol 2006; 215(1):64–70.

13

Improving the Delivery of Complex Formulations Using the DepotOne® Needle

Kevin Maynard and Peter Crocker

Imprint Pharmaceuticals Ltd., OCFI, Oxford, U.K.

INTRODUCTION

This chapter provides the background to the DepotOne® Needle, a device that can aid the injection of complex formulations such as viscous materials, pastes, gels, and particulates. DepotOne is a family of two-part hypodermic needles designed by Imprint. The technology is applicable to many therapeutic formulations and is currently being used in clinical trials for therapeutics formulated as suspensions, thick pastes and pegylated proteins.

FACTORS AFFECTING INJECTABILITY

The DepotOne needle improves the injection experience in two areas. First, it reduces the needle tip which needs to be used for injecting more viscous materials. Second, it overcomes blockages caused by many types of complex fluids. To understand the value of the DepotOne needle, it is necessary to understand the limitations of current needle technology on delivering higher viscosities/volumes and the causes of blockages of some complex formulations.

Selection of Needle Lumen Size

From a chemical engineering point of view, the size of the needle lumen required to inject a formulation with a given force is dependent on the

159

viscosity of the formulation, the volume required to inject and depth of injection. The higher the viscosity of the formulation, the larger the volume to inject and the deeper the therapy has to be delivered, the larger the needle lumen size needs to be.

However, from a patient point of view the smaller the needle, the less pain and trauma. Hence the lumen size needs to be balanced against the need to minimize the trauma.

Factors that influence patient and clinician's final choice of the size of needle to use to deliver a therapy include the frequency of injection, the injection is being delivered, the place where the injection is given and the seriousness of the disease.

The more frequently a therapy is given, the smaller the needle should be. For example, if a patient receives a one off injection then it is often acceptable to use a larger needle size as the patient has nothing to compare the pain with. However, if the patient is to receive an injection four times a day, as some diabetics do, then the use of smallest needle size is important.

The type of patient being injected also influences the size of needle that can be chosen. Small children have the same number of nerves as an adult. However, small children have these same number of nerves packed into a smaller space. Therefore, the probability of a needle blade hitting a very sensitive spot is much higher in a child than an adult and once a child has been hurt then the next injection can be very traumatic. There are reports of parents chasing their child around the room to give an insulin injection. Hence, it is important to use the smallest possible needle size in children. Elderly people frequently have much more friable veins and tissue than a middle-aged adult. The breakage of nerves and veins releases many inflammatory/pain factors. A smaller needle will reduce damage and pain and is therefore preferred for elderly patients. Other patient groups where special consideration of the needle size is required include many patients on blood-thinning agents, hemophiliacs and arthritis patients who find it difficult to put too much pressure on their thumb joints.

The setting and the disease are important factors in needle selection. A doctor in a clinic will tend to have less consideration of the needle size. However, doctors are cautious about a patient using an injection at home and particularly using a large needle at home. The disease also influences the choice of needle. Similarly, a person with an acute lethal disease will not consider the needle size as much as a person who has a chronic disease and has to continuously inject themselves.

Hence, there is a strong patient-driven tendency to reduce the size of the needle. However this, by necessity, reduces the viscosity or the volume which can be easily injected.

FORMULATION FACTORS INFLUENCING INJECTABILITY

Complex formulations such as pastes, gels, and particulates are difficult to deliver into patients. The injection can become blocked due to a large range of causes. A few of the common causes of blockages of reconstituted materials, particulates and pastes are outlined.

If a product is stored as a powder, the method of mixing of the powder with the diluent in preparation for injection will influence strongly the reconsituted product's injectability particularly for complex formulations containing particulates, polymers or pastes. There are multiple steps in the mixing process, each of which can impact on injectability.

Incorrect liquid addition can lead to dry patches and/or agglomeration of the powder particles forming lumps. Further, the solublization, particularly of polymers, can be slow leading to variable amounts of swelling. The final viscosity of the formulation of complex formulations will be dependent on the method and amount of mixing (similar to the way the thickness of whipped cream is dependent on the whipping process).

Particulates are very difficult to deliver through needles as there are multiple mechanisms via which particulates can block needles. The actual mechanism by which a specific particulate blocks a needle is dependent on a complex relationship between multiple factors. These factors include many particulate characteristics such as particle concentration, particulate shape, hardness, and surface charge in combination with the fluid characteristics such as polarity, viscosity, anion/cation species present, polymer content, and dynamics. Needle design can also strongly influence the potential for blockage. Needle characteristics such as hub shape, needle bore design, and needle entry aperture characteristics can increase or decrease the potential for blockage. One area where needle design has a large influence is on the potential for formation of soft reversible aggregates. If the needle directs the energy of delivery into concentrating the particulates then soft aggregates which block the entry aperture are easily formed.

Pastes can be characterized as being particulate powders in a small amount of water. Injectability of the paste is influenced strongly by the ratio of liquid to available binding sites on the powder and whether the product is a single or multi-phase product. A strongly hydrophilic powder with ionic surface characteristics will bind water easily. If there is insufficient liquid to bind all water binding sites, the powder particles will bind to sites on other particles, creating a pseudo-one-phase product. This product will often flow without blocking a needle although it may need significant force to deliver as the liquid phase cannot act as a lubricant. It would seem logical to add more water to the product to reduce the force of injection. However, if more water is added to the paste, all the binding sites will be bound with water and free water will exist in the paste. This excess water means that the product becomes a two-phase paste and acts more like a particulate solution. The product will compress more easily forcing the water out creating a blockage. It is not until the product becomes quite dilute and free flowing that it will unblock. This characteristic means this type of paste has a bell shaped injectability curve with the oddity of the higher concentration being more easily injected than certain lower concentrations (Fig. 1). In contrast, hydrophobic powders never bind water and a paste made from these types of powders always act in a two phase manner and hence will have a straight line injectability profile (Fig. 1).

DESIGNING A NEEDLE TO DELIVER COMPLEX FORMULATIONS

The design of a needle made to deliver the above formulations has to take account of a wide range of factors impacting on the delivery. Imprint has spent 6 years optimizing the DepotOne needle so it can deliver the aforementioned envisaged broad range of complex therapeutics. Each aspect of a needle has been examined and modeled in detail. The flow characteristics have been visualized using a wide range of different techniques including dye-based flow devices, and computation fluid dynamics. Imprint has also invested significantly in understanding in detail the multiple mechanisms of blockage of needles from a wide range of complex fluids. The result of this work is the DepotOne needle, a simple yet elegant device which has the ability to deliver many complex therapeutics. The beauty of the device is not just its simplicity yet powerful design but that it can be used exactly in the same manner as a standard needle.

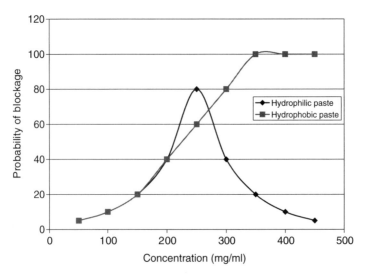

Figure 1 Examples of injectability curves of a hydrophilic and a hydrophobic paste.

DepotOne Products

The first DepotOne needle received regulatory approval in 2003. It was designed to deliver a highly viscous formulation for a rheumatoid arthritis product. Its design reduced the force to inject without compromising small needle size. The reduction in force enabled the concentration of product to be increased thus extending the duration of the product and reducing the frequency of injection. Maintaining a small needle penetration profile was important for this product as the patient population are relatively elderly and hence required a small needle size. However, the patient's thumbs can be very sensitive to applying pressure. A reduced pressure can be achieved by using a larger needle size.

The DepotOne system is now available in a number of different variants. These variants include systems to assist the delivery of particulate and paste formulations.

System Design and Operating Principles

The DepotOne needle is shown in Figure 2. It is a two-needle device with a small front end and a large back end. The blades are on the front end and the exit aperture of the needle is on the back end. Our understanding of why

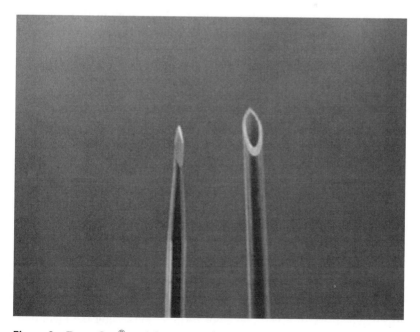

Figure 2 DepotOne® on left compared to standard needle. Note small front end.

the basic needle works is the following. As the blades are on the small front end, they are smaller than if they were on the fluidically equivalent standard needle. Hence the probability of the blades hitting something sensitive under the skin is reduced. As the aperture is on the back end of the needle, the fluidics of the needle is the same as a standard needle of similar bore size. The front end is typically 2–3 mm long. This means the fluid comes out at a slightly higher point than a needle of comparable length (measured from hub to tip). This difference by and large has no effect on the depth achieved when giving a standard injection and there have been no reports from clinical trials using the needles where this minor difference has affected the results. The extension and the receded aperture makes the DepotOne needle not suitable for delivery to specific spots such as is required in wrinkle filling injections and intravitreal injections into the eye.

The DepotOne needle is used in a similar manner to a standard needle. The tip is inserted making a small cut and the needle is pushed in stretching the skin out, up and over the top of the ramp onto the large back end of the needle. The needle tip has been especially designed to create a quality cut to ensure there is little rolling of tissue and the delivery is as smooth as possible.

There is a range of available needle sizes. The largest needle has a fluidic capacity of a 17-Ga needle and a needle tip of a 20-Ga needle. The smallest needle has a fluidic capacity of a 21-Ga needle and an entry tip of a 27-Ga needle.

Variants of the DepotOne needle have been designed to overcome certain types of blockages caused by particulates and pastes. The entry aperture, the lumen, the exit aperture, and the hub shape of these variants are redesigned to reduce particulate and paste blockages. Further, the surface topography of the needles and hubs has been modified to inhibit the initiating points of certain types of blockages.

The DepotOne needle is made using components used in most standard needles. The manufacturing techniques have been specially developed to ensure special tip performance, and to ensure that the right surface topography is obtained. A special method of applying the lubrication had to be developed that prevents skin rolling in and breaking.

The performance characteristics and safety profile of materials used in the DepotOne needle have been selected with reference to the ISO standards for needles. The testing programme included pull-out, bend, and sterility tests. Lubricants used are standard lubricants but are applied in a highly specific manner to ensure proper needle entry.

Ramp angle and shapes connecting the front end and rear end of the devices are carefully selected to ensure smooth entry with minimal catching.

PRECLINICAL DEVELOPMENT OF DepotOne

The effective delivery of a wide range of formulations using the DepotOne formulation has been tested. Figure 3 shows the time required to inject

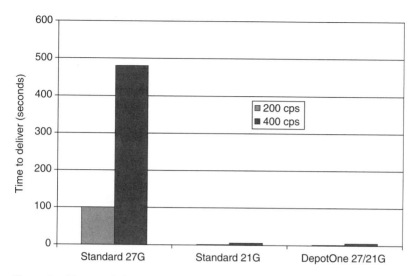

Figure 3 Time to deliver Newtonian fluids of different viscosities using 1 kg force.

Newtonian liquids of differing viscosities using a standard needle and a standard DepotOne needle. The DepotOne needle had a performance equal to a needle of the same bore size when delivering Newtonian liquids. Penetration tests showed the needle had the penetration characteristics of a needle of the smaller size of its tip. Thus for Newtonian liquids, the needle has the fluidics of a large needle yet the penetration characteristics of a small needle.

In experiments to achieve delivery of higher viscosities of Newtonian liquids, the DepotOne delivery device was modified by attaching a viscosity reducing device add-on. The add-on device reduced the time required to deliver a 30k cps fluid through an 18-G needle six-fold (Fig. 4). The combination of the viscosity reducing add-on and the DepotOne needle enabled the product to be injected through a needle with 21-G penetration characteristics in a time which was six-fold less than that necessary for delivery through a standard 18-G needle.

Particulate performance was tested with a wide range of particulates including poly(lactic-co-glycolic) acid (PLGA) particulates, and precipitates of actives. These particles had differing mechanisms of blockages. Some of these formulations blocked standard needles by settling and agglomerating at the entry aperture, some caused mid-tube blockages and others caused exit aperture blockages. Certain particulate formulations blocked all acceptable sizes of needles. (This has been shown to be the case for many particulates.) As can be seen from Figure 5, the DepotOne needle enabled delivery of higher concentrations of the PLGA particulates than could be

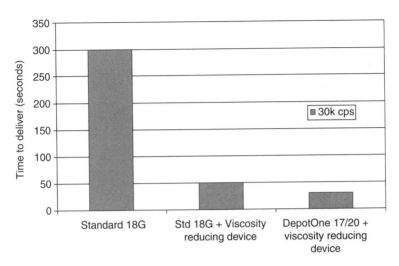

Figure 4   Delivery of Newtonian fluid of 30k cps using 2 kg force.

injected using a standard needle of larger bore size. (These results are dependent on the mixing of the particulate with the diluent being optimized to avoid dry patches and large lumps as these can clog all needles and prevent delivery.)

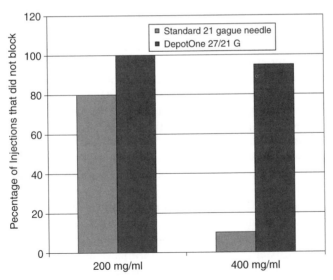

Figure 5   Delivery of a PLGA particulate solution. *Abbreviation*: PLGA, poly(lactic-co-glycolic) acid.

An important observation regarding particulate delivery was that the DepotOne needle in the standard shape as shown in the picture could enhance the delivery of particles when the particles were less than 1 μm diameter. However, when the particles were larger, e.g., between 50 and 100 μm in diameter, the standard DepotOne needle did not enhance the delivery. A modification of the needle design was required to ensure reproducible delivery without blockage.

The ability of the DepotOne needles to deliver particulates down 6-inch long needles has also been tested. The concentration of one micron sized particles that could be injected down a 27/21-Ga needle was 400 mg/mL. To achieve delivery of these concentrations of particulates through the DepotOne 27/21-Ga needle, a customized disposable powered injector was needed in addition to the DepotOne needle. The delivery of this concentration of particulates through a standard needle of larger bore (18 Ga) using the powered injector blocked, thus showing the design of the needle was important to achieve delivery. As noted before, the method of mixing of the particulate powder with the liquid diluent was important to achieve reproducible delivery.

The delivery of four pastes using the DepotOne technology has been tested. These pastes were of four differing types.

The first paste was a two-phase paste. Being a two-phase paste, the particles separated from the liquid on the application of small amounts of force. This separation meant that the paste required a very large 12-Ga bore needle (to avoid the application of high forces). This was clinically unacceptable as the wound size was so large it failed to heal. In addition, the design of standard needle hubs created areas where forces built up creating the potential for separation. Finally the back-pressure created in the tissue also induced separation creating blockages at the exit aperture of the needle.

The second paste was a high concentration protein mixture. At high concentration, the paste formed a pseudo-one-phase product and the fluid acted like a Newtonian fluid.

The last two pastes were setting pastes that needed to be injected down long (6–9 inch) needles. At the initiation of the projects for these products, the products were being injected down extremely wide bore needles (12 and 14 Ga, respectively). However, this size of bore caused significant damage to tissue, leaving behind deep wounds that would not heal properly leaving the wound open to ingress of infectious agents deep into the body. If smaller needles were used, the pastes set in the needle and blocked, regardless of what force was applied to the needle. A key need of these products was to reduce the bore size of needle required to inject the product.

The mixing method had to be optimized to achieve the optimum delivery of all paste. If not mixed properly, delivery was poorly reproducible. However, once optimum mixing was achieved, the DepotOne needle was able to enhance the delivery of the four pastes. The correct hub design enabled delivery of the separating two-phase pastes thus enabling a reduction in needle gauge. The DepotOne needle design reduced the force of injection of the one-phase paste and also reduce the size of needle that was required to deliver the setting pastes.

IN VIVO RESULTS AND CLINICAL TRIALS

The DepotOne needle is now being used to deliver a number of therapeutic products in both animal and clinical trials. The results of this work are the intellectual property of the pharmaceutical companies sponsoring the trials and as trials have not concluded we do not have definitive results to show at this time about DepotOne needles.

Initial small-scale animal and clinical trials with the DepotOne needle showed that the manufacture process of the product was extremely important. These trials showed that there was an absolute limit to the skin stretch that was necessary to allow the small cut created by the tip to stretch up over the ramp on to the barrel. This meant that the needle became more difficult to insert as larger needle barrels were used. The practical consequence of this was that the tip to barrel ratio that could be used was reduced as the needle barrel approached larger sizes.

In addition, these developmental trials indicated the tip structure was important for the level of pain that occurred. If the tip was poorly made, then the needle caused more pain than the standard needle.

The feedback from two of the animal and clinical trials as far as we have received it is summarized below.

The delivery of a setting paste has been tested using the DepotOne needle. The 12–14 Ga standard needles required to deliver this paste caused wounds which were clinically unacceptable, i.e., the wound was too large and did not heal. The products could be delivered into animals using the DepotOne needle with a special injection gun whereas the pastes blocked the standard needle of similar bore size.

The DepotOne needle product was evaluated as a potential method to deliver a particulate therapeutic product which was made up of a suspension of the precipitated active agent. This product blocked when injected into patients using a standard 21-Ga needle and the product could not be used clinically. Clinical trials delivering the product with the DepotOne needle have been carried out. No blockages have been reported in the two clinical trials carried out so far.

Other trials are proceeding and the results are shortly anticipated.

OUTLOOK AND SUMMARY

The DepotOne needle can be adapted to enhance the delivery of a variety of complex therapeutics. It has been shown to be of benefit for delivery of viscous products especially when these products are injected by arthritis patients, particulates and pastes. It is increasingly being tested for more tissue engineering products as well as the complex fluids such as pastes and precipitates already mentioned. Potential applications of the technology include facilitating the delivery of gene therapy, cell therapies, and site-directed therapies. As the device is approved in both the United States and Europe, it can be used as a "retrofitable" solution to many of the issues associated with delivery of complex fluids.

ACKNOWLEDGMENTS

The authors would like to acknowledge the contributions of their colleagues in the DepotOne team to the development of the data and comments on the chapter.

14

ReGel Depot Technology

Ramesh C. Rathi and Kirk D. Fowers

Protherics Plc, West Valley City, Utah, U.S.A.

INTRODUCTION

The design of a biodegradable thermosensitive polymer was inspired by the thermosensitive nature of nonbiodegradable pluronics or poloxamers (PEO-PPO-PEO). The sol↔gel transformation of pluronics or poloxamers is exhibited by only a subset of this group of polymers within a specific molecular weight range and hydrophilic/hydrophobic balance (1–4). It was hypothesized that block copolymers based on biodegradable and biocompatible components of polyethylene glycol (PEG) and poly (DL-lactide-co-glycolide) (PLG) with a defined molecular weight and hydrophilic/hydrophobic balance would demonstrate a similar sol↔gel transformation.

MacroMed, Inc. (recently acquired by Protherics, PLC) developed a novel drug delivery system (ReGel®), which was designed to exhibit the unique reversible thermal gelation properties (sol↔gel) of Poloxamers, but also allow biodegradation through inclusion of biodegradable PLG blocks (ABA or BAB) (5–7). The A-block consists of PLG (hydrophobic block) whereas the B-block is comprised of PEG (hydrophilic block). The polymer construct is specifically designed to attain a defined hydrophilic/hydrophobic balance, which enables it to be water-soluble (free-flowing, Sol) at or below room temperature and allows it to gel (insoluble, bioerodible Gel) when the temperature is raised to body temperature (8). A variety of ReGel polymers have been synthesized, which enables broad formulation capability.

Prior to injection, the polymer is reconstituted yielding aqueous ReGel as a free-flowing liquid below its gelation temperature with a viscosity of

<1 poise, water is 0.01 poise. The sol↔gel transition occurs without chemical modification of the triblock copolymer or active agent because ReGel is a physically formed thermally reversible hydrogel (Fig. 1). The gel state can be converted to the sol state simply by reducing the temperature below the gelation temperature of the formulation.

Release of compounds from the ReGel depot occurs through two primary mechanisms. The first mechanism is diffusion, followed by a combination of diffusion and erosion of the depot. For the original ReGel polymer, the predominant mechanism for highly water-soluble compounds is diffusion, while both mechanisms contribute significantly for moderate to nearly water-insoluble compounds. Newer generations of ReGel create depot formulations where diffusion and erosion of the depot contribute to controlled release of highly water-soluble proteins, in addition to similar release profiles for hydrophobic compounds.

Biodegradation begins following exposure to an aqueous environment, and as the PLG blocks degrade hydrolytically into lactic and glycolic acid they are eliminated through normal metabolic pathways. The degradation can be tailored to occur over 1–6 weeks, and the PEG blocks are excreted through the kidneys following diffusion from the injection site. OncoGel® (ReGel/paclitaxel), for local treatment of solid tumors, has completed a Phase I safety study and is currently in Phase II clinical trials in the United States and Europe in two indications (esophageal and neoadjuvancy-breast cancer) (9).

RESEARCH AND DEVELOPMENT

ReGel has been evaluated with a variety of active agents that are generally formulated as a 23% (w/w) aqueous solution of polymer in phosphate buffer

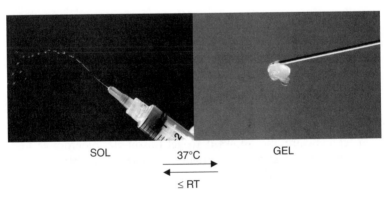

SOL   37°C   GEL
                    ⟶
                   ⟵
                   ≤ RT

Figure 1   ReGel can be injected through small gauge needles (23 Ga shown) and undergoes a thermorevisible transition from a free flowing solution to a viscous gel.

(pH 7.4) (8). In vitro stability and degradation of ReGel was studied under several conditions. The polymer weight average molecular weight (Mw) was monitored as a function of time in experiments designed to assess the stability of the ReGel polymer. The ReGel Mw was stable, and no physical property changes were observed, after storage for lessthan 2 years at -10 to $-20°C$ and for morethan 6 months at 2–8°C. At room temperature (21–25°C) the polymer degrades (i.e., Mw decreases via hydrolysis) in a near zero-order fashion over an 18-week period with eventual loss of gel integrity and complete degradation of the polymer. At 37°C, in vitro, the PLG blocks degrade (i.e., Mw decreases) completely in a near zero-order fashion over approximately 6–10 weeks (8). In all cases, the gel converts into a clear solution of water-soluble components (lactic acid, glycolic acid, and PEG 1000) as polymer degradation occurs. This biodegradation behavior is desirable and eliminates the need to retrieve the polymer carrier once the drug load has been delivered. The degradation products are well known and in the case of lactic and glycolic acid represent the same degradation products that are produced from many approved sutures and microsphere products based on biodegradable PLG polymers.

DRUG SOLUBILIZATION AND SOLUBILITY ENHANCEMENT WITH REGEL

ReGel significantly increases the solubility (up to 2000-fold) of hydrophobic drugs, such as paclitaxel and cyclosporine A (Table 1), and there is a significant improvement in the stability of paclitaxel in the ReGel formulation (Fig. 2).

ReGel maintained >95% of paclitaxel in its parent form over a 28-day stability study, while paclitaxel rapidly degraded in an aqueous environment to approximately 20% during the same time period. This study demonstrated that as ReGel hydrolytically degrades paclitaxel is stabilized within hydrophobic domains of the polymer.

Table 1 Paclitaxel or Cyclosporin A Added to 23% Solution (w/w) of ReGel at Various Concentrations

Drug	Media	Solubility (at 5°C)
Paclitaxel	Water	<5 µg/mL
	ReGel	>10 mg/mL
Cyclosporin A	Water	<5 µg/mL
	ReGel	>2 mg/mL

The equilibrium concentration was determined by high pressure liquid chromatography.

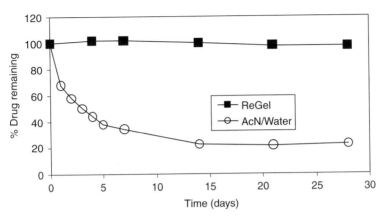

Figure 2 The stability of paclitaxel was measured at specific time points following incubation in either ReGel [23% solution (w/w)] or a 75% acetonitrile (AcN) solution at 37°C.

DELIVERY OF HYDROPHOBIC DRUGS

Protherics' proprietary polymeric drug delivery system, ReGel (7), has demonstrated broad formulation capability (8,10–12). ReGel formulations have successfully been developed for hydrophobic small molecules, peptides, and proteins. Protherics' lead ReGel formulation incorporates a hydrophobic small molecule, OncoGel (ReGel/paclitaxel), for local tumor management and is currently in a phase II trial in the United States and Europe (esophageal) and a phase II trial in Europe (neoadjuvancy breast).

The OncoGel product is stored frozen ($-20 \pm 10°C$) and has demonstrated greater than 2 years stability. OncoGel is packed in ready-to-inject syringes and thawed prior to injection. Currently, it is administered as multiple intralesional injections (based on the tumor volume) distributed evenly within the tumor, and provides local delivery of paclitaxel for up to 6 weeks. Planned studies may also place OncoGel into the resected tumor cavity. Preclinical studies using MDA-231 (human breast tumor xenografts) tumors in mice showed similar or superior efficacy with a 10-fold lower dose compared to the maximum tolerated systemic dose. This improved efficacy was accompanied by minimal side effects and no toxic deaths (8). The diffusion of paclitaxel from OncoGel was monitored in a [C14]paclitaxel biodistribution study in tumor bearing mice (8), and following injection into normal pig pancreata (13). The biodistribution study demonstrated a half-life within the tumor of approximately 3 weeks, while paclitaxel levels in plasma, urine, and distal tissues were <5% of the total dose. Distribution within the pancreas exhibited therapeutic paclitaxel levels at distances up to 3–5 cm from the depot site 14 days post-injection. The residual OncoGel depot and tissue contained paclitaxel in its parent form (13).

DELIVERY OF PEPTIDE AND PROTEIN DRUGS

ReGel has been formulated with a wide range of peptides and proteins (8,10,12). ReGel is a totally aqueous based formulation (no organic solvents) that creates a mild environment conducive to maintaining native protein structure and function.

Porcine Growth Hormone (pGH)

A ReGel/pGH formulation demonstrated a 2-week in vitro release period, which was mirrored in vivo in a bioefficacy study using hypophysectomized rats (8). Identical total pGH doses were administered either as a single ReGel/pGH injection or divided into 14 equal daily injections that exhibited similar efficacy (i.e., growth curves). Once daily injections ceased or the ReGel/pGH depot was depleted a loss in body weight was observed.

Insulin

Initial studies of ReGel/insulin formulations extended the release duration and enhanced the stability of Zn–insulin from the ReGel depot over a period of 2 weeks. Further improvement in sustaining the in vivo pharmacokinetic release profile of insulin was achieved using excess Zn as a reservoir, and a concurrent drop in blood glucose levels was demonstrated in diabetic ZDF rat studies (10).

Glucagon-Like Peptide-1

A further example of the ability of ReGel delivery systems to enhance peptide delivery was demonstrated using glucagon-like peptide-1 (GLP-1). It is known to be highly unstable in aqueous solutions in the concentration range required for efficient administration, and commonly undergoes aggregation/fibrillation. While non-complexed synthetically prepared GLP-1 is incompletely released from ReGel in 3 days (data not shown), a suspension of complexed GLP-1 in ReGel provides for complete release of the drug over a greater than 2-week period in its bioactive form (Fig. 3).

In vivo studies in ZDF rats demonstrated the ability of this formulation to significantly lower blood glucose levels over a period of 10–12 days (Fig. 4).

Cytoryn™

Interleukin 2 (IL-2) is approved for systemic administration to treat renal carcinoma and melanoma. IL-2 administration is often associated with significant toxicities, such as severe hypotension that leads to hypoperfusion of vital organs and vascular leak syndrome (14).

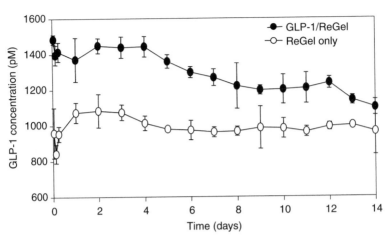

Figure 3 GLP-1 concentrations following injection of GLP-1/ReGel in ZDF diabetic rats. *Abbreviation*: GLP-1, Glucagon-like peptide-1.

Cytoryn is an immunomodulatory localized peri-tumoral delivery system based on a combination of IL-2 in ReGel. Cytoryn has undergone preclinical studies in a number of tumor cell lines demonstrating enhanced efficacy and reduced toxicity over conventional methods of IL-2 delivery (12). Through peri-tumoral delivery of Cytoryn, it was possible to increase the dose administered by 4-fold over subcutaneous doses, which enhanced the effect of IL-2 on tumor regression, while still avoiding systemic toxic effects. In vitro release experiments demonstrated that IL-2 is released over a 3- to 4-day period in fully bioactive form as measured by a cell

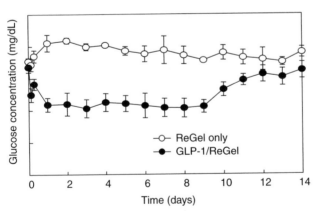

Figure 4 Glucose concentrations following injection of GLP-1/ReGel in ZDF diabetic rats. *Abbreviation*: GLP-1, Glucagon-like peptide-1.

proliferative assay, and induces lymphocyte cytotoxicity against target cells in an identical manner to reconstituted Proleukin®.

The efficacy of Cytoryn was tested in four different tumor types in tumor bearing mice. Intraperitoneally administered Cytoryn demonstrated significant antitumor response, defined as statistically increased survival versus control or Proleukin, against MethA fibrosarcoma growing as ascites in mouse peritoneum. Solid subcutaneous tumors (RD 995 squamous carcinoma, B16 melanoma, and RENCA renal carcinoma) received weekly peritumoral Cytoryn injections, and tumor size was measured periodically. Cytoryn arrested local tumor growth when administered as weekly peritumoral injections. Tumor stasis directly correlated with improved survival for all tumor types studied to date, both of which was statistically significant compared to control or Proleukin (12). Adverse effects, such as low-blood pressure associated with conventional administration of IL-2, were negligible. Pharmacokinetic data demonstrated IL-2 retention in the peritumoral region for protracted periods, significantly lower kidney excretion, and a prolonged half-life in blood as compared to peritumoral administered soluble IL-2.

Cytoryn's mechanism of action includes increased concentration near the tumor where cytotoxic T-lymphocytes that recognize tumor antigen are localized and recruitment of additional anti-tumor immune cells. Cytoryn was shown to increase lymphocyte recruitment (including CD8 lymphocytes and NK cells) into ascites and solid tumors in comparison to conventional administration of IL-2. It is likely that the prolonged release of IL-2, as demonstrated by a prolonged half-life in blood, creates a concentration gradient that allows immunologic cells to track to the site of injection/tumor.

A number of model proteins have been evaluated to determine their release kinetics as well as methods to modulate and improve both the stability and the duration of release. Additional proteins formulated in ReGel have demonstrated a range of release profiles that are dependent on the properties of ReGel and the molecular weight and solubility (i.e., glycosylation) of the protein. Typical release kinetics range from 1 to 7 days for lower molecular weight soluble proteins, and up to 4-week delivery periods for Zn-complexed proteins or less soluble peptides have been achieved with the parent ReGel polymer. Progress continues in the development of ReGel polymers capable of prolonging the release of more hydrophilic proteins.

REGULATORY STRATEGY

Although the triblock design of ReGel is new, the polymer constituents are based on well-known components (PEG and PLG) that are used in several FDA approved products. Biocompatibility and degradation pathways of PLG and PEG–PLG polymers have been established previously (15–17). Biodegradation of the ReGel polymer, in vivo, will eventually result in lactic acid, glycolic acid, PEG and low molecular weight PLG, as breakdown products that are easily metabolized or degrade into compounds that are readily and completely excreted by the kidney.

In support of the IND filed for OncoGel, a number of studies have been conducted to demonstrate the biocompatibility of ReGel. Modified FDA biocompatibility tests were performed with ReGel to demonstrate that ReGel is non-pyrogenic (LAL; endotoxin and material mediated pyrogen; rabbits), non-cytotoxic (agar overlay), non-mutagenic (Ames test; bacteria), no acute toxicity (i.p. injection in mice), and non-irritating (intracutaneous injection in rabbits).

Animals injected subcutaneously with ReGel have demonstrated that ReGel forms a transparent, semi-solid gel at the injection site that slowly degrades in the body over time. Acute and chronic inflammation (granulation tissue, macrophages, and capsule formation) were evaluated after subcutaneous injection of ReGel in rats, and ranged from no tissue response to mild inflammation over the 30-day study period. Overall histological scores of ReGel were similar to that observed with commercial PLG microspheres and resorbable sutures. GLP safety/toxicity studies were performed in rats and dogs. After subcutaneous injection of ReGel in normal tissues, histopathological readouts ranged from no tissue response to the response similar to the approved biodegradable polymers (8).

TECHNOLOGY POSITION/COMPETITIVE ADVANTAGE

ReGel, Protherics' proprietary injectable drug delivery system, is protected by several U.S. and foreign patents (5–7), and additional patents are pending. ReGel offers simplicity of formulation and distinct advantages over solvent based in situ forming gels and microspheres in the systemic as well as local delivery of sensitive molecules including proteins and peptides (18–21). These advantages include: (*i*) *simplicity*, polymer design is based on well-known biodegradable PLG and biocompatible PEG components; (*ii*) *easy fabrication*, ReGel is an aqueous solution (no organic solvents) of polymer, which can be filter sterilized; (*iii*) *ease of drug/polymer formulation*, drug formulation in ReGel is simply accomplished by physical mixing of drug with polymer solution; (*iv*) *high drug loading*, drug is directly added (dissolved or suspended) in the aqueous solution of polymer; (*v*) *reversible sol↔gel transition*, where the aqueous solution of polymer drug formulation at or below room temperature is free-flowing and easily injectable through narrow gauge needles which upon injection and in response to body temperature ($\geq 30°C$) quickly transforms into a bioerodible gel depot; (*vi*) *biodegradability*, the ReGel depot is completely eliminated from the body over a period of 1–6 weeks by a combination of dissolution and degradation to its constituents, PEG and lactic and glycolic acid, which are eliminated or metabolized in the body. As a biodegradable drug delivery depot, ReGel is designed for repeat administration (every 2–3 wk) as the polymer is degraded and eliminated from the injection site during the release period which eliminates the need for retrieval after the drug has been released.

ReGel's unique properties offer significant advantages to the pharmaceutical industry. ReGel is nontoxic, water-based, easy to administer, offers systemic or local drug delivery and has a low burst effect. In addition, it is simple and inexpensive to produce and is compatible with a wide variety of drugs. Competitive technologies that do not offer these characteristics have significant limitations in their commercial application and ability to effectively improve drug performance. There have been several products commercialized in the area of injectable depot delivery. These have been primarily 1 month or multi-month delivery products, such as Lupron Depot®. Drawbacks of existing depot technologies include difficulty in administration, and poor drug yield that is associated with the use of organic solvents and with complex manufacturing. In addition, microspheres typically produce a high burst effect losing a significant percentage of the drug upon injection. Competitive gel depot technologies have been designed to avoid some of the problems with microspheres, examples include Alzamer® developed by Alza (a subsidiary of Johnson & Johnson), Atrigel® owned by QLT Therapeutics (from the acquisition of Atrix) and the SABER™ system owned by Durect (from the acquisition of Southern BioSystems). These systems have improved on earlier drug delivery systems, but are still limited in their ability to formulate proteins due to the use of organic solvents in formulation.

FUTURE OUTLOOK

Protherics' local tumor management product, OncoGel, is a controlled release formulation of paclitaxel based on ReGel drug delivery system. OncoGel is currently in phase II clinical studies in the United States and European Union for esophageal (palliative) cancer treatment and in the European Union for breast (neoadjuvancy) cancer treatment. A phase I dose escalation study in the United States demonstrated that OncoGel could be successfully administered intralesionally to patients with solid tumors without significant systemic adverse events, and with minimal local side effects in the majority of patients (9). OncoGel was injected into 18 superficially accessible tumors found in 16 patients. There were no drug-related severe adverse events in any patient and no dose-limiting toxicities in the highest dose cohort. The majority of OncoGel-related adverse events presented at the site of the injection (e.g., injection site pain and erythema) and were of mild to moderate severity (Table 2).

No hematological, neurological or gastrointestinal adverse events, normally associated with IV administration of paclitaxel, were related to OncoGel injection. Paclitaxel levels were determined for patients in the highest three dose cohorts, and most levels were below the detection limit,

Table 2 Adverse Events Related to OncoGel as Reported in a Phase 1 Dose Escalation Study

Adverse event	Number of events	Number of patients	Maximum severity per patient
Related to study drug	5	1	Mild
Injection site pain		2	Moderate
		1	Severe
Injection site or tumor site erythema	4	4	Mild
Injection site bruising	1	1	Mild
Post-procedural discharge	1	1	Moderate
Muscle spasm	1	1	Mild

0.5 ng/mL. Only five samples were detectable, and all levels were less than 2 ng/mL. This confirms preclinical data demonstrating localization of paclitaxel at the injection site with minimal systemic exposure.

Indications of OncoGel's efficacy in the management of solid tumors were observed in patients participating in the dose-escalating clinical trial. Following a single-administration, stable disease and tumor regression were observed. Of the 14 patients evaluable by the modified WHO criteria, 6 patients had stable disease and 8 patients had progressive disease at their final assessment. Change in tumor volumes from the smallest reported tumor volume to the final assessment ranged from 56.3% reduction to 232.5% increase in volume (9).

REFERENCES

1. Bhardwaj R, Blanchard J. Controlled-release delivery system for the alpha-MSH analog melanotan-I using poloxamer 407. J Pharm Sci 1996; 85:915–9.
2. Fults KA, Johnston TP. Sustained-release of urease from a poloxamer gel matrix. J Parenter Sci Technol 1990; 44:58–65.
3. Johnston TP, Punjabi MA, Froelich CJ. Sustained delivery of interleukin-2 from a poloxamer 407 gel matrix following intraperitoneal injection in mice. Pharm Res 1992; 9:425–34.
4. Miyazaki S, Ohkawa Y, Takada M, et al. Antitumor effect of pluronic F-127 gel containing mitomycin C on sarcoma-180 ascites tumor in mice. Chem Pharm Bull (Tokyo) 1992; 40:2224–6.
5. Rathi RC, Zentner GM. Biodegradable low molecular weight triblock poly (lactide-co-glycolide) polyethylene glycol copolymers having reverse thermal gelation properties. US Patent 6,004,573, December 21, 1999.
6. Rathi RC, Zentner GM, Jeong B. Biodegradable low molecular weight triblock poly(lactide-co-glycolide) poly-ethylene glycol copolymers having reverse thermal gelation properties. US Patent 6,117,949, September 12, 2000.

7. Rathi RC, Zentner GM, Jeong B. Biodegradable low molecular weight triblock poly(lactide-co-glycolide) polyethylene glycol copolymers having reverse thermal gelation properties. US Patent 6,201,072, March 13, 2001
8. Zentner GM, Rathi R, Shih C, et al. Biodegradable block copolymers for delivery of proteins and water-insoluble drugs. J Control Release 2001; 72:203–15.
9. Vulkelja SJ, Anthony A, Berman BS, et al. Phase 1 study of escalating-dose OncoGel (Paclitaxel/ReGel) depot injection, a controlled-release formulation of paclitaxel, for local management of superficial solid tumor lesions. Anticancer Drugs, 2007; 18(3):283–9.
10. Choi S, Kim SW. Controlled release of insulin from injectable biodegradable triblock copolymer depot in ZDF rats. Pharm Res 2003; 20:2008–10.
11. Masaki T, Rathi R, Zentner G, et al: Inhibition of neointimal hyperplasia in vascular grafts by sustained perivascular delivery of paclitaxel. Kidney Int 2004; 66:2061–9.
12. Samlowski WE, McGregor JR, Jurek M, et al. ReGel polymer-based delivery of interleukin-2 as a cancer treatment. J Immunother 2006; 29:524–35.
13. Matthes K, Mino-Kenudson M, Sahani DV, et al. EUS-guided injection of paclitaxel (OncoGel) provides therapeutic drug concentrations in the porcine pancreas. Gastrointest Endosc 2007; 65(3):448–53.
14. Ognibene FP, Rosenberg SA, Lotze M, et al. Interleukin-2 administration causes reversible hemodynamic changes and left ventricular dysfunction similar to those seen in septic shock. Chest 1988; 94:750–4.
15. Okada H, Toguchi H. Biodegradable microspheres in drug delivery. Crit Rev Ther Drug Carrier Syst 1995; 12:1–99.
16. Ronneberger B, Kao WJ, Anderson JM, et al. In vivo biocompatibility study of ABA triblock copolymers consisting of poly(L-lactic-co-glycolic acid) A blocks attached to central poly(oxyethylene) B blocks. J Biomed Mater Res 1996; 30:31–40.
17. Youxin L, Vollant C, Kissel T. In vitro degradation and bovine serum albumin release of ABA triblock copolymers consisting of poly(L-(+)-lactid acide, or poly(L-(+)-lactid acid-co-glycolid acid) A blocks attached to central polyoxyethylene B-block. J Control Release 1994; 32:121–8.
18. Duncan G, Jess TJ, Mohamed F, et al. The influence of protein solubilisation, conformation and size on the burst release from poly(lactide-co-glycolide) microspheres. J Control Release 2005; 110:34–48.
19. Lee ES, Kwon MJ, Lee H, Kim JJ. Stabilization of protein encapsulated in poly (lactide-co-glycolide) microspheres by novel viscous S/W/O/W method. Intl J Pharmaccutics 2007; 331(1):27–37.
20. Berges R, Bello U. Effect of a new leuprorelin formulation on testosterone levels in patients with advanced prostate cancer. Curr Med Res Opin 2006; 22:649–55.
21. Southard GL, Dunn RL, Garrett S. The drug delivery and biomaterial attributes of the ATRIGEL technology in the treatment of periodontal disease. Expert Opin Investig Drugs 1998; 7:1483–91.

15

The Atrigel® Drug Delivery System

Eric J. Dadey

QLT USA, Inc., Fort Collins, Colorado, U.S.A.

INTRODUCTION

The recent advances in the development and commercialization of the Atrigel® delivery system are presented in this chapter. This implantable depot technology was developed by Dunn and co-workers at Southern Research Institute in Birmingham, Alabama, in 1987 (1) and was subsequently licensed in toto to Vipont Research Laboratories (which became Atrix Laboratories, Inc. in 1989 and then QLT USA, Inc. in 2004). From a composition standpoint, the Atrigel Delivery System consists of a biodegradable polymer dissolved in a biocompatible carrier. An active pharmaceutical ingredient is incorporated into the delivery system and the resulting mixture is injected into the subcutaneous space or into a local site using a standard syringe and needle. After injection and upon contact with body fluids, the polymer precipitates and traps the drug in a solid implant. The drug is then released as the implant undergoes biodegradation.

The Atrigel patent family identifies a number of biodegradable polymersthat can be incorporated in the delivery system and include polyhydroxyacids, polyanhydrides, poly(DL-lactide), and poly(lactide-co-glycolide). In general, these polymers are linear polyesters that undergo biodegradation through ester hydrolysis. In addition, the patents claim N-methyl-2-pyrrolidinone (NMP), triacetin, low-molecular weight polyethylene glycol, propylene carbonate, benzyl alcohol, and other solvents as the biocompatible carrier.

Using the Atrigel delivery system, QLT USA, Inc. has delivered a variety of drugs, ranging from small molecules to recombinant biopharmaceuticals with a duration of drug delivery ranging from 1 week to

6 months. Currently, QLT USA, Inc. has a number of FDA approved products on the market that utilize the Atrigel delivery system, including dental (ATRIDOX® ATRISORB®, and ATRISORB®-D) and pharmaceutical products (ELIGARD® 7.5 mg, ELIGARD® 22.5 mg, ELIGARD® 30 mg, and ELIGARD® 45.0 mg and several in clinical trials).

IMPLANT FORMATION AND DRUG RELEASE

The rate of drug release from Atrigel implants is controlled by a number of interdependent properties of the constituted product. For example, polymer characteristics such as (*i*) the monomer composition, (*ii*) the end-group chemistry, (*iii*) the molecular weight, and (*iv*) the polymer content of the constituted product all play a role in the release kinetics of Atrigel implants. Furthermore, (*i*) the total drug content of the constituted product, (*ii*) the hydrophilicity or hydrophobicity of the carrier, (*iii*) the solubility of the drug, (*iv*) the intermolecular interactions (van der Waals, hydrogen-bonding, and electrostatic interactions) between polymer and drug, and (*iv*) the rate of ester hydrolysis also contribute to drug release. Therefore, an understanding and optimization of these interdependent parameters is required to identify a formulation suitable for clinical development.

In general, the release of drug from Atrigel implants occurs in two stages. The first stage is associated with implant formation and involves the release of drug during the first 24 hours post injection. This initial burst is followed by the second stage during which the implant undergoes systematic biodegradation and releases drug in a linear fashion. This latter period of zero-order kinetics typically correlates to steady-state plasma concentrations of the drug and defines the sustained-release characteristics of the delivery system. Eventually, the implant completely biodegrades which is followed by resolution of the injection site.

RESEARCH AND DEVELOPMENT

Historical experience with this delivery system has demonstrated a complicated in vivo/in vitro correlation. One explanation for this complexity can be attributed to the fluid dynamics present in reservoirs (e.g., phosphate-buffered saline or a simulated biological fluid) as compared to the environment that exists in a tissue or in the subcutaneous space. Biological tissue presents a complex, dynamic environment that consists of many different molecular species and a variety of cell types that are not encountered in a two or three component system typically used for in vitro studies. Furthermore, early studies showed that in vitro release profiles are strongly influenced by such factors as the pH, ionic strength, and the hydrophilicity of the receiving medium. Therefore, the composition of the receiving medium must be selected carefully before an in vitro release profile can be used to predict the in vivo performance of an Atrigel formulation. Because of this complex correlation, formulation development and optimization typically rely on the results from in vivo studies to identify the preferred product.

From an experimental standpoint, selection of a clinical candidate is an iterative process. Various polymer, solvent, drug, and release modifier(s) combinations are injected into the subcutaneous space of rats. At specified time points postdosing, the implants are removed and the residual drug is determined by high performance liquid chromatography. The weight percent of drug released is then calculated by comparing the dose of drug each rat received to the amount of drug remaining in the corresponding implant. From these data, a release profile for each test article is generated. Depending on the slope of this release profile and the intended duration of action, the delivery system is modified to improve the burst and/or to alter the rate of drug release. Through a number of iterations, a formulation that meets the specific product criteria can be identified. Although labor intensive, this implant retrieval method is the most efficient way to identify a clinical candidate.

To date, all commercial Atrigel products exist in a two-syringe product configuration. The delivery system syringe (Syringe A) contains the solution of the biodegradable polymer in NMP. This syringe is filled with a known volume of the delivery system and terminally sterilized by gamma irradiation. For the ELIGARD products, a bulk, aqueous solution of leuprolide acetate is prepared and an aliquot is sterile filtered into syringe B. The syringe is frozen at −86°C and then lyophilized to produce a cake within the polypropylene syringe. The finished product is prepared by packaging both syringes and a needle for injection into a thermoform tray.

At the time of injection, the clinician couples both syringes through the luer-lock ends and the product is constituted by sequentially depressing each plunger and cycling the contents between both syringes. The constituted product is collected in syringe B, the syringes are decoupled, the needle is attached and the product is ready for injection.

From a manufacturing perspective, this two-syringe configuration imparts a number of distinct advantages to the product, especially for complex biologics. The sterile filtration and lyophilization step minimizes the loss of drug and increases shelf-life as compared to other sustained-release products in which the drug is incorporated into the delivery system during manufacture. Furthermore, storage of a sterile, active pharmaceutical ingredient as a lyophilized cake imparts a higher degree of stability to the drug as compared to a drug that is compounded in a specific dosage form.

REGULATORY CONSIDERATIONS

The safety of the poly(DL-lactide) and poly(lactide-co-glycolide) polymers has been studied extensively for the last 35 years and has been reported in the literature (4–6). Furthermore, the safety and toxicity profiles of NMP following parenteral and oral administration have been established (7–9). More importantly, regulatory agencies worldwide have reviewed the safety data for the combination of the biodegradable polymers and NMP and have approved their use as a sustained-release delivery system. Taken as a whole, it appears that the Atrigel delivery system is safe for use in a broad range of potential applications.

COMPETITIVE ADVANTAGES OF THE ATRIGEL® DELIVERY SYSTEM

The Atrigel delivery system offers a number of distinct advantages over currently available parenteral, sustained-release technologies. For example, the Atrigel products combine into a single, proven, and FDA-approved delivery platform (*i*) the duration of action of microspheres without the complex manufacturing process, (*ii*) the low cost and sustained-release properties of thermoreversible gels without the need for additional safety and toxicological testing of the delivery system, (*iii*) the flexibility to deliver actives over a wider range of duration of action than other in situ-forming implants, and (*iv*) the ability to remove the implant should an adverse event occur without the need for implantation with a trochar as for injectable solid implants.

The clinical benefit of the Atrigel delivery system can be appreciated from a comparison of clinical performance of three ELIGARD products. The pharmacokinetic and pharmacodynamic profiles of the 1-, 3-, and 6-month products are shown below. Figure 1 summarizes the results of the first 90 days of a 6-month open-label clinical study to evaluate the 1-month ELIGARD product in 20 patients diagnosed with adenocarcinoma of the prostate (8). Figure 2 presents the results from a 6-month clinical study to assess the safety, efficacy, and pharmacokinetics of the 3-month ELIGARD product in 117 patients (9) and Figure 3 illustrates the results from a 12-month clinical study to evaluate the performance of the 6-month ELIGARD formulation in 111 patents diagnosed with adenocarcinoma of the prostate (10). The results show that each formulation provided measurable levels of leuprolide acetate over the intended duration of action and that these levels were sufficient to suppress testosterone at or below FDA-defined serum testosterone castrate levels of 50 ng/dL. Moreover, the pharmacokinetic profiles show that serum leuprolide levels did not accumulate in the systemic circulation following chronic administration and that the steady-state serum levels were constant following multiple doses. These results show that the Atrigel delivery system can provide therapeutic levels of leuprolide acetate for 1, 3, and 6 months and by extension, can be used to develop long-acting formulations of other therapeutic agents.

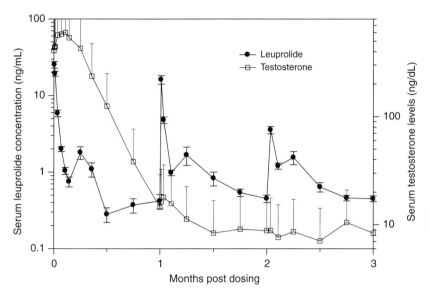

Figure 1 Pharmacokinetic and pharmacodynamic profiles of the 1-month ELIGARD® 7.5 mg product.

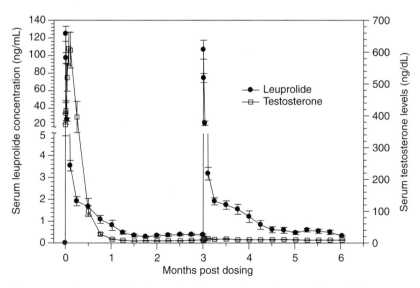

Figure 2 Pharmacokinetic and pharmacodynamic profiles of the 3-month ELIGARD® 22.5 mg product.

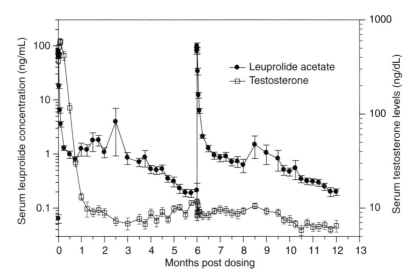

Figure 3 Pharmacokinetic and pharmacodynamic profiles of the 6-month ELIGARD® 45 mg product.

FUTURE DIRECTIONS

Currently, the commercial Atrigel products focus on the delivery of doxycycline to the periodontal pocket or the delivery of leuprolide acetate to the systemic circulation; however, future directions will expand the technology into site-specific delivery. For example, recent studies have shown that the Atrigel delivery system may be suitable for the sustained release of drugs to the eye. Preclinical studies in rabbits demonstrated that Atrigel implants were well tolerated and produced minimal and transient local effects following intravitreal, subconjunctival, and subtenon injection (11,12). Subsequent implant retrieval studies with a long-acting formulation of octreotide, an eight amino acid peptide, showed that the release profiles from intravitreal or subtenon implants were consistent with the release profile observed for subcutaneous implants. Furthermore, bioanalysis of the retina and choroid demonstrated measurable levels of octreotide for 90 days following both routes of ocular administration. These results strongly suggest that the Atrigel delivery system can be used for the local delivery of drugs to the eye.

CONCLUSIONS

Over the past decade, the Atrigel delivery system has matured from the conceptual and preclinical phase into an established sustained-release technology with approved products. Safety issues with regard to the polymers and to *N*-methyl-2-pyrrolidinone were reviewed by regulatory agencies worldwide and found acceptable for parenteral administration. It is anticipated that the flexibility of the technology coupled with the increasing need for biodegradable, sustained-release parenteral dosage forms for complex biologics will insure the commercial success of Atrigel-based products for the foreseeable future.

REFERENCES

1. Dunn RL, English JP, Cowsar DR, Vanderbilt DP. Biodegradable in situ forming implants and methods of producing the same. US Patent 4,938,763, 1990.
2. Gourlay SJ, Rice RM, Hegyeli AF, et al. Biocompatibility testing of polymers: in vivo implantation studies. Biomed Mater Res 1978; 12:219–32.
3. Cutright DE, Hunsuck EE. Tissue reaction to the biodegradable polylactic acid suture. Oral Surg 1971; 31:134–9.
4. Visscher GE, Robison RL, Argentieri GL. Tissue response to biodegradable injectable microcapsules. J Biomat Appl 1987; 2:118–31.
5. Akesson B. Nordic experts group for criteria documentation for health risks to chemicals. N-Methyl-2-pyrrolidinone (NMP). Arbete och Halsa 1994; 40:1–24.
6. Lee KP, Chromey C, Culik R. Toxicity of N-methyl-2-pyrrolidinone (NMP): teratogenic, subchronic and two-year inhalation studies. Fund Appl Toxicol 1987; 9:222–35.
7. Becci PJ, Gephart LA, Koschier FJ, Johnson WD. Subchronic feeding study in beagle dogs of N-methyl-2-pyrrolidinone. J Appl Toxicol 1982; 2:73–76.
8. Perez-Marreno R, Chu FM, Gleason D, Loizides E, Wachs B, Tyler RC. A six-month open-label study assessing a new formulation of Leuprolide 7.5 mg for suppression of testosterone in patients with prostate cancer. Clin Therapeut 2002; 24(11):1902–14.
9. Chu FM, Jayson M, Dineen MK, Perez R, Harkway R, Tyler RC. A clinical study of 22.5 MG LA-2550: A new subcutaneous depot delivery system for leuprolide acetate for the treatment of prostate cancer. J Urol 2002; 168(3): 1199–203.
10. Crawford ED, Sartor O, Chu F, Perez R, Karlin G, Garrett JS. A new 6-month subcutaneous delivery system for Leuprolide acetate for the treatment of prostate cancer. J Urol 2006; 175:533–6.
11. Margaron P, Li R, Im S, et al. Evaluation of Octreotide/Atrigel® sustained-release formulation administered intravitreally or in the sub-tenon space in the rabbit. In Proceedings of the Annual Meeting, Association for Research in Vision and Ophthalmology, Fort Lauderdale, FL, April 30–May 4, 2006.
12. Dadey E, Margaron P, Li R, et al. The compatibility and utility of the Atrigel® drug delivery system for the sustained-release of drugs to the eye. In: Proceedings of the 2nd Annual Ophthalmic Drug Development & Delivery Summit, September 19–20, San Diego, CA, 2006.

16

Enhancing Drug Delivery by Chemical Modification

Mimoun Ayoub, Christina Wedemeyer, and Torsten Wöhr
Genzyme Pharmaceuticals, Liestal, Switzerland

INTRODUCTION

Developing physiologically active substances into pharmaceutical drugs is a challenge with many obstacles, despite recent progress in the design of drug delivery systems. The therapeutic potential of hit and lead compounds is often limited due to poor oral bioavailability, short circulation half-life, and/or a generally diminished ability to penetrate biological barriers. There is a growing body of literature proposing chemical modification and prodrug concepts for overcoming several typical limitations of early drug development candidates, a selection of which is discussed in this chapter.

The prodrug design aims to modulate the physicochemical characteristics of a particular bioactive substance through structural modification, resulting in improved formulation properties and enhanced bioavailability (1). Most importantly, the modification is designed to be reversible under physiological conditions. Passive proteolysis, or enzymatic degradation, of the prodrug releases the parent molecule at the site of therapeutic action. In addition, the following parameters need to be considered when designing prodrugs:

- chemical stability under drug formulation conditions;
- chemical compatibility with drug delivery systems;
- modifying solubility for improved pharmacological properties;
- improved permeability through biological barriers, e.g., through the cell membrane;
- biodegradability of the prodrug conjugate and the pro-component.

Prodrugs are a result of reversible chemical modifications leading to improved physiochemical properties (1). The resulting prodrugs show enhanced stability and improved bioavailability. They are designed to biodegrade under the release of the parent drug, ideally only after having reached their target. Drug stability and pharmacokinetics considerations thus need to be carefully balanced. The prodrug concept is illustrated in Figure 1.

Some of the most promising and thus widely investigated conjugation approaches are highlighted in the following:

- phosphorylation,
- lipidization/lipid conjugation,
- esterifications,
- pegylations,
- glycosylations,
- cell penetrating peptides (CPPs).

PHOSPHORYLATED PRODRUGS

The use of phosphate, phosphonate and phosphinate moieties in prodrug design goes back to the early 1960s, when phosphates containing nucleoside analogues were used as cancer therapeutics. Phosphorylation offers a versatile method for modulating polarity, charge distribution, and the isoelectric point of the active ingredient. Suboptimal electric properties may negatively impact transmembrane delivery and thus therapeutic efficacy.

The phosphorylation of hydroxyl functions may also help in overcoming low solubility issues, particularly with hydrophobic substances. In the case of the Echinocandin lipopeptide, which is a cyclic peptidomimetic,

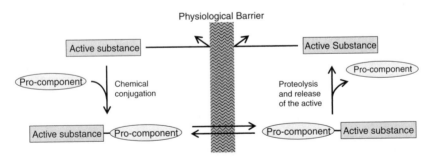

Figure 1 The reversible conjugation to the prodrug enables the transport across the physiological barrier. The peptide is released at its target site of action.

phosphorylation of the hydroxyl function of the tyrosine residue resulted in a prodrug with improved aqueous solubility, excellent hydrolytic stability, and only marginally diminished potency (3). On the other hand, passive diffusion through cell membranes is usually impeded for highly ionized drugs (2). This disadvantage can be reversed by esterification of the phosphate moiety, i.e., by neutralizing the negative phosphate charges. The result is a phosphate ester prodrug with increased stability towards endogenous phosphatases and improved cell membrane permeability (Fig. 2). Cell membrane permeability and enzymatic stability can be further altered by varying the phosphate ester function.

Montgomery et al. reported lower biological activity for the phosphate monoester than for the corresponding diester analogue due to its lower bioavailability. The phosphate diester proved to be more resistant to early enzymatic degradation and demonstrated improved cell membrane permeability (4). Furthermore, arylphosphate esters exhibited poor cell membrane permeability, presumably due to early hydrolysis of the aryl group. The impact of various alkyl phosphate esters has been investigated by McGuigan for AZT-phosphate analogues (Fig. 3). The study revealed higher activity

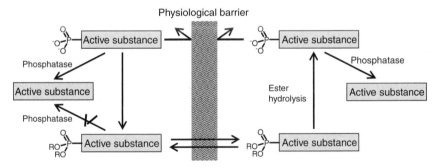

Figure 2 The phosphate charges are neutralized by esterification for enhanced cell uptake.

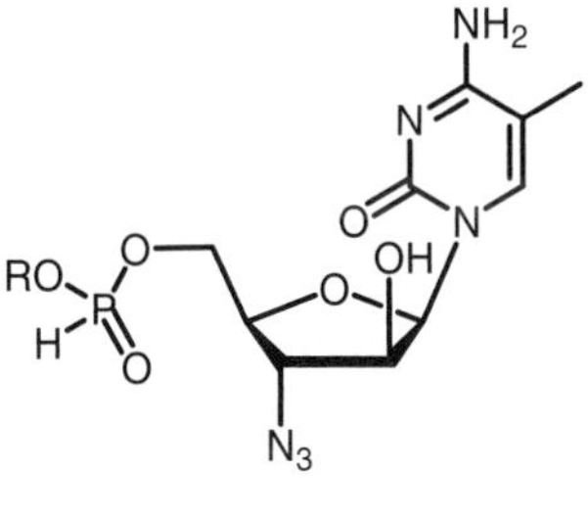

Figure 3 AZT analogues, investigation of the ester alkyl chain length on biological activity. R = Me, Et, *n*-heptyl, *n*-$C_{18}H_{37}$.

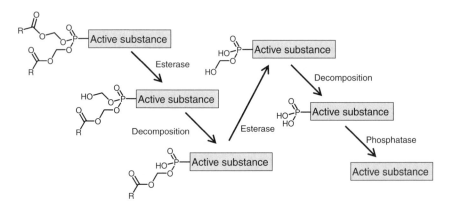

Figure 4 Degradation sequence of acyloxyalkylester prodrugs.

for short alkyl chains (< 7 carbons) than for the corresponding longer chain analogues (5).

An elegant phosphorylation strategy was proposed by Farquhar et al. for a series of molecules which have been transformed into acyloxyalkyl phosphate ester prodrugs (Fig. 4) with good cell permeation properties (6,7).

The first acylester group is cleaved through esterase activity resulting in labile hydroxylmethyl metabolite, which spontaneously decomposes into formaldehyde and a mono acyloxyalkylester intermediate. The latter undergoes the same reaction sequence leading to the dihydro phosphate analogue. The acylester phosphate prodrug strategy was applied to several antiviral therapeutics (7).

Further examples of phosphorylated prodrugs can be found in the comprehensive literature review article by Krise and Stell (8).

LIPID CONJUGATES

Polar groups of a bioactive substance promote hydrogen bonding and solvation in aqueous solutions, and exhibit concomitantly low lipid solubility leading to cell membrane permeability properties. The effect of hydrogen bond acceptors and donors can be suppressed to a certain extent by chemical conjugation. Covalently bound lipophilic groups such as fatty acids or phospholipids may increase lipid solubility and facilitate passive transport through the membrane bilayer. The resulting compound may also exhibit a lower charge density if the conjugation involves ionisable groups of the drug substance. This modification strategy increased the lipid solubility for several compounds described in the literature, e.g., kyotropin analogue (10), tyrotropin releasing hormone (11), and γ aminobutyric acid (12).

The charge distribution and density profile can be of particular importance for the delivery of peptide drugs. Some conjugation strategies for the carboxyl group of the glutamic acid residue and the positively charged amino function of the lysine side chain are depicted in Figure 5.

Lipidization is also a promising modification strategy for extending the circulation half-life of a drug substance. In the case of liraglutide, a 32-residue long glucagon-like peptide analogue in development for type 2 diabetes, palmitoylation of the lysine residue in position 20 increased the half-life from 1–2 hours to 12 hours (9). The conjugated peptide was designed to be protected against DPPIV enzymatic degradation and elimination by the kidneys, resulting in a prolonged half-life and sustained insulin stimulation.

ESTERIFICATION

Ester conjugates can be obtained either by esterification of a carboxylic group, or alternatively, by acetylation of a hydroxyl function of the active substance (Table 1 lists the commonly used, low molecular weight pro-components). Either way, the result is a less hydrophilic prodrug substance. Esterification with structurally simple pro-components is often used in the design of orally administered prodrug substances. However, the increased

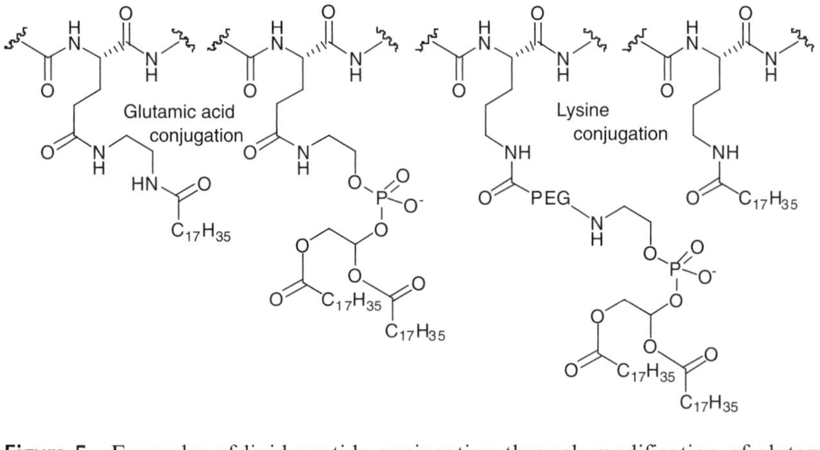

Figure 5 Examples of lipid-peptide conjugation through modification of glutamic acid and lysine residues.

Table 1   Common Pro-Components for the Esterification of Hydroxyl, Carboxyl and Amino Functions

Hydroxyl function 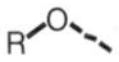	Carboxyl function 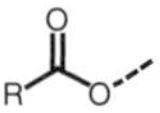	Amino function 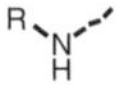

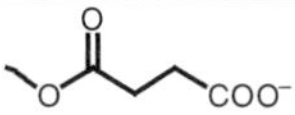

hemisuccinate (15)   cholinyl acetate   N-alkyloxycarboxamid (19)

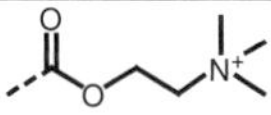

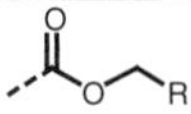

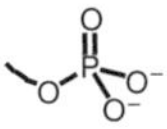

phosphate (16)   γ-dimethylamino acetates   phosphorylmethyl oxycarboxamid (20)

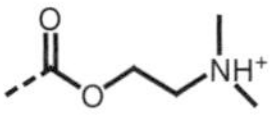

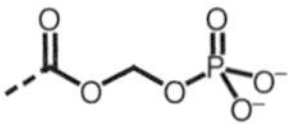

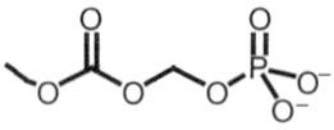

phosphorylmethyl oxycarbonate   amide linked amino acids (18)   amid linked amino acids (21)

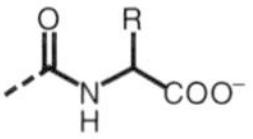

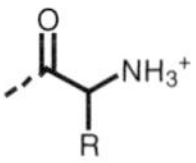

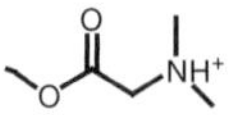

dimethylaminoacetate

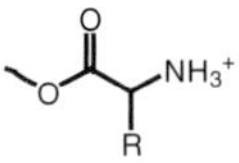

aminoacetate (17)

absorption and bioavailability of such prodrugs needs to be coordinated with the drug release kinetics. The ester group masking the carboxylic acid or hydroxyl function of the parent drug is cleaved by passive hydrolysis or by esterases.

Sibrafiban, an amidoxime ester double prodrug of a low molecular weight glycoprotein (GP)-IIb/IIIa antagonist, showed in mice a 20-fold increase in absorption compared to the parent substance (Fig. 6). The commercial drug benazepril is the ethyl ester prodrug form of the active

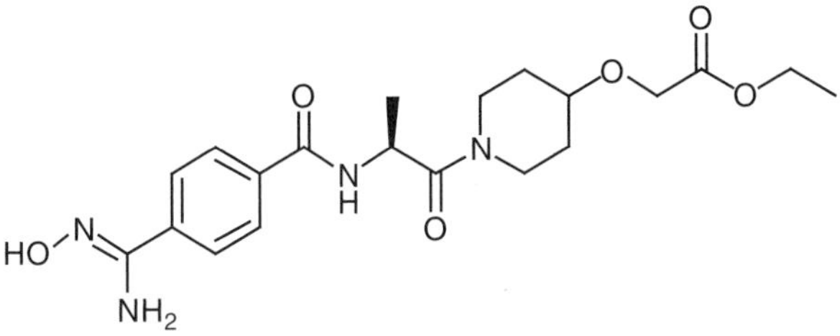

Figure 6 Sibrafiban, a double prodrug.

benazeprilat with increased oral bioavailability. Upon cleavage of the ester, the angiotensin-converting enzyme inhibiting benazeprilat is released in its hydrophylic dicarboxylat form (13). Furthermore, esterification of the tyrosine hydroxyl function of desmopressin, a vasopressing agonist, demonstrated improved bioavailablity of the parent cyclic nonameric peptide drug (14).

An interesting variation of ester prodrugs has been recently reported for peptide actives. The concept is based on the reversible insertion of an ester bond in the peptide backbone whereby the ester is formed by the hydroxyl function of the threonine or serine side chain and the carboxylic group of the preceding residue leading to the corresponding isopeptide structure (Fig. 7). Spontaneous O to N acyl transfer restores the thermodynamically more stable amid bond. In the literature, isopeptides are therefore also referred to as switch-peptides (22). The isopeptide backbone modification disrupts secondary structures and prevents peptide self-assembly, which in the case of γ-strand forming peptides, may improve its solvation and solubility properties. This effect is amplified by the presence of the ionisable amino function in the isopeptide form. Interestingly, the switch from the prodrug form to the bioactive native peptide is triggered by esterase activity. The kinetics for this O,N acyl migration have been investigated for

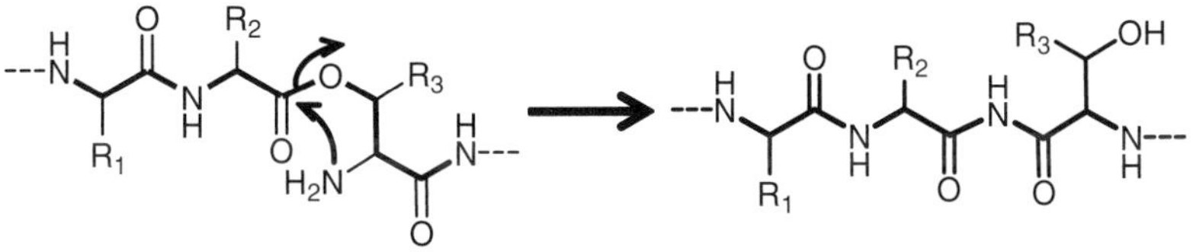

Figure 7 Transformation of isopeptides into bioactive peptide drugs via O,N acyl migration.

primary and secondary amino groups in cyclosporin A isopeptides and shown to be considerably slower for secondary amine groups (24).

The primary objectives of peptide prodrug designs are to prevent early enzymatic degradation and to facilitate the inherently limited permeation through biological barriers, particularly through the intestinal mucosa of orally administered peptide drugs. Prevention from early degradation can be achieved by chemical modifications interfering with molecular substrate/enzyme recognition. The modification is typically introduced N-terminally.

An interesting modification of the N-terminus has been reported (Fig. 8) by Amsberry and Borchardt (25). The strategy involves the esterolysis of the prodrug followed by the spontaneous lactonization of the procomponent. This concept has been extended into the design of end-to-end cyclized peptide pro-drugs (26). The pharmacological benefits of peptide cyclization include generally higher serum stability and improved bioavailability.

Interesting peptide produgs can also be obtained by a simple condensation reaction of the terminal amino function with suitable aldehydes and ketones. The resulting condensation products are either 4-imidazolidinone ring systems (27) or the enamine precursors (Fig. 9) (28). Both product types can be considered for prolonging the pharmacological effect of the

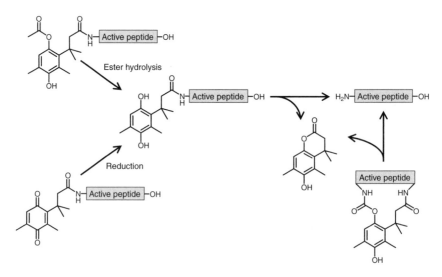

Figure 8 Peptide N-terminus modification proposed by Borchardt et al. Ester cleavage and in situ lactonization of the pro-components releases the biologically active peptide. *Source*: From Refs. 25, 26.

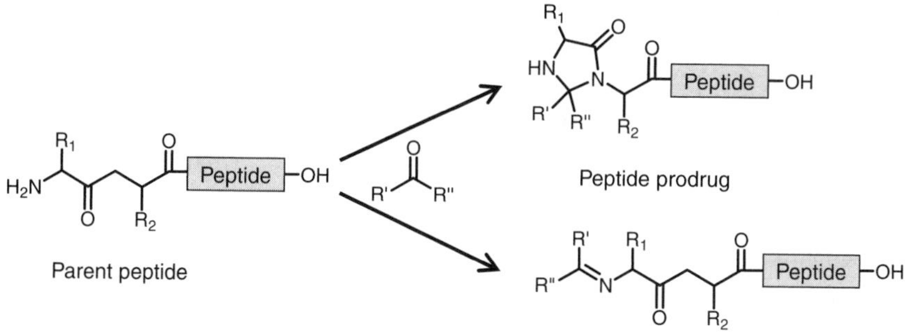

Figure 9 4-imidazolidinone and enamine peptide prodrugs.

parent peptide drug. This modification concept has been used for design of carboxypeptidase and endopeptidase resistant peptide prodrugs.

POLYMER CONJUGATION

Polymer conjugation is an interesting approach for prolonging the circulation time in the body, particularly of biologics and peptides. The increased molecular weight and bulky polymeric surface of such conjugates decrease drug elimination and enzymatic degradation rates. The advantages are less frequent or lower dose administrations, which ultimately may improve the safety profile of the drug. Alternatively, disadvantages such as low cell permeability and a possibly compromised functionality of the polymer drug conjugate limit the applicability of the approach, e.g., for targeting intracellular cancer targets.

Both naturally occurring and fully synthetic polymer components have been proposed in the literature for drug modifications. Examples include: transferrin (45), albumin (46), N-(2-hydroxypropyl)methacrylamide copolymer (47), elastin-like polypeptides (48), and various macromolecular carbohydrates (49). Most recently, the use of folate-conjugated micelle copolymers has been successfully tested in animal studies for carrying the approved anticancer agent adriamycin into cells while minimizing dose-dependent toxic effects of the drug (31).

PEGylation is one of the most thoroughly investigated drug modification approaches. This non-immunogenic, FDA approved methodology has been applied to peptide drugs, biologics and other substance classes using either polyethylene glycol (PEG) or methoxypolyethylene glycol polymers. The stabilizing and long-acting effect of PEG polymers enabled the development of a number of commercial drugs including Oncospar, PEG-Intron (32), Pegasys (33) Somavert, and Amgen's recently approved NeulastaR (granulocytes colony stimulating factor). Other PEGylated peptides, recombinant proteins, and antibody agents are currently in the development pipeline.

The bulky PEG chain shields the drug substance from enzymatic degradation without increasing the immunogenicity risk substantially, as long as the molecular weight of PEG averages in a low range. In fact, the half-life of the drug substance, and thus its inherent toxicity properties, are a function of the PEG molecular weight. A longer PEG moiety may extend the half-life of the drug conjugate, whereas drugs with low molecular weight PEG units are clearly more quickly from the circulation system. The regio/ chemo selective introduction of the PEG chain is a critical step in the development of a scalable drug substance manufacturing process (34). The development of an effective preparative HPLC purification protocol can be particularly challenging.

A number of suitable PEG conjugation synthesis approaches have been reported over the past few years (50). There is a number of commercially available PEG-reagents which are suitable for peptide or protein modifications via an amide, ester, thioester, carbamate, or carbonate linkage. One of the most commonly used reactions is that of an amino function with an activated PEG polymer N-hydroxysuccinimid ester (Fig. 10).

CELL PENETRATING PEPTIDES

Peptide drug development has become a focus again for many pharmaceutical and biotech companies over the last few years. The trend is supported by recent advances in peptide drug delivery, substantially reduced large-scale production costs, and fundamental research in endocrinology and immunology. Peptide drugs have been, and still are, developed to address antiviral and antimicrobial infections, oncology, cardiovascular diseases, obesity, allergies, metabolic diseases, and other therapeutic areas. Today, peptides are recognized as one of the most useful drug classes with enormous potential for chemical diversity which can be readily accessed and exploited for the design of highly potent and target selective low-dose drug candidates. On the other hand, low chemical and physical stability in conjunction with an inherently low bioavailability typically confine

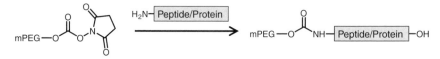

Figure 10 N-PEGylation of peptides and proteins using succinimidic active esters.

the application of peptide drugs to the treatment of severe diseases. These limitations lead to the development of numerous peptidomimetics of endogenous peptides and hormones with increased enzymatic and physical stability. A particularly interesting approach for improving bio-availability and cell penetration properties of peptide drugs in discussed in the following.

The membrane permeability of peptide drugs highly depends on sequence charge density and distribution. In general, peptides prepared and administered in their zwitter-ionic form with intramolecular base–acid parings exhibit higher trans-membrane diffusion rates in comparison to conventional salt forms. Naturally, the ionization state and global net charge of a given peptide is a function of the medium pH, which offers a simple but attractive route for improving the "drugability" of a bioactive peptide. This finding is the basis for the research on CPPs.

More than 100 cell penetrating peptide and protein sequences descri-bed in the literature to date can be potentially used as cell membrane pen-etrating drug carrier systems (35). Most CPPs have amphiphilic properties (with exceptions of poly arginine and poly lysines sequences) and carry several positive charges at the physiological pH. They can be classified in three different categories:

■ Protein transduction domain sequences are short proteinogenic sequences, which may initiate the cell internalization of the protein. The HIV-1 TAT-protein transduction domain is one of the best-described examples (36).
■ Rationally designed amphiphilic peptides with structural features similar to naturally occurring CPPs.
■ Chimeric peptides consisting of an hydrophilic peptide strand interacting with its hydrophobic counterpart (peptide design derived from different CPPs).

Chassaing and Prochiantz reported the first CPP, penetratin (37), more than a decade ago. The internalization mechanism of CPPs is still under investigation. Several mechanism models have been postulated. It appears that the CPPs bind to the cell surface by electrostatic interactions between the positive charges of the CPP and the phosphate groups of the lipidic bilayer (38). Endocytosis is also strongly suggested as a translocation mechanism.

The drug (cargo), to be transported into the cell, is attached to the CPP by means of covalent bonds such as disulphide bridge linkages between thiol functions of cysteine side chains, which are readily cleaved in the reductive environment of the cell. Alternatively, the CPP sequence can be conjugated to the bioactive peptide by simple amid and ester bonds, as well as through bi-functional (labile) linker systems (38,39) (Fig. 11).

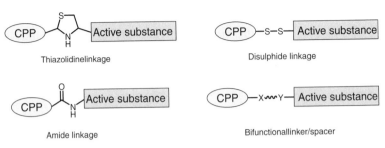

Figure 11 Commonly used conjugation systems for peptide drugs and CPPs. *Abbreviation*: CPPs, cell penetrating peptides.

Of particular interest are reversible conjugation systems that degrade after cell penetration under the release of the bioactive substance. The successful transport of DNA fragments, proteins and even phages could be achieved using CPPs conjugations.

In the case of CNS targeted drugs, the use of transport vector concepts may result in improved delivery rates across the blood–brain barrier (BBB). The transport strategy for CNS delivery is very similar to the CPP-transport methodology discussed above. Again, the drug substance is linked to a known BBB-crossing moiety, e.g., by receptor-mediated endocytosis, and the conjugate linker system can be designed to degrade as soon as the drug crosses the delivery barrier. This conjugation technology has been discussed in detail for peptide and protein drugs in previous review articles (40–42).

OTHER CHEMICAL MODIFICATIONS

The prodrug concept is not limited to the methodologies presented above. There are many other interesting chemical modification strategies described in the literature including glycosylation, which has been shown to increase membrane permeability and degradation stability (43). The glycosylated deltorphin analogues exhibiting an improved analgesic efficacy profile are mentioned here as an example (44).

The regio-selective insertion of threonine-derived ring systems, also known as pseudo-prolines, has been proposed for the reversible chemical modification of cyclosporine C, a co-metabilite of the immunosuppressant drug cyclosporine A (Fig. 12). The stability of the introduced oxazolidine ring system highly depend on the nature of the ring substituents in position C(2) of the ring system (51). Furthermore, the oxazolidine ring system exerts a temporary distortion on the bioactive cyclosporine

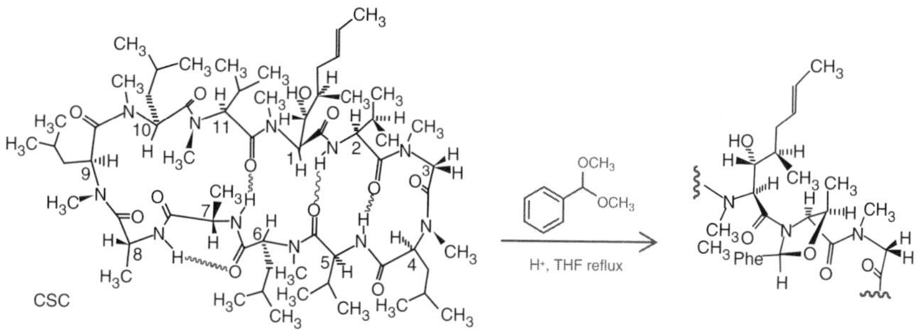

Figure 12 Acid labile modification of cyclosporine C by direct N,O acetylation of the threonine residue.

conformation, which represents an additional dimension to the prodrug design concept.

Years of extensive research in prodrug modification resulted in numerous drug delivery concepts, which are of particular interest for the modification of small molecule therapeutics. Recent peptide and protein drug development trends created a rebirth of the prodrug delivery concept. Today, the drug discovery and optimization process is mainly focused on maximizing potency and selectivity. Drug product formulation and delivery questions are usually not considered until later in the early drug development stages. We believe there is tremendous potential for improving the "drugability" of a lead compound and thus mitigating the pharmaceutical drug development risk, provided these chemical modification concepts are taken into consideration in early development stages.

REFERENCES

1. Bundgaard H. Design of Prodrugs. New York: Elsevier, 1985.
2. Posternk T. Ann Rev Pharmacol 1974; 14:23–33; Lichtenstein J, Barner HD, Cohen SS. J Biol Chem 1960; 235:457–65; Leibman KC, Heidlberger C. J Biol Chem 1995; 216:823–30; Roll PM, Weinfeld H, Caroll E, Braun GB. J Biol Chem 1956; 220:439–54.
3. Balkovec JM, Blak RM, Hammond MJ, et al. J Med Chem 1992; 35:194–8.
4. Montgomery JA, Schabel FM Jr, Skipper HE. Cancer Res 1962; 22:504–9.
5. McGuigan C, Bellevergue P, Jones BCNM, et al. Antiviral Chem Chemother 1994; 5:271–7.
6. Farquhar D, Srivastva DN, Kutesch NJ, Suanders PP. J Pharm Sci 1983; 72: 324–5.
7. McGuigan C, Nickson C, Petrik J, Karpas A. FEBS Lett 1992; 310:171–4; Lyer RP, Phillips LR, Biddle JA, et al. Tetrahedron Lett 1989; 30:7141–44;

Farquhar D. Proc Am Assoc Cancer Res 1985; 26:248; Starret JEJ, Tortolani DR, Hitchcock MJM, et al. Antiviral Res 1992; 19:267–73; Sastry JK, Nehete PN, Khan S, et al. Mol Pharmacol 1992; 41:441–5; Freed JJ, Farquhar D, Hampton A. Biochem Pharmacol 1989; 38:3193–8; Srinivas RV, Robbins BL, Connelly MC, et al. Antimicrob Agents Chemother 1993; 37: 2247–50.

8.   Krise JP, Stella VJ. Adv Drug Deliv Rev 1996; 19:287–310.

9.   Knudsen LB, Nielsen PF, Huusfeldt PO, et al. J Med Chem 2000; 43(9): 1664–69.

10. Chen P, Bodor N, Wu WM, Prokai L. J Med Chem 1998; 41:3773–81.

11. Muranishi S, Sakai A, Yamada K, Muratam MI, Takada K, Kiso Y. Pharm Res 1991; 8:649–52.

12. Shashoua VE, Jacob JN, Ridge R, Campbell A, Baldessarini RJ. J Med Chem 1984; 27:659–64.

13. Kim JS, Oberle DA, Krummel DA, Dressman JB, Fleisher D. J Pharm Sci 1994; 83:1350–56.

14. Kahns AH, Buur A, Bundgaard H. Pharm Res 1993; 10:68–74.

15. Takata J, Karube Y, Nagata Y, Matsushima Y. J Pharm Sci 1995; 84:96–98.

16. Varia SA, Schuller S, Stella VJ. J Pharm Sci 1984; 73:1074–80.

17. Fleisher D, Johnson KC, Strewart BH, Amidon GL. J Pharm Sci 1986; 75:934–9.

18. Pochopin NL, Charman WN, Stella VJ. Int J Pharm 1994; 105:169–76.

19. Nielsen LS, Slok F, Bundgaard H. Int J Pharm 1994; 102:231–9.

20. Safadi M, Oliyai R, Stella VJ. Pharm Res 1993; 10:1350–5.

21. Sakamoto F, Ikeda S, Tzukamoto G. Chem Pharm Bull 1984; 32:2241–8; Kakeya N, Nishizawa S, Nishimura KI, et al. J Antibiot 1985; 38:380–9; Beauchamp LM, Orr GF, DeMiranda P, et al. Antivir Chem Chemother 1992; 3:157–64; DeMiranda P, Burnette T. Drug Metab Dispos 1994; 22:55–8; Bentley S, Soul-Lawton J, Rolan P. Int Conf AIDS 1994; 10:127.

22. Dos Santos S, Chandravarkar A, Mandal B, et al. Biopolymers 2005; 80(4):568; Dos Santos S, Chandravarkar A, Mandal B, et al. J Amer Chem Soc 2005; 127 (34):11888–9; Oliyai R, Safadi M, Meier PG, et al. Int J Pept Prot Res 1994; 43: 239–47; Oliyai R, Stella VJ. Pharm Res 1992; 9:617–22; Oliyai R, Siahaan T, Stella VJ. Pharm Res 1995; 12:1–7 .

23. Bundgaard H, Friis GJ. Int J Pharm 1992; 82:85–90.

24. Hurley TR, Colson CE, Hicks G, Ryan MJ. J Med Chem 1993; 36:1496–8; Oliyai R, Stella VJ. Bioorg Med Chem Lett 1995; 5:2735–40.

25. Amsberry KL, Borchardt RT. J Org Chem 1990; 55:5867–77; Amsberry KL, Borchardt RT. Pharm Res 1991; 8:323–30; Amsberry KL, Gerstenberger AE, Borchardt RT. Pharm Res 1991; 8:455–61.

26. Gangwar S, Pauletti GM, Siahaan TJ, Vander Velde DG, Stella VJ, Borchardt RT. 210th ACS Annual Meeeting, August 20–24, Chicago, 1995.

27. Rasmussen GJ, Bundgaard H. Int J Pharm 1991; 76:113–22.

28. Nishihata T, Kunieda S. Preparation of enamine derivatives of peptides as prodrugs. Jpn Kokai Tokkyo Koho, 1994; 10.

29. Ni S, Stephenson SM, Lee RJ. Anticancer Res 2002; 22:2131–5.

30. Lu Y, Low PS. Adv Drug Deliv Rev 2002; 54:675–93.

31. Bae Y and Kataoka K., J Control Release 2006; 116(2):49–50.
32. Glue P, Rouzier-Panis R, Raffanel C, et al. Hepathology 2000; 32:647–53.
33. Zenzem S, Feinman SV, Rasenack J, et al. European Association for the Study of Liver, Annual meeting, Rotterdam, 2000.
34. Hooftman G, Herman S, Schacht EJ. Bioact Comp Pol 1996; 11:135–59.
35. Zorko M, Langel Ü. Adv Drug Deliv Rev 2005; 54(4):529–45.
36. Vivés E, Richard JP, Rispal C, Lebleu B. Curr Protein Pept Sci 2003; 4:125–32 (and herein cited literature); Vivés E, Lebleu B. Cell-penetrating Pept Proc Appl CRC Press USA: Boca Raton 2002; 3–21.
37. Derossi D, Joliot AH, Chassaing G, Prochiantz A. J Biol Chem 1994; 269:10444–50; Derossi D, Calvet S, Tremblau A, et al. Biol Chem 1996; 271: 18188–93.
38. Pooga M, Hällbrink M, Zorko M, Langel Ü. FASEB J 1998; 12:67–77; Soomets U, Lindren M, Gallet X, et al. Biohim Biophys Acta 2000; 1467: 165–176; Boufioux O, Basyn F, Rezsohazy R, Brasseur R. Cell-penetrating Pept Proc Appl CRC Press USA: Boca Raton 2002; 187–222.
39. Pooga M, Soomets U, Hällbrinnk M, et al. Nat Biotech 1998; 16:857–61.
40. Bickel U, Yoskikawa T, Pardridge PM. Adv Drug Deliv Rev 2001; 46:247–79; Pardridge WM. Adv Drug Deliv Rev 1999; 36:299–321; Pardridge WM, Boado RJ, Kang YS. Proc Natl Acad Sci USA 1995; 92:5592–6; Zlokovic BV. Pharm Res 1995; 12:1395–406.
41. Chbrier PE, Roubert P, Braquet P. Proc Natl Acad Sci USA 1987; 84:2078–81; Frank HJ, Pardridge WM. Diabetes 1981; 30:757–61; Frank HJ, Pardridge WM, Morris WL, Rosenfeld RG, Choi TB. Diabetes 1986; 35:654–61; Smith KR, Kato A, Borchardt RT. Biochem Biophys Res Comm 1988; 157:308–14; Speth RC, Harik SI. Proc Natl Acad Sci USA 1985; 82:6340–3.
42. Friden PM. Neurosurgery 1994; 35:294–8; Granholm AC, Backman C, Bloom F, et al. J Pharm Exp Ther 1994; 268:448–59; Pardridge WM, Kang YS, Buciak JL, Pharm Res 1994; 11:738–46; Zhang Y, Pardridge WM. Brain Res 2001; 889:49–56; Zhang Y, Pardridge WM. Stroke 2001; 32:1378–84.
43. Powell MF, Stewart T, Otvo L, et al. Pharm Res 1993; 10:1268–73.
44. Negri L, Lattanzi R, Tabacco F, et al. Med Chem 1999; 42:400-4; Tomatis R, Marastoni M, Balboni G, et al. Med Chem 1997; 40:2948–52.
45. Kratz F, Beyer U, Roth T, et al. Pharm Sci 1998; 87(3):338–46.
46. Kratz F, Muller-Driver R, Hofmann I, Drevs J, Unger CJ. Med Chem 2000; 43(7):1253–6.
47. Minko T, Kopeckova P, Kopecek J. Int J Cancer 2000; 86:1–10.
48. Furgeson D, Dreher M, Chilkoti A. J Control Release 2006; 110:362–9.
49. Fujita F, Koike M, Sakamoto Y, et al. Clin Cancer Res 2005; 11:1650–7.
50. Veronese FM, Pasut G. Drug Discovery Today 2005; 10:1415–58.
51. Keller M, Wöhr T, Dumy P, Patiny L, Mutter MC. Chem Eur J 2000; 6: 4358–63.

17

DepoFoam® Multivesicular Liposomes for the Sustained Release of Macromolecules

William J. Lambert and Kathy Los

Pacira Pharmaceuticals, Inc., San Diego, California, U.S.A.

DESCRIPTION OF DEPOFOAM®

DepoFoam® is an aqueous suspension of multivesicular liposomes (MVL). MVLs were first described by Kim and co-workers (1), where the MVLs are formed by a double emulsion process forming a water-in-oil-in-water emulsion. A typical scanning electron micrograph of an MVL particle is shown in Figure 1. The liposome particles are generally in the 10–30 μm diameter size range. The typical DepoFoam lipids® include phospholipids, cholesterol, and triglycerides. Phospholipids, such as dioleylphosphatidylcholine, comprise the major constituent of the lipid bilayer membrane. Charged phospholipids (e.g., dipalmitoylphosphatidylglycerol) can be included in the lipid bilayer membrane to help prevent aggregation of the liposomes by charge repulsion. Cholesterol is used to provide mechanical stabilization of the lipid bilayer membrane.

Each MVL particle is a honeycomb-like structure of numerous non-concentric aqueous chambers, each chamber being surrounded by a lipid membrane barrier. Unlike conventional liposomes, bilayers can meet at junctions between the nonconcentric aqueous chambers. The junctions exhibit tetrahedral coordination analogous to a gas–liquid foam (2). Because of this geometry, gaps are created in the bilayer structures at these junctions. Triglycerides such as triolein and tricaprylin provide stabilization of membrane junctions in the multivesicular liposomal structure. The lipid

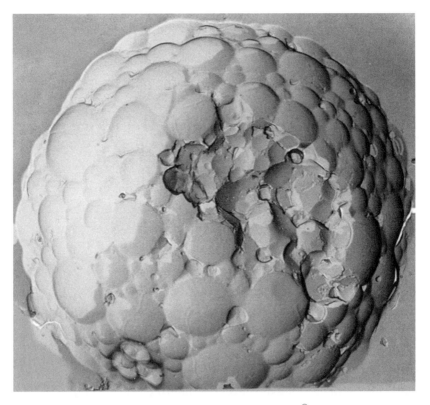

Figure 1   Scanning electron micrograph of a DepoFoam® particle.

bilayer and the membrane junctions of DepoFoam provide the sustained-release properties of the product. Drugs are gradually released from DepoFoam through reorganization of the lipids in vivo and breakdown of the particles. The rate of release is controlled primarily by the composition of the lipid layer. For example, long chain triglycerides prolong the duration of release relative to shorter chain triglycerides (3). Release rates ranging from days to weeks can be achieved to meet the needs for a specific clinical application.

COMMERCIAL USE OF DEPOFOAM®

The first commercial DepoFoam formulation was DepoCyt®, a sustained-release formulation of the chemotherapeutic agent, cytarabine. DepoCyt is used for the treatment of patients with lymphomatous meningitis, a complication of lymphoma that is characterized by the spread of cancer to the central nervous system and the formation of secondary tumors within the thin membranes surrounding the brain (4). Because of cytarabine's short half-life, a spinal injection is required twice per week. However, DepoCyt allows dosing once every 2 weeks, thus, providing significantly less invasive therapy to the patient. This product was approved by the FDA in 1999 and the EMEA in 2001.

DepoDur® uses DepoFoam technology to deliver morphine in a controlled manner for the epidural management of pain following major surgery. DepoDur reduces peak morphine plasma concentrations and extends the release of morphine for up to 48 hours (5). Thus, DepoDur is a simple alternative to continuous infusion of morphine through an indwelling epidural catheter. DepoDur received FDA approval in 2004 and MHRA (UK) approval in 2006.

RECENT CLINICAL STUDIES USING DEPOFOAM

One of the more advanced DepoFoam products in development is a formulation of the widely used local anesthetic bupivacaine, which is intended for postoperative pain management. Following local infiltration at wound sites, peripheral nerve block, epidural administration, or possibly intra-articular injection, the formulation is designed so that a single injection of DepoBupivacaine™ can provide extended pain relief. This should simplify postoperative pain management by reducing the need for repeated administration, minimizing break-through pain episodes, and reducing the need for supplemental opioid medications. In addition, the extended release allows bupivacaine to be administered with a lower maximum plasma concentration (C_{max}) relative to the solution, presumably providing a safety advantage. For example, 175 mg of DepoBupivacaine™ given epidurally leads to a C_{max} of approximately 125 ng/mL while a 3.5-fold lower dose of bupivacaine HCl solution leads to a C_{max} of 254 ng/mL (6). DepoBupivacaine has completed Phase II trials and is expected to commence its Phase III trial program immanently.

Competitive Advantage

Sustained release systems are superior to conventional administration because they (*i*) reduce side effects by reducing peak systemic levels and (*ii*) reduce the frequency of injections by providing prolonged duration of the therapeutic drug in the bloodstream. The ideal sustained release injectable formulation would have a number of positive attributes in eyes of the patient, health care provider, health care payer, manufacturer, and regulator. These attributes are ranked in Table 1 for a number of different types of controlled release formulations (+ to +++ with +++ being the best).

For patients suffering from chronic disease, tolerability is a prerequisite for successful long-term therapy. Since DepoFoam formulations

Table 1 The Ideal Sustained-Release Injectable Formulation

Attribute	Compressed pellets	Suspensions	Oil depots	Polymer implants	"Polymerization"	Traditional biodegradable microspheres	Gelling systems	Multivesicular liposomes
Well tolerated	+	+	+	+	+++	+	+	+++
≥1 Week delivery	+	+	++	+++	+	++	++	++
High loading capacity	+++	++	+	++	++	++	++	++
Little or no burst	+	+	++	+++	+	+	+	++
Low cost	+++	+++	++	+	+	++	+++	++
No modification of drug	+++	+++	+++	+++	+	+++	+++	+++
Scalable manufacture	+++	+++	+++	++	++	+	++	++
Precedented excipients	+++	+++	++	++	++	++	+	++
Commercialized	+	+++	+++	++	++	++	++	++
Ease of administration	+	+++	++	+	+++	+	+	++

are made up primarily of simple lipids and water, the system is bio-compatible and biodegradable. The lipids in the formulation enter standard catabolic pathways (7). Thus, DepoFoam is one of the best tolerated sustained release injectable formulations available today. The toleration profile of DepoFoam has been demonstrated in both animal and clinical studies, as well as in the marketplace. With the exception of intravenous delivery, DepoFoam can be utilized for nearly any parenteral administration route including subcutaneous (8), intraperitoneal (9,10), intrathecal (4), epidural (5), subconjuctival (11), and intraocular (12).

DepoFoam compares favorably to other sustained release injectable technologies in most other attributes as well. The DepoFoam formulation can be produced in a sterile and non-pyrogenic manner, is ready to use, and is generally isotonic. Since the DepoFoam particles are small and deformable, they can be easily injected through a narrow gauge needle. DepoFoam is suitable for the delivery of small molecules as well as proteins, peptides, nucleotides, carbohydrates, and vaccines. The technology can provide either site-specific or systemic delivery of the drug. The drug is typically contained in the aqueous chambers. Since the particles can occupy as much as 70% of the formulation volume, DepoFoam has a large carrying capacity for water soluble drugs. The percentage of encapsulated drug is controlled during manufacture, and can approach 100%. If a pulse of drug is desired following injection, unencapsulated drug can be set at essentially any level to deliver such a pulse.

The existence of marketed products using this technology is an obvious strong point to those considering sustained release injectable formulations for their drug. The formulation utilizes precedented excipients and the manufacture at various scales has been demonstrated (13). Thus, the acceptance of DepoFoam by regulatory authorities is simplified for new applications.

APPLICATION OF DEPOFOAM TO THE DELIVERY OF PEPTIDES, PROTEINS AND OTHER MACROMOLECULES

As seen by the above examples, DepoFoam can be used to provide extended release following injection by various routes of administration for traditional pharmaceuticals. One of the more promising applications is for macromolecules. Due to their size and hydrogen-bonding capability, macromolecules generally do not cross biological membranes well. In addition, most have poor stability in the gastrointestinal tract. Thus, most cannot be delivered by the oral route of administration. While alternative routes of administration have shown some promise for some macromolecules, most must be delivered by injection for systemic use. In addition, therapeutic macromolecules are generally cleared rapidly from the bloodstream and thus, must be administered frequently. The rapidly varying plasma levels potentially lead to poor patient compliance, adverse events at peak plasma levels, inefficient pharmacodynamics and high cost of goods.

Sustained-release technologies can overcome these drawbacks and improve the likelihood for macromolecule-based therapies to compete and succeed in the pharmaceutical marketplace. Pacira Pharmaceuticals, Inc. has assessed DepoFoam technology for therapeutics ranging from 6-residue peptides to 50 kD protein macromolecules and has demonstrated (*i*) high encapsulation efficiency (up to 95%), (*ii*) retention of peptide/protein structure and activity, (*iii*) minimal burst (3–5%) following administration during initial release phase, and (*iv*) sustained plasma levels for 1–4 weeks.

Sustained delivery of a protein with DepoFoam has been shown for myelopoietin (Leridistim) (14). Myelopoietin is a 35-kD IL-2/G-CCSF chimeric protein designed for the treatment of myelosuppression in patients following chemotherapy. In primates, the G-CSF/IL-2 chimera have been shown to enhance neutrophil and platelet regeneration (14). Like most therapeutic proteins, when administered as the unencapsulated native protein, Leridistim must be administered frequently (typically daily) to maintain efficacious levels of the protein in the bloodstream. Figure 2 shows the relationship between pharmacokinetics and pharmacodynamic efficacy in rats following a single subcutaneous injection of DepoFoam-encapsulated Leridistim. Plasma levels were elevated for between 4 and 7 days, and

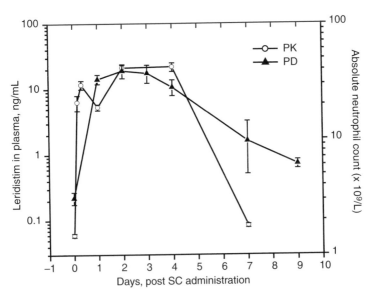

Figure 2 Plasma Leridistim levels (*open circles*) and neutrophil counts (closed triangles) in rats following subcutaneous administration of DepoFoam® encapsulated Leridistim. *Source*: From Ref. 14.

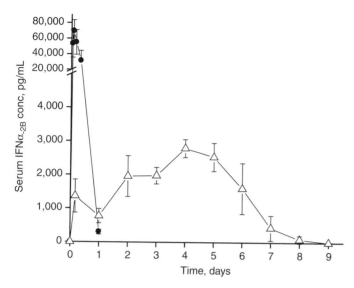

Figure 3 Plasma pharmacokinetics of IFNα-2B in rats following subcutaneous administration of DepoFoam® encapsulated IFNα-2B (160 μg dose, *triangles*) and unencapsulated IFNα-2B (100 μg dose, *circles*). *Abbreviation*: IFNα-2B, interferon alpha-2b. *Source*: From Ref. 15.

absolute neutrophil levels were elevated for 7–9 days. DepoFoam formulations with a higher triglyceride level provided even longer durations of action. For patients undergoing chemotherapy, weekly versus daily dosing represents a significant improvement in convenience and quality of life.

Figure 3 shows the plasma levels of interferon alpha-2b (IFNα-2B) following subcutaneous administration of IFNα-2B solution and DepoFoam-encapsulated IFNα-2B (15). IFNα-2B is a 19-kD protein used for the treatment of hepatitis and various cancers. IFNα treatment is often associated with flu-like symptoms which are induced by high plasma levels of interferon (16). As shown in Figure 3, peak plasma levels were significantly reduced following treatment with DepoFoam-encapsulated IFNα-2B, as compared to unencapsulated IFNα-2B. In addition, little or no burst was observed in the initial time period for the DepoFoam formulation. Finally, IFNα-2B levels were maintained for up to 7 days in the DepoFoam group, as compared to 1-day elevation in the bolus group.

CONCLUSIONS

Formulations using DepoFoam are well tolerated and have been approved for use in Europe and the United States. DepoFoam has significant potential for the sustained release of macromolecules. Myelopoietin and IFNα-2B

DepoFoam formulations with 1 week of sustained delivery and little or no burst have been demonstrated in rats.

REFERENCES

1. Kim S, Turker M, Chi E, et al. Preparation of multivesicular liposomes. Biochim Biophys Acta 1983; 728:339–48.
2. Spector MS, Zasadzinski JA, Sankaram MB. Topology of multivesicular liposomes, a model biliquid foam. Langmuir 1996; 12:4704–8.
3. Sankaram M. A lipid based depot (DepoFoam technology) for sustained release drug delivery. Progr Lipid Res 2002; 41:392–406.
4. Glantz MJ, et al. Randomized trial of a slow-release versus a standard formulation of cytarabine for the intrathecal treatment of lymphomatous meningitis. J Clin Oncol 1999; 17(10):3110–6.
5. Viscusi ER, Martin G, Hartrick CT, et al. Forty-eight hours of postoperative pain relief after total hip arthroplasty with a novel, extended-release epidural morphine formulation. Anesthesiology 2005; 102:1014–22.
6. Manvelian, G, Ardeleanu, M, Rashti N. The Pharmacokinetic Profile of an Extended-Release Liposomal Formulation of Bupivacaine (SKY0402) Administered via a Single Epidural Injection. Presented at the ASRA 31st Annual Regional Anesthesia Meeting & Workshops, Rancho Mirage, CA, April 7, 2006.
7. Kohn FR, Malkmus SA, Brownson EA, et al. Fate of the predominant phospholipid component of Depotoam drug delivery matrix. Drug Delivery 1998; 5:143–51.
8. Katre NV, Asherman J, Schaefer H, Hora M. Multivesicular liposome (DepoFoam) technology for the sustained delivery of insulin-like growth factor-I. J Pharm Sci 1998; 87:1341–6.
9. Chatelut E, Suh P, Kim S. Sustained release methotraxate for intracavity chemotherapy. J Pharm Sci 1994; 83(3):429–32.
10. Bonetti A, Kim S. Pharmakokinetics of an extended-release human interferon alpha-2b formulation. Cancer Chemother Pharmacol 1993; 333:258–61.
11. Assil KK, Weinreb RN. Multivesicular liposomes: Sustained release of the antimetabolite cytarabine in the eye. Arch Ophthalmol 1987; 105(3):400–3.
12. Howell SB. Clinical applications of a novel sustained release injectable drug delivery system: DepoFoam technology. Cancer J 2001; 7(3):219–27.
13. Pepper C, Patel M, Hartounian H. cGMP Manufacturing scale-up of a multivesicular lipid based drug delivery system. Pharm Eng 1999; Mar/Apr:8–18.
14. Langstrom MV, Ramprasad MP, Kararli TT, et al. Modulation of the sustained delivery of myelopoietin (leridistim) encapsulated in multivesicular liposomes (DepoFoam). J Control Release 2003; 89:87–99.
15. Willis R. Lipid Foams: Formulation development and characterization of DepoInterferon alpha. In: Proceedings of the Fine Particle Society Meeting in San Diego, CA, Dec. 2006.
16. Lane HC, Davey V, Kovacs JA, et al. Interferon-alpha in patients with asymptomatic human immunodeficiency virus (HIV) infection. A randomized, placebo-controlled trial. Ann Intern Med 1990; 112(11):805–11.

18

ALZAMER® Depot™ Bioerodible Polymer Technology

Guohua Chen and Gunjan Junnarkar

ALZA Corporation, Mountain View, California, U.S.A.

INTRODUCTION

With the advent of therapeutic biomolecules produced by the biotechnology industry, the need for convenient, sustained delivery of proteins and other biomolecules has greatly increased. The ALZAMER® Depot™ technology was designed to offer sustained delivery of therapeutic agents with minimal initial drug burst in a bioerodable dosage form for durations varying from days to months.

The ALZAMER Depot technology consists of a biodegradable polymer, a solvent, and formulated drug particles. The depot is injected subcutaneously or intramuscularly. The early stage drug release is predominantly from diffusion out of the system while biological fluids diffusing in, and at later stages, polymer degradation further contribute to drug release. Compared to standard injections, microspheres and other depots offer the advantages of sustained drug release, potential improvements in compliance and convenience, fewer drug concentration peaks and troughs, and dose-sparing effects (1–10). Microspheres, however, typically require complex production processes and harsh solvents that must be removed (5–14). Solution depot formulation processes tend to be simpler, typically involving only biocompatible solvents as part of the depot platform (15–22). In most published work citing depot formulations to date, water-miscible solvents tended to migrate quickly from the depot, resulting in rapid formation of a porous structure (15,17,19,20). Initial drug release from microspheres and these earlier generation depot formulations tends to

215

be rapid with up to 50% of the drug being released soon after injection (4,10,14–18).

In contrast, ALZAMER Depot technology (ALZA Corporation, Mountain View, CA) uses biocompatible solvents of low water miscibility, which slow the dynamics of phase inversion and alter the resultant morphology. The result is significantly reduced porosity of the injected depot system, thus helping to control the initial drug release. In addition, this type of depot is easy to process and can be presented in a pre-filled syringe with the drug pre-formulated into the gel, potentially enhancing convenience of use (21).

The development of ALZAMER Depot technology was initially focused on the delivery of therapeutic proteins (21), but recently it has been expanded into other therapeutic agents including peptides and small molecules (23,24).

FORMULATION DEVELOPMENT

ALZAMER® Depot™ technology consists of the biodegradable polymer poly-lactic glycolic acid (PLGA), a biocompatible solvent of low water miscibility [e.g., benzyl benzoate (BB)], and formulated drug particles. Drug stability, especially for protein and peptide drugs, is maintained by isolating the drug in a solid particle. This particle is suspended in the nonaqueous polymer/solvent depot to prevent premature exposure to water. Dose release can be adjusted by varying the initial formulation and drug loading, as well as the injection volume of the preloaded syringe.

Solvent Choice and Phase Inversion

Injectable polymer/solvent depots comprising a biodegradable polymer dissolved in a biocompatible solvent transform when injected. Since the polymer is water-insoluble, contact with water in a physiological environment causes the gel to undergo phase inversion (liquid demixing), resulting in a two-phase, gelled implant (19,20). As a result, development of the depot morphology occurs in vivo, simultaneously with release of drug, and the dynamics of phase inversion must be controlled to maintain consistent drug delivery within a specified therapeutic window.

Figure 1 shows the impact of the choice of solvent on the phase inversion process and the resultant morphology of the depot. A range of PLGAs has been tested, and the preferred polymer is a PLGA of 50/50 lactide/glycolide (L/G) ratio and a molecular weight of approximately 15,000. Figure 1A shows the morphology of a depot comprised of PLGA (L/G 50/50, M_w 16,000) and N-methylpyrrolidone (NMP), a solvent with relatively high water solubility. This system rapidly absorbs water and hardens. As predicted by the theory of phase inversion dynamics (25), a

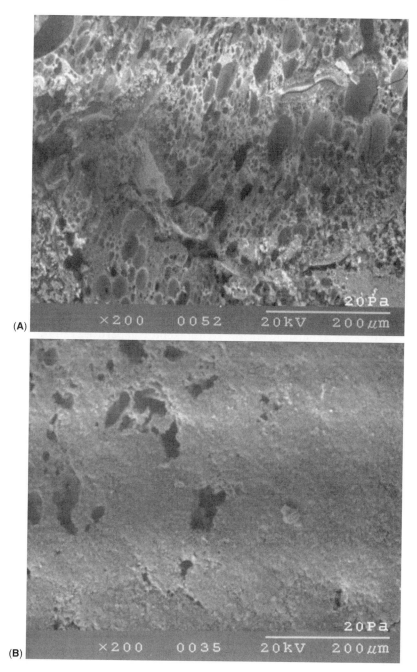

Figure 1 Gel structure after 4 days implantation (PLGA RG502/solvent, 1:1, 10% loading). (**A**) N-methylpyrrolidone; (**B**) benzyl benzoate.

highly porous matrix is formed within the injected depot. Drug residing in or near the pores is quickly released. This results in a system that releases a significant portion of the drug upon initial administration.

The ALZAMER® Depot™ technology uses solvents of low water miscibility that slow the dynamics of phase inversion and alter the resultant morphology of the injected depot system. Figure 1B shows the morphology of a depot comprised of PLGA (L/G 50/50, M_w ~16,000) and BB [insoluble in water (27)]. Slowing the phase inversion process significantly reduces the porosity of the system.

Figure 2 illustrates the effect of solvent choice and the phase-inversion process on drug release from ALZAMER® Depot™ technology. An initial drug burst is observed with the solvents triacetin and NMP; this initial burst is greatly reduced with the formulation containing BB as the solvent.

Choice of solvent also influences the time course of water absorption into the ALZAMER® Depot™. Water absorption is substantially quicker for NMP and triacetin than for BB (20).

Drug Particle Development

Formulation of the drug particles dispersed in the ALZAMER® Depot™ can also affect the initial drug release. Densified protein particles can be produced by compressing protein and stearic acid together and redispersing the compacted protein into particles of defined size. Alternatively, the addition

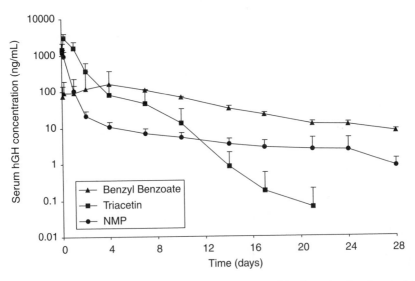

Figure 2 Effect of water solubility of solvent on hGH release in vivo (serum hGH levels in rats receiving a single depot injection). *Abbreviation*: hGH, human growth hormone.

of divalent cations to lyophilized human growth hormone (hGH) is known to decrease solubility and dissolution (14). Both techniques produce lower initial release from depot systems than from lyophilized hGH alone dispersed in the ALZAMER® Depot™ gel (21). Additionally, water absorption into the gel is slower with the densified hGH/SA particles than with the lyophilized hGH (21). Initial release can thus be moderated and engineered to remain within a specified therapeutic window. Similar techniques can be applied to peptides. For a small molecule drug, its release rate profile from the depot can be modulated by changing the hydrophobic/hydrophilic properties of drug particles, the particle size, the salt form, etc.

Drug Loading

The loading of drug in the gel can also affect the release kinetics. However, drug particle loading can be varied from 5% to 30% without inducing a significant initial drug burst and while maintaining a sustained release rate.

Choice of Biodegradable Polymer and Polymer/Solvent Ratio

The choice of biodegradable polymer is one of the critical factors that can affect the release of a drug from depot formulations. PLGA is the most commonly used biodegradable polymer. Changing the polymer molecular weight or the L/G ratio in the polymer can alter the interaction between the solvent and the polymer, resulting in alteration of the release profile and duration. The polymer solvent ratio can be varied to modulate drug release kinetics and release duration.

PRECLINICAL EVALUATION

The PLGA polymer used in ALZAMER® Depot™ technology has an extensive history of use in sutures, clips, implants, and carriers for the sustained release of various pharmaceuticals (28). The polymer is degraded by hydrolytic cleavage to form lactic and glycolic acids (i.e,. parent monomers) that are normal metabolic compounds. The solvents and other excipients used in ALZAMER® Depot™ technology were initially screened for their performance characteristics and their safety/biocompatibility profile for parenteral use.

Protein Delivery

By proper choice of solvent and formulation of protein particles, sustained delivery of protein can be achieved with ALZAMER® Depot™ with minimum initial burst (Fig. 2) (20). To demonstrate the biological activity of the delivered drug, an ALZAMER® Depot™ containing hGH was administered to hypophysectomized rats; biological activity was confirmed by assessment of body weight gain and elevations in Insulin-like Growth Factor-1 levels for 28 days (26).

The immunogenicity of a protein released from a sustained release dosage form such as ALZAMER® Depot™ was investigated by formulating native animal protein [rat growth hormone (rGH)] into the ALZAMER® Depot™, administering it into rats, and monitoring the antibody response to rGH released from the formulation. Figure 3 illustrates the antibody titer against rGH in various formulations including an aqueous rGH solution (negative control) and rGH in Freund's Complete Adjuvant/Freund's Incomplete Adjuvant (positive control) as a function of time. Elevated antibody titers were observed only with the adjuvant positive control and depot formulation containing benzyl alcohol as a co-solvent. No immune response was observed for the ALZAMER® Depot™ with BB as solvent and the aqueous solution of rGH.

Peptide Delivery

To demonstrate the feasibility of sustained delivery of peptide from the ALZAMER® Depot™, leuprolide acetate was selected as a model molecule. Figure 4 illustrates the in vivo release-rate profile of leuprolide from ALZAMER® Depot™ formulations and the pharmacodynamic effect (suppression of testosterone) of released leuprolide in rats. By selecting different biodegradable polymer compositions, ALZAMER® Depot™ formulations

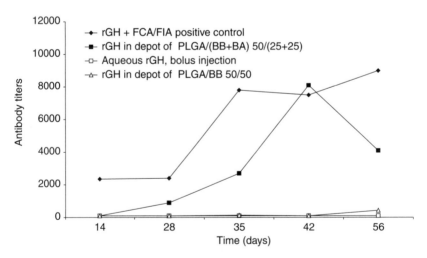

Figure 3 Antibody response to rGH released from various formulations (twice a week bolus injections of aqueous rGH solution and rGH + FCA/FIA as negative and positive controls, respectively; twice depot injections at $t = 0$ and 28 days; $n = 6$). *Abbreviation*: rGH, rat growth hormone.

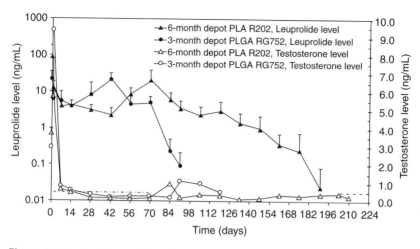

Figure 4 In vivo Leuprolide release-rate profile and testosterone suppression from both 3- and 6-month ALZAMER® Depot™ in rats (polymer/BB ratio, 55/45; leuprolide acetate loading: 8 wt%; $n = 6$). *Abbreviation*: BB, benzyl benzoate.

of leuprolide for durations of 3 and 6 months, respectively, have been achieved with pharmacodynamic effects for the intended duration.

Delivery of Small Molecules

The ALZAMER® Depot™ system can be used for sustained delivery of small molecules as well. A long-acting formulation that exhibits a rapid onset, low burst, near zero-order release profile, and acceptable drug stability was developed for delivery of an anti-psychotic compound. The rat plasma concentration of this anti-psychotic compound was monitored after subcutaneous administration of the depot formulation. Figure 5 shows that the release rate and duration can be modulated and near zero-order release without lag can be achieved by appropriate selection of polymer and drug particle size. A combination of appropriate polymer with appropriate drug particle size can be used to adjust onset of action, the duration, the C_{max}, and the plasma drug levels of the administered compound. Sustained release of another small molecule, bupivacaine, from ALZAMER® Depot™ for about 1 month was also demonstrated in vivo (24).

Other Preclinical Developments

To date, more than 100 different ALZAMER® Depot™ formulations have been tested in vivo with different animals. No remarkable adverse clinical observations or systemic signs of toxicity have been noted. Macroscopic evaluation of the subcutaneous injection sites has generally indicated mild

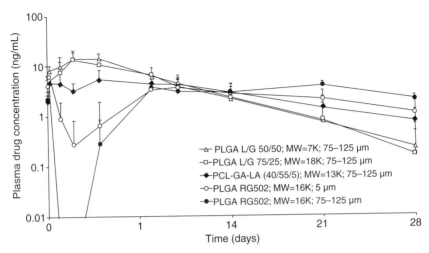

Figure 5 In vivo release profile of an anti-psychotic compound from ALZAMER® Depot™ formulation in rats via subcutaneous administration (Polymer/BB ratio, 50/ 50; drug loading: 30 wt%; $n = 5$).

irritation. Histopathologic evaluation of the injection sites revealed typical responses to the presence of a foreign body in rats, with simple fibrosis or a mild to moderate granulomatous inflammation (26). Biodegradation of the depot was observed to be partially complete after 56 days.

IN VIVO/IN VITRO CORRELATION

While significant insight can be gained from in vitro testing of depot formulations containing water-miscible solvents, the testing of depot formulations containing water-immiscible solvents is far more difficult, and the results of these types of tests do not correlate with in vivo data in a straightforward fashion. Since it is extremely difficult to reproduce in vitro the complexity of the phenomena occurring in vivo, the performance of depot formulations must often be evaluated only in vivo. A reproducible drug-release profile in vivo is achievable and has been confirmed in a large body of formulation work.

MANUFACTURING

Depot gels are manufactured using standard sizing and compounding equipment. For drugs that do not withstand terminal sterilization, aseptic manufacturing procedures are employed. As a product concept, ALZAMER® Depot™ technology is expected to be offered in convenient, prefilled syringe dosage forms with no premixing required.

KEY ADVANTAGES OF ALZAMER® DEPOT™ TECHNOLOGY

The ALZAMER® Depot™ technology presents several advantages over other depots. The low water miscibility of the solvent significantly reduces the initial burst release as compared to microsphere technology (14) or injectable depot gel using water miscible solvents such as NMP or glycofurol (15,18). The manufacturing process is much simpler than that for the microsphere technologies. The loading of drug in ALZAMER® Depot™ can be as high as 200–300 mg/mL. This loading is significantly higher than microsphere technologies, which may only load about 20–60 mg/mL. Finally, the dosage form is presented in a prefilled syringe, potentially enhancing the convenience of use.

SUMMARY AND OUTLOOK

The ALZAMER® Depot™ technology platform was designed to provide sustained delivery of pharmaceutical agents for extended periods from days to months. Use of solvents having low water miscibility controls the morphology of the injected depot via phase inversion, leading to a product with minimal initial drug burst. The release profile can be engineered by choice of depot solvent, polymer composition, formulation of the drug particle, and the loading of drug particles in the depot gel. Safety of the ALZAMER® Depot™ technology has been shown in preclinical work to date. While a useful in vitro release test that correlates with in vivo release has yet to be fully developed, a reproducible in vivo drug-release profile is achievable and has been demonstrated in a large body of formulation work. ALZAMER® Depot™ technology represents a promising new platform technology for the sustained delivery of small molecules, peptides, proteins, and other biomolecules.

ACKNOWLEDGMENTS

The authors wish to acknowledge the contributions of their colleagues on the ALZAMER® Depot™ team, especially in the Nonclinical, Analytical, and Biologics Drug Delivery Departments, and appreciate the expert assistance in the editing and formatting of this monograph.

REFERENCES

1. Lewis DH. Controlled release of bioactive agents from lactide/glycolide polymers. In: M Chasin, R Langer, eds. Biodegradable Polymers as Drug Delivery Systems. New York: Marcel Dekker, 1990: 1–41.
2. Okada H, Toguchi H. Biodegradable microspheres in drug delivery. Crit Rev Ther Drug Carrier Syst 1995; 12(1):1–99.

3. Cleland JL. Solvent evaporation processes for the production of controlled release biodegradable microsphere formulations for therapeutics and vaccines. Biotechnol Prog 1998; 14(1):102–7.

4. Toguchi H. Pharmaceutical manipulation of leuprorelin acetate to improve clinical performance. J Int Med Res 1990; 18(Suppl. 1):35–41.

5. Saltzman WM, Mak MW, Mahoney MJ, Duenas ET, Cleland JL. Intracranial delivery of recombinant nerve growth factor: release kinetics and protein distribution for three delivery systems. Pharm Res 1999; 16(2):232–40.

6. Hsu YY, Hao T, Hedley ML. Comparison of process parameters for microencapsulation of plasmid DNA in poly(D,L-lactic-co-glycolic) acid microspheres. J Drug Target 1999; 7(4):313–23.

7. Lewis KJ, Irwin WJ, Akhtar S. Development of a sustained-release biodegradable polymer delivery system for site-specific delivery of oligonucleotides: characterization of P(LA-GA) copolymer microspheres in vitro. J Drug Target 1998; 5(4):291–302.

8. Bittner B, Morlock M, Koll H, Winter G, Kissel T. Recombinant human erythropoietin (rhEPO) loaded poly(lactide-co-glycolide) microspheres: influence of the encapsulation technique and polymer purity on microsphere characteristics. Eur J Pharm Biopharm 1998; 45(3):295–305.

9. Moore A, McGuirk P, Adams S, et al. Immunization with a soluble recombinant HIV protein entrapped in biodegradable microparticles induces HIV-specific CD8+ cytotoxic T lymphocytes and CD4+ Th1 cells. Vaccine 1998; 13(18):1741–9.

10. Okada H, Doken Y, Ogawa Y, Toguchi H. Preparation of three-month depot injectable microspheres of leuprorelin acetate using biodegradable polymers. Pharm Res 1994; 11(8):1143–7.

11. Cohen S, Yoshioka T, Lucarelli M, et al. Controlled delivery systems for proteins based on poly(lactic/glycolic acid) microspheres. Pharm Res 1991; 8 (6):713–20.

12. Garcia-Contreras L, Abu-Izza K, Lu DR. Biodegradable cisplatin microspheres for direct brain injection: preparation and characterization. Pharm Dev Technol 1997; 2(1):53–65.

13. Okada H. One- and three-month release injectable microspheres of the LH RH superagonist leuprorelin acetate. Adv Drug Deliv Rev 1997; 28(1):43–70.

14. Cleland JL, Johnson OL, Putney S, et al. Recombinant human growth hormone poly(lactic-co-glycolic acid) microsphere formulation development. Adv Drug Deliv Rev 1997; 28:71–84.

15. Yewey GL, Duysen EG, Cox SM, Dunn RL. Delivery of proteins from a controlled release injectable implant. Pharm Biotechnol 1997; 10:93–117.

16. Ravivarapu HB, Moyer KL, Dunn RL. Parameters affecting the efficacy of a sustained release polymeric implant of leuprolide. Int J Pharm 2000; 194(2):181–91.

17. Jain RA, Rhodes CT, Railkar AM, et al. Comparison of various injectable protein-loaded biodegradable poly(lactide-co-glycolide) (PLGA) devices: in-situ-formed implant versus in-situ-formed microspheres versus isolated microspheres. Pharm Dev Technol 2000; 5(2):201–7.

18. Eliaz RE, Kost J. Characterization of a polymeric PLGA-injectable implant delivery system for the controlled release of proteins. J Biomed Mater Res 2000; 50(3):388–96.
19. Graham PD, Brodbeck KJ, McHugh AJ. Phase inversion dynamics of PLGA solutions related to drug delivery. J Controlled Release 1999; 58(2):233–45.
20. Brodbeck KJ, DesNoyer JR, McHugh AJ. Phase inversion dynamics of PLGA solutions related to drug delivery. Part II. The role of solution thermodynamics and bath-side mass transfer. J Controlled Release 1999; 62(3):333–44.
21. Brodbeck KJ, Pushpala S, McHugh AJ. Sustained release of human growth hormone from PLGA solution depots. Pharm Res 1999; 16(12):1825–9.
22. Jeong B, Bae YH, Kim SW. In situ gelation of PEG-PLGA-PEG triblock copolymer aqueous solutions and degradation thereof. J Biomed Mater Res 2000; 50(2):171–7.
23. Chen GH, Kleiner L, Houston P, et al. Sustained release of leuprolide acetate from ALZAMER® Depot™. Proceedings of 30th annual meeting of Controlled Release Society, Glasgow, Scotland, 2003: 406, 407.
24. Chen GH, Priebe D, Baudouin K, et al. Sustained release of a small molecule drug, bupivacaine. Proceedings of 28th annual meeting of Controlled Release Society, San Diego, USA, #6176, 2001.
25. Barton BF, Reeve JL, McHugh AJ. Observations on the dynamics of non-solvent-induced phase inversion. J Polym Sci, Polym Phys Ed 1997; 35: 569–85.
26. Bannister R, Baudouin K, Maze E, et al. Biological activity, pharmacokinetics, and safety assessment of human growth hormone (hGH) delivered via a subcutaneous depot. Toxicol Sci 2000; 54(1):407.
27. The Merck Index. 12th ed. Whitehouse Station, NJ: Merck & Co., 1996: 1162–3.
28. Physicians' Desk Reference. Oradell, NJ: Medical Economics Company, 2000; 581, 3094.

19

Pegylated Liposome Delivery of Chemotherapeutic Agents: Rationale and Clinical Benefit

Francis J. Martin

Eclipse Nanomedical, Inc., San Francisco, California, U.S.A.

INTRODUCTION

Parenterally administered nanoscale drug delivery systems, including liposomes, albumin microspheres, micellar dispersions, dendrimers, polymeric nanoparticles, and polyplexes continue to show promise in improving the profile of selected anti-tumor drugs, which, given alone, suffer from unfavorable chemistry or pharmacologic properties and/or narrow safety margins (1–11). Yet, product introductions based on these technologies have been few. This chapter will update the history of one commercial success story in this category, pegylated liposomal doxorubicin (PLD), a product marketed in the United States under the trade name Doxil® (Ortho Pharmaceuticals), and in the rest of the world as CAELYX® (Schering-Plough). The clinical niche PLD now occupies, plus the growing understanding of its pharmacologic properties, provide insight into the desirable attributes *and* limitations of a solid-tumor delivery system and shed light on key challenges developers face in striking the delicate balance required to entrap, carry, selectively deliver, and release a drug at the intended site and at active concentrations in solid tumors.

The clinical validation of PLD has inspired interest in other liposome product opportunities based on the same basic architecture. For example, camptothecin analogues, anti-angiogenesis agents, antisense oligonucleotides, and short-interfering RNA each represent rational candidates for delivery in pegylated liposomes. For such agents, pegylated liposome delivery offers protection of encapsulated drug and enhanced tumor accumulation and prolonged local drug exposure. True molecular targeting can be achieved using liposomes linked to ligands such as monoclonal antibodies (or binding fragments) or peptides directed against cell surface receptors. Properly selected ligands can influence the disposition of drug-loaded liposomes within the tumor by provoking internalization and intracellular release. Recent advances in ligand-targeted liposome design include rapid selection of phage antibody-derived single chain fragments (scFv) and peptides for targeting, and methods for introduction of ligands into preformed, drug-loaded liposomes. A targeted formulation consisting of a novel, fully humanized, single-chain antibody fragment that binds to the HER2 receptor (anti-HER2 of scFv) conjugated to PLD (Her2 PLD), currently in development, selectively binds to and internalizes in HER2-overexpressing tumor cells in vitro and in vivo. Future applications may include therapeutics tailored to treat individual patients' disease; the modular design of the targeted liposome enables a combinatorial approach in which a repertoire of ligands can be used in conjunction with a series of liposomal drugs.

CONVENTIONAL LIPOSOMES

The notion of using liposomes or other nanoparticle systems to deliver encapsulated drugs more selectively to sites of disease is particularly seductive for cancer chemotherapeutics, many of which exhibit intrinsically poor solubilities, undesirable pharmacologic properties, and narrow safety margins. The paradigm is venerable: use the particle to entrap and protect the drug (in soluble or insoluble form), carry it to sites of diseases, release it, thereby increasing the local exposure to bioavailable drug, while, at the same time, significantly reducing exposure of normal tissues (12). Since the time serious liposome pharmacologic studies began (circa 1975), countless formulations have been tested and meaningful progress, albeit slow, has been reported. Early on, it was observed that by changing drug pharmacokinetics and biodistribution (e.g., by reducing the peak levels of bioavailable drug in plasma, or by creating a drug reservoir within macrophages after liposome uptake), conventional liposomal delivery systems [which rely on a mononuclear phagocyte system (MPS) depot approach] can reduce serious drug toxicities, such as cardiotoxicity associated with doxorubicin or renal toxicity associated with amphotericin B, thereby increasing the safety margin of the drugs (13,14). Liposome administration is perceived to be low risk because the lipids used are usually extracted from natural sources, such as egg yolks or soybean oil, that have been safely used as emulsifying agents in lipid emulsions for human parenteral administration (15).

Although safer, early liposome formulations of doxorubicin were found to be no more active against implanted tumors than the same dose of unencapsulated drug. This lack of improved antitumor activity was subsequently attributed to two related biological responses. First, the liposomes themselves were often unstable when introduced into blood and quickly released much of their drug payload, presumably as a consequence of rapid interaction and destabilization by plasma proteins (16,17). Second, liposomes that survived destabilization in blood were rapidly sequestered by fixed macrophages residing in the liver and spleen (the MPS) creating a temporary drug depot in these organs (18). Following internalization by macrophages, the lipid membrane of the liposomes appears to be digested by intracellular enzymes as evidenced by the fact that the drug in "free" form returns to the central compartment in a pattern resembling a prolonged intravenous infusion. Although this model provided meaningful safety improvements, the combination of instability and MPS uptake restricted access to tumors and thus reduced the opportunity for "true" tumor targeting.

Recognition of the limited tumor-targeting potential of conventional liposomes led to the development of more stable "pure lipid" systems. Designs converged on two structural features to improve pharmacokinetics and shift tissue distribution away from the MPS and to other tissues including tumors: size and lipid matrix composition. Liposomes less than 100 nm composed of a mixture of cholesterol and an unsaturated high-phase transition lipid (such as distearoyl phosphatidyl choline or sphingomyelin) were found to be less leaky and have plasma residence times many-fold greater than earlier designs (19). Although an improvement over conventional liposomes (which typically have distribution half-lives of several minutes), the pure lipid systems failed to provide circulation times beyond about 5 hours in humans (20,21). Liposomes with longer circulation times, which are required to achieve optimal tumor accumulation (see below), required other critical innovations including more robust drug loading methods and surface modification.

PEGYLATED LIPOSOMES: FIRST GENERATION

A quantum leap forward in the quest for long-circulating liposomes was reported by Allen and Chonn (22): incorporation of a specific ganglioside (GM_1) into liposomes cut MPS uptake and prolonged the circulation time of intravenously administered liposomes (22). It was believed that the hydrophilic negatively-charged sugar residue of GM_1 (sialic acid), "shielded" by three neutral sugars, provided electrostatic stability without protein binding. In our hands, GM_1, which is derived from a complex mixture from brain tissue, was not an attractive raw material.

Pegylation

Several groups, including our own, suggested using polymers in place of the carbohydrate (23–27). PEG was everyone's first choice based on the success of protein pegylation, its safety profile and its availability in pharmaceutical quality (28,29).

Incorporation of PEG-derived lipids profoundly alters the pharmacology of liposomes. MPS uptake is slowed, and residence times increase from hours to days. A direct link was documented between long-circulation times and tumor uptake and superior anti-tumor activity in animal tumor models (Fig. 1) (30).

The structure–function relationships between PEG-derivatized phosphatidylethanolamine (PEG-PE) and liposome blood lifetime and tissue distribution have been reported in rodents and reflect the profound impact of PEG incorporation (Fig. 2). With a PEG molecular weight in the range of 1000–5000, prolonged circulation and reduced MPS uptake is achieved. After 24 hour, up to 35% of the injected dose remains in the blood and less than 10% is taken up by the two major organs of the MPS, liver, and spleen, compared with 1% and up to 50%, respectively, for liposomes without PEG-PE. Other important advantages of PEG-PE have

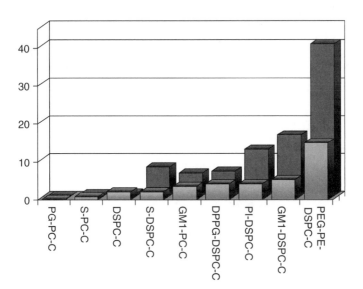

Figure 1 Correlation of blood level at 24 hr (*front bars*) and tumor uptake (*rear bars*) among formulations of similar size (circa 100 nm), but exhibiting differential circulation time in vivo. *Abbreviations*: PG, phosphatidyl glycerol; PC, egg phosphatidyl choline; C, cholesterol; DSPC, distearoyl phosphatidyl choline; GM1, brain derived ganglioside GM1; PI, phosphatidylinositol; PEG-PE, polyethylene glycol (2000)-phosphatidylethanolamine. *Source*: From Ref. 30.

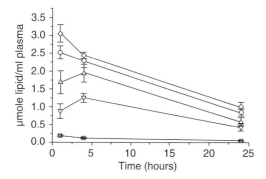

Figure 2 The effect of mol% DSPE-PEG proportion on the plasma clearance of DSPC liposomes. Liposome formulations composed of DSPC and varying amounts of DSPE-PEG; 0 mol% (□), 0.5 mol% (▽), 1 mol% (△), 2 mol% (○), and 5 mol% (◇) were administered as a single Iv bolus injection of 165 μmol/kg total lipid in female Balb/c mice (injected dose = 3.3 μmol lipid/ml plasma) (35). *Abbreviations*: DSPE, distearoyl phosphatidyl choline; PEG, polyethylene glycol.

been identified: prolonged circulation is independent of liposome cholesterol content, degree of hydrocarbon chain saturation in either the PC or the PE lipid anchor, or addition of most other negatively charged lipids (Table 1). This versatility in lipid composition is important for tailoring the formulation to specific drugs, many of which have diverse chemistries. For example, the flexibility provided by PEG to select matrix lipid components can be helpful to optimize stability and drug release rates (31).

Steric Stabilization

Steric stabilization has been proposed as a theoretical basis for the in vivo behavior of pegylated liposomes. It is believed that the hydrophilic surface layer provided by PEG reduces short-range van der Waals attraction among liposomes by physically interfering with their close approach. In qualitative terms, the steric repulsion has been described as brushing and pushing away the incoming surfaces of formed elements, macromolecules, or lipoprotein complexes (32).

The long circulation times of PEG grafted liposomes has been attributed, at least in part, to the reduced binding of protein opsonins in plasma, thus contributing to a reduced rate of macrophage-mediated liposome uptake (33). This explanation is not entirely consistent with experimental results. For example, surface force measurements between opposed lipid bilayers, one grafted with PEG and the other presenting an adsorbed protein, streptavidin, provide direct evidence for the formation of relatively strong attractive forces between PEG and this protein. Paradoxically, at low compressive loads, the forces were repulsive, but they became attractive when the proteins were

Table 1   Tissue Distribution 24 Hours After Intrarvnous Injection in Swiss-Webster Mice

| Lipid composition[a] | % Injected dose per tissue[b] | | | L + S[c]/ blood |
	Blood	Liver + spleen	total[d]	
EPG: PC: C[e]	0.7±0.3	38.9±3.8	59.3±5.9	55.6
DSPC: C(10:5)	11.0±2.6	25.7±3.4	60.0±3.4	2.3
G_{MI}: EPC:C	13±1.6	15.4±2.3	53.5±6.6	1.2
G_{MI}: DSPC: C	17.5±1.5	10.5±1.2	61.6±6.6	0.6
G_{MI}: PG:PC: C(1:1:10:5)	8.8±2.7	19.8±6.7	59.6±2.0	2.3
PEG-DSPE: DSPC: C[f]	21.5±5.9	18.0±3.8	70.3±2.0	1.2
PEG-DSPE: HSPC: C	20.5±6.1	7.2±0.6	55.1±4.9	0.4
PEG-DSPE: HEPC (IV 1): C	19.1±1.9	7.2±0.5	61.1±0.2	0.4
PEG-DSPE: PHEPC (IV 20): C	24.6±3.5	7.5±2.3	61.9±4.8	0.3
PEG-DSPE: PHEPC (IV 40): C	17.2±0.1	9.4±0.7	57.6±5.2	0.6
PEG-DSPE: EPG: C	18.6±1.8	13.0±1.0	63.4±3.3	0.7
PEG-DSPE: EPG: EPC: C (1:1:10:5)	12.5±1.3	10.2±0.6	56.5±3.3	0.8

[a]Molar ratio is 1:10:5 except where indicated; 80 nm mean diameter particle size distribution: IV value in parentheses describes degree of acyl chain unsaturation determined from iodine uptake value (19).
[b]Results are based on Ga-DF aqueous entrapped label and expressed as the mean ± S.D. from at least three animals.
[c]L + S refers to the sum of label in liver and spleen.
[d]Total is the sum of label in all organs and the remaining carcass.
[e]Data from Gabizon and Papahadjopoulos, 1988.
[f]Results obtained with nine animals.

pressed into the polymer layer at higher loads suggesting direct short-range PEG-protein interactions (34). Dos Santos et al. have reported that in the case of cholesterol-free liposomes, the total protein adsorption and protein profile was not influenced by the inclusion of PEG-modified lipids (35). However, plasma protein interactions with liposomal PEG appears to be fairly weak as protein adsorbed to liposomes exposed to plasma in vivo and in vitro is removed by washing the liposomes (by ultracentrifugal pelleting and resuspension) or column chromatography (36).

Pharmacology of Pegylated Liposomes

The pharmacology of pegylated liposomes is confounded by recently described effects that may be attributable to such protein-PEG interactions, weak or not. First, a threshold dose of lipid is needed to achieve "stealthlike" pharmacokinetics; at low dose rates, below about 0.03 μmol/kg in rabbits, rats, and humans, pegylated liposomes are eliminated more rapidly by hepatic and splenic clearance than at doses greater > 1 μmol/kg. Two related mechanisms for the dose threshold effect have been proposed: a small subpopulation of macrophages must need to be saturated in order to achieve long circulation times or a liposome-trophic opsonin, present at low levels in plasma, must be adsorbed/neutralized by a threshold number of liposomes, or both. Repeat dose experiments in rats also lead to a surprising result; fast elimination of a second dose of PLD when given within a "refractory period" of about a week of the first dose (Fig. 3) (37–40). Binding of PEG-specific IgM class antibodies secreted in response to the initial dose may responsible for this observation (41,42). Pre-incubating PEG liposomes with serum reduced the uptake of liposomes by macrophages suggesting that binding of "anti-opsonins" may play a role (43). It has been postulated the bound serum protein may provide a non-specific surface-shielding property and change the properties of the PEG, resulting in a surface that is better protected against interactions with cells (42,43).

Passive Tumor Targeting Mechanism: The EPR Effect

Greater than 90% of cancer deaths are a consequence of metastatic disease; lesions develop in normal organs as neoplastic cells, shed by primary tumors, invade and multiply, eventually leading to compromised organ function. As micrometastatic cell clusters reach several cubic millimeter in

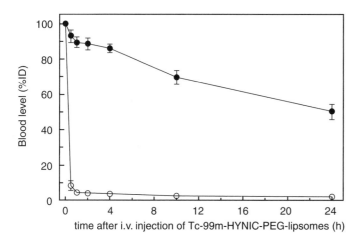

Figure 3   Blood clearance of 99mTc-labeled liposomes in rats after the first (●) or the second injection (○). The blood pool activity was determined by quantitative analysis of the scintigraphic images, by drawing regions of interest over the heart region. Blood pool activity at 2-min postinjection was set at 100%. Each point represents the mean values of six rats ± S.E. *Source*: From Ref. 40.

size, angiogenesis is needed to accommodate the metabolic needs of the tumors (44). Structural features of the angiogenic neovasculature differ greatly from that of normal tissues (45–48). Tumor vessels are irregular in shape, dilated and can exhibit bizarre transluminal projections (Fig. 4).

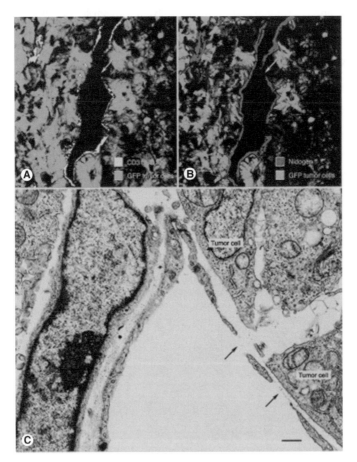

Figure 4 Basement membrane defects in regions of endothelium lacking CD31/CD105 staining. (**A**) confocal images of blood vessel in ectopic tumor with multiple sites lacking CD31/CD105 immunoreactivity. CD31/CD105 expression of tumor vessel surrounded by GFP-expressing tumor cells. CD31/CD105 immunoreactivity is not detectable in at least two sites (*arrow* and *arrowheads*). (**B**) Another confocal image of the same vessel showing the basement membrane protein nidogen, which envelopes most of the vessel including one of the CD31/CD105 defects (*arrowheads*) but is not detectable at another (*arrow*). (**C**) Electron micrograph of a tumor vessel with two endothelial gaps (*arrows*). Basement membrane is attenuated and incomplete in the region of the upper gap. Bar, 0.5 μm. *Source*: From Ref. 49.

The normal barrier properties of tumor vessels are often compromised. Endothelial cells fail to align and form continuous junctions, often with large irregular gaps interspersed among the cells. Extravascular pockets of formed elements seen in implanted tumors suggest whole-scale breakdown of the vessel integrity in these segments. The basement membrane is frequently absent or abnormally formed (Fig. 5). Tumor tissues exhibit poor lymphatic drainage (50). The combination of these anatomical defects can result in extensive leakage of blood plasma components, such as macromolecules, nanoparticles and liposomes, into the tumor tissue. Sluggish venous return in tumor tissue, (51) and the poor lymphatic clearance prolongs residence times for such drug carriers within the tumor and promotes extravasation into tumor interstitium. This phenomenon, termed the enhanced vascular permeability and retention (EPR) effect, was first introduced by Matsummura et al. in 1986 (52), has been exploited to selectively target macromolecular drugs to the site of solid tumors. It is possible to achieve very high local concentrations of polymeric drugs at the tumor site, for instance, 10- to 50-fold higher than in normal tissue within 1–2 days. The EPR effect may not act as efficiently for small drugs, macromolecules and very small nanoparticles (dendrimers, micelles) because these types of

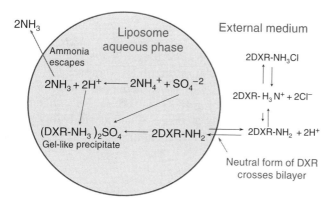

Figure 5 Illustration of mechanism of drug loading used for PLD. Liposome are first hydrated and sized in a high concentration of ammonium sulfate. The external ammonium sulfate is replaced with a nonelectrolyte (*e.g., sucrose*) and doxorubicin hydrochloride is added. A uncharged (*deprotonated*) form of doxorubicin forms externally (although the equilibrium is unfavorable). The uncharged form is lipid soluble and thus enters the liposome through the lipid bilayer; the rate is somewhat dependent on the matrix lipid composition and temperature. As doxorubicin enters the internal aqueous phase it forms an insoluble salt with sulfate ions and precipitates internally. For each mole of doxorubicin that enters, a mole of ammonia escapes the liposome. The equilibrium is driven to completion and virtually all the added doxorubicin is loaded as a precipitate.

particles are not truly trapped; they diffuse into and out of the tumor at about the same rate. This equilibrium serves to dilute the fraction that originally reached the tumor into the bloodstream (and possibly the rest of the aqueous volume of distribution of body tissues as well) where they are subject to a variety of clearance mechanisms (renal, MPS) (53).

Drug Loading and Retention

The finding that long circulation time is correlated with reduced MPS uptake and greater tumor exposure presented yet another challenge to liposome formulators: keeping the drug "on board" the liposome during the plasma distribution phase (which in humans can be 3 days or more). Drug that is lost from liposomes during this long period within the bloodstream would not benefit from the passive tumor targeting feature of the carrier. In response to this challenge, active loading methods were devised. For example, an ammonium sulfate gradient loading approach is used to load doxorubicin into PLD. Liposomes are made with a high internal concentration of ammonium sulfate. When doxorubicin is added it enters the liposome, complexes with sulfate and precipitates within the aqueous compartment of the liposome (Fig. 5). This loading is not only efficient, it provides long product shelf-life and little leakage is seen from PLD following injection (54).

THE PLD EXPERIENCE

PLD (Doxil), has been in clinical practice since the early 1990s and represents the only pegylated liposome formulation that has progressed into randomized clinical trials and approval. PLD received accelerated approval in refractory AIDS-related Kaposi's sarcoma (KS) in 1995 and was launched in the United States in early 1996. Early evidence of activity in highly pretreated ovarian cancer patients led to supplemental submissions in this indication.

PLD Pharmacology

Nonclinical PK, Tissue Distribution

In animals, pharmacokinetic advantages of PLD over unencapsulated doxorubicin include an increased area under the plasma concentration–time curve, longer distribution half-life, smaller volume of distribution, and reduced clearance. In preclinical models, PLD produced remission and cure against a broad range of implanted tumors including tumors of the breast, lung, ovaries, prostate, colon, bladder, and pancreas, as well as lymphoma, sarcoma, and myeloma. It crosses the blood–brain barrier and induces remission in tumors of the CNS. It is effective as adjuvant therapy. Increased potency over free doxorubicin was observed and, in contrast to free doxorubicin, PLD was equally effective against low- and high-growth fraction tumors (55–59).

Clinical Pharmacokinetics

Clinical pharmacokinetics of PLD have been reported for three groups of solid tumor patients, hormone resistant prostate cancer (60), metastatic breast cancer (MBC) (61) and a group of patients with various refractory malignancies (Table 2) (58,62,63). The results of these studies are summarized in Table 2. In the analysis by Hubert et al. (60), 10 prostate cancer patients were given PLD in two regimes of equal dose intensity, either $45\,mg/m^2$ every 3 weeks or $60\,mg/m^2$ every 4 weeks. AUC and Cmax increased proportionally with dose. The characteristic long distribution half-life of PLD in the range of 3 days was observed. The objectives of the Lyass et al. study (61) were to examine the toxicity profile and PK of various dose schedules of PLD in a group of MBC patients previously treated with chemotherapy. PLD PK was examined in 24 patients at the dose levels of 35, 45, 60, and $70\,mg/m^2$.

In general the pharmacokinetic profile in humans at doses between 10 and $80\,mg/m^2$ is similar to that in animals, with one or two distribution phases: an initial phase with a half-life of 1–3 hours and a second phase with a half-life of 30–90 hours. The AUC after a dose of $50\,mg/m^2$ is approximately 300-fold greater than that with free drug. Clearance and volume of distribution are drastically reduced (at least 250- and 60-fold, respectively) (64).

Dose-Limiting Toxicity, Dose Rate/Balance

On balance, the clinical safety profile of PLD compares favorably to that of doxorubicin. On the plus side, relative to equally efficacious doses of doxorubicin, PLD is less cardiotoxic, causes less alopecia, nausea, and neutropenia. The dose-limiting toxicity of PLD is palmar-plantar erythrodysesthesia (PPE) and is believed to be related to entry and accumulation of the liposomes into the skin after repeat dosing. The incidence of PPE appears to be directly related to dose rate. At a dose rate of greater than $12.5\,mg/m^2/$ wk, grade 3–4 PPE (measured by National Cancer Institute Common Toxicity Criteria) does occur in some patients after a several cycles and can lead to patient discomfort, restricted movement, and treatment delays. However, in the range of $10\,mg/m^2/wk$ clinically significant PPE (grade 3 or 4) is largely avoided while tumor response appears equivalent to doxorubicin (61,64–70).

Clinical Benefit

Encapsulating doxorubicin into pegylated liposomes profoundly alters the pharmacology of the drug. A sizable body of preclinical and clinical

Table 2 Human Pharmacokinetic Parameters of PLD for Three Groups of Sold Tumor Patients

Reference:	Gabizon et al. (143)		Hubert et al. (144)		Lyass et al. (61)				Hilger et al. (62)
Formulation	DOXIL-1[b]		DOXIL[c]		DOXIL[c]				DOXIL[c]
dose (mg/m²)[a]	25	50	45	60	35	45	60	70	60
$V_{1/2}$ (I)	4.1	5.9	4.6	4.9	3.8	3.5	4	3.5	1.75
$T_{1/2}$ α (h)	3.2	1.4	ME[d]		ME				ME
$T_{1/2}$ β (h)	45.2	45.9	74	84	78.9	86	62	80.3	60
Cl (ml/min)	1.3	1.5	0.73	0.73	0.53	0.67	0.72	0.53	0.38
AUC (mg · h/L)	609	902	1891	2778	1572	2005	2325	3724	3676
C_{max} (mg/L)	12.6	21.2	17.9	22.7	13.9	20.7	26.9	32.6	37.4

[a] Adapted from the primary reference by conversion to units shown.
[b] DOXIL-1 refers to an experimental formulation used by Gabizon et al. in a pilot PK study.
[c] DOXIL refers to the commercial formulation of pegylated personal doxorubicin.
[d] Elimination best are by monoexponential decay defined here by $T_{1/2}$ β.

pharmacologic evidence is entirely consistent with the belief that the long half-life of the drug and the small size of the liposomes leads to selective accumulation of the liposome in tumors, with release of doxorubicin in the tumor bed. The experience in humans parallels reports of accumulation of doxorubicin in animal tumor models, with observation of radiolabeled liposomes and/or doxorubicin accumulation in multiple types of solid tumors. For a review of the preclinical evidence, the reader is referred to the article by Vail et al. (58).

Two lines of evidence suggest that PLD provides meaningful clinical benefits compared to the unencapsulated drug alone: (*i*) evidence showing tumor targeting of PLD and (*ii*) randomized clinical trial outcomes documenting the clinical benefits of PLD relative to various comparators, including doxorubicin.

Clinical evidence of PLD tumor targeting: When compared to conventional doxorubicin, PLD results in an altered pharmacokinetic profile. Several reports of selective accumulation of PLD in human tumor tissue have been published.

Harrington et al. demonstrated targeting of radiolabeled pegylated liposomes of the same size and composition of PLD to several common malignancies, including breast cancer, squamous cell cancer of the head and neck, lung cancer, cancer of the cervix, and high-grade glioma. In that series, tumor uptake of the radiolabeled liposomes exceeded uptake in any of the normal tissues with the exception of RES tissues (Fig. 6) (71).

Norrthfelt reported localization of higher concentrations of doxorubicin (from PLD) in KS lesions following administration of equal doses of PLD and conventional doxorubicin, with a 5.2- to 11.4-fold higher concentration after treatment with PLD compared to treatment with conventional doxorubicin (Fig. 7) (72).

Accumulation of radiolabeled PLD was studied in patients with locally advanced sarcomas undergoing radiotherapy, with dramatic accumulation of the drug observed in each of the 7 patients studied. Similarly, relative to surrounding normal tissues, biopsy-proven higher intratumoral concentrations of doxorubicin were reported following administration of PLD in patients with breast cancer (10 patients), one patient each with ovarian cancer and hepatoma, and in three patients with liver metastases. In addition, a high concentration of doxorubicin was found in a cervical lymph node biopsied in a patient treated with PLD (73).

Selective accumulation of PLD has been reported in two breast cancer patients with osseous metastases treated with PLD. In both patients, the concentration of doxorubicin was 10-fold higher in the tumor than in the surrounding muscle (74). In addition, intense accumulation of radiolabeled PLD was demonstrated by planar and single photon emission computed

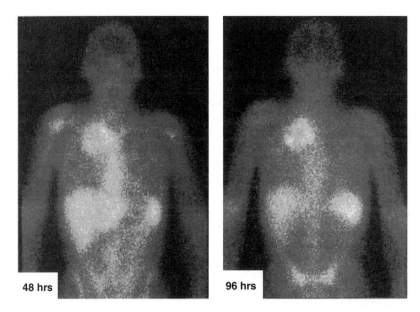

Figure 6 Gamma scintigraphic images of lung cancer patient 48 hr (*left*) and 96 hr (*right*) after given pegylated liposomes of the same size and composition of PLD but loaded with 111In-DTPA. Uptake of radioactivity is seen in normal organs including spleen, liver, and bone marrow (*ilium*). The activity visible in the central chest (*substernal*) and upper abdomen represent liposomes that are still in the circulation in the heart and major vessels at these time points. Liposome are taken up by the large tumor in the upper lobe of the left lung. The density of radioactivity is as high or higher in the tumor than any normal organ. *Source*: From Ref. 12.

tomography in 15 patients with brain metastases or glioblastoma following treatment (73,75).

   Clinical trial results: The most straightforward approach to document the clinical benefit provided by pegylated liposome delivery would be to compare the efficacy and safety of the drug in unencapsulated and encapsulated form in a randomized trial. Yet, given the appeal of such a design and the wide clinical spectrum of doxorubicin, no clinical trial, in any doxorubicin-sensitive histology, has been undertaken to compare the efficacy of single-agent PLD vs. doxorubicin administered at the same dose-rate. The reason is simple; the two drugs have different safety profiles and cannot be administered at the same dose rate. The typical dose schedule for single-agent doxorubicin is $60 \, mg/m^2$ every 3 weeks (which translates into a dose rate of $20 \, mg/m^2/wk$); the dose-limiting toxicity is generally neutropenia (absolute neutrophil count nadir at about 10–14 days, with recovery by week 3). The dose-limiting toxicity for PLD, PPE, occurs after multiple doses. Empirically it has been observed

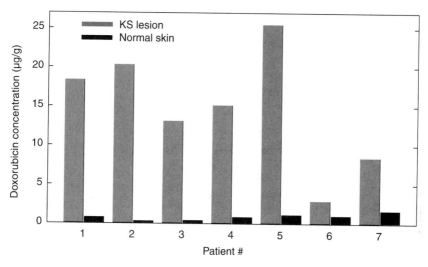

Figure 7 Selective accumulation of doxorubicin in tumor tissue vs. normal skin. Seven Kaposi's sarcoma (ks) patients underwent biopsies of normal skin and a representative cutaneous KS lesion 48 hr after receiving a 20 mg/m^2 dose of PLD and total doxorubicin was measured. *Source*: From Ref. 12.

that the most clinically significant PPE appears when PLD is given at a dose-rate exceeding 12.5 mg/m^2/wk. Below this dose rate, patients appear to tolerate the skin toxicity, sometimes benefiting from therapy for very long periods.

PLD vs. ABV in KS. PLD has indirectly been compared to doxorubicin in the AIDS KS setting (76). A total of 258 patients with advanced AIDS-KS were randomly assigned to receive either PLD (20 mg/m^2) or the combination of doxorubicin (at the same dose at PLD, 20 mg/m^2) plus bleomycin (10 mg/m^2) and vincristine (1 mg) (ABV). Both therapies were administered every 14 days for six cycles; the primary end-point was tumor response. ABV was considered the standard of care for advanced AIDS KS at the time, and doxorubicin given alone had been shown to have little activity (77). Standard response criteria, toxicity criteria, and predefined indicators of clinical benefit were examined to evaluate outcomes. Among 133 patients randomized to receive PLD, the overall response rate (ORR) was 45.9% (95% CI, 37–54%). Among 125 patients randomized to receive ABV, the ORR was 24.8% (95% CI, 17–32%). This difference was statistically significant ($p < 0.001$). In addition to objective responses, prospectively defined clinical benefits and toxicity outcomes also favored PLD.

PLD vs. doxorubicin in MBC. The closest to a head-to-head comparison of PLD to doxorubicin was the trial reported by O'Brien et al. in MBC (78). The statistical hypothesis of the trial was to demonstrate that progression-free survival (PFS) of PLD is non-inferior to doxorubicin with significantly less cardiotoxicity in first-line treatment of women with MBC. A total of 509 women with normal cardiac function at first assessment were randomized to receive either PLD ($50 \, mg/m^2$ every 4 weeks; dose-rate $12.5 \, mg/m^2/wk$) or doxorubicin ($60 \, mg/m^2$ every 3 weeks; dose-rate $20 \, mg/ m^2/wk$). Adverse cardiac events were based on predefined reductions in left ventricular ejection fraction from baseline as a function of cumulative anthracycline dose. Multigated blood-pool imaging scans were performed to measure LVEF before treatment, after $300 \, mg/m^2$ cumulative anthracycline exposure, and after every additional $100 \, mg/m^2$ of PLD and every $120 \, mg/ m^2$ of doxorubicin. A protocol-specified cardiac event was defined as a decrease of $\geq 20\%$ from baseline if the resting LVEF remained in the normal range, or a decrease of $\geq 10\%$ if the LVEF became abnormal (less than the institutional lower limit of normal). Patients were also assessed for signs and symptoms of congestive heart failure.

Median duration of therapy was similar in both arms. PLD and doxorubicin were comparable with respect to PFS [6.9 versus 7.8 months, respectively; hazard ratio (HR) = 1.00; 95% CI 0.82–1.22, Fig. 8]. Overall risk of cardiotoxicity was significantly higher with doxorubicin than PLD (HR = 3.16; 95% CI 1.58–6.31; $p < 0.001$, Fig. 9). Overall survival was similar (21 and 22 months for PLD and doxorubicin, respectively; HR = 0.94; 95% CI 0.74–1.19). Alopecia, nausea, vomiting and neutropenia were more often associated with doxorubicin than PLD. Skin and mucus

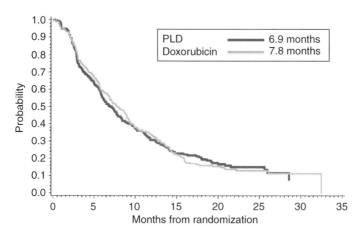

Figure 8 PFS of MBC patients randomized to receive PLD ($n = 254$ at a dose rate of $50 \, mg/m^2/month$) or doxorubicin ($n = 255$ at a dose rate of $60 \, mg/m^2$ every 3 weeks). The hazard ratio between the groups is 1.00 (95% CI 0.82–1.22) indicating that the treatments are equivalent, even though the doxorubicin dose is about 40% lower in the PLD group. *Source*: From Ref. 78.

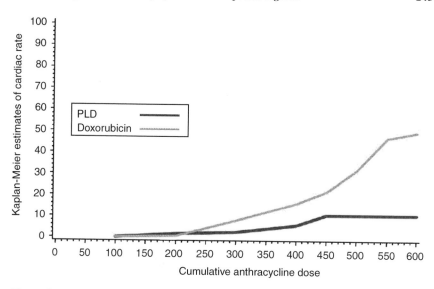

Figure 9 Rate of cardiac events vs. cumulative doxorubicin dose. Patients who had a baseline and at least one additional multigated blood pool imaging scan during treatment. Cumulative percentage of events versus cumulative anthracycline dose, protocol-defined cardiac events. HR = 3.16; 95% CI 1.58–6.31; p <0.001; PLD, n = 254; doxorubicin, n = 255. *Source*: From Ref. 78.

membrane toxicity including PPE, stomatitis and mucositis were more often associated with PLD than doxorubicin. The toxicity advantages may be related to the reduced rate of exposure of patients to doxorubicin in the PLD arm. The finding that efficacy was comparable in both the PLD and doxorubicin arms of this trial, and given that patients received about 60% less exposure to the drug in the PLD arm (by virtue of the differential dose-rates between the two arms), suggests that the shift in tissue distribution provided by pegylated liposome delivery provides a clinical benefit over the unencapsulated drug given at its active dose.

PLD vs. comparator (physicians' choice) in taxane-refractory breast cancer. Since doxorubicin has become so widely used in the adjuvant breast cancer setting, patients who relapse are not often retreated because of the risk of cumulative-dose related anthracycline-induced cardiotoxicity (79). And, although high-dose anthracyclines (i.e., $75\,mg/m^2$ doxorubicin or $90\,mg/m^2$ epirubicin) are active as single-agents in first-line treatment of recurrent breast (80), taxane combinations are currently the most often used for first-line treatment of MBC. Following taxane failure, a number of agents with known activity may be considered.

Single agent therapy such as weekly vinorelbine is active and well tolerated in this palliative setting (81). Sequential therapy with capecitabine followed by vinorelbine/cisplatin or epirubicin followed by mitomycin C have shown benefit (82,83), as have combinations including mitomycin C/vinblastine (84), cisplatin/vinorelbine (85), and oxaliplatin/vinorelbine/5-fluorouracil (86).

PLD has been compared with two common salvage regimens ("comparator") in patients with taxane-refractory advanced breast cancer (87). Again, although not a direct comparison, evidence of meaningful objective activity in the PLD arm of this study suggests that it is more beneficial than doxorubicin in this setting.

Following failure of a first- or second-line taxane-containing regimen for metastatic disease, 301 women were randomly assigned to receive PLD (50 mg/m^2 every 28 days); or one of two physicians' choice comparators, either vinorelbine (30 mg/m^2/wk) or a combination of mitomycin C (10 mg/m^2 day 1 and every 28 days) plus vinblastine (5 mg/m^2 day 1, day 14, day 28, and day 42) every 6–8 weeks. PFS and overall survival were similar for PLD and the comparator. In anthracycline-naïve patients, PFS was somewhat longer with PLD, relative to the comparator (n = 44; median PFS, 5.8 vs. 2.1 months; HR, 2.40; 95% CI 1.16–4.95; p = 0.01) (Fig. 10). The most frequently reported adverse events were nausea (2–31%), vomiting (17–20%), and fatigue (9–20%) and were similar, among treatment groups. PLD-treated patients experienced more PPE (37%; 18% grade 3, 1 patient

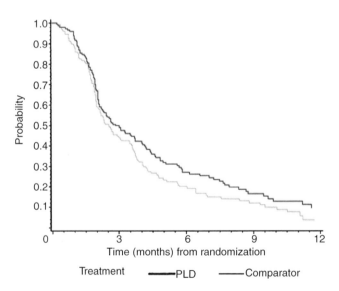

Figure 10 PFS was similar for PLD and comparator (HR = 1.26; 95% CI 0.98–1.62; p = .11; median PFS, 2.9 months vs. 2.5 months for PLD and comparator, respectively). *Abbreviation*: PLD, pegylated liposomal doxorubicin. *Source*: From Ref. 87.

grade 4) and stomatitis (22%; 5% grades 3/4). Neuropathy (11%), constipation (16%), and neutropenia (14%) were more common with vinorelbine. Alopecia was low in both the PLD and vinorelbine groups (3% and 5%). The authors conclude that PLD efficacy was comparable to that of common salvage regimens in patients with taxane-refractory MBC.

PLD vs. topotecan in ovarian cancer. Single-agent topotecan is active in epithelial ovarian carcinoma which recurs after or is unresponsive to first-line, platinum-based chemotherapy (88). In a randomized trial, PLD compared favorably to topotecan in this setting. Although the comparison is not direct, objective evidence of activity in the PLD arm of this study suggests that PLD is more active than doxorubicin which lacks single-agent activity in this setting (89).

Patients were randomized to receive either PLD $50 \, mg/m^2$ as a 1-hour infusion every 4 weeks or topotecan $1.5 \, mg/m^2/d$ for 5 consecutive days every 3 weeks. Patients were stratified prospectively for platinum sensitivity and for the presence or absence of bulky disease. The intent-to-treat population consisted of 474 patients, 239 treated with PLD and 235 with topotecan (90).

Among the intent-to-treat population there was an 18% reduction in the risk of death for patients treated with PLD (median survival 62.7 weeks for PLD and 59.7 weeks for topotecan-treated patients; HR = 1.216; 95% CI 1.000–1.478; p = 0.050). For patients with platinum-sensitive disease, there was a 30% reduction in the risk of death for the PLD-treated group (median survival 107.9 weeks for PLD and 70.1 weeks for topotecan-treated patients; HR = 1.432; 95% CI 1.066–1.923; p = 0.017). In patients with platinum-refractory disease, survival was similar between treatment groups. (Fig. 11). Long-term follow-up confirms that treatment with PLD significantly prolongs survival compared with topotecan in patients with recurrent and refractory epithelial ovarian cancer (91).

PLD in multiple myeloma. The hallmark of multiple myeloma (MM) is the accumulation of monoclonal plasma cells that secrete monoclonal immunoglobulins (or fragments thereof) that can lead to renal failure. Although doxorubicin has been shown to be active in combination regimens used to treat MM, its toxicity often limits adequate dosing. When doxorubicin is substituted with PLD in a combination regimens, meaningful safety benefits have been documented (Table 3) (92–94).

In a randomized trial designed to shown that PLD, vincristine and dexamethasone (PLDVD) has similar response with better safety relative to the same combination using doxorubicin, 192 patients with newly diagnosed, active MM were assigned to receive either combined PLD ($40 \, mg/m^2$) and vincristine ($1.4 \, mg/m^2$; maximum, 2.0 mg) as an intravenous infusion on Day 1 plus reduced-dose dexamethasone (40 mg) orally on days 1–4 (PLDVD) (n = 97 patients) or combined vincristine (0.4 mg per day) and conventional doxorubicin ($9 \, mg/m^2$ per day) as a continuous intravenous

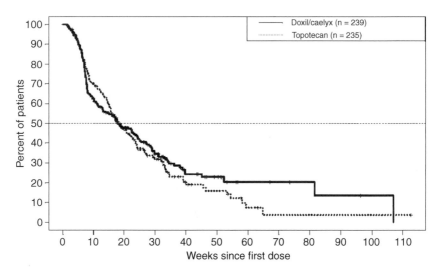

Figure 11 Kaplan–Meier curve of time to progression among advanced ovarian cancer patients randomized to receive PLD at $50\,mg/m^2$ every 4 weeks (n = 239) or topotecan at 1.5 mg for 5 consecutive days every 3 weeks (n = 235). In this intent-to-treat population, the comparison favors PLD (p = 0.05). *Note*: Curves are based on Kaplan-Meier estimates. F(t) = prob{Time to progression > t} *Abbreviation*: PLD, pegylated liposomal doxorubicin. *Source*: From Ref. 91 and \3049\$\stat\figpgm\psrand\g_tm^{2}pd.ssc MR 04FEB04.

infusion on days 1–4 plus reduced-dose dexamethasone (VAd) (n = 95 patients) for at least 4 cycles, repeated every 4 weeks. The primary endpoints were response and toxicity. Objective response rates (PLDVD, 44%; VAd, 41%), PFS (HR = 1.11; p = 0.69), and overall survival (hazard ratio, 0.88; p = 0.67) were similar between the treatment groups.

Table 3 Clinical Benefit of Substitution of Doxorubicin with PLD in VAd Regimen for Multiple Myeloma

Incidence type	No. of patients (%)		
	DVd n = 97	VAd n = 95	P^a
Neutropenia (Grade 3 or 4) or neutropenic fever	11(10.3)	23(24.2)	0.02
Documented sepsis	3(3.1)	8(8.4)	0.13
Antibiotic treatment	61(62.9)	65(68.4)	0.45
Hospitalizations for adverse events	36(37.1)	34(35.8)	0.88

[a]P values were determined with a two-sided Fisher exact test.
Abbreviations: DVd, pegylated liposomal doxorubicin, vincristine, and reduced-dose dexamethasone; VAd, doxorubicin, vincristine, and reduced-dose dexamethasone.

However, PLDVD was associated with significantly less Grade 3/4 neutropenia or neutropenic fever (10% vs. 24%; $p = 0.01$), a lower incidence of sepsis, less antibiotic and growth-factor support, less alopecia (20% vs. 44%; $p < 0.001$) but more hand-foot syndrome (25% vs. 1%; $p < 0.001$), mainly Grade 1/2 (93). PLD has also shown promise in MM when used in combination with bortezomib (95).

PEGYLATED LIPOSOMAL CAMPTHOTHECIN

Camptothecin was identified in the 1960s as a potent cytotoxin; it inhibits topoisomerase I, resulting in DNA damage and apoptosis during DNA synthesis (96). Unfortunately, the sodium salt of camptothecin failed in early clinical trials due to toxicities related to its poor water solubility (97). A number of analogues were subsequently synthesized, including topotecan and irinotecan. These derivatives were designed to be more water-soluble while retaining anti-tumor activity. Both topotecan (Hycamtin®) and irinotecan (Camptosar®) are now registered in the United States and elsewhere.

The clinical utility of camptothecins may be improved by delivery in pegylated liposomes. This class of drug has poor intrinsic chemical stability; at physiological pH in biological fluids, camptothecins are subject to rapid hydrolysis of the lactone ring that is required for anticancer activity. Stabilization or protection of this structure can in principle be achieved by liposome encapsulation, thus preserving activity until deposition in the tumor (Fig. 12). Moreover, toxicities such as myelosuppression and adverse GI effects may be reduced by liposome encapsulation.

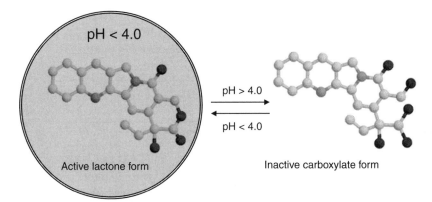

Figure 12 Scientific rationale for delivery of camptothecins using pegylated liposomes of the same size and composition as PLD. At physiological pH, camptothecins convert to an inactive carboxylate form. Encapsulation in pegylated liposomes with low internal pH preserves the drug in its active lactone form. *Abbreviation*: PLD, pegylated liposomal doxorubicin.

CKD 602 is a relatively new camptothecin analogue exhibiting anti-tumor activity similar to that of topotecan (98). Encapsulation of this compound in pegylated liposomes which are modeled after the PLD architecture offers a number of potential advantages, perhaps representing an ideal marriage between a drug and a delivery system. First, the chemical stability of CKD 602 can be preserved by adjusting the pH within the liposome (Fig. 12). In the encapsulated form, the drug can circulate without being degraded. Second, as with PLD, the polymer coating and small size of the pegylated liposomes provide passive targeting to tumor sites. Once in the tumor, the drug is slowly released from liposomes. Local release of drug in tumors is believed to occur over a period of weeks following a single administration. This release pattern is well-suited to cell cycle-specific drugs such as CKD 602, since cancer cells become exposed continuously to cytotoxic levels of drug and anti-tumor efficacy is enhanced (Fig. 13).

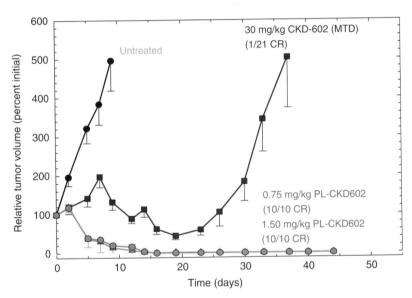

Figure 13 Tumor growth kinetics of ES-2 ovarian xenografts implanted in the flank of nude mice. Curves show untreated animals (•) or groups of mice treated with the camptothecin analogue CKD-602 given alone at its maximum tolerated dose (30 mg/kg, ■) or encapsulated in pegylated liposomes of the same composition and size as PLD at doses of 0.75 mg/kg (▲) or 1.50 mg/kg (•). Initial tumor size was ~105 mm^3 and treated animals received three weekly injections (*arrows*). The MTD of the pegylated liposomes containing CKD-602 is 2.25 mg/kg. Note the liposome encapsulated drug is active at 1/3 of its MTD (0.75 mg/kg) and provides superior efficacy (including complete responses, CR) compared to CKD-602 alone at its MTD (30 mg/kg). *Abbreviations*: PLD, pegylated liposomal doxorubicin; CR, complete responses. *Source*: From Ref. 99.

Finally, the long circulation associated with pegylated liposome encapsulation allows for relatively infrequent dosing intervals as compared with free drug.

Early clinical results for pegylated liposomal CKD-602 (PL-CKD602) appear promising (100). In a phase 1 dose-ranging study, 45 patients received PL-CKD602 once every 3 weeks. Dose levels ranged from 0.1 to 2.5 mg/m^2. Encapsulated, released, and total CKD602 (lactone + hydroxyl acid) were measured by LC-MS/MS. The majority of reported adverse events were grades 1 and 2. Frequent nonhematological toxicities were asthenia, nausea, diarrhea, vomiting, and anorexia. Dose-limiting toxicities were related to bone marrow suppression in 2/3 patients at 2.5 mg/m^2, and G3 febrile neutropenia in 1/6 pts at 2.1 mg/m^2. The maximum tolerated dose was 2.1 mg/m^2. Stable disease for ≥ 6 cycles occurred in 5 patients [hepatocellular carcinoma (CA), thyroid, prostate, 2 patients sarcoma]. Partial responses occurred in 2 patients with ovarian CA (1.7 and 2.1 mg/m^2). At 2.1 mg/m^2, the mean $\pm$ SD AUC and $t_{1/2}$ of sum total S-CKD602 were 44 $\pm$ 33 µg/mL $\pm$ h and 18 $\pm$ 8 h, respectively. In all plasma samples, > 90% of drug was encapsulated. Phase II studies of PL-CKD602 at 2.1 mg/m^2 IV once every 3 weeks are planned.

LIGAND-TARGETED PEGYLATED LIPOSOMES

Although PLD provides stable formulation, improved pharmacokinetic profile, "passive" targeting to tumor tissue, and meaningful clinical benefit to patients (101), it does not directly targets tumor cells. A second generation of pegylated liposomes is under development that incorporates ligands designed to actively target the liposomes to cells expressing the appropriate surface receptors.

HER-2 Targeted Pegylated Liposomal Doxorubicin (Her-2 PLD)

Patients with breast cancer and HER2 amplification have a poor prognosis relative to patients with lesser levels of HER2 expression (102,103). Randomized clinical trials have shown that HER2-overexpression is associated with a steep dose–response relationship to, and clinical benefit from, anthracycline-based chemotherapy. Indeed, HER2-overexpression in breast and gastric tumors is correlated with anthracycline sensitivity (104,105). HER2-mediated delivery of doxorubicin encapsulated in pegylated liposomes may represent a particularly advantageous clinical approach to treating HER2-overexpressing cancers.

A new generation of PLD that is actively targeted to the HER2 receptor has been created by incorporating scFv antibody fragments which recognize the HER2 receptor, into the surface of preformed pegylated doxorubicin liposomes (Her-2 PLD). The HER2-targeted formulation is designed to enhance the therapeutic index of doxorubicin by combining the passive tumor targeting provided by PLD with specific targeting to HER2 cell surface receptors on tumor cells.

In vitro, Her-2 PLD bind with high specificity to cancer cells that over-express HER2 and are internalized by tumor cells which express high levels (e.g., 10^6) of HER2 receptors per cell. The amplification potential of this approach is illustrated by comparing in vitro cell uptake of Her-2 PLD with that of PLD lacking the ligand; total doxorubicin uptake of Her-2 PLD is more than 700-fold higher in HER2-overexpressing than in non-overexpressing cells (106). For example, uptake of Her-2 PLD in HER2-overexpressing SKBR-3 cells in culture reaches 7.21 ± 0.45 nmol phospholipid/mg cell protein, which equates to about 23,000 liposomes per cell (107). Since each liposome can be loaded with up to 10^4 doxorubicin molecules, this approach has the potential to achieve highly productive intracellular delivery.

The therapeutic efficacy of Her-2 PLD in HER2 overexpressing xen-ograft models is impressive, including tumor inhibition, regressions of large established tumors, and pathologic complete responses at sacrifice (Fig. 14) (106). Her-2 PLD treatment is superior to conventional doxorubicin, PLD, and anti-HER2 MAb (herceptin). Her-2 PLD treatment was also sig-nificantly superior to combination treatments consisting of conventional doxorubicin + herceptin.

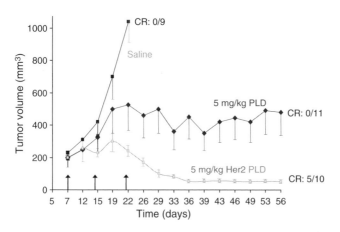

Figure 14 Nude mice were inoculated in the flank with BT-474 cells (which are highly HER2-amplified) and the tumors were allowed to grow to about 200 mm^3. Treated animal were then dosed with a liposome equivalent of 5 mg/kg doxorubicin once weekly for 3 weeks with either PLD or Her-2 PLD. Significant tumor regression is seen with clear separation of the antitumor effect of PLD and Her2-PLD with, most notably, cures in 5 out of the 10 animals in the Her2-PLD group. *Abbreviation*: PLD, pegylated liposomal doxorubicin. *Source*: From Ref. 106.

Tumor localization studies indicate a novel mechanism of drug delivery for Her-2 PLD (108). Both PLD and Her-2 PLD achieve comparably high drug levels in tumor xenografts, indicating that tumor accumulation of pegylated liposomes is not enhanced by antibody targeting. These finding further suggests that extravasation is the rate-limiting process for tumor uptake of long-circulating liposomes. Once in the tumor bed, the disposition of Her-2 PLD is different than that of liposomes lacking the ligand; Her-2 PLD is internalized by tumor cells, while non-targeted liposomes are restricted to the tumor interstitium (and tissue macrophage compartment). Electron microscopy studies suggest that binding of Her-2 PLD is followed by rapid receptor-mediated endocytosis and intracellular drug release (109). Plasma pharmacokinetics of Her-2 PLD do not differ from PLD after single and multiple dosing indicating that the ligand does not compromise long circulation time nor provoke a neutralizing antibody response (106).

Other Ligands, Drug Payloads for Targeting Pegylated Liposomes to Tumors

Ligands other than those which recognize the HER2 receptor may be useful to target drug-loaded pegylated liposomes to tumors. The strategy followed to select the internalizing ligand used in the Her-2 PLD formulation from non-immune phage libraries can potentially be applied to select ligands to target pegylated liposomes to tumor cells which overexpressed other clinically validated receptors (110,111). Peptide ligands selected from phage display libraries are also attractive in this setting (112–116). Clinical experience with monoclonal antibody products provides a number of attractive targets including growth factor receptors other than HER2, such as EGF, VEGF, integrins, and surface enzymes (117–133).

Recently, a combinatorial approach to the preparation of ligand-targeted liposomes has been introduced, termed the post-insertion technique, which is simple, flexible, and offers the potential to create "tailor-made" chemotherapeutic ligand–drug combinations for individual patients' needs. Using the approach, the ligand is first coupled to the terminus of a PEG lipid (such as PEG_{2000}-DSPE); such constructs form a micellar suspension when dispersed in buffer. When mixed with preformed liposomes at elevated temperature, individual ligand-PEG-lipid molecules transfer from micelles and quantitatively insert into the outer surface of the liposomes. Using this technique it may be possible to use a combinatorial approach to create targeted chemotherapy that is tailored to individual patients' tumors. Ligands would be selected on the basis of receptor expression status and the drug, loaded into the liposomes, selected based on its known activity against the histological type of tumor being treated (134–137).

COMPARISON TO OTHER NANO-PARTICULATE SYSTEMS

Other nanoparticle formulations of chemotherapeutics including albumin microspheres have been shown to provide patient benefit. ABI-007 (Abraxane®; Abraxis in the United States and Astra-Zeneca in the European Union) is a crosslinked albumin microsphere of about 130-nm diameter which forms a strong complex with paclitaxel. It was developed to avoid the requirement for Cremophor/ethanol as solubilizers in the commercial formulation and to exploit albumin receptor-mediated endothelial transport. In animal toxicology studies, the LD_{50} and maximum tolerated dose for ABI-007 and Cremophor-based paclitaxel were 47 and 30 mg/kg/d and 30 and 13.4 mg/kg/d, respectively. In implanted tumor models, at equitoxic dose, the ABI-007-treated groups showed more complete regressions, longer time to recurrence, longer doubling time, and prolonged survival. Enhanced endothelial cell binding and transcytosis for ABI-007 and inhibition by Cremophor in Cremophor-based paclitaxel may account in part for the greater efficacy and intratumor delivery of ABI-007 (138–140).

ABI-077 is now approved for treatment of recurrent breast cancer based on results demonstrating that ABI-007, without the Cremophor-related toxicities, can be administered safely at twice the dose intensity relative to standard paclitaxel. The higher dose leads to significantly higher response rates in MBC compared with standard paclitaxel at its recommended dose (33% vs. 19%, respectively; $p < .001$) and significantly longer time to tumor progression (23.0 vs. 16.9 weeks, respectively; $p < 0.006$). The incidence of grade 4 neutropenia was significantly lower for ABI-007 compared with standard paclitaxel (9% vs. 22%, respectively) and despite a 49% higher paclitaxel dose (141).

FUTURE DIRECTIONS

Although product introductions based on nanoscale delivery systems have been few thus far, momentum to reformulate existing drugs (i.e., those with know activity and safety profile) is mounting based on the success of PLD and ABI-077. It is likely that other drugs will benefit from these approaches. For example, the benefit provided by passive tumor targeting of pegylated liposomes loaded with mitomycin C is now being explored with promising initial results (142). An albumin microsphere formulation of docetaxel is also in development.

Perhaps the most exciting opportunity for the pegylated liposomes systems is their versatility which provides the possibility to create personalized chemotherapies. The ability to fine tune the system by insertion of ligands (or mixtures of ligands), adjust size, drug encapsulation, release rate, and surface properties are unique to liposomes. Assuming that other first generation pegylated liposome products, in addition to PLD, become available in the future (such a camptothecin, mitomycin C, taxane, cisplatin) and that that other ligand cassettes are created to insert into these liposomes, (such as antiEGFR, antiVEGFR, anti-integrins) it will be possible to rationally mix and match the ligand and drug to treat tumors exhibiting particular properties (surface receptors, drug sensitivities).

Liposomes may also serve a useful role to deliver nucleic acid-based therapeutics to systemic sites of disease. These drugs are intrinsically unstable, have poor pharmacologic properties and lack a means to enter the cellular compartment in which they are designed to act. Liposomes offer the means to encapsulate and protect such drugs, deliver them to tumors and, with a ligand on board, mediate intracellular delivery into endosomes (and perhaps caveolae or other alternative routes exploited by viruses). The current pathways relied upon for intracellular delivery may not be ideal, exposing the nucleic acids to degradation in the acidic compartment of the cell. Engineering cytoplasmic delivery of nucleic acid-based, by providing a mechanism for escape from endosomes after liposome internalization, for example, is an exciting area for future research.

REFERENCES

1. Moses MA, Brem H, et al. Advancing the field of drug delivery: taking aim at cancer. Cancer Cell 2003; 4(5):337–41.
2. Schiffelers RM, Ansari A, et al. Cancer siRNA therapy by tumor selective delivery with ligand-targeted sterically stabilized nanoparticle. Nucleic Acids Res 2004; 32(19):e149.
3. Choi Y, Baker JR, Jr. Targeting cancer cells with DNA-assembled dendrimers: a mix and match strategy for cancer. Cell Cycle 2005; 4(5):669–71.
4. Moghimi SM, Hunter AC, et al. Nanomedicine: current status and future prospects. Faseb J 2005; 19(3):311–30.
5. Sengupta S, Eavarone D, et al. Temporal targeting of tumour cells and neovasculature with a nanoscale delivery system. Nature 2005; 436(7050):568–72.
6. Duncan R. Polymer conjugates as anticancer nanomedicines. Nat Rev Cancer 2006; 6(9):688–701.
7. Schiffelers RM, Storm G. ICS-283: a system for targeted intravenous delivery of siRNA. Expert Opin Drug Deliv 2006; 3(3):445–54.
8. Socinski M. Update on nanoparticle albumin-bound paclitaxel. Clin Adv Hematol Oncol 2006; 4(10):745–6.
9. Wu G, Barth RF, et al. Targeted delivery of methotrexate to epidermal growth factor receptor-positive brain tumors by means of cetuximab (IMC-C225) dendrimer bioconjugates. Mol Cancer Ther 2006; 5(1):52–9.
10. de Wolf HK, Snel CJ, et al. Effect of cationic carriers on the pharmacokinetics and tumor localization of nucleic acids after intravenous administration. Int J Pharm 2007; 331(2):167–75.
11. Torchilin VP. Micellar nanocarriers: pharmaceutical perspectives. Pharm Res 2007; 24(1):1–16.

12. Martin FJ. Pegylated liposomal doxorubicin: scientific rationale and pre-clinical pharmacology. Oncology 1997; 11(Suppl. 11):11–20.
13. Amantea M, Bowden, et al. Population Pharmacokinetics and Renal Function–Sparing Effects of Amphotericin B. Colloidal Dispersion in Patients Receiving Bone Marrow Transplants. Antimicrob Agents & Chemo 1995.
14. Ewer MS, Martin FJ, et al. Cardiac safety of liposomal anthracyclines. Semin Oncol 2004; 31(6Suppl. 13):161–81.
15. Allen TM, Martin FJ, Advantages of liposomal delivery systems for anthra-cyclines. Semin Oncol 2004; 31(6Suppl. 13):5–15.
16. Gabizon A, Chisin R, et al. Pharmacokinetic and imaging studies in patients receiving a formulation of liposome-associated adriamycin. Br J Cancer 1991; 64(6):1125–32.
17. Conley BA, Egorin MJ, et al. Phase I and pharmacokinetic trial of liposome-encapsulated doxorubicin. Cancer Chemother Pharmacol 1993; 33(2): 107–12.
18. Liu D, Hu Q, et al. Liposome clearance from blood: different animal species have different mechanisms. Biochim Biophys Acta 1995; 1240(2):277–84.
19. Semple SC, Harasym TO, et al. Immunogenicity and rapid blood clearance of liposomes containing polyethylene glycol-lipid conjugates and nucleic Acid. J Pharmacol Exp Ther 2005; 312(3):1020–6.
20. Bellott R, Auvrignon A, et al. Pharmacokinetics of liposomal daunorubicin (DaunoXome) during a phase I–II study in children with relapsed acute lymphoblastic leukaemia. Cancer Chemother Pharmacol 2001; 47(1):15–21.
21. Krishna R, Webb MS, et al. Liposomal and nonliposomal drug pharmaco-kinetics after administration of liposome-encapsulated vincristine and their contribution to drug tissue distribution properties. J Pharmacol Exp Ther 2001; 298(3):1206–12.
22. Allen TM, Chonn A. Large unilamellar liposomes with low uptake into the reticuloendothelial system. FEBS Lett 1987; 223(1):42–6.
23. Klibanov AL, Maruyama K, et al. Amphipathic polyethyleneglycols effec-tively prolong the circulation time of liposomes. FEBS Lett 1990; 268(1): 235–7.
24. Allen TM, Hansen C, et al. Liposomes containing synthetic lipid derivatives of poly(ethylene glycol) show prolonged circulation half-lives in vivo. Biochim Biophys Acta 1991; 1066(1):29–36.
25. Klibanov AL, Maruyama K, et al. Activity of amphipathic poly(ethylene glycol) 5000 to prolong the circulation time of liposomes depends on the liposome size and is unfavorable for immunoliposome binding to target. Biochim Biophys Acta 1991; 1062(2):142–8.
26. Senior J, Delgado C, et al. Influence of surface hydrophilicity of liposomes on their interaction with plasma protein and clearance from the circulation: studies with poly(ethylene glycol)-coated vesicles. Biochim Biophys Acta 1991; 1062(1):77–82.
27. Torchilin VP, Klibanov AL, et al. Targeted accumulation of polyethylene glycol-coated immunoliposomes in infarcted rabbit myocardium. Faseb J 1992; 6(9):2716–9.

28. Zhang F. Pegylated interferons in the treatment of chronic hepatitis C. Chin Med J Engl 2003; 116(4):495–8.
29. Webster R, Didier E, et al. PEGylated proteins: evaluation of their safety in the absence of definitive metabolism studies. Drug Metab Dispos 2007; 35(1): 9–16.
30. Papahadjopoulos D, Allen TM, et al. Sterically stabilized liposomes: improvements in pharmacokinetics and antitumor therapeutic efficacy. Proc Natl Acad Sci USA 1991; 88(24):11460–4.
31. Woodle MC, Matthay KK, et al. Versatility in lipid compositions showing prolonged circulation with sterically stabilized liposomes. Biochim Biophys Acta 1992; 1105(2):193–200.
32. Lasic DD, Martin FJ, et al. Sterically stabilized liposomes: a hypothesis on the molecular origin of the extended circulation times. Biochim Biophys Acta 1991; 1070(1):187–92.
33. Cullis PR, Chonn A, et al. Interactions of liposomes and lipid-based carrier systems with blood proteins: Relation to clearance behaviour in vivo. Adv Drug Deliv Rev 1998; 32(1–2):3–17.
34. Sheth SR, Leckband D. Measurements of attractive forces between proteins and end-grafted poly(ethylene glycol) chains. Proc Natl Acad Sci USA 1997; 94(16):8399–404.
35. Dos Santos N, Allen C, et al. Influence of poly(ethylene glycol) grafting density and polymer length on liposomes: Relating plasma circulation lifetimes to protein binding. Biochim Biophys Acta 2007.
36. Moribe K, Maruyama K, et al. Estimation of surface state of poly(ethylene glycol)-coated liposomes using an aqueous two-phase partitioning technique. Chem Pharm Bull (Tokyo) 1997; 45(10):1683–7.
37. Dams ET, Laverman P, et al. Accelerated blood clearance and altered biodistribution of repeated injections of sterically stabilized liposomes. J Pharmacol Exp Ther 2000; 292(3):1071–9.
38. Laverman P, Brouwers AH, et al. Preclinical and clinical evidence for disappearance of long-circulating characteristics of polyethylene glycol liposomes at low lipid dose. J Pharmacol Exp Ther 2000; 293(3):996–1001.
39. Laverman P, Boerman OC, et al. In vivo applications of PEG liposomes: unexpected observations. Crit Rev Ther Drug Carrier Syst 2001; 18(6):551–66.
40. Laverman P, Carstens MG, et al. Factors affecting the accelerated blood clearance of polyethylene glycol-liposomes upon repeated injection. J Pharmacol Exp Ther 2001; 298(2):607–12.
41. Ishida T, Harada M, et al. Accelerated blood clearance of PEGylated liposomes following preceding liposome injection: effects of lipid dose and PEG surface-density and chain length of the first-dose liposomes. J Control Release 2005; 105(3):305–17.
42. Ishida T, Ichihara M, et al. Injection of PEGylated liposomes in rats elicits PEG-specific IgM, which is responsible for rapid elimination of a second dose of PEGylated liposomes. J Control Release 2006; 112(1):15–25.
43. Johnstone SA, Masin D, et al. Surface-associated serum proteins inhibit the uptake of phosphatidylserine and poly(ethylene glycol) liposomes by mouse macrophages. Biochim Biophys Acta 2001; 1513(1):25–37.

44. Folkman J. Angiogenesis in cancer, vascular, rheumatoid and other disease. Nat Med 1995; 1(1):27–31.

45. Skinner SA, Tutton PJ, et al. Microvascular architecture of experimental colon tumors in the rat. Cancer Res 1990; 50(8):2411–7.

46. Dvorak HF, Nagy JA, et al. Structure of solid tumors and their vasculature: implications for therapy with monoclonal antibodies. Cancer Cells 1991; 3(3): 77–85.

47. Chang YS, di Tomaso E, et al. Mosaic blood vessels in tumors: frequency of cancer cells in contact with flowing blood. Proc Natl Acad Sci USA 2000; 97 (26):14608–13.

48. McDonald DM, Foss AJ. Endothelial cells of tumor vessels: abnormal but not absent. Cancer Metastasis Rev 2000; 19(1–2):109–20.

49. di Tomaso E, Capen D, et al. Mosaic tumor vessels: cellular basis and ultrastructure of focal regions lacking endothelial cell markers. Cancer Res 2005; 65(13):5740–9.

50. Matsumura Y, Maeda H. A new concept for macromolecular therapeutics in cancer chemotherapy: mechanism of tumoritropic accumulation of proteins and the antitumor agent smancs. Cancer Res 1986; 46(12 Pt 1):6387–92.

51. Greish K, et al. Enhanced permeability and retention (EPR) effect and tumor-selective delivery of anticancer drugs. London, Imperial College Press.

52. Matsumura Y, Maeda H. A new concept for macromolecular therapeutics in cancer chemotherapy: mechanism of tumoritropic accumulation of proteins and the antitumor agent SMANCS. Cancer Res 1986; 6:193–210.

53. Seymour LW, Miyamoto Y, et al. Influence of molecular weight on passive tumour accumulation of a soluble macromolecular drug carrier. Eur J Cancer 1995; 31A(5):766–70.

54. Haran G, Cohen R, et al. Transmembrane ammonium sulfate gradients in liposomes produce efficient and stable entrapment of amphipathic weak bases [published erratum appears in Biochim Biophys Acta 1994 Feb 23;1190(1): 197]. Biochim Biophys Acta 1993; 1151(2):201–15.

55. Working PK, Dayan AD. Pharmacological-toxicological expert report. CAELYX. (Stealth liposomal doxorubicin HCl). Hum Exp Toxicol 1996; 15 (9):751–85.

56. Coukell AJ, Spencer CM. Polyethylene glycol-liposomal doxorubicin. A review of its pharmacodynamic and pharmacokinetic properties, and therapeutic efficacy in the management of AIDS-related Kaposi's sarcoma. Drugs 1997; 53(3):520–38.

57. Di Paolo, A. Liposomal anticancer therapy: pharmacokinetic and clinical aspects. J Chemother 2004; 16(Suppl. 4):90–3.

58. Vail DM, Amantea MA, et al. Pegylated liposomal doxorubicin: proof of principle using preclinical animal models and pharmacokinetic studies. Semin Oncol 2004; 31(6 Suppl. 13):16–35.

59. Allen TM, Cheng WW, et al. Pharmacokinetics and pharmacodynamics of lipidic nano-particles in cancer. Anticancer Agents Med Chem 2006; 6(6):513–23.

60. Hubert A, Lyass O, et al. Doxil (Caelyx): an exploratory study with phar-macokinetics in patients with hormone-refractory prostate cancer. Anticancer Drugs 2000; 11(2):123–7.

61. Lyass O, Uziely B, et al. Correlation of toxicity with pharmacokinetics of pegylated liposomal doxorubicin (Doxil) in metastatic breast carcinoma. Cancer 2000; 89(5):1037–47.
62. Hilger RA, Richly H, et al. Pharmacokinetics of Encapsulated as Well as Free Doxorubicin and its Metabolites After Intravenous Infusion of Caelyx. Proc Am Soc Clin Oncol 2001; 20:116a.
63. Richly H, Oberhoff C, et al. Pharmacokinetics (PK) of the liposomal encapsulated fraction (Caelyx, Doxil) as well as released doxorubicin after intravenous infusion of pegylated liposomes: PK based evidence for an indirect tumortargeting and a high systemic disposition of the released drug. Proc Am Soc Clin Oncol 2002; 21:Abs. 478.
64. Gabizon A, Shmeeda H, et al. Pharmacokinetics of pegylated liposomal Doxorubicin: review of animal and human studies. Clin Pharmacokinet 2003; 42(5):419–36.
65. Alberts DS, Garcia DJ. Safety aspects of pegylated liposomal doxorubicin in patients with cancer. Drugs 1997; 54(Suppl. 4):30–5.
66. Amantea M, Newman MS, et al. Relationship of dose intensity to the induction of palmar-plantar erythrodysesthia by pegylated liposomal doxorubicin in dogs. Hum Exp Toxicol 1999; 18(1):17–26.
67. Charrois GJ, Allen TM. Multiple injections of pegylated liposomal Doxorubicin: pharmacokinetics and therapeutic activity. J Pharmacol Exp Ther 2003; 306(3):1058–67.
68. Al-Batran SE, Meerpohl HG, et al. Reduced incidence of severe palmar-plantar erythrodysesthesia and mucositis in a prospective multicenter phase II trial with pegylated liposomal doxorubicin at 40 mg/m2 every 4 weeks in previously treated patients with metastatic breast cancer. Oncology 2006; 70(2):141–6.
69. Gabizon A, Isacson R, et al. An open-label study to evaluate dose and cycle dependence of the pharmacokinetics (PK) of pegylated liposomal doxorubicin (PLD). ASCO Annual Meeting Proceedings Part I. J Clin Oncol 2006; 24 (18S): Abs. No 2012.
70. Lorusso D, Di Stefano A, et al. Pegylated liposomal doxorubicin-related palmar-plantar erythrodysesthesia ('hand-foot' syndrome). Ann Oncol 2007.
71. Harrington KJ, Mohammadtaghi S, et al. Effective targeting of solid tumors in patients with locally advanced cancers by radiolabeled pegylated liposomes. Clin Cancer Res 2001; 7(2):243–54.
72. Northfelt DW, Martin FJ, et al. Doxorubicin encapsulated in liposomes containing surface-bound polyethylene glycol: pharmacokinetics, tumor localization, and safety in patients with AIDS-related Kaposi's sarcoma. J Clin Pharmacol 1996; 36(1):55–63.
73. Koukourakis MI, Koukouraki S, et al. High intratumoural accumulation of stealth liposomal doxorubicin (Caelyx) in glioblastomas and in metastatic brain tumours. Br J Cancer 2000; 83(10):1281–6.
74. Symon Z, Peyser A, et al. Selective delivery of doxorubicin to patients with breast carcinoma metastases by stealth liposomes. Cancer 1999; 86(1):72–8.
75. Koukourakis MI, Koukouraki S, et al. High intratumoral accumulation of stealth liposomal doxorubicin in sarcomas–rationale for combination with radiotherapy. Acta Oncol 2000; 39(2):207–11.

76. Northfelt DW, Dezube BJ, et al. Pegylated-liposomal doxorubicin versus doxorubicin, bleomycin, and vincristine in the treatment of AIDS-related Kaposi's sarcoma: results of a randomized phase III clinical trial. J Clin Oncol 1998; 16(7):2445–51.

77. Fischl MA, Krown SE, et al. Weekly doxorubicin in the treatment of patients with AIDS-related Kaposi's sarcoma. AIDS Clinical Trials Group. J Acquir Immune Defic Syndr 1993; 6(3):259–64.

78. O'Brien ME, Wigler N, et al. Reduced cardiotoxicity and comparable efficacy in a phase III trial of pegylated liposomal doxorubicin HCl (CAELYX/Doxil) versus conventional doxorubicin for first-line treatment of metastatic breast cancer. Ann Oncol 2004; 15(3):440–9.

79. Von Hoff DD, Layard MW, et al. Risk factors for doxorubicin-induced congestive heart failure. Ann Intern Med 1979; 91(5):710–7.

80. Paridaens R. Efficacy of paclitaxel or doxorubicin used as single agents in advanced breast cancer: a literature survey. Semin Oncol 1998; 25(5Suppl. 12): 3–6.

81. Zelek L, Barthier S, et al. Weekly vinorelbine is an effective palliative regimen after failure with anthracyclines and taxanes in metastatic breast carcinoma. Cancer 2001; 92(9):2267–72.

82. Joensuu H, Holli K, et al. Combination chemotherapy versus single-agent therapy as first- and second-line treatment in metastatic breast cancer: a prospective randomized trial. J Clin Oncol 1998; 16(12):3720–30.

83. Lin PC, Wang WS, et al. Sequential therapy with capecitabine followed by vinorelbine/cisplatin in patients with anthracycline/taxane-refractory metastatic breast cancer. J Chin Med Assoc 2006; 69(7):304–9.

84. Kalofonos HP, Onyenadum A, et al. Mitomycin C and vinblastine in anthracycline-resistant metastatic breast cancer: a phase II study. Tumori 2001; 87(6):394–7.

85. Gunel N, Akcali Z, et al. Cisplatin plus vinorelbine as a salvage regimen in refractory breast cancer. Tumori 2000; 86(4):283–5.

86. Delozier T, Guastalla JP, et al. A phase II study of an oxaliplatin/vinorelbine/5-fluorouracil combination in patients with anthracycline-pretreated and taxane-pretreated metastatic breast cancer. Anticancer Drugs 2006; 17(9): 1067–73.

87. Keller AM, Mennel RG, et al. Randomized Phase III Trial of Pegylated Liposomal Doxorubicin Versus Vinorelbine or Mitomycin C Plus Vinblastine in Women With Taxane-Refractory Advanced Breast Cancer. J Clin Oncol 2004; 22(19):3893–901.

88. Brogden RN, Wiseman LR. Topotecan. A review of its potential in advanced ovarian cancer. Drugs 1998; 56(4):709–23.

89. Muggia F, Lu MJ. Emerging treatments for ovarian cancer. Expert Opin Emerg Drugs 2003; 8(1):203–16.

90. Gordon AN, Fleagle JT, et al. Recurrent epithelial ovarian carcinoma: a randomized phase III study of pegylated liposomal doxorubicin versus topotecan. J Clin Oncol 2001; 19(14):3312–22.

91. Gordon AN, Tonda M, et al. Long-term survival advantage for women treated with pegylated liposomal doxorubicin compared with topotecan in a

phase 3 randomized study of recurrent and refractory epithelial ovarian cancer. Gynecol Oncol 2004; 95(1):1–8.

92. Tsiara SN, Kapsali E, et al. Administration of a modified chemotherapeutic regimen containing vincristine, liposomal doxorubicin and dexamethasone to multiple myeloma patients: preliminary data. Eur J Haematol 2000; 65(2):118–22.

93. Hussein MA, Tonda ME, et al. A phase III randomized trial of doxil, vincristine and dexamethasone (DVd) versus vincristine, adriamycin and reduced-dose dexamethasone (VAd) in the treatment of patients with newly diagnosed multiple myeloma (n-MM). Proc Am Soc Clin Oncol 2002; 21: Abs 1107.

94. Hussein MA, Wood L, et al. A Phase II trial of pegylated liposomal doxorubicin, vincristine, and reduced-dose dexamethasone combination therapy in newly diagnosed multiple myeloma patients. Cancer 2002; 95(10):2160–8.

95. Orlowski RZ, Voorhees PM, et al. Phase 1 trial of the proteasome inhibitor bortezomib and pegylated liposomal doxorubicin in patients with advanced hematologic malignancies. Blood 2005; 105(8):3058–65.

96. Garcia-Carbonero R, Paz-Ares L. Antibiotics and growth factors in the management of fever and neutropenia in cancer patients. Curr Opin Hematol 2002; 9(3):215–21.

97. Muggia FM, Creaven PJ, et al. Phase I clinical trial of weekly and daily treatment with camptothecin (NSC-100880): correlation with preclinical studies. Cancer Chemother Rep 1972; 56(4):515–21.

98. Lee JH, Lee JM, et al. Antitumor activity of 7-[2-(N-isopropylamino)ethyl]-(20S)-camptothecin, CKD602, as a potent DNA topoisomerase I inhibitor. Arch Pharm Res 1998; 21(5):581–90.

99. Yu N, Conway C, et al. STEALTH® Liposome Formulation Enhances Antitumor Efficacy of CKD-602, a Topoisomerase I Inhibitor, in Human Tumor Xenograft Models. 95th American Association for Cancer Research Annual Meeting, March 27–31, 2004, Orlando, Florida.

100. Zamboni WC, Friedland DM, et al. Final results of a phase I and pharmacokinetic study of STEALTH liposomal CKD-602 (S-CKD602) in patients with advanced solid tumors. ASCO Annual Meeting Proceedings Part I. J Clin Oncol 2006; 24(18S)2013.

101. Martin FJ. Clinical pharmacology and antitumor efficacy of DOXIL (pegylated liposomal doxorubicin). Medical Applications of Liposomes. D. D. Lasic, Papahadjopoulos, D. Amsterdam: Elsevier, 1988: 635–88.

102. Paik S, Bryant J, et al. erbB-2 and response to doxorubicin in patients with axillary lymph node-positive, hormone receptor-negative breast cancer. J Natl Cancer Inst 1998; 90(18):1361–70.

103. Ross JS, Fletcher JA The HER-2/neu Oncogene in Breast Cancer: Prognostic Factor, Predictive Factor, and Target for Therapy. Oncologist 1998; 3(4): 237–52.

104. Jarvinen TA, Tanner M, et al. Characterization of topoisomerase II alpha gene amplification and deletion in breast cancer. Genes Chromosomes Cancer 1999; 26(2):142–50.

105. Tanner M, Hollmen M, et al. Amplification of HER-2 in gastric carcinoma: association with Topoisomerase IIalpha gene amplification, intestinal type, poor prognosis and sensitivity to trastuzumab. Ann Oncol 2005; 16(2):273–8.

106. Park JW, Hong K, et al. Anti-HER2 immunoliposomes: enhanced efficacy attributable to targeted delivery. Clin Cancer Res 2002; 8(4):1172–81.

107. Kirpotin D, Park JW, et al. Sterically stabilized anti-HER2 immunoliposomes: design and targeting to human breast cancer cells in vitro. Biochemistry 1997; 36(1):66–75.

108. Park JW, Colbern G, et al. Targeted intracellular drug delivery via anti-HER2 immunoliposomes yields superior antitumor efficacy. Proc Am Soc Clin Oncol 1997; 16:430a.

109. Park JW, Hong K, et al. Pharmacodynamic and pharmacokinetic advantages of anti-p185HER2 immunoliposomes. Proc Am Soc Clin Oncol 1995; 14:420.

110. Nielsen UB, Kirpotin DB, et al. Therapeutic efficacy of anti-ErbB2 immunoliposomes targeted by a phage antibody selected for cellular endocytosis. Biochim Biophys Acta 2002; 1591(1–3):109–18.

111. Marks JD. Selection of internalizing antibodies for drug delivery. Meth Mol Biol 2004; 248:201–8.

112. Koivunen E, Arap W, et al. Identification of receptor ligands with phage display peptide libraries. J Nucl Med 1999; 40(5):883–8.

113. Li Z, Zhao R, et al. Identification and characterization of a novel peptide ligand of epidermal growth factor receptor for targeted delivery of therapeutics. FASEB J 2005; 19(14):1978–85.

114. Du B, Qian M, et al. In vitro panning of a targeting peptide to hepatocarcinoma from a phage display peptide library. Biochem Biophys Res Commun 2006; 342(3):956–62.

115. Lau D, Guo L, et al. Peptide ligands targeting integrin alpha3beta1 in non-small cell lung cancer. Lung Cancer 2006; 52(3):291–7.

116. Stevenson M, Hale AB, et al. Incorporation of a laminin-derived peptide (SIKVAV) on polymer-modified adenovirus permits tumor-specific targeting via alpha6-integrins. Cancer Gene Ther 2007; 14(4):335–45.

117. Grunicke HH. The cell membrane as a target for cancer chemotherapy. Eur J Cancer 1991; 27(3):281–4.

118. Mendelsohn J. Epidermal growth factor receptor as a target for therapy with antireceptor monoclonal antibodies. J Natl Cancer Inst Monogr 1992; (13): 125–31.

119. Rabbani SA. Metalloproteases and urokinase in angiogenesis and tumor progression. In vivo 1998; 12(1):135–42.

120. Trippett TM, Bertino JR. Therapeutic strategies targeting proteins that regulate folate and reduced folate transport. J Chemother 1999; 11(1):3–10.

121. Hu XF, Xing PX. Discovery and validation of new molecular targets for ovarian cancer. Curr Opin Mol Ther 2003; 5(6):625–30.

122. Ke CY, Mathias CJ, et al. The folate receptor as a molecular target for tumor-selective radionuclide delivery. Nucl Med Biol 2003; 30(8):811–7.

123. Rafii S, Avecilla ST, et al. Tumor vasculature address book: identification of stage-specific tumor vessel zip codes by phage display. Cancer Cell 2003; 4(5): 331–3.

124. St-Pierre Y, Van Themsche C, et al. Emerging features in the regulation of MMP-9 gene expression for the development of novel molecular targets and therapeutic strategies. Curr Drug Targets Inflamm Allergy 2003; 2(3):206–15.

125. Hamid O. Emerging treatments in oncology: focus on tyrosine kinase (erbB) receptor inhibitors. J Am Pharm Assoc (Wash DC) 2004; 44(1):52–8.

126. Mori T. Cancer-specific ligands identified from screening of peptide-display libraries. Curr Pharm Des 2004; 10(19):2335–43.

127. Beeram M, Patnaik A, et al. Raf: a strategic target for therapeutic development against cancer. J Clin Oncol 2005; 23(27):6771–90.

128. McInturff JE, Modlin RL, et al. The role of toll-like receptors in the pathogenesis and treatment of dermatological disease. J Invest Dermatol 2005; 125 (1):1–8.

129. Mendoza FJ, Espino PS, et al. Anti-tumor chemotherapy utilizing peptide-based approaches–apoptotic pathways, kinases, and proteasome as targets. Arch Immunol Ther Exp (Warsz) 2005; 53(1):47–60.

130. Srinivasan DM, Kapoor M, et al. Growth factor receptors: implications in tumor biology. Curr Opin Investig Drugs 2005; 6(12):1246–9.

131. Benson JD, Chen YN, et al. Validating cancer drug targets. Nature 2006; 441 (7092):451–6.

132. Germanov E, Berman JN, et al. Current and future approaches for the therapeutic targeting of metastasis (review). Int J Mol Med 18(6):1025–36.

133. Tucker, G. C. Integrins: molecular targets in cancer therapy. Curr Oncol Rep 2006; 8(2):96–103.

134. Iden DL, Allen TM. In vitro and in vivo comparison of immunoliposomes made by conventional coupling techniques with those made by a new post-insertion approach. Biochim Biophys Acta 2001; 1513(2):207–16.

135. Allen TM, Sapra P, et al. Use of the post-insertion method for the formation of ligand-coupled liposomes. Cell Mol Biol Lett 2002; 7(2):217–9.

136. Moreira JN, Ishida T, et al. Use of the post-insertion technique to insert peptide ligands into pre- formed stealth liposomes with retention of binding activity and cytotoxicity. Pharm Res 19(3):265–9.

137. Noble CO, Kirpotin DB, et al. Development of ligand-targeted liposomes for cancer therapy. Expert Opin Ther Targets 2004; 8(4):335–53.

138. Desai N, Trieu V, et al. Increased antitumor activity, intratumor paclitaxel concentrations, and endothelial cell transport of cremophor-free, albumin-bound paclitaxel, ABI-007, compared with cremophor-based paclitaxel. Clin Cancer Res 2006; 12(4):1317–24.

139. Gradishar WJ. Albumin-bound paclitaxel: a next-generation taxane. Expert Opin Pharmacother 2006; 7(8):1041–53.

140. Stinchcombe TE, Socinski MA, et al. Phase I and pharmacokinetic trial of carboplatin and albumin-bound paclitaxel, ABI-007 (Abraxane((R))) on three treatment schedules in patients with solid tumors. Cancer Chemother Pharmacol 2007.

141. Gradishar WJ, Tjulandin S, et al. Phase III trial of nanoparticle albumin-bound paclitaxel compared with polyethylated castor oil-based paclitaxel in women with breast cancer. J Clin Oncol 2005; 23(31):7794–803.

142. Gabizon AA, Tzemach D, et al. Reduced toxicity and superior therapeutic activity of a mitomycin C lipid-based prodrug incorporated in pegylated liposomes. Clin Cancer Res 2006; 12(6):1913–20.

143. Gabizon A, Catane R, Uziely B, et al. Prolonged circulation time and enhanced accumulation in malignant exudates of doxorubicin encapsulated in polyethylene-glycol coated liposomes. Cancer Res 1994; 54:987–92.
144. Hubert A, Lyass O, Pode D et al. Doxil (Caelyx): an exploratory study with pharmacokinetics in patients with hormone-refractory prostate cancer. Anticancer Drugs 2000; 11:123–7.

20

Dermal and Transdermal Drug Delivery

Jonathan Hadgraft and Majella E. Lane
School of Pharmacy, University of London, London, U.K.

Adam C. Watkinson
Acrux Ltd., Melbourne, Australia

INTRODUCTION

Although the skin is the most accessible organ, it is in many ways one of the most difficult to treat. This is because it has evolved to prevent the loss of water and also the ingress of xenobiotics. There are reports in the ancient Egyptian literature on the use of agents to treat the skin and some 4000 years later we are still investigating the precise nature of the barrier function (1). It is possible now to use sophisticated and sensitive techniques to examine the barrier properties at a molecular level and to use this information to optimize the structure of the drug to be delivered and the formulation in which it is presented. Unfortunately it is not as simple as this and many actives that are used on the skin, either for dermal or transdermal use, were not originally developed with the target of the skin in mind. This means that often they have the wrong characteristics for dermal delivery and it is only with judicious formulation that some activity is produced. Even though it has been known for many years that skin bioavailability is only of the order of a few percent (2) there have been few attempts to discover what happens to the rest of the applied drug.

For the majority of drugs the barrier to penetration is in the stratum corneum. This thin membrane, typically only 15 μm thick has unique properties. The major route of penetration through the stratum corneum is through the intercellular channels, which contain structured lipids organized into bilayers (3). These lipids are predominantly ceramides, unlike most biological membranes there are no phospholipids present (4). The intercellular channels can be likened to the mortar in a "brick and mortar" wall and the corneocytes are the bricks (5). The corneocytes are additionally held together with corneodesmosomes, which are broken in the desquamation process by proteolytic enzymes in the stratum corneum. If the homeostasis of this complex enzyme system is modulated in any way diseased skin, such as that found in eczema and psoriasis, is produced. If the corneodesmosomes are broken too early the "brick wall" becomes leaky and the barrier function is impaired. This can lead to the ingress of large molecules such as allergens and atopic eczema results (6).

The reason for the excellent barrier properties is thus a result of the tortuous pathway round the dead cells and the repetitive partitioning that the permeant has to undergo as it crosses the sequence of bilayers. Clearly it encounters both lipophilic and hydrophilic domains and thus a good permeant is one that is small, has a balanced partition coefficient and good solubility in both water and oils. Hence the transdermally delivered compounds, nicotine and nitroglycerin are "good" permeants (7). Even though these are "good" permeants the bioavailability from a transdermal patch is far from 100%.

The normal dose of a dermally applied agent is of the order of $2 \, mg/cm^2$ (8), this forms a film approximately 20 m thick on the skin surface. It is a very dynamic system with any solvents present permeating into the skin or evaporating. This can leave the active on the skin surface in a crystalline state and therefore unavailable for permeation. Alternatively if the active does not crystallize it can become supersaturated and permeation into the stratum corneum is enhanced (9). The stability of the supersaturated state will depend on the presence of anti-nucleant polymers. The presence of the solvent in the skin can also modify the solubility properties of the skin and hence modulate permeation (10). However, the solvent in the skin may only be transient as it will diffuse into the deeper tissue and be removed by the blood supply. Very few publications have examined the significance of the solvent on the skin properties particularly at the low dosing levels experienced clinically.

There are thus a significant number of challenges in the delivery of drugs into and through the skin. Dermatologic disorders are prevalent in a large percentage of the population and it is a problem that appears to be increasing with time. The number of children who suffer from atopic eczema has risen exponentially over the past 5 decades from 5% to 30% (11). Also as the life expectancy of the population increases there is a large number of people suffering from skin disorders. This has a significant impact on the quality of life (12) and one that should be addressed.

When the skin is diseased the barrier function may be compromised and delivery is facilitated. In this event the dose applied has to be sufficient to be therapeutically effective but not large enough to have systemic significance. As the disease state is treated, delivery will become harder to achieve and any formulation has to take this into account. The formulation also has to be elegant and have good patient acceptability. For example, dermal preparations should have good cosmetic appeal and transdermal systems should be thin and discreet with high drug loading. Silicones, which are frequently used in cosmetics to improve the feel of the product, are slowly being used in the pharmaceutical arena with some 35 products now containing silicones.

Recent advances in transdermal delivery, in particular with regard to polymer selection and design, have produced extremely thin devices with very high drug loading. If drug loading is high the devices will be close to saturation and long-term stability has to be considered. Metered dose spray delivery systems have been produced in which there is no polymer film and patient acceptability is very high (13).

Until recently the only transdermally delivered drugs were compounds that had been delivered via other routes of administration and therefore significant safety data were available before development. Rotigotine has now been launched onto the market and this is the first instance of a new chemical entity (NCE) that has been delivered first by the transdermal route (14). Now that the regulatory hurdles are known it is anticipated that a number of other NCEs will be delivered transdermally with the consequent benefits that this route provides.

There remains the problem in transdermal delivery that the barrier function precludes the passive delivery of more than a few mg per day and this is for an "ideal" permeant. For larger biotech molecules the problems are significantly greater and it is likely that only techniques, which physically breach the stratum corneum, will permit the delivery of higher doses or high molecular weight species.

An additional problem, which may be exacerbated by the occlusive nature of normal transdermal systems, is the ability of the agent to promote skin toxicity, which may manifest itself as an irritant or allergic response. It is noteworthy that clonidine shows an incidence of skin toxicity when it is delivered transdermally but the significance of this is not sufficient to stop the product being commercially successful (15).

Finally the skin is not a "dead" barrier. Proteases in the stratum corneum can break down proteins or peptides that are delivered transdermally (16,17). Phases I and II enzymes are present in the viable tissue and can also metabolize diffusing drugs (18). For example, it has been estimated that a substantial fraction of transdermally delivered nitroglycerin may be metabolized before it reaches the systemic circulation (19).

ENHANCEMENT STRATEGIES

Over the past decades a number of strategies has been examined to enhance the permeation of dermal and transdermal drugs. These can be largely categorized as being passive in which no external energy source is used to promote the permeation or active where an external energy source such as an electrical current or ultrasound facilitates absorption or causes breaches in the barrier. Many of the enhancement strategies feature in some form or other in the subsequent chapters in this book.

PASSIVE ENHANCEMENT

Formulation Effects (Delivery to and into the Stratum Corneum)

The activity state or chemical potential of the drug is most important and, as mentioned above, it is possible for components of a topical formulation to evaporate. This dynamic situation will leave a residual phase on the skin surface from which the drug may crystallize or become supersaturated. If the former occurs, then the drug may become unavailable. If the latter occurs, then drug permeation will be promoted. In the case of a transdermal system, delivery through the device to the skin surface can be adjusted so that it is at a comparable rate to diffusion through the skin. In this way if the patch is applied to a particularly permeable site drug delivery will be limited by the patch. This can be important for drugs with a narrow therapeutic window such as fentanyl and clonidine.

Formulation Effects (Diffusion Through Stratum Corneum)

It is generally recognized that hydrated skin is more permeable than dry skin and any formulation that has an occlusive effect on the stratum corneum is likely to promote absorption (20). Even though this is a relatively simple concept the precise reasons why hydrated skin is more permeable remains unclear.

Formulation components will diffuse into the stratum corneum and can influence the barrier properties. They can do this in a variety of ways. Some can intercalate into the lipids in the intercellular channels and modify the fluidity of the bilayers (10). These penetration enhancers increase the diffusion rate through the skin. Typically they have a polar headgroup and a long alkyl chain (e.g., oleic acid). Other penetration enhancers are incorporated into the skin and modify the solubility properties of the skin; they will affect the partition of the drug in a favorable way between the skin and the formulation (10). The residence time of the enhancer in the skin is an important determinant of its effectiveness. For example, small solvent molecules such as propylene glycol act as good enhancers but they will diffuse out of the stratum corneum rapidly compared with a more lipophilic molecule such as isopropyl myristate (21). It is also possible to obtain synergistic effects with combinations of enhancers.

Transfer through the skin can also be influenced by the use of vesicular systems and nanoparticulates. The precise mechanism by which these act is still debated in the literature and is considered in subsequent chapters.

The surfactants in some microemulsion systems may reorganize to form nanostructured films on the skin surface, which may also intercalate with the lower bilayers of the skin. It has been suggested that some nano-particles accumulate in the hair follicles, considering their size and esti-mating their diffusion coefficient suggests that the delivery to the lower regions of the follicle is via a mechanical rather than a passive diffusion process (22).

PHYSICAL ENHANCEMENT

One of the techniques that has been available for many decades is ion-tophoresis or the application of a small electric current to drive charged molecules through the skin. Commercially available products are now on the market and it can be anticipated that more will follow. It is possible to modulate the delivery of the drug using iontophoresis as the amount of drug delivered is proportional to the current. Delivery can therefore be ramped or pulsed if this is appropriate for therapy. Patient controlled analgesia is also possible with the additional benefit of a safety element using electronic control of the total amount of analgesic delivered. Although predominantly used for the delivery of charged species iontophoresis (through electro-osmosis) can also facilitate the delivery of uncharged but water soluble entities (23). This process has been used in the development of an electronic device for monitoring the amount of glucose in the blood (24). In this case the process is called reverse iontophoresis and is also under development for other biological markers, for instance compounds used to assess renal impairment (25).

Electroporation and ultrasound have also been examined as potential sources of energy to promote percutaneous penetration. There are some reports in the literature concerning clinical studies on ultrasound and animal studies in the case of electroporation. It is also possible to couple enhancement strategies, examples being electroporation plus iontophoresis, and ultrasound and chemical permeation enhancers (26).

Breaching the stratum corneum barrier can also be achieved by "shooting" particles though the skin, by employing thermal methods or radiofrequency radiation, both of which create microchannels, and laser ablation. These have been reported to varying degrees in the literature but few clinical studies described. It is also possible to use microneedles both of a synthetic nature and those derived from natural sources. These will be discussed in later chapters. The different techniques can be refined to allow penetration to different depths within the skin and it is possible to avoid the nervous system and the delivery is therefore pain free.

Based on the method used to deliver an active into the skin, its interaction with the local components of the skin must be taken into account and local toxicity examined. In addition, if the barrier of the skin is compromised, it may be possible for other unwanted exogenous compounds to be absorbed. Safety issues associated with this need to be considered. It is possible that the barrier function is only modulated for a short period of time but the recovery of the barrier will have to be monitored and also repeated application to the same site considered.

COMMERCIAL CONSIDERATIONS

Transdermal drug delivery represents a small but significant proportion of the world pharmaceutical market. In 2005 global pharmaceutical sales stood at approximately $540 billion, of which about 20% can be attributed to sales involving specialized drug delivery technology. Of this 20% about $13 billion worth of sales came from transdermal products. This is expected to grow to somewhere in the region of $22 billion by 2010 and $32 billion by 2015. As with most pharmaceuticals the largest single market for transdermal products is in the United States, which represents nearly 50% of the global market.

For many years Johnson & Johnson's (J&J) Duragesic™ fentanyl patch dominated the transdermal market and global sales peaked at in excess of $2 billion in 2004. By 2006, after patent expiration and the advent of generic competition, sales of Duragesic™ were still greater than $1.2 billion. Despite the massive sales of Duragesic™ patches, only 2 generic versions of these delivery systems have appeared in the United States since the expiration of the patents protecting the product. This is in part due to J&J's vigorous protection of their market share and the initial confusion caused by the submission of a citizen's petition to FDA aimed at blocking generic approvals. Despite these moves by J&J, Mylan Technologies gained approval for their fentanyl patch in January 2005 and Lavipharm followed with another in August 2006. Interestingly, in September 2005, Noven had an NDA for a generic fentanyl patch turned down by FDA on the grounds of its high fentanyl content relative to Duragesic. Perhaps a more significant advance that occurred between the approval of these generic transdermal systems was the European Union and FDA approval of Alza's iontophoretic delivery system for fentanyl, Ionsys, in January and May 2006 respectively. This was and, at the time of writing still is, the first 'dial a dose' iontophoretic system to reach the market. At present the product has a fairly limited indication relative to that of the fentanyl transdermal patches i.e. the management of acute moderate to severe post-operative pain in a hospital setting only.

The sales figures associated with transdermal fentanyl are unquestionably impressive and will ensure that the drug has a place in the pipeline of many drug delivery companies for years to come. Despite the dedication of much of the drug delivery world to reformulating a single opioid, there have been several other interesting and novel transdermal product launches over the last few years.

In relatively rapid succession, 2006 saw the approval of three new passive transdermal delivery systems. A rotigotine patch (Neupro™) for use in Parkinson's disease was launched in the European Union by Schwarz in early 2006 and subsequently approved by the U.S. FDA in May 2007. Initial EU sales amounted to approximately $13 million in 2006 with Q1 sales of $3.3 million in 2007. The Emsam® patch contains a monoamine oxidase inhibitor, selegiline, and is indicated for major depressive disorder. Emsam™ was approved by the FDA in February 2006 and has accrued sales of some $18 million since its launch by Bristol-Myers Squibb in April of that year. Emsam™ represents the fruition of a joint venture, Somerset Pharmaceuticals, between Mylan Laboratories and Watson Pharmaceuticals. After significant work by Noven and Shire, April 2006 saw the FDA approval of Daytrana™, Noven's methylphenidate patch for ADHD (attention deficit hyperactivity disorder). This product was launched in the US by Shire in June 2006 and has seen sales in excess of $25 million since that time. Less recently, Oxytrol (oxybutynin for overactive bladder) was approved by FDA in Q1 2003 and launched by Watson in Q2 of the same year. In its first 12 months of sales it realised about $30 million and has sold in the region of $40 million per annum since then. It is probably too early to pass judgment on how these products will ultimately fair in the market place but it seems unlikely that their sales will match those of fentanyl.

Older transdermal products that still yield significant sales exist in the form of a contraceptive patch (Ortho Evra™ launched in 2001), HRT patches and gels (launched from the mid-1980s onwards), nicotine patches (launches from the early 1990s onwards), a clonidine patch (Catapress™, approved in the United States in 1990) and several testosterone gels (launched from 2000 onwards). Ortho Evra sales dipped because the greater dose of ethinyl estradiol delivered by the patch (than by oral contraceptives) has been linked with an increased risk of thromboembolism. Despite these safety concerns and the inevitable associated litigation, the patch remains on the market in the United States and has sales of more than $400 million per annum. HRT patch sales slowed for the same reason that all HRT therapies did after the women's health initiative (WHI) study reported an increased risk of breast cancer as well as heart disease, blood clots and stroke. A more recent interpretation of the data from this study and a better understanding of the differences between transdermally and orally delivered estrogens seems set to reverse this trend and the decline in sales has now halted. It remains to be seen how these very different issues will affect ongoing sales figures of these products. Transdermal testosterone therapy for male hypogonadism is an interesting prospect for the future as, despite formulations that require less than ideal dosing regimens, it does represent a market of about $600 million. As some of the improved formulations currently in development hit the market it will be interesting to see if these already significant sales increase further.

Although reasonably successful, the majority of recent product launches have not demonstrated initial sales to suggest they may reach those achieved by transdermal fentanyl. So, why the disparity between the fentanyl story and that of some of the more recent transdermal launches discussed earlier?

The launch of Duragesic represented a sea change in the way in which pain could be controlled and the control of pain is a huge part of the modern medical world. Prior to the launch of Duragesic, fentanyl was administered by injection and, by virtue of its short half life, was inconvenient to administer effectively to maintain appropriate pain relief. The advent of Duragesic allowed the continuous delivery of varying doses of fentanyl to be administered in a way that did not require patient hospitalization, or even the presence of a physician. It represented an enormous leap forward in the amelioration of pain in a population that otherwise did not need to be kept in hospital thus appealing to both patients, doctors and those responsible for healthcare budgets. It "ticked all of the boxes" in a very impressive manner. From a harsh commercial perspective, an analysis of other current transdermal products does not produce as emphatic an argument for their potential as that associated with fentanyl. Hence, the advent of transdermal fentanyl can be regarded as a great leap forward in drug delivery and, whilst most other transdermal products represent significant improvements in their respective areas of medicine, their impact is arguably smaller.

What of the future? There will, no doubt, be further launches of transdermal products and these will continue to sell in reasonable numbers with acceptable profits to their manufacturers and the investors that support them. However, it will take a company with a very good understanding of both its own technology and the clinical benefits of its application to devise and launch a transdermal product that may ultimately match the commercial success of Duragesic. This is not a unique challenge in the pharmaceutical industry but it will require an intelligent and pragmatic blend of commercial and scientific knowledge and expertise to achieve.

RELATED ISSUES

In many ways delivery of actives into and through the nail is similar to skin permeation, however the barrier is even more significant, which is why it is very difficult to treat nail disorders topically. The rational basis for the formulation of nail products has its roots in the understanding of the basic physicochemical properties that control the diffusion process and it may be that some of the physical techniques that have been used to breach the dermal barrier will also be appropriate for ungual delivery.

Wound tissue and its healing is also an important issue in topical delivery. In an open wound, delivery to the target site is relatively facile but systemic absorption needs to be considered so that the doses used are appropriate locally but not sufficient to cause unwanted systemic effects. As the wound heals, delivery to the local environment becomes more difficult and it is probable that "smart" systems are required that will deliver the active at a rate dependent on the integrity of the tissue.

THE FUTURE

Our understanding of the skin has improved significantly over the past few years. This is predominantly a result of advances in the instrumentation available to probe the barrier properties of the skin at a molecular level. It is also a result of our biological understanding of the processes involved in the homeostasis of the barrier. With this increase in knowledge it should be possible to design both actives and formulations that can deliver better to both the skin and, if required, to the systemic circulation. Safety issues are paramount and it will be easier to address these at an early stage of any development program with an increased awareness of the barrier structure and properties, from both a physicochemical and biochemical perspective, at a molecular level.

REFERENCES

1. Ebbell B. The Papyrus Ebers. The Greatest Egyptian Medical Document. Copenhagen: Levin & Munksgaard, 1937:135.
2. Feldmann RJ, Maibach HI. Regional variation in percutaneous penetration of ^{14}C cortisol in man. J Invest Dermatol 1967; 48:181–3.
3. Cornwell PA, Barry BW, Stoddart CP, Bouwstra JA. Wide-angle X-ray diffraction of human stratum corneum effects of hydration and terpene enhancement treatment. J Pharm Pharmacol 1994; 46:938–50.
4. Wertz PW. Epidermal Lipids. Semin Dermatol 1992; 11:106–13.
5. Michaels AS, Chandrasekaran SK, Shaw JE. Drug permeation through human skin: theory and in vitro experimental measurement. Am Inst Chem Eng J 1975; 21:985–96.
6. Cork MJ, Robinson DA, Vasilopoulos Y, et al. New perspectives on epidermal barrier dysfunction in atopic dermatitis: gene-environment interactions. J Allergy Clin Immunol 2006; 118(1):3–21.
7. Hadgraft J. Pharmaceutical aspects of transdermal nitroglycerin. Int J Pharm 1996; 135:1–11.
8. Surber C, Davis AF. Bioavailability and bioequivalence. In: Walters KA, ed. Dermatological and Transdermal Formulations. New York: Marcel Dekker, 2002: 401–98.

9. Pellett MA, Roberts MS, Hadgraft J. Supersaturated solutions evaluated with an in vitro stratum corneum tape stripping technique. Int J Pharm 1997; 151:91–8.

10. Hadgraft J. Passive enhancement strategies in topical and transdermal delivery. Int J Pharm 1999; 184:1–6.

11. Thestrup-Pedersen K. Atopic eczema. What has caused the epidemic in industrialised countries and can early intervention modify the natural history of atopic eczema? J Cosmet Dermatol 2003; 2(3–4):202–10.

12. Finlay Y. Measures of the effect of adult severe atopic eczema on quality of life. J Eur Acad Dermatol Venereol 1996; 7(2):149–54.

13. Thomas BJ, Finnin BC. The transdermal revolution. Drug Discov Today 2004; 9:697–703.

14. Reynolds NA, Wellington K, Easthorpe SE. Rotigotine in Parkinson's disease. CNS Drugs 2006; 11:973–81.

15. Prisant LM. Transdermal clonidine skin reactions. J Clin Hypertens 2002; 4:136–8.

16. Brattsand M, Egelrud T. Purification, molecular cloning and expression of a human stratum corneum trypsin-like serine protease with possible function in desquamation. J Biol Chem 1999; 274:30033–40.

17. Sondell B, Thornell LE, Egelrud T. Evidence that stratum-corneum chymotryptic enzyme is transported to the stratum-corneum extracellular-space via lamellar bodies. J Invest Dermatol 1995; 104:819–23.

18. Steinstrasse I, Merkle HP. Dermal metabolism of topically applied drugs: pathways and models reconsidered. Pharm Acta Helv 1995; 70:3–24.

19. Wester RC, Noonan PK, Smeach S, Kosobud L. Pharmacokinetics and bioavailability of intravenous and topical nitroglycerin in the rhesus monkey: estimate of percutaneous first-pass metabolism. J Pharm Sci 1983; 72:745–8.

20. Barry BW. Dermatological Formulations. P 172. New York: Marcel Dekker, 1983: 480.

21. Trottet L, Merly C, Mirza M, Hadgraft J, Davis AF. Effect of finite doses of propylene glycol on enhancement of in vitro percutaneous permeation of loperamide hydrochloride. I J Pharm 2004; 274(1–2):213–9.

22. Lademann J, Richter H, Teichmann A, et al. Nanoparticles–An efficient carrier for drug delivery into the hair follicles. Eur J Pharm Biopharm 2007; 66(2):159–64.

23. Guy RH, Kalia YN, Delgado-Charro MB, Merino V, Lopez A, Marro D. Iontophoreis, electrorepulsion and electroosmosis. J Control Rel 2000; 64:129–32.

24. Garg SK, Potts RO, Ackerman NR, Fermi SJ, Tamada JA, Chase HP. Correlation at fingerstick blood glucose measurements with GLucoWatch biographer glucose results in young subjects with type 1 diabetes. Diabetes Care 1999; 22:1708–14.

25. Degim IT, Ilbasmis S, Dundaroz R, Oguz Y. Reverse iontophoresis: a noninvasive technique for measuring blood urea level. Pediatr Nephrol 2003; 18(10):1032–7.

26. Mitragotri S. Synergistic effect of enhancers for transdermal delivery. Pharm Res 2000; 17:1354–9.

21

ALZA Transdermal Drug Delivery Technologies

Rama Padmanabhan, J. Bradley Phipps, Michel Cormier, Janet Tamada, and Jay Audett
ALZA Corporation, Mountain View, California, U.S.A.

J. Richard Gyory
Transform Pharmaceuticals, Lexington, Massachusetts, U.S.A.

Peter E. Daddona
Zosano Pharma, Fremont, California, U.S.A.

INTRODUCTION

Challenges in transdermal drug delivery are largely associated with the impermeability of the skin barrier. The stratum corneum, the uppermost epidermal layer of the skin comprising a matrix of highly ordered lipid lamellae, serves as the principal barrier to the permeation of chemicals that come in contact with the skin. In addition to the matrix composition, the tortuosity of the intercellular pathways through the stratum corneum also limits the ingress of permeants. Passive transdermal drug delivery is generally limited to lipophilic and low molecular weight compounds (1,2). ALZA Corporation (Mountain View, CA) has explored strategies to enhance skin permeability for a wide array of compounds through the use of chemical permeation enhancers, an electric field to facilitate transport of charged molecules, and mechanical formation of microscopic transport channels through the skin to deliver, in particular, high molecular weight compounds (3–5). This review focuses on three ALZA-developed transdermal delivery technologies: (*i*) D-TRANS® incorporates means to improve, sustain, and control passive transdermal transport, (*ii*) E-TRANS® uses low levels of electrical current to actively transport a broad range of drugs through intact skin, and (*iii*) Macroflux® creates superficial pathways through the skin barrier allowing transport of macromolecules.

Transdermal drug delivery has a long history dating back thousands of years to the use of plasters and poultices. Topical drug formulations are the simplest types of transdermal drug delivery. These systems utilize a vehicle, such as a gel or cream, to facilitate passive penetration of drug into the skin to produce a pharmacological response. Advanced passive transdermal systems, such as D-TRANS systems, incorporate a separate drug reservoir and/or rate-controlling membrane that can release drug into the bloodstream at a controlled rate over precise periods of time ranging from 1 day to 1 week (3,6). Their functionality is analogous to that of a continuous IV or subcutaneous (SC) infusion.

Active transport facilitated by an electric potential enhances delivery of polar, hydrophilic, and charged molecules. According to Banga (7), the use of an electric field to enhance delivery across the skin was first described by Veratti in 1747. Leduc is generally recognized as an important early contributor to the field because of his comprehensive study of the delivery of ionic substances published in 1908 (8). Applying recent innovations in microelectronics and battery technology, iontophoretic systems have evolved from large bench-top nonambulatory units for local topical drug administration to small patch-like devices for systemic delivery of charged drugs including peptides (9–11).

Although electrotransport technology broadens the range of drugs that can be delivered transdermally, transport of high molecular weight molecules has relied primarily on physical methods of permeation enhancement. Several methods of mechanically-assisted transport have been examined, including sandpaper abrasion or tape stripping of the skin (12,13), laser ablation (14), and ultrasound (15). In general, these techniques are limited by their inability to control the rate of drug absorption or are cumbersome and expensive. Advances in our understanding of the skin and its barrier properties have led to improved methods of mechanical disruption involving the formation of microchannels. Macroflux transdermal technology creates superficial pathways through the skin barrier layer allowing consistent and controlled delivery of large and/or highly charged molecules, such as therapeutic proteins and vaccines (16).

DESCRIPTION OF THE TECHNOLOGIES

D-TRANS® Transdermal Therapeutic Systems

D-TRANS transdermal technologies provide rate-controlled passive delivery of drugs via a patch resembling a small adhesive bandage placed on the surface of intact skin. The steady-state flux of drug-per-unit-area of stratum corneum, J, across the effective thickness of stratum corneum, L, is given by $D \cdot K \cdot C_v / L$, where D is the drug diffusion coefficient, K is the drug partition coefficient between vehicle and stratum corneum, and C_v is the drug concentration in the vehicle.

While currently available transdermal drug delivery systems display a wide array of designs, they consist of two basic types: membrane-controlled and matrix (6). A schematic of these designs is shown in Figure 1. Older membrane-controlled systems consist of a backing layer, a drug reservoir, a rate-controlling membrane, and an adhesive covered by a peelable liner. The drug reservoir may consist of drug in liquid or gel form, referred to as form–fill–seal (FFS), or drug dispersed in a polymeric material. Examples of membrane-controlled FFS systems include ALZA-developed products Duragesic® and Testoderm-TTS® for the delivery of fentanyl and testosterone, respectively. More recent matrix systems contain a backing layer, a polymeric drug reservoir, an adhesive, and a peelable liner. In some cases, the system contains only the backing layer and the drug in the adhesive, which is covered by a peelable liner. Matrix systems currently marketed include 3M Pharmaceuticals' Climara® for the delivery of 17β–estradiol, Elan's nicotine delivery system Prostep®, Schwarz Pharma's Neupro® for Parkinson's disease, Somerset Pharmaceuticals' Emsam® for depression, Noven Pharmaceuticals' Daytrana® for attention deficit hyperactivity disorder (ADHD), as well as the ALZA-developed scrotal testosterone patch

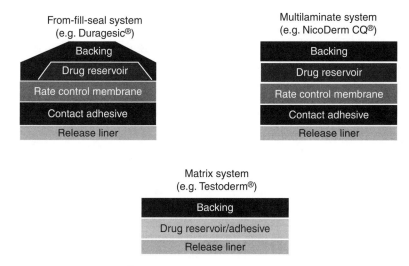

Figure 1 D-TRANS® technology: three structural types for optimal delivery: membrane-controlled Duragesic® FFS system, NicoDerm® multilaminate system, and Testoderm matrix system. *Abbreviation*: FFS, form–fill–seal.

Testoderm®. The choice of system design for a given drug depends on several factors, including the solubility and stability of the drug and excipients in the various components, and the drug's release kinetics from the device and through the skin (3,6). Matrix systems are desirable because their simplicity reduces manufacturing costs and their thinner device design may allow greater patient comfort. However, formulation challenges are greatest with this design, especially in the drug-in-adhesive systems, as the adhesive must serve multiple functions including housing the drug and controlling its release while maintaining adhesion to the skin (6).

A major limitation of transdermal drug delivery is the low percutaneous permeability of many drugs. In addition, the potential for irritation or sensitization can be challenging when developing transdermal drug delivery systems. Much research has focused on chemical permeation enhancers that alter the structure and dynamics of the stratum corneum (17). Permeation enhancers can affect drug transport in several ways, i.e., by increasing drug solubility within the matrix, increasing drug solubility within the skin lipid structure, increasing diffusivity of the drug through the system matrix or skin lipid structure, or modify the partitioning of drug between system components and the skin. These effects can be additive so that the incorporation of multiple permeation enhancers, each having a different influence on drug transport, can maximize the transport of drug (18). The challenge is to formulate permeation enhancer combinations and compositions that yield the best overall enhancement of flux with an acceptable level of irritation.

E-TRANS® Transdermal Therapeutic Systems

Electric fields assist transdermal drug delivery through mechanisms referred to as electrotransport and electroporation. Electrotransport uses a low-level electrical current to facilitate transport of charged and neutral therapeutic substances noninvasively across intact skin, whereas, electroporation uses short high voltage pulses to create transient aqueous pores in lipid bilayers of the skin to facilitate delivery of macromolecules (19,20). The rate of delivery in electrotransport systems is expressed by the Nernst–Planck equation, which includes terms for passive diffusion, electromigration, and bulk convection. Since electromigration is the dominant mechanism for delivery of a charged drug, transport is related to the electric current according to Faraday's principle, $N = t_d \cdot I \cdot M / z_d \cdot F$, where N is the total rate of delivery (mol/sec), t_d is the transport number (the fraction of charge carried by the drug), I is the current applied across the skin, M and z_d are the molecular weight and charge of the drug molecule, respectively, and F is Faraday's constant. Since the rate of drug delivery is proportional to the applied electrical current, electrotransport systems have the potential to provide precise dosing as well as patterned and on-demand delivery (21).

An electrotransport drug delivery system typically consists of electronic components, including control circuitry and a power supply (such as a battery) connected to a pair of electrodes in contact with ionically conductive reservoirs that, in turn, are in contact with the skin (Fig. 2). The reservoirs contain either the drug (for the donor electrode assembly) or a pharmacologically inactive electrolyte (for the counter electrode assembly). The donor electrode delivers the drug into the body and the counter electrode closes the electrical circuit. These different electronic and chemical components must be manufactured, stored, and ultimately function together to meet therapeutic, functional, and user needs. Electrotransport systems can be designed to be modular or completely integrated. In modular system designs, the user attaches single- or multiple-day disposable drug patches containing the reservoirs and electrodes to a single- or multiple-day use controller comprising the power source and electronic circuitry (22). In integrated systems, all components are fully integrated into a single disposable system eliminating assembly at the point of use. IONSYS™ (E TRANS fentanyl 40 µg), which was developed by ALZA Corporation and received approval in the United States in May 2006, is a fully integrated, non-reusable system for patient-controlled transdermal delivery of fentanyl for the management of post-surgical pain. Figure 3 is an illustration of a modular electrotransport system with a controller and disposable drug unit, while Figure 4 displays an exploded view of IONSYS, an integrated E TRANS system.

Macroflux Transdermal Technology

Macroflux technology is a novel transdermal drug delivery method that is being developed for use with several transdermal delivery systems (5,16). The system combines a drug coated titanium microprojection array screen fixed onto an adhesive patch. Macroflux patch application systems are

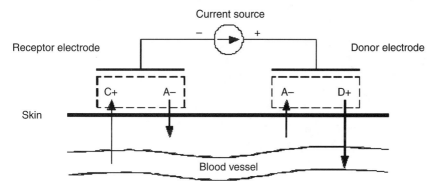

Figure 2 Schematic diagram of electrotransport device on skin indicating the flow of ions in response to an applied voltage.

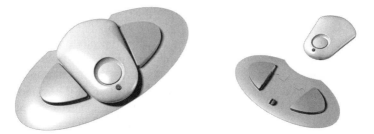

Figure 3 A modular electrotransport system with controller and disposable drug unit. The drug unit also contains electrodes. Conductive snaps make mechanical and electrical attachment between disposable unit and controller.

easy to use and require no special training. As shown in Figure 5, the drug-coated ready-to-use patch is held in a retainer ring and is applied to the skin using a reusable, spring-loaded, impact applicator. The titanium microprojection array creates superficial pathways through the stratum corneum layer. The shape of the microprojections, which is organized into arrays for up to 1000 projections/cm^2, is highly uniform. The projections are

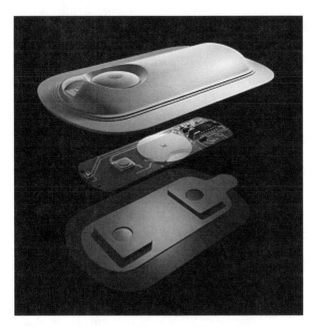

Figure 4 Exploded view of representative single-use electrotransport system showing major components: top housing, printed circuit board assembly, and bottom housing (containing reservoirs for placement of electrodes and hydrogels with adhesive laminate).

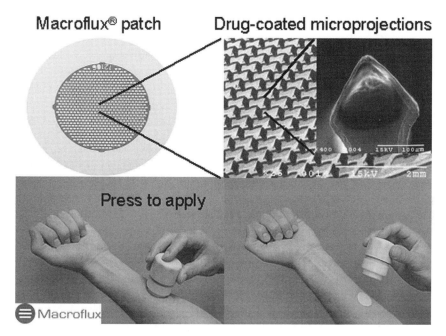

Figure 5 Macroflux transdermal patch technology.

generally less than 200 µm long to avoid penetration into the dermis. When the applicator is pressed onto the skin, it self actuates to release and apply the patch with the correct force and timing (in milliseconds) ensuring consistent patch application and uniform penetration of the microprojections. Once the drug-coated microprojections are inserted into the skin, interstitial fluid dissolves the dry drug coating, allowing diffusion of drug to the adjacent capillary beds for rapid and efficient absorption into the systemic circulation. In addition to direct dry-coating of drug on the microprojection array for bolus delivery, uncoated Macroflux systems can be integrated with a drug reservoir for continuous passive or iontophoretic delivery or they can be used to pretreat a skin site for application of a topical drug formulation (5,45). Drug delivery via Macroflux systems can be optimized for dose delivery of target therapeutics by controlling the area of the patch (1–10 cm^2), the amount of drug loaded per microprojection, the design of the microprojection (density, length, and shape), and drug solubility.

RESEARCH AND DEVELOPMENT

High-Throughput Adhesive Enhancer Formulation Screening

The use of chemical permeation enhancers has been expanded by the development of a high-throughput testing platform that enables testing of large numbers of potential adhesive matrix formulations simultaneously. Table 1 shows the number of different formulations possible based on the number of enhancers used in combination and the level of adhesion at which each enhancer is tested. Newsam et al. describes one approach where a single piece of full-thickness skin is exposed to drug in multiple liquid vehicles for a set period of time and drug penetration into tissue at each application site is quantified (23). This method allows the determination of the partitioned compound into the tissue as a function of vehicle composition but does not enable direct determination of flux from commercially viable transdermal patches. An alternative approach used by ALZA scientists and described by Cima et al. (24) utilizes miniaturized transdermal adhesive patches each having a unique and controllable composition. These patches are arranged in a standard 384 or 1536 microtiter plate layout allowing for simultaneous testing of up to 1536 prototype formulations containing a wide range of enhancer combinations. The magnitude of simultaneous testing with this approach increases the likelihood that a formulation with an acceptable rate of delivery and adequate adhesion, stability, and biocompatibility will be identified. Figure 6 displays the results of a screening assay testing 18 permeation enhancers in every combination of unary (18), binary (153), and ternary (816) formulations (total 997) for rate of flux of risperidone from an acrylate adhesive through human cadaver epidermis. The figure demonstrates that the high flux formulations are predominantly those containing three different enhancers.

In Vivo/In Vitro Evaluation

For passive transdermal systems, in vitro methods are employed to duplicate the behavior of living tissue for screening purposes as well as a means of

Table 1 Total Number of Possible Adhesive Matrix Formulations by Number of Enhancers Selected and Number of Levels of Adhesion at which Each Enhancer Is Tested

No. of enhancers	No. of levels	No. of unary	No. of binary	No. of ternary	Total no. of formulations
10	1	10	45	120	175
	2	20	180	960	1,160
	3	30	405	3,240	3,675
25	1	25	300	2,300	2,625
	2	50	1,200	18,400	19,650
	3	75	2,700	62,100	64,875
50	1	50	1,225	19,600	20,875
	2	100	4,900	156,800	161,800
	3	150	11,025	529,200	540,375

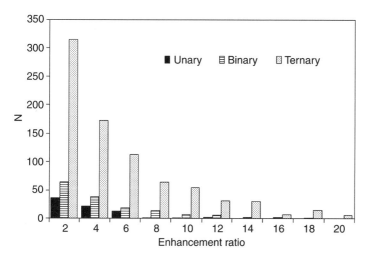

Figure 6 A histogram of the ER (measured flux of enhanced formulation divided by the measured flux of unenhanced formulation) for risperidone delivered from an acrylate adhesive. Histogram bins are sums of all formulations within a given ER range. *Abbreviation*: ER, enhancement ratio.

quality control to compare formulations to ensure batch-to-batch uniformity (25). For both passive and electrotransport systems, reasonable in vitro/in vivo correlations have been observed for several compounds with differing molecular weights, charges and solubilities (4,25–27). While the absolute in vivo transdermal transport rates for many compounds under identical conditions have been reported to be generally higher than that obtained in vitro, the in vitro electrotransport rates can be matched by proper selection of receptor solution ionic strength (28). ALZA has developed an automated method with robotic actuation of dosing, the system functionality test apparatus (SFTA), as a quality control measure to monitor batch-to-batch uniformity for the integrated IONSYS system (29). Figure 7 shows the fentanyl amount delivered per dose period by IONSYS using SFTA. The data demonstrate good correlation between in vitro fentanyl dose delivered by SFTA and in vivo fentanyl dose absorbed as a function of current.

E-TRANS Integrated Systems

Clinical studies have evaluated the pharmacokinetics, tolerance and clinical utility of E-TRANS fentanyl for the management of acute pain. The IONSYS system, which employs E-TRANS delivery technology for patient-controlled

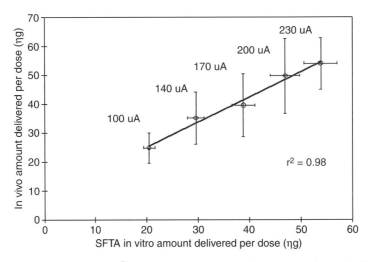

Figure 7 E-TRANS® transdermal fentanyl delivery: mean fentanyl dose (ng) delivered in vitro using the SFTA for IONSYS™ and in vivo fentanyl dose absorbed as a function of the amount of applied current. *Abbreviation*: SFTA, system functionality test apparatus.

analgesia (PCA) of postoperative pain, is a self-contained, noninvasive, preprogrammed, single-use device. The system, applied to the patient's upper outer arm or chest, delivers a 40-μg dose of fentanyl over a 10-minute period. Each device provides a maximum of 80 doses for up to 24 hours, whichever occurs first. IONSYS has a pharmacokinetic profile similar to an IV infusion of fentanyl (30,31). Viscusi et al. (32) compared the efficacy and safety of PCA using IONSYS and an IV infusion pump delivering 1 mg morphine with a 5-minute lockout and a limit of 10 doses per hour (intravenous patient-controlled analgesia; IV PCA). In total, 636 postoperative adult patients were randomized to IONSYS (316 patients) or IV PCA (320 patients). Patient assessment of pain control at 24 hours (poor, fair, good, or excellent) was the primary efficacy end point. In addition, patients indicated their pain intensity on a 100-mm visual analog scale (VAS), with 0 mm corresponding to "no pain" and 100 mm to the "worst possible pain." Respiratory rate was the primary measure of systemic safety. As shown in Figure 8, the distribution of patient assessment of pain control over a 24-hour period was very similar for IONSYS and IV PCA. This similarity between treatments was confirmed by the VAS measurements (Fig. 9). Adverse events reported during the study were typical for opioid treatment of postoperative pain. As shown in Figure 10, the incidence of opioid-related adverse events was similar between the two treatment groups. No patient treated with IONSYS experienced clinically relevant respiratory depression (CRRD), defined as a respiratory rate of 4 per minute or less with moderate sedation. One patient using IV PCA

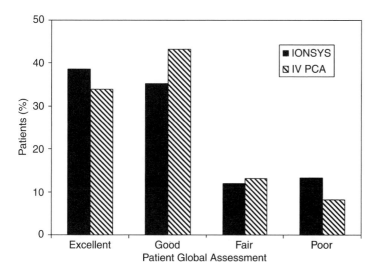

Figure 8 Comparison of patient assessment of pain control at 24 hours for IONSYS™ and IV PCA with morphine. *Abbreviation*: IV PCA, intravenous patient-controlled analgesia.

was given rescue medication for CRRD and was withdrawn from the study. Application site reactions occurred in 6.3% of IONSYS patients and were mild to moderate in all but one case. No skin reaction required treatment and all resolved within 4 weeks. Viscusi et al. (32) concluded that IONSYS and IV PCA are therapeutically equivalent.

The IONSYS design offers several advantages over currently available IV PCA devices, including noninvasive drug delivery, preprogrammed dosing, recessed dosing button to minimize unintentional dose activation, and immediate drug administration on demand. The IONSYS system circumvents many of the shortcomings associated with IV PCA devices, such as complications associated with programming errors and mechanical problems associated with assembly and maintenance.

Strategies for Enhancing Biocompatibility

Several transdermal drug delivery systems have been reported to produce clinical adverse dermatologic reactions (33). Irritant or allergic skin reactions to a number of drugs from different therapeutic classes have also been observed in preclinical studies (34). Since many drugs infrequently produce a dermatological response when taken orally, it is likely that the reactions observed following transdermal delivery are due to high drug concentrations achieved locally in the skin. Strategies to minimize these local side effects have been reviewed (34–36). A dermatologic reaction to

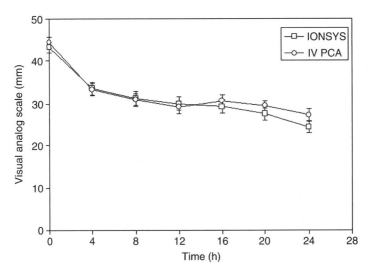

Figure 9   Comparison of patient assessment of pain using a VAS (0 mm is defined as no pain and 100 mm as the worst possible pain) for IONSYS™ and IV PCA with morphine. Mean values are plotted with standard error. *Abbreviations*: VAS, visual analog scale; IV PCA, intravenous patient-controlled analgesia.

a particular transdermal system can have various underlying causes; therefore, different approaches have been developed to address the problem. The number of different strategies that have been reported is an indication of the ubiquity of the problem and demonstrates the need for predictive

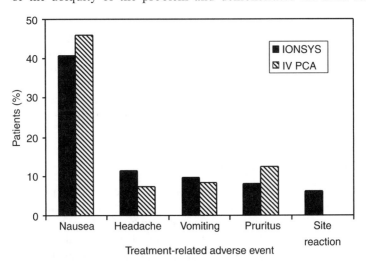

Figure 10   Comparison of treatment-related adverse events with prevalence greater than 5% for IONSYS™ and IV PCA with morphine. *Abbreviation*: IV PCA, intravenous patient-controlled analgesia.

models of skin irritation and sensitization (37). Mitigation approaches target irritation caused by the system, including irritation resulting from an electric current as well as irritation caused by the drug. Approaches to mitigate drug-induced irritation include the co-delivery of vasoactive substances to decrease local drug concentrations, modification of the drug's physicochemical properties (e.g., salification or use of a prodrug), and co-delivery of an immunosuppressive or anti-inflammatory agent to inhibit the inflammatory response. Inhibition of local inflammatory responses resulting from transdermal systems have been observed by pretreating or co-delivering low potency corticosteroids. For example, Figure 11 demonstrates that electrotransport of the anti-emetic drug metoclopramide (MCP) co-delivered with hydrocortisone (HC) caused less skin irritation in human subjects than electrotransport of MCP without HC (38). Since any co-delivered dermatologic reaction inhibitor will have to have demonstrated local safety and an absence of systemic effects for approval of the final product, strategies actually developed for commercial use may be limited to a few practical applications such as the use of preapplication or coformulation with corticosteroids (39).

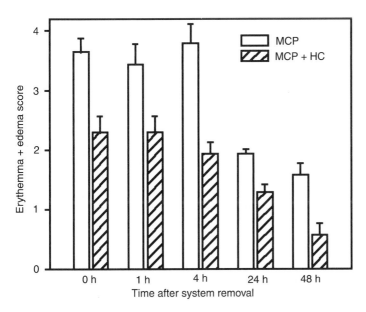

Figure 11   Reduction of irritation to MCP by coadministration of HC. Skin irritation (as measured by the sum of the erythema and edema scores) was evaluated at different time points after 4-hour electrotransport of MCP or MCP + 0.5% HC. Mean values are plotted with standard error. *Abbreviations*: MCP, metoclopramide; HC, hydrocortisone.

Manufacturing

The hybrid character of the E-TRANS technology, with a pharmaceutical component and an electronic/medical device component, presents a number of unique challenges not commonly encountered by conventional pharmaceutical products. The manufacturing of IONSYS involves an assembly of discrete components interlinked with a drug formulation procedure. Five major steps comprise the final assembly process: gel formation and mixing, bottom housing assembly, gel curing, joining, and laminating. The assembly, joining, and laminating steps involve unit operation and scale linearly, whereas, gel formulation, mixing, and curing steps involve chemical processes and scale nonlinearly. To merge these two types of processes, the chemical operations are performed as batch processes. The appropriate batch size for the overall finished product was determined by competing factors arising from both components of this hybrid. The chemical processes present scale limitations, such as gel pot life, while the discrete electronic components present issues of traceability and cost. Therefore, the chemical processes are taken directly to commercial scale in all respects, while the discrete unit operation processes are taken to a commercial production rate but are only demonstrated at a fraction of commercial volume.

Regulatory Issues

In the United States, integrated and modular E-TRANS systems with a reusable controller are regulated as new drugs by the U.S. Food and Drug Administration under the Center for Drug Evaluation and Research, with device consult by the Center for Devices and Radiological Health. In the European Union, while the integrated E-TRANS system requires only drug approval, the reusable concept requires both drug and device approvals. The electronic components of an E-TRANS system must be in conformance with harmonized standards for medical-electronic devices. To comply with medical directives, the systems undergo design verification tests such as electromagnetic interference, electrostatic discharge and environmental stress tests including shock and vibration tests.

Macroflux Systems

Macroflux systems have been tested in preclinical and clinical studies using drug-coated microprojection arrays for bolus delivery as well as integrated systems with a hydrophilic passive reservoir for continuous delivery (40). Delivery of antisense oligonucleotide (preclinical) (5), desmopressin (clinical phase 1) (41,42), and parathyroid hormone (PTH) (clinical phase 1) (43) have been evaluated. Macroflux delivery of desmopressin (an antidiuretic peptide, 1200 MW) was evaluated in an exploratory clinical feasibility study (42). A Macroflux patch with a 2-cm^2 array coated with 25 µg desmopressin was applied to the upper arm for 15 minutes and compared with desmo-pressin IV infusion (30 and 15 µg) in a randomized crossover study of 20 normal healthy volunteers. As shown in Figure 12, desmopressin was rapidly absorbed following Macroflux patch application, with peak concentration achieved by 25 minutes. Mean absorption (5.5 µg) was within the dose range (2–8 µg) for desmopressin antidiuretic effects. Increases in factor VIII release (a biomarker) indicated that the absorbed drug was pharmacologically active. Topical effects and pain perception were scored none to mild.

An initial proof-of-concept study compared Macroflux patch coated with 30 µg of recombinant human PTH (teriparatide), a 3400-MW peptide (1–34), to SC FORTEO® (teriparatide) 40 µg (43). As shown in Figure 13, systemic plasma levels of teriparatide following administration of Macroflux and FORTEO were comparable. Bioavailability of Macroflux was 86.1% relative to FORTEO. Urinary cAMP increased markedly within 2 hours for both the transdermal and SC routes of administration, indicating that transdermally delivered teriparatide was biologically active. Based on the findings from this proof-of-concept study in humans, Macroflux technology appears to provide a well-tolerated and clinically feasible route of admin-istration for peptides.

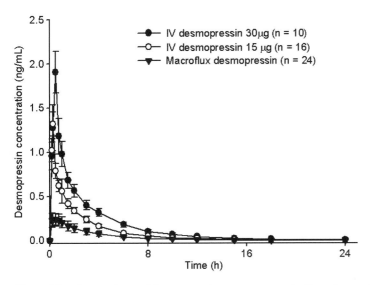

Figure 12 Comparison of desmopressin serum concentrations (mean ± SD) follow-ing administration of desmopressin by IV infusion (30 and 15 µg, 1 µg/min) or coated microneedle array (25 µg). Time 0 indicates the beginning of drug administration or injection. The microneedle array wearing time was 15 minutes.

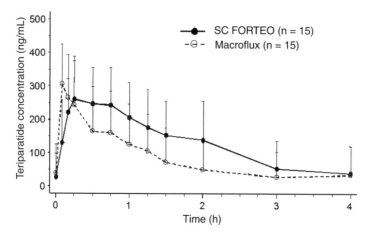

Figure 13 Comparison of plasma concentrations of teriparatide following administration with Macroflux® and SC delivery of FORTEO®. Data are expressed as mean ± SD. *Abbreviation*: SC, subcutaneous.

FUTURE DIRECTIONS

The electronic control in E-TRANS technology offers the potential for personalized medicine with complex patterned and modulated drug delivery, similar to that achievable by infusion pumps. The feasibility of delivering discrete pulses of the decapeptide, luteinizing hormone releasing hormone (LHRH), using E-TRANS technology has been established in human subjects (19). Eight healthy male volunteers received one 15-minute electrotransport pulse every 2 hours for 8 hours at a current of 0.8 mA (0.1 mA/cm² current density) from an 8 cm² hydrogel formulation, which included 15 mM LHRH as the hydrochloride salt. Plasma LHRH and resultant luteinizing hormone (LH) concentrations are shown in Figure 14. Shown for reference is the LHRH plasma concentration profile resulting from IV administration of a single 5-µg bolus dose. These results demonstrate that pulsatile delivery of LHRH is possible using feasible electrotransport conditions. The plasma LHRH profile obtained with E-TRANS systems is comparable with that obtained following IV bolus administration, with sharp peaks and valleys and a rapid decline to negligible baseline values between electrotransport pulses. The extent of variability in the E-TRANS LHRH delivery data was comparable with that obtained following IV administration.

    Another area of future development is poration and transdermal drug delivery combination technologies, which may provide expanded capability for delivery of higher molecular weight drugs. An example is Macroflux technology combined with E-TRANS technology. A 100-µA/cm² iontophoresis system was used in combination with Macroflux to deliver the therapeutic protein human growth hormone (hGH) in vivo to hairless guinea

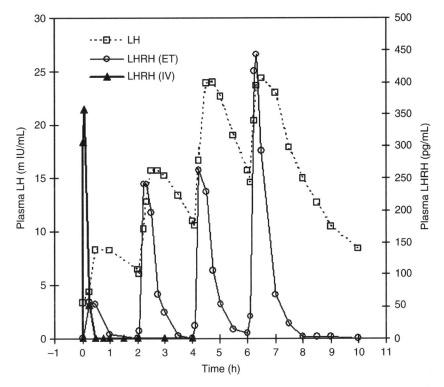

Figure 14 Mean plasma LHRH concentrations in healthy male volunteers receiving E-TRANS® LHRH (0.1 mA/cm², 15-minute dose every 2 hours for 8 hours) and an IV LHRH bolus (5 μg). Mean plasma LH resulting from the E-TRANS LHRH treatment also plotted ($n = 8$). *Abbreviations*: LHRH, luteinizing hormone releasing hormone; LH, luteinizing hormone. *Source*: From Ref. 19.

pigs (HGPs) (44). The protein, hGH, was formulated at 1 mM in a hydrogel and delivered from the cathodic electrode. When the system was applied to HGP skin and activated, Macroflux technology enabled electrotransport of hGH. Pharmacokinetic calculations revealed systemic absorption of hGH at 24 ± 2 and 39 ± 6 μg, respectively, for 1- and 4-hour delivery. When the same electrotransport conditions were used to deliver hGH without Macroflux technology, no significant hGH blood levels were detected (Fig. 15). Combination electroporation and iontophoresis has also been used to enhance transport of peptides, including LHRH, vasopressin, neurotensin, and calcitonin. For transdermal delivery, electroporation is applied to the skin to create pathways through the lipid bilayers of the stratum corneum. In in vitro human cadaver skin studies, application of an electroporative voltage pulse prior to iontophoresis increased the transport number of the peptides from 2- to 10-fold compared to iontophoresis alone (45).

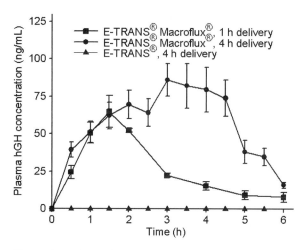

Figure 15 Plasma levels of hGH obtained from E-TRANS® with Macroflux® treatment compared to E-TRANS® alone. Data are expressed as mean ± SEM ($n = 3 - 6$). *Abbreviation*: hGH, human growth hormone.

In addition to drug delivery, E-TRANS and Macroflux technologies also have applications for sampling analytes in biological fluids. The Macroflux system is minimally invasive and provides access to the interstitial fluid. Iontophoresis can be used in reverse as an extraction technique for sampling. For example, glucose can be extracted from interstitial fluid through the skin by electroosmotic flow, which is convective solvent flow caused by passage of iontophoretic current (46). The extracted glucose amount can be quantitatively determined by an electrochemical sensor located in situ in the device. This concept has been used in a commercial glucose monitoring product, the GlucoWatch® Biographer (47). Iontophoresis, with its ability to control the dose of drug delivered by electronic control, is uniquely suited for feedback delivery systems. Such systems would combine sensing technology with drug delivery to achieve automated feedback control. An example is an artificial pancreas, in which delivery of insulin is continually adjusted based on glucose readings. Ultimately iontophoresis can be incorporated into "smart" systems, providing automatic control of delivery profiles.

REFERENCES

1. Shaw JE, Chandrasekaran SK. Controlled topical delivery of drugs for systemic action. Drug Metab Rev 1978; 8(2):223–33.
2. Guy RH, Hadgraft J. Selection of drug candidates for transdermal drug delivery. In: Hadgraft J, Guy RH, eds. Transdermal Drug Delivery. New York: Marcel Dekker, Inc., 1989:59–81.

3. Gale R, Hunt J, Prevo ME. Transdermal drug delivery, passive. In: Mathiowitz E, ed. Encyclopedia of Controlled Drug Delivery. New York: J Wiley & Sons, Inc., 1999:975–91.
4. Phipps JB, Padmanabhan RV, Lattin GA. Iontophoretic delivery of model inorganic and organic drug ions. J Pharm Sci 1989; 78(5):365–9.
5. Lin W, Cormier M, Samiee A, et al. Transdermal delivery of antisense oligonucleotides with microprojection patch (Macroflux) technology. Pharm Res 2001; 18(12):1789–93.
6. Venkatraman S, Gale R. Skin adhesives and skin adhesion: 1. Transdermal drug delivery systems. Biomaterials 1998; 19(13):1119–36.
7. Banga AK. Electrically Assisted Transdermal and Topical Drug Delivery. Bristol: Taylor and Fransis, 1998.
8. Leduc S. Electric Ions and Their Use in Medicine. Liverpool: Rebman Ltd., 1908.
9. Gupta SK, Bernstein KJ, Noorduin H, et al. Fentanyl delivery from an electrotransport system: Delivery is a function of total current, not duration of current. J Clin Pharmacol 1998; 38(10):951–8.
10. Gupta SK, Southam MA, Sathyan G, et al. Effect of current density on pharmacokinetics following continuous or intermittent input from a fentanyl electrotransport system. J Pharm Sci 1998; 87(8):976–81.
11. Kalia YN, Naik A, Garrison J. Iontophoretic drug delivery. Adv Drug Deliv Rev 2004; 56(5):619–58.
12. Tse FL, Laplanche R. Absorption, metabolism, and disposition of [14C]SDZ ENA 713, and acetylcholinesterase inhibitor, in mini pigs following oral, intravenous, and dermal administration. Pharm Res 1998; 15(10):1614–20.
13. Kompaore F, Dupont C, Marty JP. In vivo evaluation in man by two noninvasive methods of stratum corneum barrier function after physical and chemical modifications. Int J Cosm Sci 1991; 13:293–302.
14. Nelson JS, McCullough JL, Glenn TC, et al. Mid-infrared laser ablation of stratum corneum enhances in vitro percutaneous transport of drugs. Invest Dermatol 1991; 97(5):874–9.
15. Mitragotri S, Blankschtein D, Langer R. Ultrasound-mediated transdermal protein delivery. Science 1995; 269(5225): 850–3.
16. Matriano JA, Cormier M, Johnson J. Macroflux microprojection array patch technology: A new and efficient approach for intracutaneous immunization. Pharm Res 2002; 19(1):63–70.
17. Walters KA. Penetration enhancers and their use in transdermal therapeutic systems. In: Hadgraft J, Guy RH, eds. Transdermal Drug Delivery. New York: Marcel Dekker, Inc., 1989:197–246.
18. Karande P, Mitragotri S. High throughput screening of transdermal formulations. Pharm Res 2002; 19(1):655–60.
19. Scott ER, Phipps JB, Gyory JR, et al. Electrotransport systems for transdermal delivery: A practical implementation of iontophoresis. In: Wise D, ed. Handbook of Pharmaceutical Controlled Release Technology. New York: Marcel Dekker Inc., 2000:617–59.
20. Tamada J. Transdermal drug delivery, electrical. In: Mathiowitz E, ed. Encyclopedia of Controlled Drug Delivery. New York: J Wiley & Sons, Inc., 1999:966–73.

21. Lattin GA, Padmanabhan RV, Phipps JB. Electronic control of iontophoretic drug delivery. Ann NY Acad Sci 1991; 618:450–64.
22. Subramony JA, Sharma A, Phipps JB. Microprocessor controlled transdermal drug delivery. Int J Pharm 2006; 317(1):1–6.
23. Newsam JM, Feygin I, Mitragotri S, et al. Apparatus and methods for evaluating the barrier properties of a membrane. Int. Pub. No. WO 2205/012549 A2, Int. Pub. Date: Feb 10, 2005.
24. Cima MJ, Chen H, Gyory JR, et al. System and method for optimizing tissue barrier transfer of compounds. US Patent 6,758,099, July 6, 2004.
25. Transdermal delivery systems, general drug release standards. In: USP 24 (NF 19) US Pharmacopeia and National Formulary. Rockwell: The United States Pharmacopeial Convention, Inc., 1999:1947–51.
26. Padmanabhan RV, Phipps JB, Lattin GA, et al. In vitro and in vivo evaluation of transdermal iontophoretic delivery of hydromorphone. J Control Rel 1990; 11:123–5.
27. Gyory R, Phipps JB, Padmanabhan R. Comparison of in vitro and in vivo iontophoretic transport rates of several therapeutic compounds. In: Couvreur P, Duchene D, Green P, Junginger HE, eds. Transdermal Administration, A Case Study, Iontophoresis. Paris: Editions de Sante, 1997:351–4.
28. Phipps JB, Gyory R. Transdermal ion migration. Adv Drug Deliv Rev 1992; 9: 137–76.
29. Gao H, Lin H, Scott E, et al. Automated in vitro drug delivery and functionality test for electrotransport transdermal systems. The Pittsburgh Conference on Analytical Chemistry and Applied Spectroscopy, New Orleans, Louisiana, March, 2001; Poster #299.
30. Gupta SK, Hwant S, Southam M, et al. Effects of application site and subject demographics on the pharmacokinetics of fentanyl HCl patient-controlled transdermal system (PCTS). Clin Pharmacokinet 2005; 44 (Suppl. 1):25–32.
31. Sathyan G, Zomorodi K, Gidwani S, et al. The effect of dosing frequency on the pharmacokinetics of a fentanyl HCl patient-controlled transdermal system (PCTS). Clin Pharmacokinet 2005; 44(Suppl. 1):17–24.
32. Viscusi ER, Reynolds L, Chung F, et al. Patient-controlled transdermal fentanyl hydrochloride vs intravenous morphine pump for postoperative pain: a randomized controlled trial. J Am Med Assoc 2004; 291(11):1333–41.
33. Patil SM, Hogan DJ, Maibach HI. Transdermal drug delivery systems: Adverse dermatologic reactions. In: Marzuli FN, Maibach HI, eds. Dermatotoxicology. 5th ed. Bristol: Taylor & Francis, 1996:389–96.
34. Kydonieus AF, Wille JJ. Biochemical Modulation of Skin Reactions: Transdermals, Topicals, Cosmetics. New York: CRC Press, 2000.
35. Phipps B, Cormier M, Gale B, et al. Transdermal drug delivery. In: Wnek G, Bowlin G, eds. Encyclopedia of Biomaterials and Biomedical Engineering. New York: Marcel Dekker, Inc., 2004:1677–89.
36. Cormier M, Johnson B. Skin reactions associated with electrotransport. In: Couvreur P, Duchene D, Green P, Junginger HE, eds. Minutes, Transdermal Administration, A Case Study, Iontophoresis. Paris: Editions de Santé, 1997: 50–7.

37. Chester A, Lin WQ, Prevo M, et al. Predictive toxicology methods for transdermal delivery systems. In: Zhai H, Wilhelm K-P, eds. Dermatotoxicology. 7th ed. New York: Taylor & Francis, 2007.
38. Cormier M, Chao ST, Gupta SK, et al. Effect of transdermal iontophoresis codelivery of hydrocortisone on metoclopramide pharmacokinetics and skin-induced reactions in human subjects. J Pharm Sci 1999; 88(10):1030–5.
39. Tamada JA, Davis TL, Leptien AD, et al. The effect of preapplication of corticosteroids on skin irritation and performance of the GlucoWatch G2 Biographer. Diabetes Technol Ther 2004; 6(3):357–67.
40. Daddona P. Macroflux® transdermal technology development for the delivery of therapeutic peptides and proteins. Drug Del Tech 2002; 2:54–7.
41. Cormier M, Johnson B, Ameri M, et al. Transdermal delivery of desmopressin using a coated microneedle array patch system. J Control Rel 2004; 97(3): 503–11.
42. Sathyan G, Weyers R, Daddona P, et al. Apparatus and method for transdermal delivery of desmopressin. US Patent Application 2006, 0093658.
43. Ameri M, Cormier M, Maa YF, et al. Apparatus and method for transdermal delivery of parathyroid hormone agents. US Patent Application 2005, 0256045.
44. Cormier M, Daddona PE. Macroflux® technology for transdermal delivery of therapeutic proteins and vaccines. In: Rathbone ML, Hadgraft J, Roberts MS, eds. Modified Release Drug Delivery Systems. New York, Basel: Marcel Dekker, Inc., 2002: 589–98.
45. Potts RO, Bommannan DB, Wong O, et al. Transdermal peptide delivery using electroporation. In: Sanders LM, Hendren RW, eds. Protien Delivery–Physical Systems. New York: Plenum Publishing, 1997:213–38.
46. Tamada JA, Bohannon NJV, Potts RO. Measurement of glucose in diabetic subjects using noninvasive transdermal extraction. Nat Med 1995; 1(11): 1198–201.
47. Tamada JA, Garg S, Jovanovic L, et al. Non-invasive glucose monitoring: comprehensive clinical results. J Am Med Assoc 1999; 282(19):1791–888.

22

Microneedles for Drug Delivery

Mark R. Prausnitz

*School of Chemical and Biomolecular Engineering, Georgia Institute
of Technology, Atlanta, Georgia, U.S.A.*

Harvinder S. Gill

*The Wallace H. Coulter Department of Biomedical Engineering at Georgia Tech and
Emory University, Georgia Institute of Technology, Atlanta, Georgia, U.S.A.*

Jung-Hwan Park

Kyungwon University, Seoul, Korea

INTRODUCTION

Transdermal drug delivery is an attractive method of administration drug
(1,2). Delivery across the skin circumvents the enzymatic degradation, poor
intestinal absorption, and first-pass liver effect associated with oral delivery.
It also avoids the pain and inconvenience of injections. In addition,
drug delivery across the skin readily lends itself to sustained or modulated
delivery from a passive or active patch. For these reasons, transdermal
drug delivery represents a multi-billion dollar market, which has significant
impact on medical practice.

Despite these advantages, transdermal delivery is currently limited to a
small group of drugs that share a narrow set of common characteristics.
Successful transdermal drugs have low molecular weight ($< 500\,\mathrm{Da}$), have an
octanol–water partition coefficient much greater than one, require low
doses, and cause little or no skin irritation. Very few drugs can cross skin at
useful rates because the stratum corneum, which is the outer 10–20 μm of
the skin, is an excellent barrier.

To overcome the stratum corneum barrier, a variety of chemical and
physical techniques have been developed to create nanometer-scale

disruptions to stratum corneum structural organization and thereby increase skin permeability. Chemical approaches, involving solvents, surfactants and other compounds, have had varied success, where increased skin permeability has often been associated with increased skin irritation and has often been applicable only to small molecules (3). Physical approaches, such as iontophoresis, electroporation, and ultrasound, have perturbed stratum corneum structure and have provided electrophoretic and possibly convective driving forces (4). These methods have been more effective to increase skin permeability to macromolecules and can be designed to avoid irritation.

These chemical and physical methods to disrupt stratum corneum on the nanometer scale, however, have had limited clinical impact. This is, in large part, because the increases in transdermal transport are still not sufficient for many drugs under clinically acceptable conditions. Moreover, the physical methods typically require a device with a power supply, which adds cost and complexity.

Recent research suggests that the approach to disrupting skin on the nanometer scale may be too mild. Micron-scale skin disruption should make skin much more permeable, yet still be safe and well tolerated by patients. Given that almost all conventional drugs, proteins, DNA and vaccines are sub-micron in size, creating holes of microns dimensions in the stratum corneum should permit delivery of a broad range of compounds. Yet, micron-scale disruption is unlikely to have significant safety or cosmetic concerns. The skin barrier is routinely breached during common experiences of minor abrasion, shaving, dry skin, and hypodermic injection, yet infection rarely occurs. This is because the skin is designed to prevent entry of pathogens, even in the presence of minor stratum corneum defects.

This observation leads to the hypothesis that micron-scale disruption of stratum corneum can dramatically increase skin permeability to a broad variety of compounds without significant safety concerns. Prompted by this idea, a number of methods to disrupt stratum corneum on the micron scale have been developed, including thermal ablation, microdermabrasion, and microneedles. Microneedles represent an especially attractive approach, because microneedle devices can be very simple and need not involve a power supply or other costly components. Microneedles are typically solid or hollow needles measuring microns in size that painlessly pierce across the stratum corneum to transport drugs into the skin for local or systemic delivery.

Although microneedles were already described in a 1976 patent (5), the first paper to demonstrate microneedles for transdermal delivery was not published until 1998 (6). This delay was in large part due to the unavailability of microfabrication methods to make needles of such small dimensions. However, the microelectronics revolution provided a workshop of instrumentation designed specifically to make micron, and sub-micron, structures, which have now been adapted to make microneedles. For this reason, the first microneedles were etched from silicon wafers, although more recent efforts have emphasized FDA-approved metals and polymers (7,8).

The first uses of microneedles involved piercing the skin with an array of solid microneedles to make the stratum corneum more permeable, after which a drug formulation or patch was applied to the treated site, i.e., the "poke-and-patch" method. Solid microneedles have also been coated with drug formulations that dissolve off within the skin after microneedle insertion, i.e., "coat-and-poke." The "poke-and-release" approach involves making microneedles out of dissolving or degrading polymers that encapsulate drug, which then release drug within the skin with predetermined kinetics. Finally, fabrication of hollow microneedles facilitates micro-infusion of a liquid drug formulation by the "poke-and-flow" method, which is more akin to a minimally invasive injection than a transdermal patch. Some of these microneedle scenarios have been the subject of previous reviews (7–17).

As discussed in the following sections, a variety of different microneedle designs and delivery scenarios have been studied and shown to deliver a breadth of different compounds in vitro and in vivo. This review seeks to provide a comprehensive review of the peer-reviewed literature on microneedles studied for transdermal delivery. We have not, however, included work presented only in conference proceedings or other non-peer-reviewed literature and have also not included the relatively large literature that primarily addresses fabrication issues in the absence of directly assessing drug delivery capabilities.

THE POKE-AND-PATCH APPROACH

Solid microneedles have been fabricated by a number of methods to pierce the skin and thereby increase skin permeability. The first needles were prepared by plasma etching tapered spikes into silicon wafers to produce needles measuring tens to hundreds of microns in length, tens of microns in base radius, and approximately 1 μm in tip radius (Figs. 1A,1B) (6,18,19). More recently, metal and polymer microneedles have been fabricated with similar dimensions, although tip radius has tended to be less sharp (e.g., 1–10 μm) (20–22).

In vitro studies have demonstrated that skin permeability can be increased by up to 10,000-fold after microneedle treatment for delivery of compounds including calcein, insulin, bovine serum albumin, and latex nanoparticles as big as 100 nm in diameter (Figs. 1A–1D) (6,18,19,22). Residual holes in the skin were measured to be 6 μm in radius, which is smaller than microneedle base dimensions, probably due to partial skin recoil after microneedle removal. Theoretical analysis indicated that

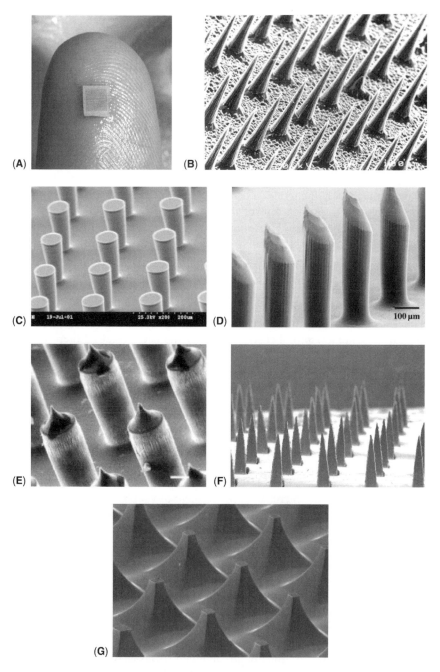

Figure 1 Representative microneedles investigated for the poke-and-patch approach. Silicon microneedle array containing 400 microneedles, each 150 μm in

(Caption continued on facing page)

increased skin permeability could be fully explained by diffusion through the water-filled holes created by microneedle penetration (18). Additional studies have demonstrated increased skin permeability after piercing with small hypodermic needles as a model for microneedles (23,24).

In addition to the delivery of inert model compounds, DNA delivery has been studied using living skin obtained from human surgical procedures and maintained by tissue culture techniques (Fig. 1E). Using these ex vivo methods, plasmid DNA was shown to be delivered and to express a reporter gene (i.e., β-galactosidase) at the sites of needle penetration (25–27).

In vivo delivery has been studied in the context of insulin delivery to diabetic, hairless rats (Fig. 1F) (21). After piercing the skin with an array of microneedles, insulin was delivered across the skin for a 4-hour period. Blood insulin levels increased and glucose levels decreased by as much as 80%, indicating delivery of bioactive protein. Increased delivery of an antisense oligonucleotide was also demonstrated after piercing hairless guinea pig skin with microneedles in vivo (13).

Using a related approach, liquid formulations of DNA, protein, and live, attenuated virus vaccines against hepatitis B, anthrax, and Japanese encephalitis, respectively, were applied to the skin of animal models. Then, blunt-tipped microneedles were scraped across the skin (Fig. 1G) (28–30). The antigen formulations were deposited in the micron-scale troughs created in the skin and induced strong immune responses that were, in most cases, at least as good as hypodermic injection. In a separate study, a tattoo machine was used to pierce the skin and drive a liquid DNA formulation into the skin for transfection (31).

Using a combined approach with iontophoresis, hairless guinea pigs in vivo were first pierced with microneedles and then an antisense oligonucleotide formulation was applied to the skin in the presence of an electric field (20). Pretreatment with microneedles before iontophoresis increased transdermal delivery by 100-fold compared to iontophoresis alone. Similar results were found for delivery of human growth hormone to hairless guinea pigs in vivo (13) and dextrans across hairless rat skin in vitro (32).

Figure 1 (*continued*) length on an area $< 0.1 \, cm^2$ shown (**A**) at low magnification resting on a forefinger and (**B**) at high magnification. (**C**) Columnar, silicon microneedles measuring 150 m in length with a base diameter of 80 μm. (**D**) Polymer microneedles made of polyglycolic acid measuring 600 μm in length with a base diameter of 100 μm and a tip diameter of 10 μm. (**E**) Silicon microneedles measuring 150 μm in length with a base diameter of about 50 μm. (**F**) Stainless steel microneedles measuring 1000 μm in length with a base width of 200 μm and a thickness of 50 μm. (**G**) Silicon "microenhancer" array containing flat-tipped, pyramidal microstructures measuring 150 μm in length used to scrape the skin. *Source*: From Refs. 6, 19, 21, 22, 25, 28, 66.

Increased skin permeability due to microneedles has also been exploited as a means to extract interstitial fluid from the skin to assay glucose levels as a non-invasive monitoring method. Data from hairless rats, as well as a small number of human subjects, indicated that up to a few microliters could be extracted within a few minutes and that glucose levels measured in the extracts correlated well with blood glucose levels (33,34).

A similar poke-and-patch approach has also been employed to pierce microneedles into the vascular wall using a modified balloon catheter to increase drug penetration in vitro (35). Microneedles have also been employed to transfect nematodes with plasmid DNA (36). Although microneedle dimensions varied for these applications and the anatomy of the transport barrier was quite different, microneedle-based delivery was nonetheless highly effective.

THE COAT-AND-POKE APPROACH

In addition to using microneedles to increase skin permeability, microneedles have also been used to carry drugs into the skin through the holes they create. To accomplish this, metal microneedles have been coated with drug formulations using dip coating methods. Water-based, room-temperature processes that use only FDA-approved excipients have been shown to coat microneedles with a broad range of compounds, including small molecules, proteins, plasmid DNA, virus particles, and polymer nanoparticles (Fig. 2A) (37). Coating formulations have been optimized (*i*) to form uniform coatings by adding surfactants that lower surface tension to facilitate microneedle wetting with coating solution and (*ii*) to form thick coatings by adding thickening agents that increase viscosity to cause a larger volume of coating solution to adhere to microneedles during drying (38). Coatings with up to 1 mg of drug per array can be achieved.

Another coating method involves the use of chitosan to coat the base substrate to which the microneedles are attached and thereby provide a drug reservoir for release across the skin using a variation on the poke-and-patch method (Fig. 2J) (39). Using a different approach, acupuncture needle tips were coated with microporous calcium phosphate, after which the micropores were filled with trehalose that could serve to stabilize proteins (40).

Coated microneedles have been used to deliver drugs and vaccines in vivo. Desmopressin was delivered to hairless guinea pigs and found to have up to 85% bioavailability (Figs. 2K–2L) (41). Ovalbumin administered as a model antigen to hairless guinea pigs developed strong antibody responses that were up to 50-fold greater than intramuscular or subcutaneous delivery of the same dose (42,43). This can be explained by the highly immunogenic dendritic cells found in the skin (44). More recently, coated

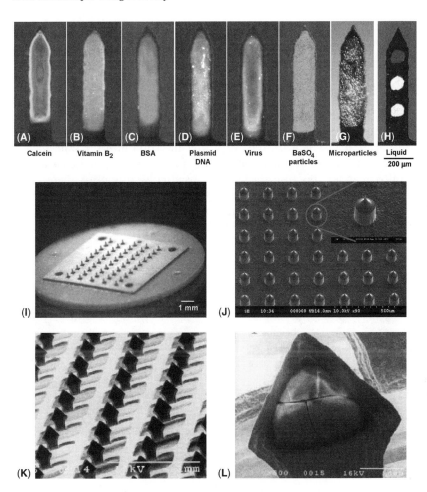

Figure 2 Representative microneedles investigated for the coat-and-poke approach. Individual stainless steel microneedles each about 700 μm in length, 160 μm in width and 50 μm in thickness coated with solid films containing: (**A**) calcein, (**B**) vitamin B_2, (**C**) bovine serum albumin conjugated with Texas Red, (**D**) plasmid DNA conjugated with YOYO-1, (**E**) modified vaccinia virus–Ankara conjugated with YOYO-1, (**F**) 1-μm diameter barium sulfate particles, (**G**) 10-μm diameter latex particles, and (**H**) liquid formulations containing red, yellow or green dye each filled exclusively into the three circular pockets of the microneedles (**I**) Prototype microneedle device containing a stainless steel microneedle array of 50 microneedles with an integrated adhesive film to stick to the skin. (**J**) Silicon microneedles measuring 130 μm in length with a base diameter of 80 μm and a tip radius of < 1 μm that were coated with chitosan films containing calcein and bovine serum albumin. (**K, L**) Titanium microneedles measuring 200 μm in length with 170 μm width at the arrow head and a thickness of 35 μm that were coated with desmopressin. *Source*: From Refs. 37, 38, 39, 41.

microneedles have been used for ocular delivery, demonstrating delivery of pilocarpine and other model compounds into the rabbit eye in vivo (45).

THE POKE-AND-RELEASE APPROACH

As a novel alternative to coated microneedles, drugs have been encapsulated within microneedles made of polymers and polysaccharides for rapid or sustained release in the skin. In this way, after insertion into the skin, microneedles can dissolve or degrade, which thereby releases encapsulated drug in a controlled manner. Because the needles eventually disappear, there is no biohazardous sharp waste, which facilitates safe disposal. Microneedles have been made in this way by filling micro-molds with molten matrix material along with dissolved or suspended drug particles, which solidify after cooling.

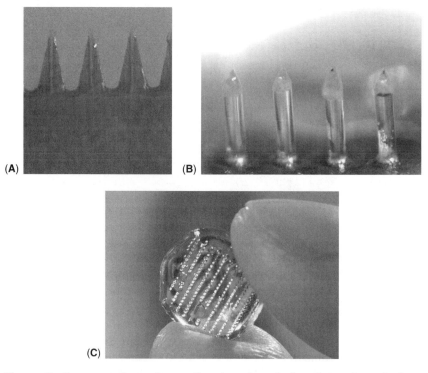

(A)

(B)

(C)

Figure 3 Representative microneedles investigated for the poke-and-release approach. (**A**) Microneedles made of maltose, measuring 500 μm in length, and encapsulating 10 wt% calcein as a model drug. (**B**) Bevel-tip, polymer microneedles made of PLGA, measuring 600 μm in length, and encapsulating calcein within their tips. (**C**) A complete 20 × 10 array of polymer microneedles made of PLGA. *Source*: From Refs. 46, 49.

One design for rapidly dissolving microneedles involves a maltose-based matrix that encapsulated sodium salicylate and ascorbate-2-glicoside (Fig. 3A) (46). Molten maltose was solidified by a process related to that used to make hard candies. Maltose microneedles were inserted into the skin of human subjects in vivo and found to dissolve within 5 minutes with no adverse reactions. Using a different fabrication process to model micro-needles, millimeter-scale needles were made out of dextrin that encapsulated erythropoietin and insulin and shown to effectively deliver these compounds to mice in vivo (47,48)

Degradable microneedles can also be used for controlled release delivery over time. Toward this end, microneedles have been fabricated out of polylactic-co-glycolic acid (PLGA) to encapsulate a model small molecule and protein (Fig. 3B and 3C) (49). Controlled release was demonstrated in vitro for times ranging from hours to months, depending on the encapsulation formulation.

THE POKE-AND-FLOW APPROACH

In contrast to solid microneedles, hollow microneedles provide additional capabilities as well as complications. Hollow microneedles enable delivery of liquid formulations (that may already be approved for injection), which can be administered much more rapidly and with modulated flow rates, if needed. However, hollow microneedles are more complex to fabricate, given their inherently weaker and more sophisticated geometry, and have posed difficulties to achieve large flow rates.

Hollow microneedles have been fabricated by a number of etching and molding methods and shown to deliver insulin and diclofenac to rats in vivo, which established the feasibility of this approach (Fig. 4A) (18,50). Another study demonstrated microneedle injection of methyl nicotinate in human subjects (Fig. 4B) (51). Additional research has shown that delivery using microneedles can be precisely targeted to the epidermis or to specified depths in the dermis, which is of interest for dermatological, vaccine, and research purposes (Fig. 4C) (52).

Despite these successes, only microliter volumes of fluid were delivered into the skin in these studies. In fact, one study reported an inability to deliver any detectable amounts of fluid into skin using microneedles (19). To address this problem, fluid flow through microneedles was measured experimentally and modeled theoretically, which showed that fluid delivery using microneedles is not primarily limited by flow through the micro-needles themselves, but is limited primarily by the resistance to flow out of the microneedles and into skin (53). Partially retracting microneedles after insertion into the skin was found to increase flow rates by up to an order of magnitude (54). Retraction allowed the skin, which was deformed during

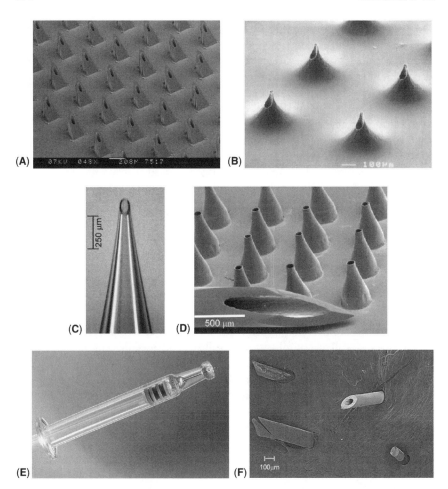

Figure 4 Representative microneedles investigated for poke-and-flow approach. (**A**) Hollow, silicon microneedles measuring 350 μm in length and containing a 70 μm-wide bore. (**B**) Hollow, silicon microneedles measuring 200 μm in length and having a lumen diameter of 40 μm. (**C**) Hollow, glass microneedle with a tip opening effective radius of 30 μm. (**D**) Hollow, metal microneedles measuring 500 μm in length shown next to a 27-gauge hypodermic needle. Hollow, metal microneedle measuring 1.5 mm in length (**E**) incorporated into an intradermal injection device and (**F**) pierced across swine skin. *Source*: From Refs. 50, 51, 54, 56, 67.

microneedle insertion, to recoil back toward its original position and thereby relieve skin compaction and increase local flow conductivity (55).

Manufacturing and delivery using microneedles can also be facilitated by using larger needles. Small hypodermic needles measuring 1–3 mm in length have been used to vaccinate mice and rabbits against anthrax (29) and nonhuman primates against Japanese encephalitis (Figs. 4E and 4F) (30). Another simplification is the use of hollow microneedles for passive delivery (i.e., without pressure-driven flow), which has been shown to deliver insulin to diabetic rats (Fig. 4D) (56).

Hollow microneedles have also been developed for delivery to cells and tissues other than skin. In combination with electrical stimulation using microneedles, neuro-active chemicals have been administered to neural tissue (57). Brain slice cultures have been perfused using microfluidic microneedle devices (58). Hollow microneedle arrays have been used to deliver genetic materials into animal and plants cells (59).

For diagnostic applications, hollow microneedles have been used to withdraw blood (60) and to extract interstitial fluid for glucose monitoring (61). Microneedles have been modified to perform microdialysis for continuous medical monitoring (62).

OTHER CONSIDERATIONS

Successful drug delivery also requires that microneedles be strong enough to insert into the skin without breaking. An experimental and theoretical study indicated that the force to insert microneedles into the skin of human subjects depended primarily on needle tip sharpness, whereas microneedle strength depended on multiple geometric and materials properties (63). Optimized solid and hollow microneedles were found to have insertion forces many fold smaller than failure forces, which provides a large margin of safety. Insertion forces, as well as skin deformation during microneedle insertion, have been reduced by insertion at high velocity (64), insertion with a drilling motion (52), and insertion with vibration (65).

Microneedles have generally been described as painless and non-irritating. One study found that microneedles caused essentially no pain other than the sensation associated with pressing against the skin during insertion (66). Another study similarly reported little or no pain, as well as little or no skin irritation, associated with microneedles (28).

CONCLUSIONS

In conclusion, a number of different microneedle delivery approaches have been investigated in vitro, in animals, and in humans. Poke-and-patch provides a simple method to enable sustained delivery of hydrophilic drugs and macromolecules from a transdermal patch. Coat-and-poke provides bolus delivery of sub-milligram doses in a patient-friendly manner that may replace some injections. Poke-and-release offers bolus or sustained delivery from microneedles that dissolve or degrade in the skin and then disappear. Poke-and-flow enables rapid and modulated delivery using a more sophisticated microneedle system. To achieve these goals, microneedles can be designed not to break and not to cause pain or irritation. Overall, microneedles hold promise to be a widely useful method for minimally invasive delivery of drugs, proteins and vaccines.

REFERENCES

1. Guy RH, Hadgraft J, eds. Transdermal Drug Delivery. New York: Marcel Dekker; 2003.
2. Prausnitz MR, Mitragotri S, Langer R. Current status and future potential of transdermal drug delivery. Nat Rev Drug Discov 2004; 3(2):115–24.
3. Williams AC, Barry BW. Penetration enhancers. Adv Drug Deliv Rev 2004; 56 (5), 603–18.
4. Cross SE, Roberts MS. Physical enhancement of transdermal drug application: is delivery technology keeping up with pharmaceutical development? Curr Drug Deliv 2004; 1(1):81–92.
5. Gerstel MS, Place VA. Drug delivery device. U.S. Patent No. 3,964,482; 1976.
6. Henry S, McAllister DV, Allen MG, et al. Microfabricated microneedles: a novel approach to transdermal drug delivery. J Pharm Sci 1998; 87(8):922–5.
7. McAllister DV, Allen MG, Prausnitz MR. Microfabricated microneedles for gene and drug delivery. Annu Rev Biomed Eng 2000; 2:289–313.
8. Reed ML, Lye W-K. Microsystems for drug and gene delivery. Proc IEEE 2004; 92(1):56–75.
9. Prausnitz M, Ackley D, Gyory J. Microneedles for transdermal drug delivery. In: Rathbone M, Hadgraft J, Roberts M, eds. Modified Release Drug Delivery Systems. New York: Marcel Dekker; 2003; 513–22.
10. Greystone Associates. Microneedle Drug Delivery: Technology, Markets, and Prospects. Amherst, NH: Greystone Associates; 2004.
11. Prausnitz MR. Microneedles for transdermal drug delivery. Adv Drug Deliv Rev 2004; 56:581–7.
12. Prausnitz M. Assessment of microneedles for transdermal drug delivery. In: Bronaugh R, Maibach H, eds. Percutaneous Absorption. New York: Marcel Dekker; 2005; 497–507.
13. Cormier M, Daddona PE. Macroflux technology for transdermal delivery of therapeutic proteins and vaccines. In: Rathbone MJ, Hadgraft J, Roberts MS, eds. Modified-Release Drug Delivery Technology. New York: Marcel Dekker; 2003; 589–98.
14. Prausnitz M, Mikszta J, Raeder-Devens J. Microneedles. In: Smith E, Maibach H, eds. Percutaneous Penetration Enhancers. Boca Raton, FL: CRC Press; 2005; 239–55.
15. Birchall JC. Microneedle array technology: the time is right but is the science ready? Expert Rev Med Devices 2006; 3(1):1–4.
16. Coulman S, Allender C, Birchall J. Microneedles and other physical methods for overcoming the stratum corneum barrier for cutaneous gene therapy. Crit Rev Ther Drug Carrier Syst 2006; 23(3):205–58.
17. Sivamani RK, Liepmann D, Maibach HI. Microneedles and transdermal applications. Expert Opin Drug Deliv 2007; 4(1):19–25.

18. McAllister DV, Wang PM, Davis SP, et al. Microfabricated needles for transdermal delivery of macromolecules and nanoparticles: fabrication methods and transport studies. Proc Natl Acad Sci USA 2003; 100:13755–60.

19. Teo MA, Shearwood C, Ng KC, et al. In vitro and in vivo characterization of MEMS microneedles. Biomed Microdevices 2005; 7(1):47–52.

20. Lin W, Cormier M, Samiee A, et al. Transdermal delivery of antisense oligonucleotides with microprojection patch (Macroflux) technology. Pharm Res 2001; 18(12):1789–93.

21. Martanto W, Davis S, Holiday N, et al. Transdermal delivery of insulin using microneedles in vivo. Pharm Res 2004; 21:947–52.

22. Park J-H, Allen MG, Prausnitz MR. Biodegradable polymer microneedles: fabrication, mechanics and transdermal drug delivery. J Control Release 2005; 104:51–66.

23. Verbaan FJ, Bal SM, van den Berg DJ, et al. Assembled microneedle arrays enhance the transport of compounds varying over a large range of molecular weight across human dermatomed skin. J Control Release 2007; 117(2):238–45.

24. Wu XM, Todo H, Sugibayashi K. Effects of pretreatment of needle puncture and sandpaper abrasion on the in vitro skin permeation of fluorescein isothiocyanate (FITC)-dextran. Int J Pharm 2006; 316(1–2):102–8.

25. Chabri F, Bouris K, Jones T, et al. Microfabricated silicon microneedles for nonviral cutaneous gene delivery. Br J Dermatol 2004; 150(5):869–77.

26. Coulman SA, Barrow D, Anstey A, et al. Minimally invasive delivery of macromolecules and plasmid DNA via microneedles. Current Drug Delivery 2006; 3:65–75.

27. Birchall J, Coulman S, Pearton M, et al. Cutaneous DNA delivery and gene expression in ex vivo human skin explants via wet-etch micro-fabricated microneedles. J Drug Target 2005; 13(7):415–21.

28. Mikszta JA, Alarcon JB, Brittingham JM, et al. Improved genetic immunization via micromechanical disruption of skin-barrier function and targeted epidermal delivery. Nat Med 2002; 8(4):415–9.

29. Mikszta JA, Sullivan VJ, Dean C, et al. Protective immunization against inhalational anthrax: a comparison of minimally invasive delivery platforms. J Infect Dis 2005; 191(2):278–88.

30. Dean CH, Alarcon JB, Waterston AM, et al. Cutaneous delivery of a live, attenuated chimeric flavivirus vaccine against Japanese encephalitis (ChimeriVax)-JE) in non-human primates. Hum Vaccin 2005; 1(3):106–11.

31. Eriksson E, Yao F, Svensjo T, et al. In vivo gene transfer to skin and wound by microseeding. J Surg Res 1998; 78(2):85–91.

32. Wu XM, Todo H, Sugibayashi K. Enhancement of skin permeation of high molecular compounds by a combination of microneedle pretreatment and iontophoresis. J Control Release 2007; 118(2):189–95.

33. Wang P, Cornwell M, Prausnitz M. Minimally invasive extraction of dermal interstitial fluid for glucose monitoring using glass microneedles. Diabetes Technol Ther 2005; 7:131–41.

34. Vesper HW, Wang PM, Archibold E, et al. Assessment of trueness of a glucose monitor using interstitial fluid and whole blood as specimen matrix. Diabetes Technol Ther 2006; 8(1):76–80.

35. Reed ML, Wu C, J K, et al. Micromechanical devices for intravascular drug delivery. J Pharm Sci 1998; 87(11):1387–94.
36. Hashmi S, Ling P, Hashmi G, et al. Genetic transformation of nematodes using arrays of micromechanical piercing structures. BioTechniques 1995; 19(5): 766–70.
37. Gill HS, Prausnitz MR. Coated microneedles for transdermal delivery. J Control Release 2007; 117(2):227–37.
38. Gill HS, Prausnitz MR. Coating formulations for microneedles. Pharm Res 2007; 24(7):1369–80.
39. Xie Y, Xu B, Gao Y. Controlled transdermal delivery of model drug compounds by MEMS microneedle array. Nanomedicine 2005; 1(2):184–90.
40. Shirkhanzadeh M. Microneedles coated with porous calcium phosphate ceramics: effective vehicles for transdermal delivery of solid trehalose. J Mater Sci Mater Med 2005; 16(1):37–45.
41. Cormier M, Johnson B, Ameri M, et al. Transdermal delivery of desmopressin using a coated microneedle array patch system. J Control Release 2004; 97(3): 503–11.
42. Matriano JA, Cormier M, Johnson J, et al. Macroflux microprojection array patch technology: a new and efficient approach for intracutaneous immunization. Pharm Res 2002; 19(1):63–70.
43. Widera G, Johnson J, Kim L, et al. Effect of delivery parameters on immunization to ovalbumin following intracutaneous administration by a coated microneedle array patch system. Vaccine 2006; 24(10):1653–64.
44. Glenn GM, Kenney RT. Mass vaccination: solutions in the skin. Curr Top Microbiol Immunol 2006; 304:247–68.
45. Jiang J, Gill HS, Ghate D, et al. Coated microneedles for drug delivery to the eye. Invest Ophthalmol Vis Sci 2007; 48(9):4038–43.
46. Miyano T, Tobinaga Y, Kanno T, et al. Sugar micro needles as transdermic drug delivery system. Biomed Microdevices 2005; 7(3):185–8.
47. Ito Y, Hagiwara E, Saeki A, et al. Feasibility of microneedles for percutaneous absorption of insulin. Eur J Pharm Sci 2006; 29(1):82–8.
48. Ito Y, Yoshimitsu J, Shiroyama K, et al. Self-dissolving microneedles for the percutaneous absorption of EPO in mice. J Drug Target 2006; 14(5):255–61.
49. Park JH, Allen MG, Prausnitz MR. Polymer microneedles for controlled-release drug delivery. Pharm Res 2006; 23(5):1008–19.
50. Gardeniers JGE, Luttge R, Berenschot JW, et al. Silicon micromachined hollow microneedles for transdermal liquid transport. J MEMS 2003; 6(12): 855–62.
51. Sivamani RK, Stoeber B, Wu GC, et al. Clinical microneedle injection of methyl nicotinate: stratum corneum penetration. Skin Res Technol 2005; 11(2): 152–6.
52. Wang PM, Cornwell M, Hill J, et al. Precise microinjection into skin using hollow microneedles. J Invest Dermatol 2006; 126(5):1080–7.
53. Martanto W, Smith MK, Baisch SM, et al. Fluid dynamics in conically tapered microneedles. AICHE J 2005; 51:1599–607.
54. Martanto W, Moore JS, Kashlan O, et al. Microinfusion using hollow microneedles. Pharm Res 2006; 23(1):104–13.

55. Martanto W, Moore JS, Couse T, et al. Mechanism of fluid infusion during microneedle insertion and retraction. J Control Release 2006; 112(3):357–61.
56. Davis SP, Martanto W, Allen MG, et al. Transdermal insulin delivery to diabetic rats through microneedles. IEEE Trans Biomed Eng 2005; 52:909–15.
57. Chen J, Wise KD. A multichannel neural probe for selective chemical delivery at the cellular level. IEEE Trans Biomed Eng 1997; 44:760–9.
58. Choi Y, McClain MA, Laplaca MC, et al. Three dimensional MEMS microfluidic perfusion system for thick brain slice cultures. Biomed Microdevices 2007; 9(1):7–13.
59. Chun K, Hashiguchi G, Toshiyoshi H, et al. Fabrication of array of hollow microcapillaries used for injection of genetic materials into animal/plant cells. Jpn J Appl Phys Part 2 1999; 38:279–81.
60. Tsuchiya K, Nakanishi N, Uetsuji Y, et al. Development of blood extraction system for health monitoring system. Biomed Microdevices 2005; 7(4):347–53.
61. Smart WH, Subramanian K. The use of silicon microfabrication technology in painless blood glucose monitoring. Diabetes Technol Ther 2000; 2(4):549–59.
62. Zahn JD, Trebotich D, Liepmann D. Microdialysis microneedles for continuous medical monitoring. Biomed Microdevices 2005; 7(1):59–69.
63. Davis SP, Landis BJ, Adams ZH, et al. Insertion of microneedles into skin: measurement and prediction of insertion force and needle fracture force. J Biomech 2004; 37:1155–63.
64. Rousche PJ, Normann RA. A method for pneumatically inserting an array of penetrating electrodes into cortical tissue. Ann Biomed Eng 1992; 20(4):413–22.
65. Yang M, Zahn JD. Microneedle insertion force reduction using vibratory actuation. Biomed Microdevices 2004; 6(3):177–82.
66. Kaushik S, Hord AH, Denson DD, et al. Lack of pain associated with microfabricated microneedles. Anesth Analg 2001; 92:502–4.
67. Mikszta J. Cutaneous or mucosal delivery of anthrax rPA provides protection against inhalational anthrax. Innovative Administration Systems for Vaccines Meeting, Rockville, MD (http://wwwhhsgov/nvpo/meetings/dec2003/Contents/ThursdayAM/Mikszta/Miksztapdf) 2003.

23

Transfersome®: Self-Optimizing and Self-Driven Drug-Carrier, for Localized and Transdermal Drug Delivery

Gregor Cevc

IDEA AG, Munich, Germany

INTRODUCTION

The skin (cutis) is not only the largest organ, with a total weight around 3 kg and a surface of approximately $2.0\,m^2$ in humans, it is also the best and most easily accessible body part. Transcutaneous drug delivery has therefore been tried innumerable times. The problem with the approach is that most drugs cannot successfully diffuse through (permeate) intact skin. This is due to special structural, biochemical, and physiological properties of the organ, especially in its outermost 8–30 μm thin layer (the stratum corneum), which has evolved into the primary skin barrier, one of the best in nature (Fig. 1, left).

Consequently, various methods have been developed to lower the skin permeability barrier. The most classical and invasive one is use of injections, over time, through smaller and smaller needles. It is now possible to penetrate the skin with micro-engineered needle(s) to just a depth of a few 10 μm. This permits well controlled and number limited creation of pores through the cells (largely corneocytes) in the outer skin layers. The functionally related skin poration with impacting particles or droplets, with high voltage electric or thermal pulses, or with sonoporation, is less well controlled in one or more aspects; so is the stratum corneum abrasion with mechanical or radio-frequency wave means (1). Despite their potential benefits, none of these methods is broadly practiced to date, owing to the resulting skin

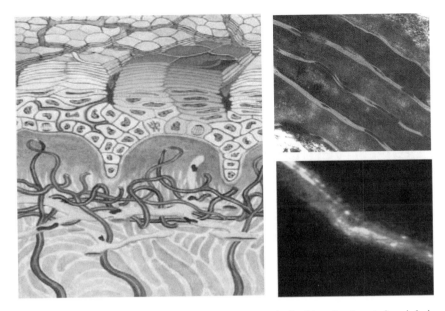

Figure 1 The skin (*left panel*) is an evolutionary optimized barrier, located mainly in the stratum corneum near the organ surface. This prevents material transport through this barrier, which is a combination of an anatomical barricade, consisting of cells arranged in a tile-like fashion, and a bio/chemical obstacle, in the form of tightly packed lipidic seals attached to the cells (dark bands in the upper right panel; electron micrograph). Possible routes through the skin pursue the path of lowest resistance between or along such hindrances (bright bands in the lower right panel; light micrograph). However, such "virtual channels" need first to be opened up to become effective. This requires application of special vehicles, such as Transfersomes®, on the skin.

irritations, inconvenience, and/or high cost of usage, but also due to their technical complexity and limited deliverable drug dose. The marketed pharmaceutical products for intra- or transcutaneous drug delivery thus still comprise small molecules (<450 Da) and rely on the oldest noninvasive procedure for lowering skin permeability barrier: employment of chemicals that act as skin permeation enhancers by partly extracting and/or fluidizing lipids in the stratum corneum (2).

Aiming at peripheral subcutaneous tissue as a therapeutic target poses an additional problem. The small, free molecules that have crossed the stratum corneum are inevitably channeled by cutaneous blood capillaries into systemic circulation, thus effectively forming the secondary skin barrier. Such diversion is welcome for systemic therapy but severely hampers local drug accumulation in peripheral target tissues. [The fact that total area of cutaneous blood vessels exceeds the skin surface area by 200–500% (3)

highlights the challenge.] Alternative and better methods for drug delivery across the skin are therefore much needed for systemic as well as local noninvasive treatment.

HISTORICAL DEVELOPMENT

To permit noninvasive transcutaneous delivery of drugs with unfavorable transport properties, such as relatively high molecular weight substances, different skin perforation (poration) methods were tested. Moreover, to improve control over drug delivery kinetics and/or depth, particulate carriers (liposomes, nanoparticles, etc.) were used on the skin. While the former approach is reasonably efficient (4) but may be poorly tolerated, the latter fails to demonstrate significant skin penetration (5). It is now clear that only few colloids can overcome the skin barrier and help expand the range of drugs deliverable through the skin. The conventional submicroscopic particles or vesicles [micro- or nanoparticles, micro- and nano-emulsions, niosomes, standard lipid vesicles (liposomes)], for example, remain confined to skin surface (6,7). The reason is that normal skin only contains tiny pores (<0.5 nm) that are too narrow to let such undeformable "vehicles" pass (8); possible exceptions are cutaneous shunts, such as pilosebaceous units or corneocyte-cluster junctions (9).

To transport a drug through the skin efficiently with a carrier, the latter must reversibly create and without breaking adjust itself[a] to the resulting pore in a skin. The only well-known and successfully tested kind of transcutaneous drug carriers are fluid and unusually adaptable, multicomponent vesicles, so-called Transfersome®[b] carriers (7). Any such special vesicle can diminish its cross section by reversible and form-dependent components demixing within the vesicle-forming bilayer (Fig. 2, top). This self-optimization allows the vesicle to adjust shape to pores in a filter (13) or to widened pores in the skin (Fig. 2, bottom) and then to penetrate the latter along transcutaneous moisture gradient (14). The gradient drives the carrier into the body and leads the vesicle through lowest resistance pathways in the skin, i.e., through the imperfectly adjoined and/or packed, hydrophilic surfaces of corneocytes or intercorneocyte lipid layers in the stratum

---

[a] Formulations which do not take into account, and compensate for, the drying induced concentration changes on non-occluded skin are likely to result in vesicle aggregation and fusion on the skin or else in vesicle disintegration or breaking on or in the skin. This probably explains the discrepancy between results obtained by our group and other researchers in the field (10–12).

[b] Transfersome® is a trademark of IDEA AG. All other related vesicles (e.g., highly fluid liposomes, ethosomes), which reportedly can transport drugs across the skin, contain several bilayer components as well and therefore could arguably rely on a similar mechanism of action. To be really efficient, however, such transcutaneous carriers must be sufficiently deformable and stable, which is the case with few, if any, such vesicles.

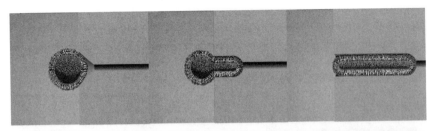

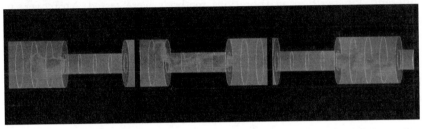

Figure 2 The highly flexible and permeable bilayer of a Transfersome® vesicle changes its local composition in response to local vesicle deformation (*upper panel*). In reality, a deformed vesicle can take less regular nonspherical form under influence of thermal motion, which helps the carrier to find its way into and through a narrow pore (*lower panel*).

corneum (Fig. 1, right bottom) (8,9). All this happens without adversely or irreversibly affecting the skin barrier.

Due to its unique barrier penetration mechanism and transport driving force, an ultradeformable, self-optimizing vesicle can deliver the drug molecules it carries into a body in a controllable manner: the cargo is (*i*) either deposited to a high concentration in a depot in viable skin (15); (*ii*) delivered into skin and deep subcutaneous tissues (16); or (*iii*) potentially transported into systemic blood circulation (17–19). The carrier penetration depth, and thus local reach of corresponding drug delivery, depends on vesicle adaptability and, for an optimized carrier, the locally applied drug dose per area (Table 1). A number of publications and patents (PCT/EP91/01596; EP 0475160; PCT/EP96/04526; PCT/EP98/06750; PCT/EP98/05539) describe how this can be done (7,8,12,16).

DESCRIPTION OF THE TECHNOLOGY

Modern carrier-mediated transdermal drug delivery started with the work on liposomes (20) or niosomes (6) applied on the skin. The tested liposomes were mainly made of phosphatidylcholine supplemented with cholesterol (20), to stabilize lipid bilayer of the vesicle and to prevent drug leakage or vesicle aggregation. More recently, liposomes prepared from skin lipids were introduced (22).

Table 1   Depth of Drug Delivery: Controlled by Applied Dose per Area

Drug dose		AUC[a] in muscles		
Per area (mg/cm^2)	Total (mg)	Superficial (µg/h/g^1)	Deep (µg/h/g^1)	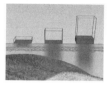
0.17	17	147	97	
0.50	50	278	266	
1.50	50	440	429	

[a]AUC gives the area-dose dependent recovery of the drug in porcine muscles ($n = 4$) measured and calculated over 0–8 hours time period (superficial: 0–1.5 cm depth; deep: 1.5–3 cm depth), following the drug application in ultradeformable carrier, Transfersome.

Niosomes have a similar morphology, but are made of nonionic surfactants, typically alkyl-polyoxyethelene ethers, mixed with cholesterol or cholesteryl-sulphate for improved stability (6,21).

The specially designed, self-optimizing, ultra-adaptable carriers for transcutaneous delivery normally also have vesicular form and comprise phosphatidylcholine (7–9,13). However, such ultradeformable aggregates also contain at least one additional component (e.g., alkyl- or acyl-polyoxyethylene, polysorbate, bile salt, glycolipid, etc.) to controllably destabilize the vesicle's lipid bilayer and make it more easily deformable. Figure 2 illustrates the phenomenon. Proper choice and balance of the carrier components is the key to obtaining not only adequately deformable but also sufficiently stable aggregates. The latter need is often neglected or underestimated, but can make or break the success of an application in vivo, especially after partial drying of the carrier suspension on the skin which inevitably changes the actual carrier composition.

Ensuring good carrier stability under osmotic stress is indeed not easy, as the outermost skin layer, the stratum corneum, is normally quite dry. The reason is that this skin part consists of flat and partly overlapping corneocytes organized in stacks, made tight by intercellular lipids (Fig. 1, right top). Such cellular organization and sealing makes the skin nearly impermeable to all but the rather small lipophilic molecules (with a size-dependent skin permeability) and water (which can cross the organ at a rate of merely < 0.5 mg h^{-1} cm^{-2}).

Some cell–cell or cell–lipid contacts are less tight, however (9). At such places, and/or where the lipidic seals are imperfect, a large number of tiny (< 0.5 nm) hydrophilic pores exists (Fig. 1, lower right). Such pores can be opened into 20–30 nm wide hydrophilic pathways (9) by applying unidirectional pressure on them. Nonocclusive epicutaneous administration of the superficially hydrophilic, highly deformable carriers (Transfersome vesicles) exerts such pressure and triggers the following motional sequence (14): transfersome under dehydration stress seeks water; the water-searching vesicle enters and crosses the skin barrier through the pores, through which water normally evaporates in the opposite direction. This allows the vesicle ultimately to enter the water rich viable skin parts where the osmotic driving force ceases to be important.

A carrier vesicle is at least 2 × and typically 4–6 × larger than opened channels across the stratum corneum. A vesicle can therefore trespass such potential pathways only if the carrier size, following vesicle deformation in at least one direction, effectively becomes smaller than the widened pore diameter. High vesicle membrane flexibility and high vesicle bilayer permeability in the pore are both preconditions for this (13). (Relatively high bilayer permeability is needed to allow excess intra-vesicular water to escape from the deformed carrier and the excess drug on the vesicle outside to enter into the carrier.) More conventional vesicles (liposomes, niosomes) fail to fulfil one or both of these necessary conditions for successful carrier passage through skin barrier (6,7).

Drug delivery and biodistribution following epicutaneous application of ultradeformable carriers starts in the well-hydrated viable skin tissue. Small and water soluble drugs must first leak out or dissociate from the carrier to diffuse further into blood (7), which is required for systemic treatment (17). The larger released drugs or the carriers themselves, which are both unable to enter directly into cutaneous blood vessels, are transported further by intercellular fluid flow, bypassing cutaneous clearance. This brings the carriers and the associated drug into deep regions below application site (16), unless they are taken up through fenestrations into lymph capillaries through which the vesicles can finally reach systemic blood circulation (7) and then may end up in the liver (23). In case of free drugs, the first transport step (trans-barrier diffusion) is followed promptly by the second one (cutaneous clearance). Transfersome® overcomes the skin intact, i.e., as very large entity, and is therefore distributed differently. This is most prominent after peripheral tissue saturation with the carriers, when the applied dose per body weight is very high. Before that, an increase in epicutaneously applied carrier dose mainly influences the maximum local depth to which carriers can penetrate (Table 1).

Ultradeformable vesicles loaded with agents of different molecular size and lipophilicity (lidocaine, tetracaine, cyclosporin, diclofenac, tamoxifen, etc.) (23) were shown in early preclinical models to cross the skin barrier well. In addition, polypeptides such as calcitonin, insulin, interferon-α and –γ, Cu–Zn superoxide dismutase (24), serum albumin (25), or dextran were delivered across the skin with ultradeformable carriers (23). Furthermore, several low molecular weight drugs associated with specially designed ultradeformable carriers were applied on human skin, in framework of phase I (26) to phase III (27) clinical trials, with aim of achieving high overall efficiency of delivery as well as high local and low systemic drug concentrations.

RESEARCH AND DEVELOPMENT

Transfersome® Preparation

Ultradeformable carriers can be prepared relying on published and patented procedures (13–17,19). For example, phosphatidylcholine (e.g., from soybean SPC) is mixed in ethanol with a biocompatible surfactant. Suitable buffer is added to the mixture to yield a suspension of vesicles with total lipid concentration 15 wt%. The suspension is then homogenizes e.g., sonicated, frozen and thawed 2–3 times, to catalyse vesicle growth, and finally brought to the preferred vesicle size by pressure homogenization, ultrasonication or some other pharmaceutically stable mechanical method. The final vesicle size, as determined with the dynamic light scattering, is of the order of 100 nm for a typical Transfersome®. No general formula or manufacturing method exists for making "the Transfersome, " owing to need to adjust the vesicle composition individually to each drug and its specific payload, considering high bilayer adaptability and stability as two crucial selection parameters (13). However, empty vesicles prepared from 8.7 wt% SPC, 1.3 wt% sodium cholate and up to 8.5 vol% ethanol in pH = 7.5 phosphate buffer will cross the skin quite well, as will 4/1–3/1 mixtures of SPC and polysorbate.

Transfersome® Characterization

In vitro measurements can be used to gauge relative ability of the given carrier preparation to penetrate artificial nano-porous barriers, mimicking the skin with regard to its narrow, but already widened, hydrophilic pores (13). For the purpose, membrane filters with fixed pore size (best: 20–30 nm) are used. Different pressures are applied over the filter, Δp, to drive the tested vesicle suspension through the pores with a pressure dependent flux density, $j(\Delta p) = \phi (\Delta p)/Area$, or rate, which define the barrier penetrability, $P(\Delta p)$, to the vesicle (Fig. 3). Such rate sensitivity, expressed in terms of activation energy, can be described by the following equation:

$$P(\Delta p) = P_{max}[1 - \mathrm{erf}\,(\Delta p^*/\Delta p)^{0.5} + (4\Delta p^*/\pi\Delta p)^{0.5}\,\exp(-\Delta p^*/\Delta p)]$$

where erf is error function. P_{max} is the maximum barrier penetrability achievable, which is directly measurable using a relatively high flux driving pressure or solubilized vesicles, i.e., mixed micelles. Δp^* is the only adjustable model parameter in the equation, and describes resistance of the tested system to trans-barrier transport in terms of driving pressure. $1/\Delta p^*$ thus defines the characteristic narrow, constant size, pore penetrability, and thus the carrier's composition dependent adaptability. The carrier's size stability before, during, and post-pore passage is easily checked or confirmed by dynamic light scattering, after flow-dependency correction (17) (Fig. 4).

In vivo methods for studying ultradeformable vesicle migration across the skin mainly rely on tissue biopsy punches, for deep tissues, or the

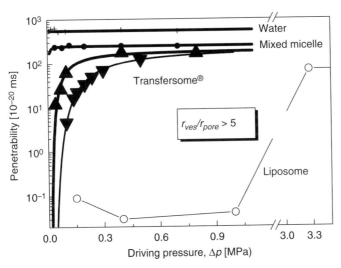

Figure 3 Transfersome® vesicles cross a barrier with pores several times smaller than the carriers diameter under osmotic or hydrostatic stress. In contrast, liposomes are confined to the application side, even under pressure, unless they are broken through the narrow pore. *Source*: From Ref. 13.

vacuum-pulled skin blisters, for cutaneous investigations. Ideally, any specimen should be taken from a living subject or animal, unless the latter can be sampled immediately post mortem. In vitro experiments most often give false positive or negative results. For example, even a poor carrier comprising membrane destabilizer, such as surfactant of certain kind, can increase skin permeability in vitro; on the other hand, even an excellent carrier, designed for deep local delivery, can lower transcutaneous drug diffusion in case of extensive drug-vesicle association. In vivo-in vitro comparison can resolve the dilemma (Fig. 5).

For intracutaneous delivery studies or the tests involving relatively superficial tissues the residual lipid suspension should be eliminated carefully from the skin with a dry cotton swab (15). More voluminous peripheral tissue samples should be sliced into convenient number of individual specimen allowing penetration profile determination (16). Labelled carriers (7) or drugs (17) as well as spectroscopic or chromatographic methods for the extracted drug analyses are nearly always useful for the purpose.

In an illustrative experiment, ultradeformable vesicles were labelled with ^{3}H-phosphatidylcholine and applied on intact murine skin or else injected subcutaneously. The carrier derived radioactivity was measured as a function of time in the blood, dermis, three different muscles, kidney, liver, spleen, and several other organs. A raise in the muscle, kidneys, and blood counts was accompanied by decline in radioactivity of the skin. After one day, essentially

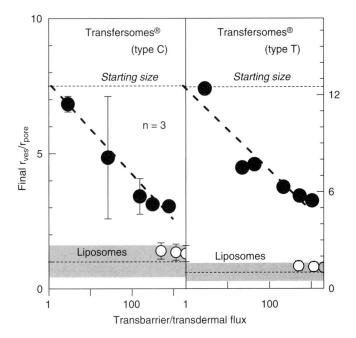

Figure 4 Ultradeformable vesicle size after crossing of narrow pores in a semi-permeable barrier as a function of relative transport rate. *Source*: From Ref. 17.

the same radioactivity biodistribution was found for the injected and epicutaneously applied ultradeformable carriers. The vesicle derived label appeared in the blood 4 hours after test formulation application and increased in concentration over time, to reach a plateau after 6–10 hours. To study the carrier mediated drug delivery through the skin, in vivo experiments were carried out using ^{3}H- or ^{14}C-labeled drugs associated with the carriers. This showed that the lipophilic low molecular weight drugs, such as testosterone (MW = 288) or triamcinolone acetonide (MW = 434.5), appear in the blood at times comparable to those measured for the carriers. Similar results were found with the highly water soluble calcitonin, heparin or dextran, with respective molecular weights of 3432, 7500, or 70,000. These substances and serum albumin (MW = 64,000) were transported through the skin equally successfully indicating lack of molecular size effect on the carrier-mediated drug delivery through the skin. Indeed, serum albumin was recovered in blood with a distribution profile similar to that of testosterone, as judged on basis of ^{125}J- or ^{3}H-radioactivity measurements.

Preclinical experiments were also done with insulin in mixed phosphatidylcholine-bile salt carriers prepared and tested by independent groups (17–19). All published results confirm feasibility of noninvasive transcutaneous transport of the biologically active polypeptide by the

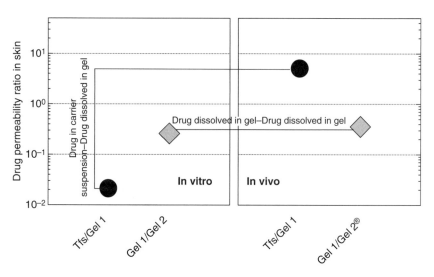

Figure 5 Comparison of drug transport rate through a mammalian skin in vitro and in vivo based on the results measured with a conventional topical NSAID gel or the corresponding pharmaceutical formulation based on ultradeformable carriers. *Abbreviations*: NSAID, nonsteroidal anti-inflammatory agent, Tfs, ultradeformable vesicle.

carriers moving through intact skin in vivo. Some of the data collected in our own, early human experiments with regular, commercial recombinant human insulin (Actrapid®, Novo-Nordisk) associated with a preparation of 90–110 nm large vesicles are illustrated in Ref. 19. In preclinical experiments, we prepared the carriers with ^{125}I-labeled insulin which has been applied on murine skin. We subsequently measured distribution of the carrier derived insulin radioactivity throughout the body with autoradiography (17). We detected the highest concentration of insulin-derived radioactivity in urine, followed by gastrointestinal tract, other soft tissues, and the blood. No significant differences was seen between biodistribution results of an epicutaneous and subcutaneous application, except that the lag time was prolonged by 4–6 hour for the epicutaneous versus subcutaneous group. In humans we observed and reported 2–30% lowering of the blood glucose level, starting approximately 2 hour after an epicutaneous application of insulin in ultradeformable carriers [Transfersulin (17)]. In contrast, the analogously prepared and used insulin in the related mixed lipid micelles or liposomes suspension did not change the blood glucose level significantly. Further related experiments are needed before final conclusion about therapeutic value of the treatment under real life conditions can reached. However, only little doubt exists that ultradeformable vesicles can transport polypeptide of the size of insulin (MW = 5808) through intact skin.

Regulatory Issues

Around 100 first generation products based on conventional transdermal drug-delivery technology are now on the market, but only few were added over the last few years. Likewise, only three topical, lipid containing products were introduced in pharmaceutical markets to date, despite intensive related research going on in academia over the last 25 years.

The most advanced colloid-based transcutaneous drug-delivery system, Transfersome® carrier, is well advanced and has already been scrutinized by several national and international regulatory bodies. No based on such carriers product is as yet commercialized but the first marketing approval from the Swiss regulatory authority is now available; registration in other European countries should follow in not too distant future.

The underlying product, a carrier based analgesic for local pain and inflammation treatment, contains a potent nonsteroidal anti-inflammatory agent (NSAID) associated with the ultradeformable carriers (Dractin®). It has been tested successfully in nearly four thousand patients, including some treated for over 1.5 years, confirming vastly superior drug distribution profile in preclinical experiments as well as a well differentiated and beneficial therapeutic profile in human clinical studies. The pharmacokinetic characteristics of the product are broadly similar to those measured and published for another NSAID in ultradeformable carrier, diclofenac in Transfersome® (Fig. 5). In either case, much higher NSAID concentration is deposited into deep muscular tissue by the carriers compared with a conventional gel, simultaneously ensuring very flat depth-profile of delivery. We measured similar distribution profiles for different NSAIDs delivered transcutaneously with ultradeformable carriers.

Position and Advantages of the Technology

Intact skin has long been considered an interesting but very restrictive port of entry into the body. This was seen as a natural limitation, a difficult to overcome consequence of biological barrier optimization. ultradeformable carriers can pass through this obstacle without causing damage to it, and thus overcome the problem of non-invasive transcutaneous delivery into blood or deep subcutaneous tissues. In contrast, standard topical drug formulations, such as hydrogels, ointments or cremes, but also more modern recipes involving liposomes, are all of limited usefulness for controlled drug delivery across the skin either into systemic blood circulation or else into peripheral tissues. An addition of chemical skin permeation enhancers can improve the situation in the first but not in the second of these two aspects, but only for small drugs. Skin poration using electrical fields, ultrasound, thermal injury or various ballistic methods (e.g., powder-jection, high velocity micro-droplet impact) suffers from long skin recovery period, brings the danger of body infection through the resulting lesions, and also cannot deliver a large quantity of any drug. The same is true for mini-pumps which introduce small wounds in the skin through which a drug is continuously infused into body.

Ultradeformable vesicles therefore stand alone as a versatile and efficient, but also extremely gentle, kind of noninvasive drug carriers. They can carry various agents with different sizes, structure, molecular weight, and polarity either through the primary skin barrier in the stratum corneum or beyond the secondary, dissipative barrier of cutaneous blood plexus. The ultradeformable, stable carries developed by IDEA AG are made with standard manufacturing methods of pharmaceutically acceptable ingredients, which need to be combined in judicious fashion that is optimized on a case by case basis.

Ultradeformable vesicles moreover require unconventional thinking in application design and use of analytical methods to potentially affect drug biodistribution. The latter phenomenon can be used for region-specific targeting into skin or deep subcutaneous tissues, as is exemplified in Figure 6.

Epicutaneously applied ultradeformable vesicles can ensure sustained localized drug release, in which either the carrier and/or the skin surface acts as drug reservoirs. The ultradeformable carriers cannot be used for achieving high and rapid drug concentration peak, however, unless the skin at the application site is administration target.

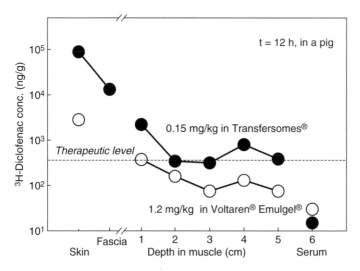

Figure 6 Direct transcutaneous delivery of an NSAID, diclofenac, into porcine muscles by conventional commercial gel, Voltaren® Emulgel® or a suspension of ultradeformable vesicles, Transfersome®. The latter deposits the drug more efficiently and uniformly into target tissue, compared with systemic drug concentration. *Abbreviation*: NSAID, nonsteroidal anti-inflammatory agent. *Source*: From Ref. 16.

Ultradeformable vesicles applied on the skin in a small quantity are "consumed" relatively rapidly and cause drug deposition nearly exclusively in the skin proper. A 100–1000 times higher amount of epicutaneously administered carriers tends to favor systemic delivery. Intermediate doses have an intermediate effect. No other system reported in the literature to date offers a similar versatility and controllability of non-invasive local drug delivery.

FUTURE DIRECTIONS

No drug delivery system has been perfected in a single step. Likewise, the Transfersome® technology is expected to evolve further. This relates to potential use of self-regulating, ultradeformable carriers in devices (patches; electrically controlled epicutaneous reservoirs), and in design of formulations with additional special features, allowing, e.g., targeting of cellular subsets. The nearest term goal that remains to be reached is expansion of the positive experiences with NSAID targeting into peripheral tissues to other drugs with similar therapeutic demands.

REFERENCES

1. Mitragoni S. Breaking the skin barrier. Adv Drug Del Rev 2004; 555–711.
2. Hadgraft J Lane ME. Passive transdermal drug delivery systems: Recent considerations and advances. Am J Drug Del 2006; 4:153–60.
3. Cevc G, Vierl U. Spatial distribution of cutaneous microvasculature and local drug clearance after drug application on the skin. J Control Release 2007; 118: 18–26.
4. Prausnitz MR. Microneedles for transdermal drug delivery. Adv Drug Del Rev 2004; 56:581–7.
5. van den Bergh BAI, Vroom J, Gerritsen H, Junginger HE, Bouwstra JA. Interactions of elastic and rigid vesicles with human skin in vitro: Electron microscopy. Biochim Biophys Acta 1999; 1461:155–73.
6. Schreier H, Bouwstra J. Liposomes and niosomes as topical drug carriers: Dermal and transdermal drug delivery. J Control Release 1994; 30:1–15.
7. Cevc G. Drug delivery across the skin. Exp Opin Invest Drugs 1997; 6:1887–37.
8. Cevc G. Lipid vesicles and other colloids as drug carriers on the skin. Adv Drug Del Rev 2004; 56:675–11.
9. Schätzlein A, Cevc G. Non-uniform cellular packing of the stratum corneum and permeability barrier function on intact skin: A high-resolution confocal laser microscopy study using highly deformable vesicles (Transfersomes®). Brit J Dermatol 1998; 138:583–2.
10. van Kuijk-Meuwissen ME, Junginger HE, Bouwstra JA. Interactions between liposomes and human skin in vitro, a confocal laser scanning microscopy study. Biochim Biophys Acta 1998; 1371:31–9.
11. Godin B, Touitou E. Ethosomes: New prospects in transdermal delivery. Crit Rev Ther Drug Carrier Syst 2003; 20:63–2.
12. Benson HAE. Transfersomes for transdermal drug delivery. Exp Opinion Drug Delivery 2006; 3:727–37.

13. Cevc G, Schätzlein A, Richardsen H, Vierl U. Overcoming semi-permeable barriers, such as the skin, with ultradeformable mixed lipid vesicles, Transfersomes®, liposomes or mixed lipid micelles. Langmuir 2003; 19:10753–63.
14. Cevc G, Gebauer D. Hydration driven transport of deformable lipid vesicles through fine pores and the skin barrier. Biophys J 2003; 84:1010–24.
15. Cevc G, Blume G. Hydrocortisone and dexamethasone in ultra-deformable drug carriers, Transfersomes®, have an increased biological potency and reduced therapeutic dosages. Biochim Biophys Acta 2004; 1663:61–3.
16. Cevc G, Blume G. New, highly efficient formulation of diclofenac for the topical, transdermal administration in ultradeformable drug carriers, Transfersomes. Biochim Biophys Acta 2001; 1514:191–5.
17. Cevc G, Gebauer D, Stieber J, Schätzlein A, Blume G. Ultraflexible vesicles, Transfersomes®, have an extremely low pore penetration resistance and transport therapeutic amounts of insulin across the intact mammalian skin. Biochim Biophys Acta 1998; 1368:201–5.
18. Guo J, Ping Q, Zhang L. Transdermal delivery of insulin in mice by using lecithin vesicles as a carrier. Drug Delivery 2000; 7:113–6.
19. Cevc G. Transdermal drug delivery of insulin with ultradeformable carriers, Transfersomes®. Clin Pharmacokinet 2003; 42:461–4.
20. Mezei ML. Liposomes as a skin drug delivery system. In: Breimer DD, Speiser P, eds. Topics in Pharmaceutical Sciences. Amsterdam: Elsevier, 1985: 345–58.
21. Hofland HEJ, Vander Geest R, Bouwstra JA, Bodde HE, Junginger HE. Estradiol permeation from non-ionic surfactant vesicles through human stratum corneum in vitro. Pharm Res 1994; 11:659–4.
22. du Plessis WN, Müller JDG. The influence of in vivo treatment of skin with liposomes on the topical absorption of a hydrophilic and a hydrophobic drug in vitro. Int J Pharm 1994; 103:R1–R5.
23. Cevc G. Transfersomes®, liposomes and other lipid suspensions on the skin: permeation enhancement, vesicle penetration and transdermal drug delivery. Crit Rev Ther Drug Carrier Syst 1996; 13:257–8.
24. Simoes SI, Delgado TC, Lopes RM, et al. Developments in the rat adjuvant arthritis model and its use in therapeutic evaluation of novel non-invasive treatment by SOD in Transfersomes. J Control Release 2005; 103:419–4.
25. Paul A, Cevc G. Non-invasive administration of protein antigens. Epicutaneous immunization with the bovine serum albumin. Vaccine Res 1995; 4:145–4.
26. Fesq H, Gloeckner A, Abeck D, et al. Improved risk-benefit ratio for a triamcinolone acetonide Transfersome® formulation in comparison to a commercial triamcinolone acetonide formulation. Br J Dermatol 2003; 149:611–9.
27. Cevc G, Schätzlein A, Richardsen H. Ultradeformable lipid vesicles can penetrate the skin and other semi-permeable barriers intact. Evidence from double label CLSM experiments and direct size measurements. Biochim Biophys Acta 2002; 1564:21–30.

24

Advances in Wound Healing

Michael Walker and Steven Percival

*ConvaTec Wound Therapeutics™, Global Development Centre,
Deeside, Flintshire, U.K.*

INTRODUCTION

Invariably, any interruption of the epidermal barrier, whether by accident, warfare, disease or even surgery results in the formation of a wound. Consequently, throughout history the simple act of covering that wound, by whatever means, to effectively duplicate the function of the epidermis, has been understood as a way of protecting the wound from the potentially harmful external environment. In this chapter, the emphasis will be on the recalcitrant nonhealing or "chronic" wound (e.g., leg ulceration). These wounds present an enormous health problem and costs continue to spiral. Present health care costs are thought to be >US$1 billion annually in the United States alone (1). The pathology of these wounds is complex and beyond the scope of the present chapter, but increasingly, commonalities are presented across the three major wound types (e.g., venous ulcers, diabetic ulcers and pressure sores). Each wound may be represented by a combination of factors, which on their own can be deleterious, and if these factors are found collectively they are likely to result in prolonged wound chronicity and increased health care costs.

This chapter briefly highlights some of the most historically significant advances in wound healing and then focuses on more recent advances as our knowledge of wound pathophysiology has increased. Finally, a brief overview of future opportunities (including gene therapy) is given.

HISTORICAL DEVELOPMENT

Cave drawings from around 20,000 to 30,000 years ago, have been found in Spain that suggest man's initial awareness of wound healing (2). Similarly it would appear that man has been concerned with wound formation ever since he first learned to write. In Manjo's book *The Healing Hand* there are recorded observations on wounds in Sumerian cuneiform script, which is generally accepted as the first form of syllabic writing developed around 2400 B.C. (3). Figure 1 highlights these and other significant events relating to wound treatments that have unfolded throughout history.

Various medicaments have been recorded since early Egyptian times and in the Edwin smith surgical papyrus the words *awy* (thought to be a form of suture, or piece of thread) and *ydr* (a type of steri-strip, use of lined strips to hold a wound together) have been found (2,4). However, Hippocrates is credited with one of the earliest mentions of chronic wounds through his recognition of a possible relationship between leg ulceration and venous disorders (5). Along with Celsus and Galen the writings of these gentlemen became the major medical references of the day (6). In the tenth century Avicenna believed that in order to cure an ulcer it was necessary to prevent the efflux of dangerous humors (7) and this concept became widespread and was upheld until the eighteenth century. During the Renaissance period anatomy in particular advanced through the work of Leonardo de Vinci, and subsequently Versalius, who vigorously challenged the old Galen dogma (8). Other studies looking at varicose veins suggested that compression therapy may be an answer and Guy de Chauliac is credited with the application of lead plates to treat leg ulceration (9).

There were many subsequent advances during the eighteenth and nineteenth centuries, including the findings of Hunter, the association between thrombosis and phlebitis (10) and Gay's understanding of clot formation and post-thrombotic recanalisation (11). Who described Gay also recorded the fact that ulceration could occur in the absence of varicose veins and introduced the term venous ulcer (11). Perhaps one of the most significant findings of this era was the discovery of chemical preservatives and disinfectants during the nineteenth century. This helped create a better understanding of the nature of infection and inflammation that subsequently led to an increased control of wound infection, and the introduction of antiseptics containing carbolic acid in operation theaters, which led to a significant reduction in death rates associated with surgery (2).

More recently the pioneering work of Winter in the early 1960s transformed modern thinking of wound healing and introduced the concept of moist wound healing (12), which has subsequently led to a plethora of modern wound dressings and other forms of topical products. Ultimately the best dressing is skin itself, but this is not often a practical solution and therefore the remainder of this chapter will try to provide information of

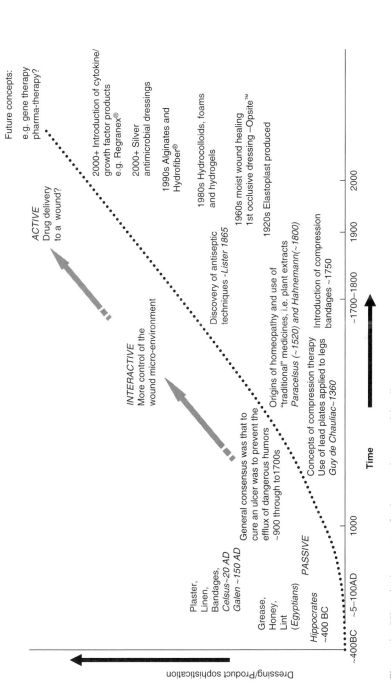

Figure 1 Historical aspects of advances in wound healing.

new concepts and possible topical treatments that are emerging as our knowledge of the complex events that take place in a chronic wounds increases.

Any form of wound healing treatment is going to require careful and considered interventions and this can lead to difficulties in setting up suitable clinical trails and incur huge expenses. Hence, there has not been a particularly fast growth in new treatment options. Due to the complexity of the wound pathophysiology, the major emphasis has been on the development of dressings and their ability to modulate the wound environment (13), and also by the introduction of antimicrobial agents (e.g., silver). However, there are very few treatments than can be offered that may be considered as a result of a pharmacological action. With a greater understanding of wound pathophysiology and, in particular, the role microorganisms play as causative agents of infections, much work has been done searching for chemicals with selective toxicity for infectious agents rather than nonspecific inhibitors, e.g., antiseptic and disinfectants. Traditional medicines using plant extracts are presently under consideration, as well as skin substitutes and tissue sealants. Along with these, this chapter will outline some of the more recent studies that have been or are presently under investigation into the use of growth factor and cytokine products, and the possibility of future use of gene therapy.

ANTISEPTICS AND DISINFECTANTS

The discovery of chemical preservatives and disinfectants during the ninteength century and a better understanding of the nature of infection and inflammation have led to increased control of wound infection. In 1865, John Lister used carbolic acid in operation theaters, significantly reducing death rates associated with surgery. Later, when it was found that microorganisms were the causative agents of infections, researchers began to search for chemicals with selective toxicity for infectious agents rather than nonspecific inhibitors, e.g., antiseptic and disinfectant. Some of the main chemicals or substances used in wound care include chlorhexidine, honey, hydrogen peroxide, iodine, and, most recently, ionic silver (14).

Chlorhexidine: Discovered in 1946, chlorhexidne was introduced into clinical practice as an antiseptic in hand wash and surgical scrub in 1954. A recent assessment of several animal and human studies showed that it is associated with few adverse effects on healing (15).

Honey: Honey has been used for a long time and has been claimed to possess antibacterial activity and able to promote healing (16). In vitro studies with cell lines exposed to honey solutions have demonstrated modulation of monocytic cell activity; it is speculated that this is likely to influence the wound healing process (17,18), though it is not yet fully explained.

Hydrogen peroxide: Widely used as an oxidising agent, an antiseptic, and disinfectant, hydrgenperoxide uses free radicals that react with lipids, proteins and nucleic acids to affect cellular constituents nonspecifically. Sleigh and Linter (19) reported that air emboli is formed when it is used in cleaning wounds, yet studies in animals and humans failed to find any negative effects on wound healing.

Iodine: Considered to affect protein structure by oxidizing S–H bonds of cysteine and methionine, iodine reacts with the phenolic groups of tyrosine and N–H groups in amino acids to block hydrogen bonding. It also prevents hydrogen bonding by reacting with bases of nucleotides and alters membrane structure by reacting with C=C bonds in fatty acids. It has a broad spectrum of activity against bacteria, mycobacteria, fungi, protozoa, and viruses. Although many authors have stated that resistance to iodine is not a problem, reports of resistance are limited to one (20).

Silver: The role of silver as an antimicrobial agent in inhibiting microorganisms has been recognized since the late nineteenth century (14). It is especially used in treating burn wounds (21). Metallic silver itself is not reactive, silver ions in aqueous environments exert antimicrobial activity, depending on the intracellular accumulation of low concentrations of silver ions. These ions intensely bind to negatively charged components in proteins and nucleic acids and subsequently affect the bacterial cell walls, membrane and nucleic acids structure, which then affect viability (14). Skin discoloration and irritation associated with the use of silver nitrate is well documented (22); absorption of silver, systemic distribution, and excretion in urine has also been reported (23).

TRADITIONAL MEDICINES

It is suggested that early use of natural elements was a reaction to the extensive overuse of bleeding and cupping, a well know practice used in the eighteenth century. However, the understanding of using these types of medicines is much older and may have gained substantial impetus based on the studies of Paracelsus in the fifteength century and subsequently Hahnemann in the eighteength century (24). Both these gentlemen independently used laws of similar and small doses preferring to let nature subsequently intervene (24).

More recently there has been another surge of interest in this area, with many plant extracts now under consideration for wound healing (Table 1). Invariably these have involved aqueous (26) or alcoholic (25,34,35) to utilize either polyphenolic extracts (30), polysaccharides (27), or flavonoids (28), although the vast majority of these studies have only been performed on animals.

Table 1 Outlining Traditional Medicines and Their Involvement in Wound Healing

Traditional medicine	Extract medium	Species	Wound healing effect	Ref.
Terminata arjuna bark	Hydroalcohol	Rat	FT dermal wounds	25
Acalypha langinia	Aqueous	Diabetic rats	FT wounds	26
Opuntia fincus-India cladodes	Lyophilized polysaccharide	Rat	FT wounds	27
Calendula officinalis	Ointment	Humans	Lower leg ulcers/venous ulcer re-epithelialization	28
Tumeric (compared with honey)	Paste	Rats	FT wounds	29
Green tea phenols	Anti-oxidants, anti-aging	Humans	FT wounds	30
Butea monosperma bark	Alcohol extraction	Rats	FT wounds	31
Punica granatum (pomegranate)	Alcohol extraction	Rats	FT wounds	32
Ocimum oil	Essential oil–carrier	Rabbits	FT wounds	33
Terminatie chebula	Alcohol extraction	Rats	*Staphylococcus aureus* infected wounds	34
Tragia involcrata	Alcohol extraction	Rats	FT wounds	35
Cinnamonium zeylanicum	Alcohol extraction	Rats	Used for burns treatments and	36
Moist exposed burn ointment	Ointment	Humans	reduced scarring	37,38

Abbreviation: FT, full thickness.

SKIN SUBSTITUTES

If a wound is to be grafted with a skin substitute or autografting from the same patient, the wound must first be debrided. Debridement involves the removal of dead or necrotic tissue form the wound bed. The major forms of debridement are presented in Table 2. Once the wound has been debrided it may be treated with split-thickness autografts, allografts, xenografts or nonbiological grafts (e.g., epidermal equivalents, and/or dermal equivalents (39). The introduction of cultured keratinocyte sheets began in 1980s (40), and while these cultured cells may not provide a substantial dermal replacement they can release multiple cytokines that may help the host response to healing (41). Dermal replacements that are used include AlloDerm®, used as a template for regenerating viable epidermis and TransCyte, approved by the FDA for second- and third-degree burns (41). Others include Integra® Dermal Regenerative Template (41), Dermagraft® (42) and Apligraft® (43).

TISSUE SEALANTS AND PLATELET GELS

One way of providing good tissue adhesion is through the use of fibrin-based glued or biologically inert glues (e.g., octylcyanoacrylate-based glues) (39). As a "natural" glue, fibrin acts by polymerizing thrombin, fibrinogen and calcium. FDA-approved tissue sealants based on donor or cryo-precipitated autologous fibrinogen include Tisseel® and ViGuard (40), as well as Hemaseel for certain surgical procedures (44). Platelet gels are the latest advancement in this area and are much more likely to reduce the risk of disease transmission than from donor derived blood products (44). Like the tissue sealants, these types of products are generally aimed at reducing the need for sutures. Products include Procuren® Autogel™ and SafeBlood®.

CYTOKINES AND GROWTH FACTORS

Much research over the last few years has focused on the area of growth factors, but with a greater understanding of the highly proteolytic environment

Table 2 Aspects of Debridement

Classification/type	Characteristics
Surgical	Nonselective, but fast
Mechanical	Wet-to-dry dressings, hydrotherapy, irrigation
Autolytic	Wound bed clears itself, promoted by wound dressings, e.g., alginates, hydrocolloids, Hydrofiber®
Chemical/enzymatic	Digests/disrupts proteins, e.g., bromelain, collagenase, papain urea

that is the chronic wound (1), it is perhaps not surprising that few growth factor products have been successful (Table 3). In the late 1990s the first approved growth factor-based product to be marketed was Regranex®, a platelet-derived growth factor, produced as the recombinant human (rh) PGDF-BB form know as becaplermin (45). Subsequently, several other products have now been marketed or are under preclinical investigation.

GENE THERAPY—THE FUTURE?

Recent advances in the ability to introduce genetic material into cells and thereby alter protein synthesis (e.g., gene therapy) has led to the suggestion that these techniques may be useful in wound healing (68). However, one of the biggest challenges appears to be that most techniques provide only temporary transgene expression, which may not be practical for many treatments, but this may make it suitable for chronic wound therapy (69). Due to its general availability, skin is a good target organ for gene therapy as it can be reached directly by either injection or topical delivery and therefore does not have the concerns related with systemic delivery systems (69). Another potential delivery system is through the use of scaffold matrices or skin substitutes, although it has been suggested that one disadvantage of these types of techniques is a lower rate of transfection (69).

Alternatively in years to come it may be possible to regulate transgene expression such that certain genes may be "switched-on," while others are "switched-off," depending on the environmental needs of the wound (70). In particular this may be one way in which growth factors may be effective in reducing excessive proteolytic activity by inhibitors or down-regulators (e.g., block the cells from translating certain proteins) (71,72). Presently there is at least one delivery system (e.g., KeraPac™ device) that uses human keratinocytes grown on micro-carrier beads to control growth factor delivery, which has an extended shelf life of one month and is presently in phase II clinical trials (73).

It would appear therefore that this therapy has many potential applications and may one day provide new and novel wound treatments, but there is still much research to be done to identify specific target molecules. However, there is a generally acknowledged increase in our understanding of wound pathophysiology (1,74), the search for suitable pharmacological agents is often prohibitively expensive and beyond the capabilities of most companies except the major pharmaceutical giants (74). Financial constraints are also seen to be a problem with physicians and caregivers and unless products are reimbursed then they often do not even make a hospital formulary or become covered by health providers (e.g., Medicaid or Medicare in the United States.) (75).

Table 3 List of Growth Factors and Cytokines Used in Wound Healing

Growth factors/ cytokines	Product name	Treatment	Ref.
Granulocyte-macrophage colony-stimulating factor	LEUKINE®	Chemotherapy/radiotherapy plus bone marrow transplantation and improving olfactory wounds	39,46,47
rh-Basic fibroblast growth factor	Trafarmin	Skin ulcers in Japan	39
Recombinant form of keratinocyte growth factor(gf-2)	Repifermin	Promotion of re-epithelialization	48
rh-Keracinocyte growth factor	Palifermin	Mucositis in the GI tract, plus reduced oral ulcerative mucositis	49,50
rh-Vascular endothelial growth factor	Telbermin	Diabetic foot ulcers presently in Phase II trials	51
rh-Platelet-derived growth factor	Regranex	Diabetic foot ulcers	
Combined human growth factors with cytokines		Case studies looking at photoxicity	52–54
Tumour necrosis factor-alpha antibody–infliximab		8 patients with chronic ulcers	55
Platelet-derived growth factor		Full thickness neurotropic foot ulcers (safety and efficacy study)	56
Nerve growth factor		Neurotrophic corneal ulcers (efficacy study)	57
Fibroblast growth factor/chitosan		Db/db healing impaired diabetic mice	58
Epidermal growth factor		Full thickness wounds in mice	59–61
basic-Fibroblast growth factor		Case studies (3)—human ischaemic ulcers	
Thymosin-β_4		Mice wounds	
TGF-β (isomeric forms $\beta_1\beta_2\beta_3$)		Human scarring, venous ulcers, pressure sores	62–66
Rh lactoferrin–talactoferrin		In Phase II trials for up-regulation of cytokines (e.g., IL-18)	67

Abbreviation: rh, recombinant human.

Finally, due to the multifactorial complexities that often present in a chronic wound, it is unlikely that any one single therapeutic treatment will provide the answer. Rather there is a need to obtain a balance between best possible clinical care/practice and affordable quality products that may lead to a healing of wounds or at least an improved quality of life for individual patients.

REFERENCES

1. Mustoe TA, O'Shaughessy, Kloeters O. Chronic wound pathogenesis and current treatment strategies: A unifying hypothesis. Plast Reconstr Surg 2006; 117(Suppl. 7):35S–41S.
2. Gottrup F, Leaper D. Wound healing: Historical aspects. EWMA J 2004; 4(2): 21–32.
3. Manjo G. The healing hand: Man and Wound in the Ancient World. Cambridge: Harvard University Press, 1975: 47 pp.
4. Reed BR, Clark RAF. Cutaneous tisue repair: Practical implications of current knowledge. II. J Am Acad Dermatol 1985; 13:919–41.
5. Hippocrates. De ulcerbis and Decarnibus. In: Adams F, ed. The Genuine Works of Hippocrates, London: Sydenham Society, 1849.
6. Nordenskiöld E. The History of Biology—a Survey. London: Kegan Paul, Trench and Trauber, 1929: 99 pp.
7. Avicenna. De ulceribus, Liber IV. Quoted by Underwood M. In: A Treatise on Ulcers of the Legs. London: Matthews, 1783.
8. Kirkpatrick JJR, Curtis B, Naylor I. Back to the future for wound care? The influences of Padua on wound management in Renaissance Europe. Wound Rep Reg 1996; 4:326–34.
9. Scholz A. Historical aspects. In: Westerhof W, ed. Leg Ulcer: Diagnosis and Treatment, Amsterdam: Elsvier, 1993: pp. 5–15.
10. Hunter J. Observations on the inflammation of the internal coats of veins 1775. In: Palmer JI, ed. The Works of John Hunter. London: Longman, Rees, Orme and Longman, 1837; pp. 581–6.
11. Gay J. On varicose disease of the lower extremities and its allied disorders. Lettsomian Lectures of 1867, London: Churchill.
12. Winter GD. Formation of the scab and re-epithelialisation of superficial wounds in the skin of the young domestic pig. Nature 1962; 193:293–4.
13. Bishop SM, Walker M, Rogers AA, et al. Importance of moisture balance at the wound-dresing interface. J Wound Care 2003; 12:125–8.
14. Cooper R. A review of the evidence for the use of topical antimicrobial agents in wound care. Available online: http://www.worldwidewounds.com/2004/february/Cooper/Topical-Antimicrobial-Agents.html
15. Drosou A, Falabella A, Kirsner RS. Antiseptics on wounds: an area of controversy. Wounds 2003; 15(5):149–66.
16. Molan PC. The role of honey in the management of wounds. J Wound Care 1999; 8(8):415–8.
17. Tonks AJ, Cooper RA, Price AJ, et al. Stimulation of TNF-alpha release in monocytes by honey. Cytokine 2001: 14(4):240–2.

18. Tonks AJ, Cooper RA, Jones KP, et al. Honey stimulates inflammatory cytokine production from monocytes. Cytokine 2003; 21(5):242–7.
19. Sleigh JW, Linter SP. Hazards of hydrogen peroxide. Br Med J Clin Res Ed 1985; 291:1706.
20. Mycock G. Methicillin/antiseptic-resistant *Staphylococcus aureus*. Lancet 1985; 2(8461):949–50.
21. Klasen HJ. A historical review of the use of silver in the treatment of burns, II: Early uses. Burns 2000; 26(2):117–30.
22. Walker M, Cochrane CA, Bowler PG, et al. Silver deposition and tissue staining associated with wound dressings containing silver. Ostomy/Wound Manage 2006; 52:42–50.
23. Lansdown AB. Silver. 2: Toxicity in mammals and how its products aid wound repair. J Wound Care 2002; 11(5):1731–7.
24. Morrell M. Hahnemann's debt to alchemy. http://www.homeoint.org/morrell/articles/pm_alchem.htm.
25. Chaudhari C, Megi S. Evaluation of phytoconstituents of Terminalia arjuna for wound healing activity in rats. Phytother Res 2006; 20:799–805.
26. Perez Gutierrez RM, Vagras SR. Evaluation of the wound healing properties of Acalypha langiana in diabetic rats. Fitoterapia 2006; 77:286–9.
27. Trombetta D, Puglia C, Perri D, et al. Effect of polysaccharides from *Opuntia ficus-indica* (L.) cladodes on the healing of dermal wounds in the rat. Phytomedicine 2006; 13:352–8.
28. Duran V, Matic M, Jovanovc M, et al. Results of the clinical examination of an ointment with marigold (Calendula officinalis) extract in the treatment of venous leg ulcers. Int J Tissue Res 2005; 27:101–6.
29. Kundu S, Biswas TK, Das P, et al. Tumeric (Curuma longa) rhizone paste and honey show similar wound healing potential: a preclinical study in rabbits. Int J Low Extrem Wounds 2005; 4:205–13.
30. Hsu S. Green tea and the skin. J Am Acad Dermatol 2005; 52:1049–59.
31. Sumitra M, Manikandan P, Suguna L. Efficacy of Butea monosperma on dermal wound healing in rats. Int Biochem Cell Biol 2005; 37:566–73.
32. Murthy KN, Reddy VK, Veigas JM, et al. Study on wound healing activity of Punica granatum peel. J Med Food 2005; 7:256–9.
33. Orafidiya LO, Agbani EO, Abereoje OA, et al. An investigation into the wound healing properties of essential oil of Ocium gratissimum linn. J Wound Care 2003; 12:331–4.
34. Suguna L, Singh S, Sivakumar P, et al. Influence of Terminalia chebula on dermal wound healing in rats. Phytother Res 2002; 16:227–31.
35. Perumal Sam R, Gopalakrishnakone P, Sarumathi M, et al. Wound healing potential of Tragia involucrate extracts in rats. Fitoterapia 2006; 77:300–2.
36. Kamath JV, Rana AC, Chowdhury AR. Pro-healing effect of Cinnamomum zeylanicum bark. Phytother Res 2003; 17:970–2.
37. Zhang HQ, Yip TP, Hui I, et al. Efficacy of moist exposed burn ointment on burns. J Burn Care Rehab 2005; 26:247–51.
38. Atiyeh BS, Amm CA, El-Musa KA. Improved scar quality following primary and secondary healing of cutaneous wounds. Aesthetic Plast Surg 2003; 27:411–7.

39. Meier K, Nanney LB. Emerging new drugs for wound repair. Expert Opin Emerging Drugs 2006; 11:23–37.
40. O'Connor NE, Mulliken JB, Banks-Schegel S, et al. Grafting of burns with cultured epithelium prepared from autologus epidermal cells. Lancet 1981; 1:75–8.
41. Balasubramani M, Kumar TR, Babu M. Skin substitutes: a review. Burns 2001; 27:534–44.
42. Purdue GF, Hunt JL, Still JM, et al. A multi-center clinical trial of a biosynthetic skin replacement. Dermagraft-TC, compared with cryopreserved human cadaver skin for tempory coverage of excised burn wounds. J Burn Care Rehab 1997; 18:52–7.
43. Falanga V, Margolis D, Alvarez O, et al. Rapid healing of venous ulcers and lackm of clinical rejection with an allogenic cultured human skin equivalent. Arch Dermatol 1998; 134:293–300.
44. Limova M. New therapeutic options for chronic wounds. Derm Clin 2002; 20: 357–63.
45. Pierce GF, Mustoe TA, Altorock BW, et al. Role of platelet-derived growth factor in wound healing. J Cell Biochem 1991; 45:319–26.
46. Jyung R, Wu L, Pierce GF, et al. Granulocyte-macrophage colony-stimulating factor and granulocyte colony-stimulating factor: differential action on incisional wound healing. Surgery 1994; 115:325–34.
47. Malik IA, Zahid M, Haq S, et al. Effect of subcutaneous injection of granulocyte-macrophage colony-stimulating factor (MG-CSF) on healing of chronic refractory wounds. Eur J Surg 1998; 164:737–44.
48. Robson MC, Phillips TJ, Falanga V, et al. Randomized trial of topically applied repifermin (recombinant human keratinocyte growth factor-2) to accelerate wound healing in venous ulcers. Wound Repair Regen 2001; 9:3347–52.
49. Spielberger R, Stigg P, Bensinger W, et al. Palifermin for oral mucositis after intensive therapy for hematologic cancers. N Engl J Med 2004; 351:2590–8.
50. http://www.clinicaltrials/gov/ct/show/NCT00000431?order=1 Preliminary testing of new treatment for chronic leg wounds. National Institute of Arthritis and Musuloskeletal and Skin Diseases (NIAMS) and National Gene Vector Laboratory, 2005.
51. http://www.clinicaltrials/gov/ct/show/NCT69446?order=1 RhVEGT (Telbermin) fro induction of healing of chronic, diabetic foot ulcers. Genentech, 2005.
52. Smeill JM, Wieamn J, Steed DL, et al. Efficacy and safety of becaplermin (recombinant human platelet-derived growth factor-BB) in patients with non-healing lower extremity diabetic ulcers: a combined analysis of four randomized studies. Wound Repair Regen 1999; 7:335–46.
53. Weiman TJ, Smeill JM, Su Y. Efficacy and safety of a topical gel formulation of recombinant human platelet-derived growth factor-BB (becaplermin) in patients with chronic neuropathic diabetic ulcers. Diabetes Care 1998; 21:822–7.
54. Gold MH, Biron J. A novel skin cream containing a mixture of human growth factors and cytokines for the treatment of adverse events associated with photodynamic therapy. J Drugs Dermatol 2006; 5:796–8.
55. Streit M, Beleznay Z, Braathen LR. Topical application of the tumour necrosis factor-alpha antibody infliximab improves healing of chronic wounds. Int J Wound 2006; 3:171–9.

56. Steed DL. Clinical evaluation of recombinant human platetet-derived growth factor for the treatment of lower extremity ulcers. Plast Recontr Surg 2006; 117 (Suppl. 7):143S–149S.
57. Cellini M, Bendo E, Bravetti GO, et al. The use of nerve growth factor in surgical wound ehaling of the cornea. Ophthalmic Res 2006; 38:171–81.
58. Obara K, Ishiahar M, Fujita M, et al. Acceleration of wound healing in healing impaired db/db mice with a photocrosslinkable chitosan containing fibroblast growth factor-2. Wound Repair Regen 2005; 13:390–7.
59. Babul A, Gonal B, Dincer S. The effects of EGF application in gel form on histamine content of experimentally induced wound in mice. Amino Acids 2004; 27:321–6.
60. Draper BK, Komurasaki T Davidson MK, et al. Topical epiregulin repair of murine excisional wounds. Wound Repair Regen 2003; 11:188–97.
61. Noguchi M, Eishi K, Yamachika S, et al. Three cases of ischemic ulcer due to arteriosclerosis obliterans responding to basic fibroblast growth factor spray. Heart Vessels 2004; 19:252–6.
62. Malinda KM, Sidhu GS, Mani H, et al. Thymosin-β_4 accelerates wound healing. J Invest Dermatol 1999; 113:364–8.
63. Philip D, Goldstein AL, Kleinman HK. Thymosin-β_4 promotes angiogenesis, wound healing, and hair follicle development. Mech Ageing Develop 2004; 125: 113–5.
64. Shah M Foremna DM, Ferguson MWL. Neutralisation of TGF-β_1 and TGF-β_2 or exogenous addition of TGF-β_3 to cutaneous rat wounds reduces scarring. J Cell Sci 1995; 108:985–1002.
65. Robson MC, Philips LG, Cooper DM, et al. Safety and effect of TGF-$\beta_2$for treatment of venous stasis ulcers. Wound Repair Regen 1995; 3:157–67.
66. Hirshberg J, Coleman J, Marchant B, et al. TGF-β_3 in the treatment of pressure ulcers: a preliminary report. Adv Skin Wound Care 2001; 14:91–5.
67. http://www.agennix.com/contentpages/lactoferrinscience.htm Agennix website, 2005.
68. Davison JM, Krieg T, Eming SA. Particle-mediacted gene therapy of wounds. Wound Repair Regen 2000; 8:452–9.
69. Petrie NC, Yao F, Eriksson E. Gene therapy in wound healing. Surg Clin N Am 2003; 83:597–616.
70. Yao F, Eriksson E. A novel tetracycline-inducible viral replication switch. Gene Ther 1999; 10:419–27.
71. Eriksson E. Gene transfer in wound healing. Adv Skin Wound Care 2000; 13(Suppl. 2):20–2.
72. Lindblad WI. Genetherapy in wound healing—2000 a promising future. Wound Repair Regen 2000; 8:441–2.
73. http://www.keracure.com/keraspac.asp KerCure website, KerPac Product Information 2005.
74. Chen WYJ, Rogers AA, Walker M, et al. A rethink of the complexity of chronic wounds—implications for treatment. ETRS Bull 2003; 10:65–9.
75. Victor-Vega C Desai A, Montesnos MC. Adenosine A2A receptor antagonists promote more rapid wound healing that recombinant human platelet-derived growth factor (Becaplermin gel). Inflammation 2002; 26:19–24.

25

Ultrasound-Mediated Transdermal Drug Delivery

Samir Mitragotri

*Department of Chemical Engineering, University of California,
Santa Barbara, California, U.S.A.*

Joseph Kost

*Department of Chemical Engineering, Ben Gurion University of the Negev,
Beer-Sheva, Israel*

INTRODUCTION

Transdermal drug delivery offers several advantages over traditional drug delivery systems such as oral delivery and injection, especially in regard to protein delivery (1). Transdermal drug delivery, however, suffers from the severe limitation that the permeability of the skin is very low. Therefore, it is difficult to deliver drugs across the skin at a therapeutically relevant rate. A possible solution to this problem is to increase the permeability of the skin using physicochemical driving forces, referred to as penetration enhancers, e.g., chemical enhancers and electric fields (2). In this chapter, we describe the use of low-ferquency ultrasound ($20 \, \text{kHz} < f < 100 \, \text{kHz}$) for delivering drugs across the skin.

HISTORICAL DEVELOPMENT

Ultrasound under a variety of conditions has been used for enhancing transdermal drug transport (3–25). This phenomenon is referred to as sonophoresis. Some of the earliest studies of sonophoresis were performed using hydrocortisone. Fellinger and Schmid (26) reported successful treatment of polyarthritis of the hands digital joints using hydrocortisone ointment with sonophoresis. Since that time, several sonophoresis studies have been reported using more than 10 drugs. Among the various frequencies that have been used for sonophoresis, therapeutic frequencies (1–3 MHz) correspond to the most commonly used conditions employed in over 90% of previous studies (27). Typical enhancements induced by therapeutic ultrasound are less than 10-fold and are observed mostly for low-molecular weight drugs. We have shown that ultrasound at a frequency of 20 kHz enhances transdermal transport of drugs more effectively than therapeutic ultrasound, a phenomenon referred to as low-frequency sonophoresis (16,28). Low-frequency ultrasound has a clear advantage over therapeutic sonophoresis in that cavitational effects, which are responsible for low-frequency sonophoresis, are inversely proportional to ultrasound frequency (29). In view of this, we focus on sonophoresis in the low frequency regime ($20 \, kHz < f < 100 \, kHz$).

DESCRIPTION OF THE TECHNOLOGY

Low-frequency sonophoresis corresponds to the use of ultrasound at a frequency lower than 100 kHz for sonophoresis. Low-frequency sonophoresis can be divided into two types: (*i*) continuous application of ultrasound during drug delivery and (*ii*) pretreatment of skin using ultrasound prior to drug delivery. We discuss each of them in the following sections.

Continuous Sonophoresis

This approach corresponds to simultaneous application of drug and ultrasound to the skin. This method enhances transdermal transport in two ways: (*i*) enhanced diffusion through structural alterations of the skin and (*ii*) convection induced by ultrasound. Indeed, application of low-frequency ultrasound at 20 kHz enhances transdermal transport of various low-molecular weight drugs as well as of high-molecular weight proteins such as insulin across human skin. Skin permeability during low-frequency sonophoresis measured in vitro using human cadaver skin is up to 1000-fold higher than that in the absence of ultrasound (28). Transdermal transport enhancement decreases after ultrasound is turned off. Thus, this method of enhancement may be used to achieve a temporal control over transdermal transport. Ultrasound conditions used for this type of sonophoresis correspond to low intensity (about $1 \, W/cm^2$) and low duty cycle (e.g., 10%). This method has been tested in vitro using human cadaver skin and in vivo using rat and pig skin using a variety of low- as well as high-molecular weight solutes (16,28). In particular, this method has been tested in vivo for transdermal insulin delivery and in vitro for delivery of erythropoeitin and γ-interferon. Although this method may be used to achieve a temporal control over skin permeability, it requires that the patients use a wearable ultrasound device for drug delivery.

Pretreatment

In this method, a short application of ultrasound is used to permeabilize skin prior to drug delivery. The skin remains in a state of high permeability for several hours. Drugs can be delivered through permeabilized skin during this period. Ultrasound conditions used for this type of sonophoresis correspond to relatively high intensities and low application times. Specifically, it has been shown that ultrasound (20 kHz, 7 W/cm^2) increases skin permeability by up to 100-fold for a period exceeding 10 hours (21,30). This method has been tested for delivery of several low- as well as high-molecular weight solutes. Specifically, it has been shown that macromolecules including insulin and low-molecular weight heparin can be delivered across rat skin in vivo (30,31). In this approach, the patient does not need to wear the ultrasound device. Instead, the device can be placed on the skin for a short time followed by the placement of a patch.

RESEARCH AND DEVELOPMENT

In this chapter, we primarily discuss pretreatment type of low-frequency sonophoresis. In this method, a short application of ultrasound is used to permeabilize skin. Skin remains permeable for extended times (24 hours). Enhanced skin permeability is monitored using skin conductivity. Skin conductivity is an excellent indicator of its permeability (21). This occurs since the lipid bilayers of the stratum corneum, which offer electrical resistance to the skin, also resist transdermal transport of molecules. The relationship between skin permeability and skin conductivity can be mathematically explained based on the mechanism of low-frequency sonophoresis (32). Application of low-frequency ultrasound produces cavitation, which in turn disorders lipid bilayers of the skin. This leads to the formation of aqueous channels in the skin (28). Current carrying ions as well as drugs can permeate through these channels. Therefore, the transport pathways for the drugs during low-frequency sonophoresis are the same as those for the current carrying ions. Hence, the correlation between skin conductivity and skin permeability is fundamentally understandable. Quantitative aspects of this correlation are discussed elsewhere (32).

The increase in skin conductivity varies with the total energy, E, of ultrasound [$E=I\tau$, where, I is ultrasound intensity (W/cm^2) and τ is the net exposure time (seconds)] delivered to the skin. There exists a threshold of ultrasound energy, $E_{threshold}$ below which no significant change in the electrical conductivity of skin is observed. For rat skin (in vivo), this threshold is about 10 J/cm^2 (20). After application of an ultrasound dose of 1000 J/cm^2, the skin conductivity showed an enhancement of 60-fold over the conductivity of untreated skin. The threshold energy for enhancement in pigskin was about 10 times higher compared to rat skin (20). The threshold energy required for conductivity enhancement can be reduced by about 10-fold by combining low-frequency ultrasound with chemical enhancers such as surfactants, e.g., 1% w/v sodium lauryl sulfate (33).

Skin remained in a state of elevated conductivity for prolonged times. Note that the skin permeability would eventually recover to its baseline value. For example, experiments on type I diabetic volunteers have shown that a 2-minute application of ultrasound (20 kHz, $\sim$7 W/cm^2) significantly increased skin permeability for about 15 hours, after which skin permeability decreased to its baseline permeability within 24 hours (34).

Effect of ultrasound pretreatment on macromolecule transport has assessed in vivo in rodents for low molecular weight heparin (LMWH), insulin, and vaccines, among others. Transdermal LMWH delivery was measured by monitoring aXa activity in the blood while transdermal insulin delivery was monitored using blood glucose values. No significant aXa activity was observed when LMWH was placed on non-treated skin. However, significant amount of LMWH was transported transdermally after ultrasound pretreatment. aXa activity in the blood increased slowly for about 2 hours, after which, it increased rapidly before achieving a steady state after 4 hours at a value of about 1 U/ml (30). Effect of transdermally delivered LMWH was observed well beyond 6 hours in contrast to intravenous or subcutaneous injections, which resulted only in transient biological activity.

Effect of ultrasound on transdermal insulin delivery was also measured. In these experiments, skin was permeabilized using low-frequency ultrasound (20 kHz, $\sim$7 W/cm^2). Insulin (500 U/ml) was placed on permeabilized skin. Blood glucose levels were subsequently measured. Blood glucose level of rats decreased by about 80% when insulin was applied on ultrasound-treated site, thus suggesting that a significant dose of insulin was delivered across the skin. In contrast, no effect on blood glucose level was observed when insulin was placed on untreated site.

Ultrasound has also been used to deliver a vaccine (tetanus toxoid) in mice. In the absence of ultrasound no immune response was observed after topical application of the vaccine. However, significant IgG titers were observed in mice pretreated with 100 J/cm^2 ultrasound followed by topical application of tetanus toxoid. The immune response generated by ultrasonic immunization increased with increasing ultrasound dose. Two possible mechanisms explain why pretreatment of skin with low-frequency ultrasound prior to contact with the antigen vaccine enhances the immune response. First, ultrasound pretreatment results in increased delivery of the vaccine thus enabling sufficient amount of vaccine to enter the skin in order to activate the skins immune response. However, a comparison of the response obtained by transcutaneous and subcutaneous immunization showed that IgG titers elicited by sonophoretic transcutaneous immunization were almost 10-fold higher per dose compared to subcutaneous injections. The second mechanism involves activation of Langerhans and immune cells of the skin that effectively capture the antigen and present it to the immune system. Results showed mild activation of LCs after ultrasound application alone and a strong activation after ultrasonic tetanus toxoid delivery.

The delivery rate of drugs by pretreatment sonophoresis can be further enhanced by providing additional driving forces (additional ultrasound or iontophoresis) that may induce convection through ultrasound-pretreated skin. For example, application of low-intensity ultrasound (~1 W/cm^2) on ultrasonically pretreated skin induced an additional 21-fold enhancement of transdermal mannitol transport compared to that due to pretreatment alone (29). The enhancement induced by additional ultrasound decreased immediately after turning ultrasound off. Application of iontophoresis also induced additional enhancement across ultrasound-pretreated skin. Specifically, transdermal heparin transport after 1-hour iontophoresis across ultrasound-pretreated skin was 15-fold higher compared to that induced by ultrasound alone (24).

Enhanced skin permeability by ultrasound application may be used for delivery of various therapeutic agents. With a typical permeability achieved after ultrasound pretreatment, an insulin dose of about 1 U/hr can be delivered through a patch having an area of 10 cm^2 and containing insulin solution at a concentration of 100 U/ml. This dose is comparable to a typical baseline insulin dose for a type I diabetic patient (16). This dose can be further increased by providing additional application of low-intensity ultrasound. Sonophoretic drug delivery method can also be used for several other drugs including leutinizing hormone releasing hormone. Sonophoresis also has the potential for transcutaneous immunization. Further work in this area should focus on optimization of ultrasound parameters for increasing the delivery rates, performing detailed safety studies, and tests on human volunteers.

Relatively few clinical studies have been conducted to investigate drug delivery with low-frequency sonophoresis. Recently, Kost et al. (34) reported on the use of low-frequency sonophoresis for topical delivery of local anesthetic, EMLA. Rapid onset of topical anesthetics is impeded by low permeability of the stratum corneum. Topical anesthesia is required for procedures such as venipuncture, intravenous catheterization, skin biopsy and other cutaneous procedures. The study was a randomized, double blinded, placebo-controlled crossover trial of the onset and efficacy of cutaneous anesthesia provided by EMLA cream with and without ultrasound exposure. EMLA cream placed on ultrasound-treated site resulted in statistically significant less pain than the placebo cream at each time point.

The onset of cutaneous anesthesia after ultrasound pretreatment was rapid. After only 5 minutes of EMLA application to permeated skin, and the level of anesthesia provided was comparable to that of EMLA cream applied to intact skin for 60 minutes. The same effect was observed after 10 and 15 minutes of EMLA application on permeated skin. No significant cutaneous changes were observed due to ultrasound application in any patients. A few cases of moderate pallor or moderate needle marks, and several cases of mild pallor, redness, piloerection, and needle marks were noted. All resolved without treatment. There were no clinically significant changes in vital signs compared before and after the procedure.

Low-frequency sonophoresis also has applications in diagnostics. Specifically, a sample of interstitial fluid can be extracted through ultrasonically pretreated skin for diagnostic purposes (34). This method has been tested in vitro, in vivo in animals as well as in human volunteers. Using rat as an animal model, it was shown that low-frequency ultrasound (20 kHz, ~7 W/cm^2) can quickly permeabilize skin. Glucose was extracted through sonicated site using vacuum (10 in Hg). The first extraction flux was used for calibration and subsequent fluxes were used for prediction of blood glucose levels. The relationship between reference glucose levels and sonophoretically predicted glucose levels was excellent (mean relative error of 17%) (34). This method was also tested on type I human volunteers. Once again, the correlation between predicted and measured glucose values was excellent (mean relative error of 23%). Similar strategies may be used to non-invasively measure other analytes including electrolytes and blood gas. Initial safety studies indicated that ultrasound did not induce adverse effects on the skin. Specifically, no damage or irritation was observed by visual inspections. More recently, several clinical studies have performed on diabetic volunteers where ultrasound was used to permeabilize skin and glucose was collected by diffusion instead of vacuum through permeabilized skin. Glucose flux through sonicated site has been shown to correlate well with blood glucose values and sonophoretically extracted glucose can be used to predict blood glucose values after one-point calibration.

TECHNOLOGY POSITION AND FUTURE DIRECTIONS

Low-frequency sonophoresis offers an effective method for enhancing skin permeability. Enhanced skin permeability may be used for the purpose of drug delivery as well as diagnostics. Therapeutic doses of drugs such as insulin can be delivered through permeabilized skin. Enhanced skin permeability may also be used to extract glucose across the skin. Extracted glucose may be measured and used to predict blood glucose levels. These two methods may someday be combined to develop a self-regulated closed-loop delivery device for drugs such as insulin. Such devices may noninvasively deliver and monitor drugs (such as insulin) and maintain the desired drug concentration in the body.

Several other strategies including the use of chemicals (35,36) and electric fields (37,38) have been suggested for noninvasive transdermal drug delivery and/or diagnostics. Low-frequency sonophoresis offers an advantageous method compared to these methods in that the enhancements are high and applicable to a wide variety of molecules (hydrophilic/lipophilic, charged/uncharged, high/low molecular weight). At the same time, this method requires a more sophisticated device compared to other methods. Additional research and development are necessary before low-frequency sonophoresis can be applied in clinical practice. Specifically, attention should be focused on device development and safety assessment.

REFERENCES

1. Bronaugh RL, Maibach HIE. Percutaneous Absorption: Mechanisms–Methodology–Drug delivery. New York: Marcel Dekker, 1989.
2. Prausnitz M. Reversible skin permeabilization for transdermal delivery of macromolecules. Crit Rev Ther Drug Carrier Syst 1997;14(4):455–83.
3. Kost J. Ultrasound for controlled delivery of therapeutics. Clin Mater 1993; 13:155–61.
4. Tachibana K. Transdermal delivery of insulin to alloxan-diabetic rabbits by ultrasound exposure. Pharm Res 1992; 9:952–4.
5. Novak EJ. Experimental transmission of lidocaine through intact skin by ultrasound. Arch Phys Med Rehab 1964; May:231–2.
6. Cameroy BM. Ultrasound enhanced local anesthesia. Am J Orthoped 1966; 8:47.
7. Benson HAE, McElnay JC, Harland R. Use of ultrasound to enhance percutaneous absorption of benzydamine. Phys Ther 1989; 69(2):113–8.
8. Benson HAE, McElnay JC, Hadgraft J. Influence of ultrasound on the percutaneous absorption of nicotinate esters. Pharm Res 1991; 9:1279–83.
9. Bommannan D, Menon GK, Okuyama H, Elias PM, Guy RH. Sonophoresis. II. Examination of the mechanism(s) of ultrasound-enhanced transdermal drug delivery. Pharm Res 1992; 9(8):1043–7.
10. Ciccone CD, Leggin BQ, Callamaro JJ. Effects of ultrasound and trolamine salicylate phonophoresis on delayed-onset muscle soreness. Phys Ther 1991; 71(9):666–78.
11. Griffin JE, Echternach JL, Proce RE, Touchstone J. Patients treated with ultrasonic driven hydrocortisone and with ultrasound alone. Phys Ther 1967; 47(7):600–1.
12. Johnson ME, Mitragotri S, Patel A, Blankschtein D, Langer R. Synergistic effect of ultrasound and chemical enhancers on transdermal drug delivery. J Pharm Sci 1996; 85(7):670–9.
13. Levy D, Kost J, Meshulam Y, Langer R. Effect of ultrasound on transdermal drug delivery to rats and guinea pigs. J Clin Invest 1989; 83:2974–8.

14. McElnay JC, Matthews MP, Harland R, McCafferty DF. The effect of ultra-sound on the percutaneous absorption of lingocaine. Br J Clin Pharmacol 1985; 20:421–4.

15. McElnay JC, Kennedy TA. The influence of ultrasound on the percutaneous absorption of fluocinolone acetonide. Int J Pharm 1987; 40:105–10.

16. Mitragotri S, Blankschtein D, Langer R. Ultrasound-mediated transdermal protein delivery. Science 1995; 269: 850–3.

17. Mortimer AJ, Trollope BJ, Roy OZ. Ultrasound-enhanced diffusion through isolated frog skin. Ultrasonics 1988; 26:348–51.

18. Tachibana K, Tachibana S. Use of Ultrasound to Enhance the local anesthetic effect of topically applied aqueous lidocaine. Anesthesiology 1993; 78(6):1091–6.

19. Kost J, Levy D, Langer R. Ultrasound as a Transdermal Enhancer. In: Bronaugh R, Maibach HI, eds. Percutaneous Absorption: Mechanisms–Methodology–Drug Delivery. New York and Basel: Marcel Dekker Inc., 1989; 595–601.

20. Mitragotri S, Coleman M, Kost J, Langer R. Transdermal analyte extraction using low-frequency ultrasound. Pharm Res 2000; 17:466–70.

21. Mitragotri S, Farrell J, Tang H, Terahara T, Kost J, Langer R. Determination of the threshold energy dose for ultrasound-induced transdermal drug delivery. J Control Release 2000; 63:41–52.

22. Mitragotri S, Blankschtein D, Langer R. Sonophoresis: Enhanced transdermal drug delivery by application of ultrasound. In: Swarbrick J, Boylan J eds, Encyl. Pharm. Tech. 1996:103–22.

23. Mitragotri S, Langer R, Kost J. Ultrasound for modulation of skin properties. In: Wise D, ed. Biomaterials Engineering and Devices: Human Applications. 1999: 843–54.

24. Le L, Kost J, Mitragotri S. Synergistic effect of ultrasound and iontophoresis on transdermal drug delivery: applications to heparin delivery. Pharm Res 2000; 17:1151–4.

25. Mitragotri S, Ray D, Farrell J, et al. Enhancement of transdermal transport using ultrasound and surfactants. Proc Int Symp Control Rel Bioact Mater 1999; 26:176–7.

26. Fellinger K, Schmidt J. Klinik and Therapies des Chromischen Gelen-kreumatismus. Vienna, Austria: Maudrich, 1954; 549–52.

27. Mitragotri S, Blankschtein D, Langer R. An explanation for the variation of the sonophoretic transdermal transport enhancement from drug to drug. J Pharm Sci 1997; 86(10):1190–2.

28. Mitragotri S, Blankschtein D, Langer R. Transdermal drug delivery using low-frequency sonophoresis. Pharm Res 1996; 13(3):411–20.

29. Gaertner W. Frequency dependence of acoustic cavitation. J Acoust Soc Am 1954; 26:977–80.

30. Mitragotri S, Kost J. Transdermal delivery of heparin and low-molecular weight heparin. Pharm Res In Press.

31. Mitragotri S, Kost J. Low-frequency sonophoresis: A non-invasive method for drug delivery and diagnostics. Biotech Progress 2000; 16:488–92.

32. Tang H, Mitragotri S, Blankschetin D, Langer R. Theoretical description of transdermal transport of hydrophilic permeants: Application to low-frequency sonophoresis. J Pharm Sci 2001; 90:543–66.

33. Mitragotri S, Ray D, Farrell J, et al. Synergistic effect of ultrasound and sodium lauryl sulfate on transdermal drug delivery. J Pharm Sci 2000; 89: 892–900.

34. Kost J, Mitragotri S, Gabbay R, Pishko M, Langer R. Transdermal extraction of glucose and other analytes using ultrasound. Nat Med 2000; 6:347–50.

35. Phillips CA, Michniak BB. Transdermal delivery of drugs with differing lipophilicities using Azone analogs as dermal penetration enhancers. J Pharm Sci 1995; 84(12):1427–33.

36. Walters KA. Penetration enhancers and their use in transdermal therapeutic systems. In: Hadgraft J, Guy RH, eds. Transdermal Drug Delivery: Developmental Issues and Research Initiatives. New York: Marcel Dekker, 1989; 197–233.

37. Guy RH, Kalia Y, Delgado-Charro M, Merino V, Lopez A, Marro D. Iontophoresis: Electrorepulsion and electroosmosis. J Controlled Release 2000; 64(1–3):29–32.

38. Prausnitz MR, Bose V, Langer R, Weaver JC. Electroporation of mammalian skin: A mechanism to enhance transdermal drug delivery. Proc Natl Acad Sci USA 1993; 90:10504–8.

26

Lipid Nanoparticles with Solid Matrix for Dermal Delivery: Solid Lipid Nanoparticles and Nanostructured Lipid Carriers

Eliana B. Souto

Health Sciences Department, Fernando Pessoa University, Porto, Portugal

Rolf D. Petersen and Rainer H. Müller

Department of Pharmacy, Free University of Berlin, Berlin, Germany

INTRODUCTION

Topical and dermatological dosage forms are in many cases applied onto the skin for protection purposes. The protective aspects of those applications are passive, rather than active, even though they cannot be regarded simply in terms of placebo effect. In a number of physiological skin conditions, a more positive treatment is required, using active ingredients with definite pharmacological activity. The degree of penetration and absorption of a particular drug/active ingredient will depend on the vehicle of such formulations. Penetration implies only that a drug passes through the epidermis and reaches the underlying dermis; while percutaneous absorption includes both skin penetration of the drug, and also its absorption into the bloodstream possibly with pharmacological action at sites far removed from the application spot. A fast absorption into the blood stream in the case of a drug intended to have a predominantly local effect, is usually a disadvantage. On the other hand, eventual dispersal of the drug or its metabolic residues and excretion via the bloodstream are required to obviate toxic accumulation. Thus, the effect of a drug depends upon its rate of penetration, its rate of pharmacological action and excretion. These complex relationships are dependent on the type of topical and dermatological formulations applied onto the skin.

Lipid materials are used in a variety of topical pharmaceutic and cosmetic applications. This is due to the solubility for a variety of compounds in these materials, no dermal irritation, and extremely low acute and chronic toxicities. During the last decades, several research papers have been published describing the use of lipid-based carriers for dermal administration, e.g., liposomes (1,2), oil-in-water (o/w) emulsions (3), multiple (w/o/w) emulsions (4), and microemulsions (5,6). More recently, with the aim of increasing the physicochemical stability of the system and the loaded drug or active ingredient, solid lipid nanoparticles (SLN) (7) and nanostructured lipid carriers (NLC) (8) have been developed. SLN and NLC are carrier systems based on a solid matrix, which is composed of lipid materials having a melting point higher than the body and room temperatures. Due to their solid character, these particles immobilize the incorporated drugs/active ingredients, preventing their leakage and protecting sensitive drugs from hostile external environmental. Furthermore, SLN and NLC are thermodynamically stable against coalescence due to the presence of surfactant molecules onto their surface, providing steric and/or electrostatic stabilization. Being composed of biodegradable and physiological materials (fats and waxes) SLN and NLC can be prepared avoiding the use of organic solvents or other toxic additives minimizing the toxicological risk (9). Additionally, lipids are likely to minimize the danger of allergic contact dermatitis that might be induced by direct contact with the drug/active ingredient (10).

The morphological differences between SLN and NLC reside on the lipid organization within their matrix. SLN are formed with solid lipids only and these can decrease both the encapsulation efficiency and the loading capacity for active compounds due to the recrystallization process during storage time. NLC have been developed to overcome such drawbacks (8), because they are composed of a blend of solid and liquid lipids in a ratio that is also solid at body and room temperatures. NLC have also the advantage of allowing the modulation of the drug release. Figure 1 shows the differences between SLN and NLC matrices.

When producing lipid nanoparticles using highly pure solid lipids only (i.e., SLN), nanoparticles form relatively perfect lipid crystals, then recrystallizing after being prepared by a hot homogenization process, or during precipitation when using the microemulsion technique. This means that the loading capacity of these carriers can be limited, especially when high drug loadings are required. Mixing especially very different molecules, such as long chain acylglycerols of the solid lipid with short chain acylglycerols of the liquid lipid, creates crystals with many imperfections (i.e., NLC). Apart from

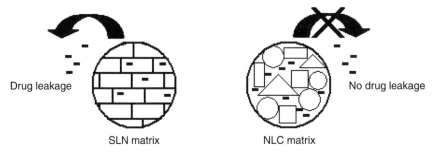

SLN matrix   NLC matrix

Figure 1 Morphological differences between the matrices of SLN and NLC. The SLN matrix is compared to a brick wall structure and leakage of the incorporated compound molecules is likely to occur, while with NLC, having a nanostructured matrix, leakage is less likely to occur. *Abbreviations*: SLN, solid lipid nanoparticles; NLC, nanostructured lipid carriers.

localizing drug in between fatty acid chains or lipid lamellae, these imperfections provide a space for additional loading of active molecules. These latter can be incorporated in the particle matrix in a molecular dispersed form, or be arranged in amorphous clusters. The type of the selected lipids used for preparation of nanoparticles also seems to be responsible for their physical shape. In case of highly pure lipids, such as tristearin or cetyl palmitate, the nanoparticles have a more cubic shape. On the contrary, in case of using rather polydispersed mixtures, which are preferentially used for cosmetic products, the lipid nanoparticles obtain a nice spherical shape. When using identical lipid molecules the cubic shape occurs because they can build up a crystal like a dense brick wall. In case of larger and smaller, and simultaneously differently shape "stones" (crystallizing molecules), the creation of a spherical structure is possible.

For both systems (i.e., SLN and NLC) three types of lipid particles have been described in the literature.

SLN can be of (*i*) homogeneous matrix model, (*ii*) drug enriched shell model, or (*iii*) drug enriched core model. The homogeneous matrix model shows the drug or active ingredient dissolved within the lipid matrix, being molecularly dispersed in the SLN core or present in form of amorphous clusters. The SLN drug enriched shell model (11,12), shows a drug-free (or drug-reduced) lipid core covered by an outer shell of enriched with drug. The drug enriched core model (13,14) shows the opposite, i.e., a core enriched with drug which is covered by a lipid shell.

NLC can be of (*i*) imperfect crystal model, (*ii*) amorphous model, or (*iii*) multiple model. The imperfect crystal model is defined by a matrix with many crystal imperfections creating vacancies where drug molecules can be accommodated in between the lipid lamellae. The amorphous model is created when mixing special lipids that do not recrystallize after cooling.

The multiple model is defined having very small oil nanocompartments created inside the solid lipid matrix of the nanoparticles by a phase separation process (15).

ROLE OF LIPIDS IN DERMAL DELIVERY

The skin is particularly effective as a selective barrier for penetration (or elimination) of a diverse range of substances (37). The epidermis is, in fact, the major layer of this control, and its principal barrier function resides almost entirely in the stratum corneum (38). In fact, most of small water-soluble non-electrolytes can diffuse into the capillary system as thousand times more rapidly when the epidermis is absent, damaged or diseased than when it is present and intact. For a compound absorbed percutaneously, the process is a sequence of deposition onto the stratum corneum, diffusion through the living epidermis and the passage through the upper part of the papillary dermis. The viable tissues may metabolize it, particularly the epidermis, which contains most of the catabolic enzymes.

The dermis contains many permeable capillaries that it is highly probable that most molecules enter the microcirculation soon after leaving the epidermis. Thus, the average total residence time of a drug species in the dermal aqueous phase may only be of the order of a minute. The deeper layers of the dermis in general should not influence percutaneous absorption.

The lipid organization of the stratum corneum is highly responsible for the transport properties of the skin. The polar head groups of the lipids are gathered in layers with the non-polar chains pointed in opposite directions forming layers of methyl groups in the plane where the hydrocarbon ends. Not all the lipids are positioned with their polar groups localized in the polar layer. In fact, some of them are actually localized in the region between the methyl groups. A layered structure, such as that in the lipid part of the stratum corneum, is not a perfectly organized array of layers parallel to the skin surface but, instead, a series of dislocations always occur. Therefore, the diffusion coefficient is the gross one for a partially organized lamellar structure. When a drug molecule moves onto the intact skin delivered from a vehicle, it first contacts with the hydrolipidic mantle, cellular debris, bacteria, and other exogenous materials which cover the skin. In general, a molecule may penetrate to the viable tissue below the horny layer via two potential routes of entry to the subepidermal tissue, i.e., transepidermal route and transappendageal route.

The actual pathway for penetration via pilosebaceous apparatus could be through the hair fiber itself, through the outer root sheath of the hair into the viable cells of the follicle, or through the air-filled canal and into the sebaceous gland (39). The route for the sweat duct may be through either the lumen or the walls to below the epidermis and through the thin ring of

Table 1 Examples of Drugs and Active Ingredients Incorporated into Lipid Nanoparticles of Different Composition Intended for Topical and Dermatological Applications

Drug active ingredient	Organic phase composition	Water phase composition	Refs.
Alpha lipoic acid	Triacylglycerols and partial acylglycerols of C_8-C_{18} fatty acids	Sodium cocoamphoacetate in water	(16)
Ascorbyl palmitate	Glycerol behenate and non-hydrogenated soybean lecithin	Poloxamer 188 in water	(17)
BMDBM[a]	Glycerol tristearate	Hydrogenated phosphatidylcholine in phosphate buffer solution (0.2M, pH 7.4)	(18)
Clotrimazole	Glycerol palmitate and Miglyol®812[c]	1,1,4,4-tetramethylbuthylphenol in water	(14,19)
Curcuminoids	Stearic acid and glycerol monostearate	Poloxamer 188 and dioctyl sodium sulfosuccinate in water	(20)
DEET[b]	Stearic acid, glycerol behenate, glycerol palmitate or glycerol monostearate	Tween 20 in aqueous solution of n-butanol	(21,22)
Ferulic acid	Cetyl palmitate	Polyglycerol methylgluco distearate in water	(23)
Ibuprofen	Glycerol palmitostearate	Poloxamer 188 in water	(24)
Indomethacin	Glycerol behenate and Miglyol®812[c]	Poloxamer 188 in water	(25)
Inorganic sunscreens TiO_2, $BaSO_4$, or $SrCO_3$	Carnuba wax and Decyl oleate	Tween 80, Simethicone and methylisothiazoline in water	(26–28)
Isotretinoin	Glycerol palmitostearate	Tween 80 in water	(29)

(Continued)

Table 1 Examples of Drugs and Active Ingredients Incorporated into Lipid Nanoparticles of Different Composition Intended for Topical and Dermatological Applications (*Continued*)

Drug active ingredient	Organic phase composition	Water phase composition	Refs.
Ketoconazole	Glycerol behenate and α-tocopherol	Poloxamer 188 and sodium deoxicholate in water	(30)
Nicotinamide	Glycerol behenate and Miglyol®812[c]	Poloxamer 188 and sodium deoxicholate in water	(31)
Podophyllotoxin	Glycerol palmitate and soybean lecithin	Poloxamer 188 in water	(32)
Retinol	Crystallized palm oil and egg phosphatidylcholine	Tween 80 in water	(33)
Triptolide	Glycerol tristearate or stearic acid	PEG400MS in aqueous solution of thiomerosal	(34)
Ubidecarenone	Cetyl palmitate and Miglyol®812[c] or Labrasol®[d]	polyglycerol methylgluco distearate in water	(35)
Valdecoxib	Glycerol dilaurate and propylene glycol monocaprylate	PEG 35 castor oil, diethylene glycol monoethyl ether and macrogol 15 hydroxy stearate in water	(36)

[a]Buthyl-methoxydibenzoylmethane.
[b]N,N-diethyl-m-toluamide.
[c]Mixture of liquid mono-, di-, and triacylglycerols.
[d]PEG-8 caprylic/capric triacylglycerols.

keratinized cells. Dense capillary networks closely envelope the bases of both the sweat ducts and the hair follicles. Most molecules reaching these highly permeable vascular regions would immediately sweep into the systemic circulation.

The dermal delivery of a drug or active ingredient when encapsulated into SLN or NLC depends obviously on the lipid composition of the skin as well as on the different materials used to prepare the solid matrix of the particles (Table 1). Ideally, SLN and NLC should be composed of materials resembling the skin's composition. Table 2 shows an overview of the complex mixture of esterified and free fatty acids found in acylglycerols of the hydrolipid mantle of the skin.

The majority of lipids used to produce SLN and NLC are similar to those existing in the human skin structure, showing therefore biocompatibility and biodegradability. This decreases the risk of both chronic and acute toxicity of SLN and NLC. Furthermore, these materials also figure in the composition of many topical pharmaceutics and cosmetic products existing on the market.

Triacylglycerols

Triacylglycerols of high melting point (>50°C), such as glycerol tripalmitate (14,40–44) and glycerol tristearate (43,45–49), are used to produce SLN, creating a relatively perfect crystalline matrix, which is stabilized by surfactant molecules in aqueous dispersion. These solid lipid matrices can be highly stable against coalescence, however, as mentioned above during storage time drug expulsion can occur due to the tendency revealed by such lipids to transform via the β', into the more stable β polymorphic form. Transition into a more stable triacylglycerols polymorph is usually related to a rearrangement of the triacylglycerol molecules with increasing the

Table 2 Fatty Acid Composition of the Hydrolipidic Mantle of the Skin

Fatty acid	% Weight
Palmitic acid (C16:0)	25.0
6-Hexadecenoic acid (C16:1)	22.0
8-Octadecenoic acid (C18:1)	9.0
Myristic acid (C14:0)	7.0
Pentadecenoic acid (C15:1)	4.0
Stearic acid (C18:0)	3.0
Oleic acid (C18:1)	2.0
Heptadecanoic acid (C17:0)	1.0
Linoleic acid (C18:2)	0.5
220 other fatty acids	26.5

lattice density (50,51). The type of crystal polymorph obtained and the kinetics of the transitions may thus have important consequences for the stability of the dispersion, as well as for the drug loading. Studies about the influence of surfactants on the crystallization process provide deeper insights into the type of interaction of the dispersed lipid with the surfactant used for the steric stabilization.

Triacylglycerols of lower melting point such as glycerol trilaurate (52–69) and glycerol tricaprate (52,70–72) are also reported in SLN technology however, instead of solid matrices supercooled melts can be obtained. Supercooled melts are not lipid suspensions, rather systems similar to o/w emulsions (73). They describe a phenomenon that lipid crystallization may not occur although the sample is stored at a temperature below the melting point of the lipid. These systems are not unusual in lipid nanoparticles preparation (74). The main reason for the formation of supercooled melts is the size dependence of crystallization processes. In order to start, crystallization requires a critical number of crystallization nuclei (75). This critical number of molecules is less likely to be formed in small droplets and therefore, the tendency for the formation of supercooled melts increases with decreasing of the droplet size. The range of supercooling (difference of temperatures between the melting and crystallization points) can reach 30–40°C in lipid dispersions (53). The amount of supercooling (difference between melting and crystallization temperatures) is different for each particular lipid. When working with triacylglycerols of high melting point and high crystallization temperature (pure lipid), the addition of lipid molecules with small-chain length will decrease the melting point of the mixture, as well as the crystallization temperature. This means that the amount of supercooling will increase, i.e., increases the difference between the melting and crystallization temperatures. The same is valid for the opposite, i.e., if working with lipid materials of low crystallization temperature, the addition of long-chain length molecules will decrease the amount of supercooling. The presence of supercooled melts can be assessed by imaging analysis, NMR, DSC, and X-ray diffraction.

Mixtures of Mono-, Di-, and Triacylglycerols

When using crude mixtures of mono-, di-, and triacylglycerols, both SLN and NLC can be produced. Very special lipids such as hydroxyoctacosanylhydroxystearate, isopropylmyristate, and dibutyl adipate, are able to create solid particles of amorphous structure, i.e., NLC of amorphous model, which can avoid the occurrence of recrystallization of lipid under cooling and during shelf life, minimizing drug expulsion during storage time (76).

To produce SLN using mixtures of mono-, di-, and triacylglycerols several lipid bases existing on the market can be used, such as Witepsol®

(partial acylglycerols and fatty acids of C_{10}–C_{18}) (77–82), Softisan® (triacylglycerols and partial acylglycerols of C_8–C_{18} fatty acids) (16) Compritol® (mono-, di-, and triacylglycerols of glyceryl behenate) (30,83–87), and Imwitor® (40–50% of glycerol monostearate) (42,44,88). Examples of other acylglycerol mixtures are the glycerol palmitostearate (43,45–49), the diacylglycerol monocitrate monostearate (89,90), and stearylamine (91).

Hard Fatty Acids and Waxes

Hard fatty acids are highly pure compounds that can be selected to produce SLN. Examples are stearic acid (92–95), palmitic acid (96,97), behenic acid (89,90), and capric acid (96). These lipids recrystallize mainly in the most stable polymorphic form β.

Waxes are also suitable to produce SLN because they recrystallize in a metastable polymorphic form, which remains unchanged during storage time. The main waxes used in SLN technology are cetyl palmitate (23,35,44,86,98–100), beeswax (68,101,102), and carnauba wax (103,104). They can be use solely or added to other lipids to increase the melting point of the solid matrix.

Liquid Lipids (Oils)

Liquid lipids are used to produce NLC. When mixing solid lipids with sufficient amounts of liquid lipids (oils) the NLC of imperfect crystal model can be obtained. Due to the different chain lengths of the fatty acids and the mixture of mono-, di-, and triacylglycerols, the matrix of NLC is not able to form a highly ordered structure (15), creating available spaces for the drug.

Oils that can be used to produce NLC are glycerol monooleate, glycerol monostearate, and mixture of mono-, di-, and triacylglycerols of caprylic and capric acids (Miglyol812). When mixing solid lipids with oils [e.g., medium (105) and long chain triacylglycerols (84), oleic acid (94)] in such a ratio that the solubility of the oil molecules in the solid lipid is exceeded the NLC of multiple model can be created. During the cooling of the nanoemulsion the lipid droplets reach the miscibility gap (40°C), the oil precipitates forming tiny oil droplets in the melted solid lipid. Subsequent solidification of the solid lipid leads to fixation of the oily nanocompartments. The advantage of this NLC model is the increase of the loading capacity for drugs that usually show higher solubility in liquid lipids than in solid lipids (101,106).

Other Lipids

Other lipids include less defined crude mixtures such as cacao butter (107), and other compounds such as cholesterol (11,63,108) and paraffin (99,101,109,110).

METHODS FOR LIPID NANOPARTICLE PRODUCTION

SLN and NLC of narrow size range and coated with suitable emulsifying agents can be produce by several techniques. These are: (*i*) the high pressure homogenization (HPH) technique developed by Müller and Lucks (111); (*ii*) the microemulsion-based technique developed by Gasco (90), (*iii*) the solvent emulsification–evaporation technique described by Sjöström and Bergenståhl (112), (*iv*) the solvent displacement technique described by Fessi et al. (113), (*v*) the emulsification–diffusion technique developed by Quintanar-Gerrero and Fessi (114), and (*vi*) the phase inversion-based technique described by Heurtault et al. (115,116).

The production of lipid nanoparticles by HPH can be performed using the hot or the cold homogenization process. In both cases, the drug/active ingredient is dissolved or dispersed in the melted lipid previously to HPH (73,117). In the hot HPH, two different phases are prepared at the same temperature, i.e., the lipid phase consisting of melted lipid mixed with drug/active ingredient, and the aqueous phase consisting of a hot solution where the emulsifying agent is dissolved. Both phases are mixed by high speed stirring or by ultrasonication breaking the large droplets of the internal lipid phase into smaller ones for the production of a pre-emulsion. This pre-emulsion is passed through the high pressure homogenizer applying a pressure of 500 bar for 1–3 cycles yielding a nanoemulsion. The obtained nanoemulsion is cooled, solidified forming the aqueous dispersion of lipid nanoparticles. In the cold HPH the lipid melt containing the drug/active ingredient is first cooled and solidified under dry ice or liquid nitrogen. After solidification, the lipid mass is ground by means of ball or mortar milling to yield lipid microparticles in a diameter range around 50–100 μm. The lipid microparticles are dispersed in a cold emulsifying solution under stirring to produce a macro-suspension. This suspension is passed through the high-pressure homogenizer at/or below room temperature and the microparticles are broken to form nanoparticles.

For the production of lipid nanoparticles via microemulsion technique, the lipid phase is melted at approx. 60–70°C and an o/w surfactant/co-surfactant containing aqueous phase is prepared at the same temperature (90,118). Both lipid and aqueous phases are added and admixed to produce a microemulsion, which is kept at higher temperatures. Lipid nanoparticles are obtained when the hot microemulsion is diluted into excess of cold water (0–4°C) leading to a "breaking" of the microemulsion, converting it into an ultra-fine nanoemulsion, which recrystallizes forming the nanoparticles.

The production of lipid nanoparticles by solvent evaporation in o/w emulsions also requires a lipid phase, which is prepared by solubilizing the lipid material in a water-immiscible organic solvent, such as cyclohexane, chloroform, or methylene chloride. Then, the drug/active ingredient is dissolved or dispersed in this phase (119,120). This organic phase is emulsified by mechanic stirring in an aqueous solution containing an o/w surfactant. Upon evaporation of the organic solvent from the obtained o/w emulsion under mechanical stirring or reduced pressure, a nanoparticle dispersion is formed by precipitation of the lipid in the aqueous medium.

In the solvent displacement technique, the lipid material is dissolved in a semi-polar water-miscible solvent, such as ethanol, acetone, or methanol, where the drug/active ingredient is also dissolved or dispersed (82,121–124). An o/w surfactant containing aqueous phase is also prepared. The organic phase is injected into the aqueous phase under magnetic stirring. A violent spreading is observed because of the miscibility of both phases. Droplets of solvent of nanometer size are formed from the o/w interface. These droplets are rapidly stabilized by the surfactant molecules being in the aqueous phase, until diffusion of the solvent is complete and lipid precipitation has occurred. Removal of solvent can be performed by distillation, and lipid nanoparticles are formed after total evaporation of the water-miscible organic solvent.

In the emulsification–diffusion technique, partially water soluble solvents are used, such as benzyl alcohol (125) or tetrahydrofuran (126). The solvent is first saturated with water to ensure the initial thermodynamic equilibrium between those two liquids (water and solvent). The lipid is dissolved in the saturated solvent producing an organic phase where the drug/active ingredient is added. This organic phase is emulsified, under vigorous stirring, in an aqueous solution containing the emulsifying agent obtaining an o/w emulsion. Adding water to the system under moderate mechanical stirring, causes solvent diffusion into the external phase and the lipid starts precipitating. The organic solvent can be afterwards removed by distillation or ultra-filtration. After the organic solvent being totally removed, an aqueous dispersion of lipid nanoparticles is formed.

The phase inversion-based technique is based on two steps (115,116). The first step consists of magnetic stirring of all the components (lipid, surfactant, and water) in the correct proportions, which need to be previously defined for each formulation. Three cycles of heating and cooling from room temperature to 85°C and back to 60°C are subsequently applied at a rate of 4°C/min. This thermal treatment will cause the inversion of the emulsion. In a second step, dilution under cooling conditions will occur. The temperature of the system before the dilution can be determined at the beginning of the inversion process. An irreversible shock induced by dilution with cold water to the mixture maintained at the previously temperature of cooling dilution will break the system. This fast cooling dilution process with cold distilled water (approaching 0°C), leads to lipid nanoparticles. A slow magnetic stirring is applied to avoid nanoparticle aggregation.

PROPERTIES OF LIPID NANOPARTICLES FOR DERMAL DELIVERY

Smoothness, Adhesiveness, and Occlusion

Having a solid matrix and a spherical-like shape, lipid nanoparticles reveal excellent smoothing and lubricating properties. These characteristics are important requisites of formulations intended for skin administration. Furthermore, lipid nanoparticle dispersions are sufficiently viscous (or fluid) to be easily applied onto the skin, and sufficiently elastic to adhere and self-immobilize onto the skin. One of the aims of topical and dermatological products is to reduce the desire to scratch that may increase the skin damage. The mechanical barrier and lubricating effect of lipid nanoparticles protect and support the skin, which is particularly useful in case of skin irritation and allergic reactions.

Lipid nanoparticles can also provide controlled hydration of the horny layer of epidermis. The degree of hydration achieved with such formulations depends on the type of lipids and emulsifying agents used for the production of lipid nanoparticles. These factors influence both the index of recrystallinity and the size of the nanoparticles (67,69). As mentioned before, highly crystalline nanoparticles can be produced using very pure lipids such as glycerol tripalmitate and tristearate, creating a high skin occlusiveness (due to film formation onto the skin), and therefore high emolliency. On the other hand, if using lipids of low melting temperatures, or high crude mixtures, supercooled melts can be produced under cooling, obtaining systems which do not show occlusive properties (69). Composed of solid and hydrophobic nanoparticles, this monolayered film has occlusion properties on the skin retarding the loss of moisture due to evaporation (67). Moisture barrier properties have been experimentally demonstrated by the different degree of occlusion, depending on the size of the applied particles (127).

The occlusion produced by the typical ointment formulations does not ensure rapid hydration, particularly if the horny layer is excessively dry. It is then desirable to use a preparation capable of supplying water. Lipid nanoparticle dispersions are suitable for the purpose because when applied onto the skin, the pressure leads to fusion of the particles forming a dense film. This fusion is promoted by capillary forces involved during water evaporation (128).

Under aging the dermis loses much of its elasticity. The skin stretched by muscular movement then fails to shrink back to its normal smoothness and wrinkles are formed (129). Due to their hydration properties, it can be assumed that lipid nanoparticles may enhance skin elasticity (68,130), and further be used to formulate anti-aging products. A consequence of occlusiveness of lipid nanoparticles, may also be the increase of skin penetration of active ingredients (131).

Whitening Properties

The whitening effects of lipid dispersions allow weaken the coloration of colored actives such as coenzyme Q10, which is yellow (132), or drugs and actives that can turn into colored intermediate products during the shelf life (vitamin C). If incorporation of those actives into lipid nanoparticles is achieved, a whitening effect is obtained which is considered more appealing to the customer.

Chemical Stabilization of Drugs and Active Ingredients

The solid matrix of lipid nanoparticles has the advantage that it is able to stabilize the drug/active ingredients which are chemically labile against degradation by other species, e.g., water or oxygen. This is achieved in optimized formulations, i.e., that do not show drug leakage during storage time due to polymorphic transformations of the lipid matrix. Thus, the choice of the lipid plays an important role because the drug/active ingredient must be solubilized or at least retained within the lipid matrix during storage time. It has been published that the enhancement of chemical stability of several drugs and active ingredients by incorporation into lipid nanoparticles, e.g., retinol (99,103), tretinoin (99), retinyl palmitate (99), ascorbyl palmitate (133–135), ferulic acid (23), and coenzyme Q10 (35,131,136,137).

Controlled Release and Skin Penetration

Drug/active ingredient release has to be taken into account whether it is required to take effect on direct contact with the skin's surface, or when the drug has to penetrate the epidermis to reach the dermis. The release profile will be dependent on the method of production of lipid nanoparticles, the composition of the formulation (i.e., composition and concentration of surfactant), the solubilizing properties of the emulsifying agent for the drug/ active, in addition to the solubility and concentration of the drug/active in the lipid matrix (oil/water partition coefficient). These factors influence the inner structure of the particle and therefore the rate of release of incorporated ingredient (15,117,132,138). Depending on the matrix structure, the release profiles can vary from very fast release, medium release or extremely prolonged release. One can achieve controlled release profile using SLN of homogeneous matrix, or the drug enriched core model where diffusion takes place through the lipid shell that covers the drug core. NLC show more flexibility in controlling the release, being usually faster than SLN of similar composition.

The majority of the substances applied onto the skin will only have a superficial action, i.e., they are not intended for deeper skin penetration and absorption. Controlling the drug/active release, lipid nanoparticle dispersions will also control the rate of penetration of drug/active into the skin. Modulation of release and active penetration into certain layers of the skin can be achieved as a consequence of, e.g., the creation of supersaturated systems (15). These systems can be obtained by the incorporation of lipid nanoparticles into topical formulations (creams, ointments, emulsions, and gels). The increase in saturation solubility will lead to an increased diffusion pressure of the drug/active into the skin. During shelf life, the active remains encapsulated within the lipid matrix, particularly NLC because these preserve the polymorphic form. After application of supersaturated cream onto the skin, and due to an increase in temperature and water evaporation, increasing the thermoactivity, the lipid matrix transforms from a more unstable polymorph to a more ordered polymorph leading to the release of active into a system already saturated with the same active, and thus creating a supersaturation effect. Penetration studies have been performed using, e.g., tocopherol and its derivatives (68,131), retinoids (101,139), molecular sunscreens (98,140), and coenzyme Q10 (131). It has been evaluated that the delivery rate of a non-steroid anti-inflammatory drug from conventional hydrogels in comparison to lipid nanoparticle formulations. When applying drug-loaded lipid nanoparticles-based gels the anti-inflammatory effect was over twofold higher than of conventional hydrogels (34). An improved drug uptake has also been observed for the topical corticosteroid prednicarbate when delivered by means of SLN (81). Due to their occlusive properties, lipid nanoparticles can increase skin penetration of corticosteroids. This is of major importance because these substances are associated to skin atrophy when applied topically.

In some special circumstances, a prolonged release of the drug/active but with little penetration may be desired. This is the case of particulate and molecular sunscreens, due to the side effects they show if penetration into the skin occurs (141). It has been reported that the penetration rate of such substances reduced when incorporated into SLN, in comparison to traditional o/w emulsions (140). In addition, lipid nanoparticles proved to have a synergistic effect of the UV scattering when used as vehicles for molecular sunscreens (103,142), which may reduce the concentration of the molecular sunscreen, consequently its potential side effects, as well as the costs of formulation of expensive sunscreens. In addition, lipid nanoparticles can be explored to formulate sunscreen products with lower and medium sun protection factor (103).

The prolonged release properties of lipid nanoparticles have also been explored with perfumes and fragrances. The aim was to achieve a once-a-day application using lipid nanoparticles instead of typical o/w emulsions (143,144). This property can also be advantageous for the delivery of insect repellents to be applied onto the skin, such as lemon oil (145–147).

CONCLUSIONS

Lipid nanoparticle technology has proven to be an effective approach to formulate drug/active ingredients for several topical and dermatological purposes. Advantages of SLN and NLC reside on their biodegradability and biocompatibility with the skin, in addition to properties such as chemical stabilization of drugs/actives, and controlled release profiles. The aqueous dispersions of lipid particles in the nanometer range also show occlusiveness, which contributes for the skin hydration enhancement, adhesiveness, and smoothness. The loading capacity of such particles for a particular drug/active can be optimized by selecting the suitable lipid material and emulsifying agents, i.e., it depends mainly on the miscibility of the drug/active in the lipid. It can range from about 4% (e.g., ferrulic acid) (23), 25% (e.g., tocopherol) (148), or even up to 50% and more, in case of well lipid miscible lipophilic molecules (e.g., tocopherol and coenzyme Q10). "Super-loaded" NLC were developed having a sunscreen loading of 70% (103). In this case, a liquid sunscreen was used as the oily component in the NLC formulation, and cetyl palmitate was added to create a solid matrix.

The first two cosmetic products based on lipid nanoparticle technology were introduced to the market by Rimpler GmbH in Wedemark/ Hannover, Germany. In October 2005 the products NanoRepair Q10 cream and NanoRepair Q10 Serum were introduced to the cosmetic market revealing the success of this research field.

REFERENCES

1. Jain S, Jain N, Bhadra D, et al. Transdermal delivery of an analgesic agent using elastic liposomes: preparation, characterization and performance evaluation. Curr Drug Deliv 2005; 2(3):223–3.
2. Singh B, Mehta G, Kumar R, et al. Design, development and optimization of nimesulide-loaded liposomal systems for topical application. Curr Drug Deliv 2005; 2(2):143–53.
3. Teichmann A, Jacobi U, Weigmann HJ, et al. Reservoir function of the stratum corneum: development of an in vivo method to quantitatively determine the stratum corneum reservoir for topically applied substances. Skin Pharmacol Physiol 2005; 18(2):75–80.
4. Gallarate M, Carlotti ME, Trotta M, et al. On the stability of ascorbic acid in emulsified systems for topical and cosmetic use. Int J Pharm 1999; 188(2): 233–41.
5. Kreilgaard M. Influence of microemulsions on cutaneous drug delivery. Adv Drug Deliv Rev 2002; 54(Suppl. 1):S77–98.
6. Park ES, Cui Y, Yun BJ, et al. Transdermal delivery of piroxicam using microemulsions. Arch Pharm Res 2005; 28(2):243–8.
7. Müller RH. Polydispersität elektrophoretische Beweglichkeit hochdisperser Systeme, in PhD Thesis. 1983; Kiel Universität: Kiel.

8. Müller RH, Mäder K, Lippacher, et al. Fest-flüssig (halbfeste) Lipidpartikel und Verfahren zur Herstellung hochkonzentrierter Lipidpartikeldispersionen. 1998; PCT application PCT/EP00/04565.
9. Souto EB, Almeida AJ, Müller RH Feasibility studies of lipid-based carriers? for dermal applications. in 14th International Workshop on Bioencapsulation & COST 865 meeting, Lausanne, Switzerland, 5–7 October, P-27. 2006.
10. Cevc G, Blume G. New, high efficient formulation of diclofenac for the topical administration in ultradeformable drug carriers, transfersomes. Biochim Biophys Acta 2001; 1514:191–205.
11. zur Mühlen A. Feste Lipid-Nanopartikel mit prolongierter Wirkstoffliberation: Herstellung, Langzeitsabilität, Charakterisierung, Freisetzungsverhalten und Mechanismen, in PhD Thesis. 1996, Freie Universität Berlin: Berlin.
12. Lukowski G, Werner U. Investigation of surface and drug release of solid lipid nanoparticles loaded with acyclovir. Intern Symp Control Rel Bioact Mater 1998; 25:425–8.
13. Westesen K, Bunjes H. Koch MHJ. Physicochemical characterization of lipid nanoparticles and evaluation of their drug loading capacity and sustained release potential. J Control Release 1997; 48:223–36.
14. Souto EB, Wissing SA, Barbosa CM, et al. Development of a controlled release formulation based on SLN and NLC for topical clotrimazole delivery. Int J Pharm 2004; 278(1):71–7.
15. Müller RH, Radtke M, Wissing SA. Solid lipid nanoparticles (SLN) and nanostructured lipid carriers (NLC) in cosmetic and dermatological preparations. Adv Drug Deliv Rev 2002; 54:S131–55.
16. Souto EB, Muller RH, Gohla S. A novel approach based on lipid nanoparticles (SLN®) for topical delivery of alpha-lipoic acid. J Microencapsul 2005; 22(6):581–92.
17. Kristl J, Volk B, Gasperlin M, et al. Effect of colloidal carriers on ascorbyl palmitate stability. Eur J Pharm Sci 2003; 19(4):181–9.
18. Iannuccelli V, Sala N, Tursilli R, et al. Influence of liposphere preparation on butyl-methoxydibenzoylmethane photostability. Eur J Pharm Biopharm 2006; 63(2):140–5.
19. Souto EB, Muller RH. Investigation of the factors influencing the incorporation of clotrimazole in SLN and NLC prepared by hot high-pressure homogenization. J Microencapsul 2006; 23(4):377–88.
20. Tiyaboonchai W, Tungpradit W, Plianbangchang P. Formulation and characterization of curcuminoids loaded solid lipid nanoparticles. Int J Pharm 2007; 337(1–2):299–306.
21. Iscan Y, Wissing SA, Hekimoglu S, et al. Solid lipid nanoparticles (SLN) for topical drug delivery: incorporation of the lipophilic drugs N,N-diethyl-m-? toluamide and vitamin K. Pharmazie 2005; 60(12):905–9.
22. Iscan Y, Hekimoglu S, Sargon MF, et al. DEET-loaded solid lipid particles for skin delivery: in vitro release and skin permeation characteristics in different vehicles. J Microencapsul 2006; 23(3):315–27.
23. Souto EB, Anselmi C, Centini M, et al. Preparation and characterization of n-dodecyl-ferulate-loaded solid lipid nanoparticles (SLN). Int J Pharm 2005; 295(1–2):261–8.

24. Casadei MA, Cerreto F, Cesa S, et al. Solid lipid nanoparticles incorporated in dextran hydrogels: A new drug delivery system for oral formulations.?Int J Pharm 2006; 325:140–6.
25. Ricci M, Puglia C, Bonina F, et al. Evaluation of indomethacin percutaneous absorption from nanostructured lipid carriers (NLC): in vitro and in vivo studies. J Pharm Sci 2005; 94 (5):1149–59.
26. Villalobos-Hernandez JR, Muller-Goymann CC. Novel nanoparticulate carrier system based on carnauba wax and decyl oleate for the dispersion of? inorganic sunscreens in aqueous media. Eur J Pharm Biopharm 2005; 60(1):113–22.
27. Villalobos-Hernandez JR, Muller-Goymann CC. Physical stability, centrifugation tests, and entrapment efficiency studies of carnauba wax-decyl oleate nanoparticles used for the dispersion of inorganic sunscreens in aqueous media. Eur J Pharm Biopharm 2006; 63(2):115–27.
28. Villalobos-Hernandez JR, Muller-Goymann CC. Sun protection enhancement of titanium dioxide crystals by the use of carnauba wax nanoparticles: The synergistic interaction between organic and inorganic sunscreens at nanoscale. Int J Pharm 2006; 322(1–2):161–70.
29. Liu J, Hu W, Chen H, et al. Isotretinoin-loaded solid lipid nanoparticles with skin targeting for topical delivery. Int J Pharm 2007; 328(2):191–5.
30. Souto EB, Mehnert W, Muller RH. Polymorphic behaviour of Compritol888 ATO as bulk lipid and as SLN and NLC. J Microencapsul 2006; 23(4):417–33.
31. Souto EB, Teeranachaideekul V, Junyaprasert VB, et al. Encapsulation of nicotinamide into nanostructured lipid carriers. in 15th International Symposium on Microencapsulation. 2005; Parma, Italy, 18–21 September 2005.
32. Chen H, Chang X, Du D, et al. Podophyllotoxin-loaded solid lipid nanoparticles for epidermal targeting. J Control Release 2006; 110(2):296–306.
33. Jee JP, Lim SJ, Park JS, et al. Stabilization of all-trans retinol by loading lipophilic antioxidants in solid lipid nanoparticles. Eur J Pharm Biopharm 2006; 63(2):134–9.
34. Mei Z, Wu Q, Hu S, et al. Triptolide loaded solid lipid nanoparticle hydrogel for topical application. Drug Dev Ind Pharm 2005; 31(2):161–8.
35. Teeranachaideekul V, Souto EB, Junyaprasert VB, Müller RH: Cetyl palmitate-based NLC for topical delivery of coenzyme Q(10)—development, physicochemical characterization and in vitro release studies. Eur J Pharm Biopharm 2007; 67(1):141–8.
36. Joshi M, Patravale V. Formulation and evaluation of nanostructured lipid carrier (NLC)-based gel of valdecoxib. Drug Dev Ind Pharm 2006; 32:911–8.
37. Gurny R, Teubner A. Dermal and transdermal drug delivery—New insights and perspectives, ed. R. Gurny, Teubner, A. 1993, Stuttgart: Wissenschaftliche Verlagsgesellschaft mbH.
38. Bouwstra JA, Honeywell-Nguyen PL, Gooris GS, et al. Structure of the skin barrier and its modulation by vesicular formulations. Prog Lipid Res 2003; 42(1):1–36.
39. Barry BW. Dermatological Formulations—Percutaneous Absorption. New York Marcel Dekker, 1983.

40. Bunjes H, Drechsler M, Koch MH, et al. Incorporation of the model drug ubidecarenone into solid lipid nanoparticles. Pharm Res 2001; 18(3):287–93.

41. Souto EB, Wissing SA, Barbosa CM, et al. Evaluation of the physical stability of SLN and NLC before and after incorporation into hydrogel formulations. Eur J Pharm Biopharm 2004; 58(1):83–90.

42. Reddy LH, Adhikari JS, Dwarakanath BS, et al. Tumoricidal effects of etoposide incorporated into solid lipid nanoparticles after intraperitoneal administration in Dalton's lymphoma bearing mice. Aaps J 2006; 8(2):E254–62.

43. Reddy LH, Vivek K, Bakshi N, et al. Tamoxifen citrate loaded solid lipid nanoparticles (SLN): preparation, characterization, in vitro drug release, and pharmacokinetic evaluation. Pharm Dev Technol 2006; 11(2):167–77.

44. Kumar VV, Chandrasekar D, Ramakrishna S, Kishan V, Rao YM, Diwan PV. Development and evaluation of nitrendipine loaded solid lipid nanoparticles: Influence of wax and glyceride lipids on plasma pharmacokinetics. Int J Pharm 2007; 335(1–2):167–75.

45. Manjunath K, Venkateswarlu V. Pharmacokinetics, tissue distribution and bioavailability of nitrendipine solid lipid nanoparticles after intravenous and intraduodenal administration. J Drug Target 2006; 14(9):632–45.

46. Bunjes H, Koch MH. Saturated phospholipids promote crystallization but slow down polymorphic transitions in triglyceride nanoparticles. J Control Release 2005; 107(2):229–43.

47. Manjunath K, Venkateswarlu V. Pharmacokinetics, tissue distribution and bioavailability of clozapine solid lipid nanoparticles after intravenous and intraduodenal administration. J Control Release 2005; 107(2):215–28.

48. Illing A, Unruh T. Investigation on the flow behavior of dispersions of solid triglyceride nanoparticles. Int J Pharm 2004; 284(1–2):123–31.

49. Venkateswarlu V, Manjunath K. Preparation, characterization and in vitro release kinetics of clozapine solid lipid nanoparticles. J Control Release 2004; 95(3):627–38.

50. Hagemann JW. Thermal behaviour and polymorphism of acylglycerides, in Crystallization and polymorphism of fats and fatty acids. Garti N, Sato K, eds. New York: Marcel Dekker, 1988.

51. Sato K. Crystallization of fats and fatty acids, in Crystallization and Polymorphism of Fats and Fatty Acids. Surfactant Science Series, Garti N, Sato K, eds. New York: Marcel Dekker, 1988.

52. Domb AJ. Long acting injectable oxytetracycline-liposphere formulation. Int J Pharm 1995; 124:271–8.

53. Westesen K, Bunjes H. Do nanoparticles prepared from lipids solid at room temperature always possess a solid lipid matrix? Int J Pharm 1995; 115:129–31.

54. Bunjes H, Westesen K, Koch MHJ. Crystallization tendency and polymorphic transitions in triglyceride nanoparticles. Int J Pharm 1996; 129:159–73.

55. Bunjes H, Koch MHJ, Westesen K. Effect of particle size on colloidal size solid triglycerides. Langmuir 2000; 16:5234–41.

56. Heiati H, Phillips NC, Tawashi R. Evidence for phospholipids bilayer formation in solid lipid nanoparticles formulated with phospholipid and triacylglyceride Pharm Res 1996; 13:1406–10.

57. Heiati H, Tawashi R, Shivers RR, et al. Solid lipid nanoparticles as drug carriers. I. Incorporation and retention of the lipophilic prodrug 3'-azido-3'-deoxythymidine palmitate. Int J Pharm 1997; 146:123–31.
58. Heiati H, Tawashi R, Phillips NC. Solid lipid nanoparticles as drug carriers. II. Plasma stability and biodistribution of solid lipid nanoparticles containing the lipophilic prodrug 3'-azido-3'-deoxythymidine palmitate in mice. Int J Pharm 1998; 174:71–80.
59. Heiati H, Tawashi R, Phillips NC. Drug retention and stability of solid lipid nanoparticles containing azidothymidine palmitate after autoclaving storage and lyophilization. J Microencapsul 1998; 15:173–84.
60. Schwarz C, Mehnert W. Freeze-drying of drug-free and drug-loaded solid lipid nanoparticles (SLN). Int J Pharm 1997; 157:171–9.
61. Schwarz C, Mehnert W. Solid lipid nanoparticles (SLN) for controlled drug delivery II. Drug incorporation and physicochemical characterization. J Microencapsul 1999; 16:205–13.
62. Mehnert W, zur Mühlen A, Dingler A, et al. Solid lipid nanoparticles (SLN)—ein neuartiger Wirkstoff-Carrier für Kosmetika und Pharmazeutika. II. Wirkstoff-Inkorporation, Freisetzung und Sterilizierbarkeit. Pharm Ind 1997; 59: p. 511–514.
63. zur Mühlen A, Schwarz C, Mehnert W. Solid lipid nanoparticles (SLN) for controlled drug delivery—Drug release and release mechanism. Eur J Pharm Biopharm 1998; 45:149–55.
64. Müller RH, Olbrich C. Solid lipid nanoparticles: phagocytic uptake, in vitro cytotoxicity and in vitro biodegradation. 2nd Comunication. Drugs made in Germany 1999. 42:75–9.
65. Unruh T, Bunjes H, Westesen K. Observation of size-dependent melting in lipid nanoparticles. J Phys Chem 1999; 103:10373–77.
66. Unruh T, Bunjes H, Westesen K, et al. Investigations on the melting behaviour of triglyceride nanoparticles. Colloid Polym Sci 2001; 279:p.?398–403.
67. Wissing S, Lippacher A, Müller RH. Investigations on the occlusive properties of solid lipid nanoparticles (SLN). J Cosmet Sci 2001; 52 (5):313–24.
68. Wissing SA. SLN als innovatives Formulierungskonzept für pflegende und protective dermale Zubereitungen, in PhD Thesis. 2002, Freie Universität Berlin: Berlin.
69. Wissing SA, Müller RH. The influence of the crystallinity of lipid nanoparticles on their occlusive properties. Int J Pharm 2002; 242:377–9.
70. Lim S-J, Kim C-K. Formulation parameters determining the physicochemical characteristics of solid lipid nanoparticles loaded with all-trans retinoic acid. Int J Pharm 2002; 243:135–46.
71. Bekerman T, Golenser J, Domb A. Cyclosporin nanoparticulate lipospheres for oral administration. J Pharm Sci 2004; 93(5):1264–70.
72. Lim S-J, Lee M-K, Kim C-K. Altered chemical and biological activities of all-trans retinoic acid incorporated in solid lipid nanoparticles powders. J Control Release 2004; 100:53–61.
73. Mehnert W, Mäder K. Solid lipid nanoparticles—Production, characterization and applications. Adv Drug Deliv Rev 2001; 47:165–96.

74. Bunjes H, Siekmann B, Westesen K. Emulsions of supercooled melts—A novel drug delivery system, in Submicron Emulsions in Drug Targeting and Delivery, S.E. Benita, Editor. 1998, Harwood Academic Publishers: Amsterdam. 175–204.

75. Boistelle, R, Fundamentals of nucleation and crystal growth. In: Garti N, Sato K, eds. Crystallization and Polymorphism of Fats and Fatty Acids. Surfactant Science Series. New York: Marcel Dekker, 1988: 189–226.

76. Müller RH, Radtke M, Wissing SA. Solid lipid nanoparticles (SLN) and nanostructured lipid carriers (NLC) in cosmetic and dermatological preparations. Adv Drug Deliv Rev 2002; 54(Suppl. 1):S131–55.

77. Siekmann B, Westesen K. Submicronized parenteral carrier systems based on solid lipids. Pharm Pharmacol Lett 1992; 1:123–6.

78. Westesen K, Siekmann B, Koch M.HJ. Investigations on the physical state of lipid nanoparticles by synchroton radiation X-ray diffraction. Int J Pharm 1993; 93:189–99.

79. Ahlin P, Kristl J, Šmid-Kobar J. Optimization of procedure parameters and physical stability of solid lipid nanoparticles in dispersions. Acta Pharm 1998; 48:259–67.

80. Ahlin A, Sentjurc M, Strancar J, et al. Location of lipophilic substances and ageing of solid lipid nanoparticles studied by EPR. STP Pharma Sci 2000; 10:125–32.

81. Maia CS, Mehnert W, Schaller M, et al. Drug targeting by solid lipid nanoparticles for dermal use. J Drug Target 2002; 10(6):489–95.

82. Schubert MA, Muller-Goymann CC. Solvent injection as a new approach for manufacturing lipid nanoparticles–evaluation of the method and process parameters. Eur J Pharm Biopharm 2003; 55(1):125–31.

83. Souto EB, Muller RH. SLN and NLC for topical delivery of ketoconazole. J Microencapsul 2005; 22(5):501–10.

84. Souto EB, Wissing SA, Barbosa CM, et al. Comparative study between the viscoelastic behaviors of different lipid nanoparticle formulations. J Cosmet Sci 2004; 55(5):463–71.

85. Borgia SL, Regehly M, Sivaramakrishnan R, et al. Lipid nanoparticles for skin penetration enhancement-correlation to drug localization within the particle matrix as determined by fluorescence and parelectric spectroscopy. J Control Release 2005; 110(1):151–63.

86. Weyhers H, Ehlers S, Hahn H, et al. Solid lipid nanoparticles (SLN)–effects of lipid composition on in vitro degradation and in vivo toxicity. Pharmazie 2006; 61(6):539–44.

87. Hu LD, Tang X, Cui FD. Preparation of solid lipid nanoparticles loaded with all-trans retinoic acid and their evaluation in vitro and in vivo. Yao Xue Xue Bao 2005; 40(1):71–5.

88. Luo Y, Chen D, Ren L, et al. Solid lipid nanoparticles for enhancing vinpocetine's oral bioavailability. J Control Release 2006; 114(1):53–9.

89. Cavalli R, Caputo O, Carlotti ME, et al. Sterilization and freeze-drying of drug-free and drug-loaded solid lipid nanoparticles. Int J Pharm 1997; 148:47–54.

90. Gasco MR. Solid lipid nanospheres from warm micro-emulsions. Pharm Tech Eur 1997; 9:52–8.
91. Heydenreich AV, Westmeier R, Pedersen N, et al. Preparation and purification of cationic solid lipid nanospheres—effects on particle size, physical stability and cell toxicity. Int J Pharm 2003; 254:83–7.
92. Ruckmani K, Sivakumar M, Ganeshkumar PA. Methotrexate loaded solid lipid nanoparticles (SLN) for effective treatment of carcinoma. J Nanosci Nanotechnol 2006; 6(9–10):2991–5.
93. Wang Y, Wu W. In situ evading of phagocytic uptake of stealth solid lipid nanoparticles by mouse peritoneal macrophages. Drug Deliv 2006; 13(3): 189–92.
94. Hu FQ, Jiang SP, Du YZ, et al. Preparation and characterization of stearic acid nanostructured lipid carriers by solvent diffusion method in an aqueous system. Colloids Surf B Biointerfaces 2005; 45(3–4):167–73.
95. Chen DB, Yang TZ, Lu WL, et al. In vitro and in vivo study of two types of long-circulating solid lipid nanoparticles containing paclitaxel. Chem Pharm Bull (Tokyo) 2001; 49(11):1444–7.
96. Gasco MR, Cavalli R, Carlotti ME. Timolol in lipospheres. Die Pharmazie 1992; 47:119–21.
97. Bondi ML, Fontana G, Carlisi B, et al. Preparation and characterization of solid lipid nanoparticles containing cloricromeme. Drug Deliv 2003; 10:245–50.
98. Wissing SA, Muller RH. Solid lipid nanoparticles (SLN)—a novel carrier for UV blockers. Pharmazie 2001; 56(10):783–6.
99. Jenning V, Gohla SH. Encapsulation of retinoids in solid lipid nanoparticles (SLN®). J Microencapsul 2001; 18(2):149–58.
100. Jenning V, Gohla S. Comparison of wax and glyceride solid lipid nanoparticles (SLN®). Int J Pharm 2000; 196(2):219–22.
101. Jenning V. Feste Lipid-Nanopartikel (SLN) als Trägersystem für die dermale Applilkation von Retinol, PhD thesis. 1999, Freie Universität Berlin: Berlin.
102. Jenning V, Gohla S. Comparison of wax and glyceride solid lipid nanoparticles (SLN®). Int J Pharm 2000; 196:219–22.
103. Saupe A. Pharmazeutisch-kosmetische Anwendungen Nanostrukturierter Lipidcarrier (NLC): Lichtschutz und Pflege, PhD thesis. 2004, Freie Universität Berlin: Berlin.
104. Xia Q, Saupe A, Souto EB, Müller RH, Nanostructured lipid carriers (NLC) as a novel carrier for sunscreen formulations. Int J Cosmetic Sci 2007; 29: 473–82.
105. Hu FQ, Jiang SP, Du YZ, et al. Preparation and characteristics of monostearin nanostructured lipid carriers. Int J Pharm 2006; 314(1):83–9.
106. Jenning V, Schäfer-Korting M, Gohla S. Vitamin A-loaded solid lipid nanoparticles for topical use: drug release properties. J Control Release 2000; 66: 115–26.
107. Kim B-D, Na K, Choi H-K. Preparation and characterization of solid lipid nanoparticles (SLN) made of cacao butter and curdlan. Eur J Pharm Sci 2005; 24:199–205.
108. zur Mühlen A, zur Mühlen E, Niehus H, et al. Atomic force microscopy studies of solid lipid nanoparticles. Pharm Res 1996; 13:1411–6.

109. Olbrich C, Bakowsky U, Lehr C-M, et al. Cationic solid-lipid nanoparticles can efficiently bind and transfect plasmid DNA. J Control Release 2001; 77: 345–55.

110. Schöler N, Hahn H, Müller RH, et al. Effect of lipid matrix and size of solid lipid nanoparticles (SLN) on the viability and cytokine production of macrophages. Int J Pharm 2002; 231:167–76.

111. Müller RH, Lucks J-S. Azneistoffträger aus festen Lipidteilchen—feste Lipid Nanosphären (SLN). 1996, European Patent 0605497: Germany.

112. Sjöström B, Bergenståhl B. Preparation of submicron drug particles in lecithin-stabilized o/w emulsions. I. Model studies of the precipitation of cholesteryl acetate. Int J Pharm 1992; 88:53–62.

113. Fessi C, Devissaguet J-P, Puisieux F, et al. Process for the preparation of dispersible colloidal systems of a substance in the form of nanoparticles. 1992; US Patent 5,118,528.

114. Quintanar-Gerrero D, Fessi H, Alléman E, et al. Pseudolatex preparation using a novel emulsion-diffusion process involving direct displacement of partially-water-miscible solvents by distillation. Int J Pharm 1999; 188:155–64.

115. Heurtault B, Saulnier P, Pech B, et al. Nanocapsules lipidiques, procédé de préparation et utilisation comme médicament. 2000, French Patent: W0 01/64328 A1: France.

116. Heurtault B, Saulnier P, Pech B, et al. A novel phase inversion-based process for the preparaion of lipid nanocarriers. Pharm Res 2002; 19:875–80.

117. Müller RH, Mäder K, Gohla S. Solid lipid nanoparticles (SLN) for controlled drug delivery—A review of the state of art. Eur J Pharm Biopharm 2000; 50:161–77.

118. Gasco MR. Method for producing solid lipid microspheres having a narrow size distribution. 1993, US Patent 5 250 236: Italy.

119. Sjöström B, Bergenståhl B, Kronberg B. A method for the preparation of submicron particles of sparingly water-soluble drugs by precipitation in oil-in-water emulsions. II: Influence of the emulsifier, the solvent, and the drug substance. J Pharm Sci 1993; 82:584–9.

120. Sjöström B, Kronberg B, Carlfors J. A method for the preparation of submicron particles of sparingly water-soluble drugs by precipitation in oil-in-water emulsions. I: Influence of emulsification and surfactant concentration. J Pharm Sci 1993; 82:579–83.

121. Dubes A, Parrot-Lopez H, Abdelwahed W, et al. Scanning electron microscopy and atomic force microscopy imaging of solid lipid nanoparticles derived from amphiphilic cyclodextrins. Eur J Pharm Biopharm 2003; 55:279–82.

122. Dubes A, Parrot-Lopez H, Shahgaldian P, et al. Interfacial interactions between amphiphilic cyclodextrins and physiologically relevant cations. J Colloid Interface Sci 2003; 259:103–11.

123. Hu FQ, Hong Y, Yuan H. Preparation and characterization of solid lipid nanoparticles containing peptide. Int J Pharm 2004; 273:29–35.

124. Hu FQ, Yuan H, Zhang HH, et al. Preparation of solid lipid nanoparticles with clobetasol propionate by a novel solvent diffusion method in aqueous system and physicochemical characterization. Int J Pharm 2002; 239:121–8.

125. Trotta M, Debernardi F, Caputo O. Preparation of solid lipid nanoparticles by a solvent emulsification-diffusion technique. Int J Pharm 2003; 257:153–60.

126. Shahgaldian P, Gualbert J, Aïssa K, et al. A study of the freeze-drying conditions of calixarene based solid lipid nanoparticles. Eur J Pharm Biopharm 2003; 55:181–4.

127. Wissing SA, Muller RH. Cosmetic applications for solid lipid nanoparticles (SLN). Int J Pharm 2003; 254(1):65–8.

128. Wissing SA, Müller RH. A novel sunscreen system based on tocopherol acetate incorporated into solid lipid nanoparticles. Int J Cosmet Sci 2001; 23:233–43.

129. Thivolet J, Nicolas JF. Skin ageing and immune competence. Br J Dermatol 1990; 122(Suppl. 35):77–81.

130. Wissing SA, Müller RH. The influence of solid lipid nanoparticles on skin hydration and viscoelasticity - in vivo study. Eur J Pharm Biopharm 2003; 56:67–72.

131. Dingler A. Feste Lipid-Nanopartickel als kolloidale Wirkstoffträgersysteme zur dermalen Applikation, in PhD Thesis. 1998, Freie Universität Berlin: Berlin.

132. Müller, RH, Mehnert, W, Souto, EB. Solid lipid nanoparticles (SLN) and nanostructured lipid carriers (NLC) for dermal delivery, In: Bronaugh L, ed. Percutaneous Absorption. New York: Marcel Dekker, 2005: 719–38.

133. Teeranachaideekul V, Souto EB, Müller RH, et al. Effect of surfactant on the physical and chemical stability of ascorbyl palmitate-loaded NLC system. in AAPS Annual Meeting and Exposition. 2005; Nashville, USA, November 6–10, #M1256.

134. Uner M, Wissing SA, Yener G, et al. Solid lipid nanoparticles (SLN) and nanostructured lipid carriers (NLC) for application of ascorbyl palmitate. Pharmazie 2005; 60(8):577–82.

135. Uner M, Wissing SA, Yener G, et al. Skin moisturizing effect and skin penetration of ascorbyl palmitate entrapped in solid lipid nanoparticles (SLN) and nanostructured lipid carriers (NLC) incorporated into hydrogel. Pharmazie 2005; 60(10):751–5.

136. Teeranachaideekul V, Souto EB, Junyaprasert VB, et al. Long-term physical stability of Q10-loaded NLC at different storage conditions. 2005; AAPS Annual Meeting and Exposition Nashville, USA, November 6–10, #M1255.

137. Müller RH, Dingler A. Feste Lipid-Nanopartikel (Lipopearls™) als neuartiger Carrier für kosmetische und dermatologische Wirkstoffe. Pharm Zeit Dermo 1998; 49:11–5.

138. Eliana, B. Souto, Rainer H. Müller, Lipid nanoparticles (SLN and NLC) for drug delivery. In: Kumar R, Tabata Y, Domb AJ, eds. Nanoparticles for Pharmaceutical Applications. 2005, American Scientific Publishers. Chapter 5, 2007; 103–22.

139. Jenning V, Gysler A, Schafer-Korting M, et al. Vitamin A loaded solid lipid nanoparticles for topical use: occlusive properties and drug targeting to the upper skin. Eur J Pharm Biopharm 2000; 49(3):211–8.

140. Wissing SA, Müller RH. In vitro and in vivo skin permeation of sunscreens from solid lipid nanoparticles (SLN™), supercooled melts and emulsions. in Proc. 4th World Meeting APGI/APV 1135–6. 2002; Florence.

141. Mariani E, Neuhoff C, Bargagna A, et al. Synthesis, in vitro percutaneous absorption and phototoxicity of new benzylidene derivatives of 1,3,3-trimethyl-2-oxabicyclo(2.2.2)octan-6-one as potential UV sunscreens. Int J Pharm 1998; 161:65–73.

142. Müller RH, Mäder K, Wissing S. Mittel mit UV-Strahlung absorbierender und/oder reflektierender Wirkung zum Schutz vor gesundheitsschädlicher UV-Strahnung und Stärkung dern natürlichen Hautbarriere, in Deutsche—Patentenanmeldung Nr. 199 32 156.6 (P 51102). PCT-application PCT/EP00/06534 (P 53516). 2000.

143. Hommoss A, Souto EB, Müller RH. Assessment of the release profiles of a perfume incorporated into NLC dispersions in comparison to reference nanoemulsions. in AAPS Annual Meeting and Exposition. 2005; Nashville, USA, November 6–10, #M1238.

144. Wissing SA, Mäder K, Müller RH. Solid lipid nanopartices (SLN™) as a novel carrier system offering prolonged release of the perfume Allure (Chanel). In Proc Int Symp Control Rel Bioact Mater 2000; 27:311–2.

145. Wissing SA, Mäder K, Müller RH. Prolonged efficacy of the insect lemon oil by incorporation into solid lipid nanoparticles (SLN™). in Proc. 3rd World Meeting APGI/APV, 2000; 439–40. Berlin.

146. Yaziksiz-Iscan Y, Wissing SA, Müller RH, et al. Different production methods for solid lipid nanoparticles (SLN) containing the insect repellent DEET. in Proc. 4th World Meeting APGI/APV, 2002; 789–90. Florence.

147. Yaziksiz-Iscan Y, Hekimoglu S, Sargon MF, et al. In vitro release and skin permeation of DEET incorporated solid lipid nanoparticles in various vehicles. in Proc. 4th World Meeting APGI/APV, 2002; 1183–4. Florence.

148. Dingler A, Hildebrand G, Niehus H, et al. Cosmetic anti-aging formulation based on vitamin E-loaded solid lipid nanoparticles. In Proc Intern Symp Control Rel Bioact Mater 1998; 25:433–4.

27

LidoSite®—Vyteris Iontophoretic Technology

Lakshmi Raghavan and Ashutosh Sharma

Vyteris, Inc., Fair Lawn, New Jersey, U.S.A.

INTRODUCTION

Iontophoresis is based on the principle that a drug can be transported across the skin, which acts as a barrier against entry of foreign objects, under the application of a mild electric current. The quantity and distribution of delivered drug is dependent on several factors which include (*i*) molecular weight of the drug molecule, (*ii*) its ionic charge, (*iii*) concentration of drug, and (*iv*) amount of applied charge, which is dependent on the intensity (amplitude) and duration of applied current. In iontophoretic drug delivery, the flux is directly proportional to the applied current, thereby allowing modulation of drug delivery by controlling the amplitude of applied current and its duration. This precise control of the charge applied can be used to control the drugs to be delivered as topical, or if they are to be pushed deeper into the skin for systemic delivery. Several reviews on iontophoresis and its applications have been published in literature (1–8).

Iontophoretic delivery systems can also be precisely programmed to deliver different dose delivery profiles by controlling the timing of switching on and off of the current. For example, the drug delivery profile can be accurately programmed to mimic that of intravenous infusion or to release the drug for rapid onset. The system can also be preprogrammed to automatically release the drug at regularly timed intervals, avoiding problems of patient compliance with multiple doses or can be programmed to deliver a bolus of drug on demand. These examples are shown in Figure 1.

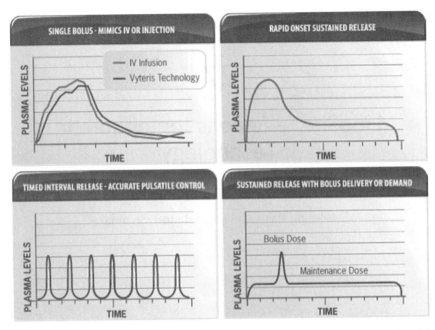

Figure 1 Examples of drug delivery profiles that can be achieved with iontophoresis.

Iontophoretic systems have several advantages which include: (*i*) expand the range of drugs available for transdermal delivery and provide enhanced skin transport; (*ii*) allow rapid onset and offset of delivery profile; (*iii*) are programmable; (*iv*) provide continuous delivery for drugs with short half-life; (*v*) avoid the hepatic "first pass" elimination; and (*vi*) eliminate the inconveniences associated with parenteral therapy.

With all the potential benefits of iontophoretic technology, the approaches in the past have had limited success due to complex delivery systems, which were large and costly and had the propensity to cause skin irritation. These early systems were not easy to use because the drug patches were not prefilled with the drug and the current amplitude and duration had to be adjusted by the clinician at the time of use. In addition, the drug formulations used in these early systems were not developed and/or optimized for iontophoretic delivery. More recently, two companies, Vyteris Inc. (Fair Lawn, NJ) and ALZA Corporation (a Johnson & Johnson Company, Mountain View, CA) have developed small, convenient, simple, prefilled iontophoretic drug delivery systems which are optimized for iontophoresis. These new systems have small electronic controller units (which can be separate or integrated as a part of the patch) and can be easily worn or attached to the body, are easy to operate, and can be preprogrammed to handle simple as well as complex drug delivery profiles.

IONTOPHORESIS THEORY

A simple schematic iontophoretic setup is shown in Figure 2, which depicts the movement of ions through the skin during iontophoresis. When an electric current is applied to the system, positively charged drug ions from the positive reservoir, which is in contact with a positive electrode (anode), migrate into the skin, while biological anions (primarily chloride) travel from the body into the positive reservoir. At the same time, anions from the negative reservoir, which is in contact with a negative electrode (cathode), migrate into the skin, while biological cations such as Na^+ and K^+ flow from the body into the negative or return electrode reservoir. As noted earlier, in iontophoresis the flux is proportional to the applied charge (which is determined by integrating the applied current over time). The drug flux, J, during iontophoresis can be expressed as below, which is derived from Faraday's Law:

$$J = t^*I^*M/Z^*F$$

where t is transport number of the drug, M is molecular weight of the drug ion, Z is charge of the drug ion, I is the current density applied, and F is Faraday's constant. The transport number t is determined by expressing the charge carried by drug ion as a fraction of the total transported charge, and is a unique attribute for each drug ion.

HISTORY OF IONTOPHORESIS

Claims of medication transfer by electricity have been made as early as 1745 (9,10), however, Munck truly demonstrated in 1879 the ability to deliver

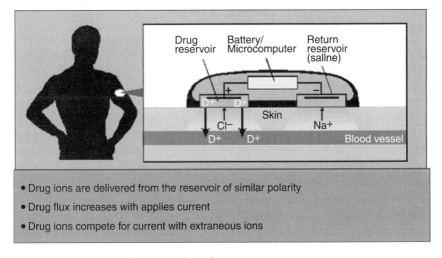

• Drug ions are delivered from the reservoir of similar polarity

• Drug flux increases with applies current

• Drug ions compete for current with extraneous ions

Figure 2 Schematic of an iontophoretic system.

ions by delivering strychnine into a rabbit with an electric current (10). The first scientific experiments relating to the mechanism of iontophoresis were performed by LeDuc in 1908 (11) Using two rabbits placed in series, he introduced strychnine into one and cyanide into the other, each depending on the polarity. He was able to determine which ions were introduced by observing the signs preceding death. Until 1924, since that study, numerous studies were devoted to ophthalmological iontophoresis. Iontophoresis was virtually discarded until the early 1940s when it was again used experimentally for the transfer of penicillin and sulfadiazine into the infected eyes of animals with results that were reported as successful. Historically several drugs have been administered using iontophoresis for several indications some of which include pain management, neurodegenerative conditions, and cardiovascular diseases (3). Until recently, this technology was considered cumbersome and unsuitable for commercial applications. However, the development of electronics and battery technologies has enabled the development of iontophoretic technology not only to deliver small molecules but also large peptides.

VYTERIS IONTOPHORETIC TECHNOLOGY: LIDOSITE®

In developing an iontophoretic drug delivery system, careful considerations should be made in the selection of: electrode material, drug reservoir, drug formulation, duration of iontophoresis, and current density applied. In Vyteris' LidoSite system for topical delivery of lidocaine (a local anesthetic), the electrode material for the system is comprised of Ag/AgCl, which prevents pH drifts during the electrochemical reaction at the electrode and produces chloride ion at the cathode. The drug reservoir consists of a polymer-based hydrogel providing adherence to the skin and easily adapting to the contours of the body.

An ideal topical anesthetic for minimizing the pain associated with needlesticks (during cannulation or venipuncture) or pain associated with minor dermal surgical procedures should be easy to apply, safe, and rapidly effective (12). Several topical formulations of local anesthetics have been developed, such as a eutectic mixture of local anesthetics (EMLA) cream (13), which contains a combination of lidocaine (2.5%) and prilocaine (2.5%), and ElaMax (14), a liposomal lidocaine formulation. While both formulations have been shown to be effective in reducing the pain associated with venipuncture and venous cannulation (15) EMLA cream requires at least 1 hour from application to provide effective anesthesia, while ElaMax requires 30 minutes. In addition, many patients still experience significant pain despite the use of these anesthetics (16).

LidoSite was developed to fulfill an unmet need for an advanced drug delivery system in the applications of topical anesthetics. A major concern among patients, both adult and children is the management of pain associated with procedures such as catheter insertions and blood draws. In fact a recent survey (covering 6 month period) conducted (17) showed that about 15 million adults and 5 million children aged over five suffer from either needle-phobia or high discomfort when faced with the prospect of getting a needle injection or a blood draw procedure. A product capable of alleviating or reducing the fear of pain associated with these procedures would help the patients as well as healthcare professionals to overcome public health challenges. Such a product should be easy to use, have a fast onset of action and be broadly applicable to a large variety of patients including pediatric patients.

The LidoSite Topical System is a drug–device combination product consisting of a LidoSite Patch ("drug") and a LidoSite Controller ("medical device"),which is battery powered and regulates the current applied. In developing such a system, challenges with regards to developing an in vitro test method for a topical application, establishing an in vitro/in vivo correlation, and performing toxicology studies were encountered and addressed.

The development of an in vitro drug release test for the LidoSite patch was challenging because of the small amount of drug released during the 10-minute application and to measure drug released from the patch when current is applied rather than drug released passively. A customized perforated barrier membrane has been developed with characteristics to allow current to pass during application consistently yet minimize passive drug flux.

An in vivo study was conducted (prior to the development of an in vitro test) using radio labeled compounds and detection techniques to determine the amounts of lidocaine and epinephrine delivered to the skin of anesthetized pigs using the LidoSite system. The results indicate that only a small amount of lidocaine (467 μg) and epinephrine (2.5 μg) are delivered.

On the issue of toxicity, since both lidocaine and epinephrine are safe and effective therapeutic agents within therapeutic labeling, and have a long history of use, their systemic and topical effects are well documented. Based on these data and discussions with the regulatory agency, a preclinical testing plan was developed that focused primarily on dermal effects (i.e., local irritation and sensitization) during and following topical iontophoretic delivery.

In small clinical trials, lidocaine iontophoresis has been shown to provide effective dermal anesthesia for needlesticks in 7–15 minutes. The LidoSite Topical Anesthetic System (Fig. 3) developed by Vyteris, Inc. (Fair Lawn, NJ) is a small, easy to use, iontophoretic lidocaine delivery system composed of a drug-filled patch connected to a controller. The patch is a one-time use disposable drug product, which contains a 5-cm^2 circular drug reservoir (anode) that delivers lidocaine and epinephrine to the skin, and an oval return reservoir (cathode) containing electrolytes. The portable

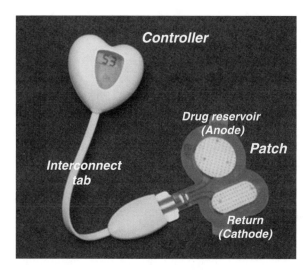

Figure 3   LidoSite® lidocaine iontophoretic drug delivery system.

controller, which is the more expensive component of the system, can be reused approximately 100 times before it is rendered unusable. It contains a non-replaceable battery that provides up to hundred 10-minute applications of direct current at 1.77 mA, and uses discrete analog circuitry to control the delivery of current to the patch. An embedded microprocessor is primarily intended to monitor the current application during controller operation and to control the system indicators. To accomplish these tasks, the micro-processor is programmed to run as a time source. Delivery is initiated by pressing the "On" button, which allows the device to detect skin at the patch site. Once started, the profile proceeds through three stages of ramp up, constant current delivery, and ramp down.

The controller incorporates both visual and audio indicators to inform the user about the system status. A green light-emitting diode (LED) is used to indicate normal conditions, while activation of a yellow LED alerts the user to an abnormal condition. The controller also has an internal beeper that sounds at the end of every delivery or self-check function. A liquid crystal display (LCD) shows the number of patches used with a given controller.

In most iontophoretic systems, iontophoresis is measured as total charge delivered in milliampere-minutes units. The total charge delivery using the lidocaine system is 17 mA-min, which achieves relatively rapid and effective analgesia, as well as minimizes irritation at the site of application. The drug formulation contains lidocaine and epinephrine. The addition of epinephrine improves the analgesic effect, presumably because of its vaso-constrictor activity. The pH of the drug formulation is 4.5 at which both lidocaine and epinephrine are both positively charged. The lidocaine drug delivery system (Fig. 3), consists of a controller and a drug patch connected through an interconnect tab. The patch is made up of a drug containing reservoir (circular anode) and a return reservoir (oval cathode), both containing Ag/AgCl electrodes under their respective reservoirs.

Two prospective, randomized, double-blind, placebo-controlled trials were conducted to assess the analgesia provided during venipuncture and intravenous cannulation. (18). The first trial utilized a 10 cm visual analog scale (VAS) to assess pain experienced by 270 subjects ≥18 years of age. The mean (±SD) VAS score was lower in the lidocaine system group (0.8 ± 1.5 cm) than in the placebo group (2.5 ± 2.3 cm) ($p < 0.001$). The second trial utilized a weighted nine face integrated scale (NFIS) to evaluate the pain experienced by 256 pediatric subjects ages 5–17 years. The mean weighted NFIS score was lower for the subjects treated with lidocaine system compared with those treated with placebo. Two additional clinical studies have demonstrated better pain control during surgical removal of superficial skin lesions using laser surgery and incisional/excisional surgery, when lidocaine system was applied prior to surgery.

REGULATORY ASPECTS OF IONTOPHORETIC TECHNOLOGY

From a regulatory point of view, a prefilled iontophoretic product falls into a growing class of new medical products called combination (drug–device) products (19). These iontophoretic systems contain a drug prefilled patch and a controller that controls all aspects of drug delivery, and has built-in fail-safe mechanisms as a part of the control circuitry. On the other hand, the patch and controller can be integrated into one system or be separated into a patch (a drug product) and a controller (a medical device) under the U.S. Food and Drug Administration (FDA) regulations.

Separation of the drug and controller provides for several advantages which include: (i) controller can be a reusable device thereby being more cost-effective per use; (ii) since controller is a medical device, future changes to the controller can be easily incorporated without changing the patch design which may require more extensive testing. A separate controller and patch requires submissions to two separate centers at the FDA. A 510(k) Premarket Notification application is required for the controller and is submitted to Center for Devices and Radiological Health, and a New Drug Application is required for the patch and is submitted to Center for Drug Evaluation and Research. In contrast, an integrated patch/controller system requires a single NDA and maybe more user friendly since it eliminates a step of connecting the patch to the controller. Due to a growing number of products falling in this new category of combination drug–device products, the FDA has established an Office of Combination Products, whose role includes helping the industry in navigating the regulatory pathway associated with these novel products/technologies.

The lidocaine drug delivery system developed by Vyteris, Inc. is being targeted as a topical anesthetic to achieve local dermal analgesia on intact skin, prior to venous cannulation, IV puncture, or local dermal procedures. The underlying technology developed as a part of the lidocaine drug delivery system provides several features, which are desirable such as programmability and noninvasiveness, and can be used to develop delivery systems for delivering other therapeutic drugs requiring local or systemic delivery.

FUTURE POTENTIAL OF IONTOPHORETIC TECHNOLOGY

The FDA approval of iontophoretic products such as LidoSite (17) and IONSYS (20) has encouraged others in the industry to develop commercial products. Companies like NuPathe (Conshohocken, PA), Dharma Therapeutics (Seattle, WA), and Transport Pharmaceuticals Inc. (Framingham, MA) are some of the companies with iontophoretic drug products in various stages of development. The progress made by Vyteris in delivery of a peptide to treat female infertility opens other avenues for the application of iontophoretic technology. Combination of iontophoretic technology with other complementary technologies that impair the stratum corneum, will expand its application further into delivering of large therapeutic doses and/or larger molecules (larger protein and peptides). As innovative materials and formulations are developed, and further advances are made in the manufacturing of these products, it is not far to imagine that iontophoretic products will become more mainstream in the coming years.

REFERENCES

1. Burnette RR. Iontophoresis. In: Hadgraft J, Guy RH, eds. Transdermal Drug Delivery. Developmental Issues and Research Initiatives. New York: Marcel Dekker, 1989:247–91.
2. Tyle P. Iontophoretic devices for drug delivery. Pharm Res 1986; 3:318–26.
3. Kalia YN, Naik A, Garrison J, Guy RH. Iontophoretic drug delivery. Adv Drug Deliv Rev 2004; 56:619–58.
4. Pikal MJ. The role of electroosmotic flow in transdermal iontophoresis. Adv Drug Deliv Rev 1992; 9:201–37.
5. Degado-Charro MB, Guy RH. Iontophoresis: applications in drug delivery and noninvasive monitoring. In: Hadgraft J, Guy RH, eds. Transdermal Drug Delivery. New York: Marcel Dekker, 2003: 199–225.
6. Sage BH, Rivere JR. Model systems in iontophoresis transport efficacy. Adv Drug Deliv Rev 1992; 9:265–87.
7. Phipps JB, Gyory JR. Trandermal ion migration. Adv Drug Deliv Rev 1992; 9: 137–76.

8. Scott ER, Phipps B, Gyory R, Padmanabahan RV. Electrotransport system for transdermal drug delivery: a practical implementation of iontophoresis. In: Wise DL, ed. Handbook of Pharmaceutical Controlled Release Technology. New York: Marcel Dekker, 2000: 617–59.
9. Chien YW, Banga AK. Iontophoretic (transdermal) delivery of drugs: overview of historical development. J Pharm Sci 1989; 78:353–4.
10. Banga AK. Electrically Assisted Transdermal and Topical Drug Delivery. Bristol: Taylor & Francis Group, 1998.
11. Leduc S. Electric Ions and their Uses in Medicine. London: Rebman, 1908.
12. Lener EV, Bucalo BD, Kist DA, Moy RL. Topical anesthetic agents in dermatologic surgery. Dermatol Surg 1997; 23:673–83.
13. www.astrazeneca.com
14. www.ferndalelabs.com
15. Eichenfield LF, Funk A, Fallon-Friedlander S, Cunningham BB. A clinical study to evaluate the efficacy of ELA-Max (4% liposomal lidocaine) as compared with eutectic mixture of local anesthetics cream for pain reduction of venipuncture in children. Pediatrics 2002; 109:1093–9.
16. Kleiber C, Sorenson M, Whiteside K, Gronstal BA, Tannous R. Topical anesthetics for intravenous insertion in children: a randomized equivalency study. Pediatrics 2002; 110:758–61.
17. TVG Study, Vyteris Inc. 2006, www.vyteris.com
18. Zempsky WT, Sullivan J, Paulson DM, Hoath SB. Evaluation of a low-dose lidocaine iontophoresis system for topical anesthesia in adults and children: a randomized, controlled trial. Clin Ther 2004; 26:1110–9.
19. www.fda.gov
20. www.alza.com

28

Nail Delivery

Darren M. Green, Keith R. Brain, and Kenneth A. Walters

An-eX Analytical Services Ltd., Cardiff, U.K.

INTRODUCTION

The human nail can be afflicted by several disease states including parony-
chia, psoriasis and infections due to bacteria, viruses or fungi. Whilst rarely
life threatening, these generate self-consciousness and psychological stress.
Approximately 50% of all problems result from fungal infections, onychomycoses, and the prevalence of these may be as high as 27% in Europe (1)
and 10% in the United States (2). There are many treatment regimens, but
the most common involves oral dosing with antifungal agents such as terbinafine or itraconazole (3). Experimental techniques for investigation of the
penetration and distribution of chemicals into and through the nail plate
demonstrated that it is possible to deliver drugs to the nail following topical
application and led to the development of newer more effective topical products and regimens for treatment of onychomycoses and other nail diseases
(4–9). This chapter describes nail structure and chemical composition, provides an overview of our knowledge of permeation of molecules through the
nail plate, and reviews selected clinical studies designed to determine the efficacy of topical treatment of onychomycoses.

NAIL STRUCTURE

The nail plate is composed of layers of flattened keratinized cells fused into a
dense but somewhat elastic mass. Nail plate cells grow distally from the
matrix at a rate of about 0.1 mm per day. During keratinization, cells
undergo shape and other changes similar to those experienced by the epidermal cells forming the stratum corneum. There are three very tightly knit

keratinized layers, a thin outermost dorsal lamina, a thicker intermediate lamina and an innermost ventral layer (10). Keratins in hair and nail are classified as "hard" trichocyte keratins.

As a cornified epithelial structure, the chemical composition of the nail plate has many similarities to hair (11). The major components are keratin proteins with small amounts (0.1–1.0%) of lipid, the latter presumably located in the intercellular spaces. The nail contains significant amounts of phospholipid, mainly in the dorsal and intermediate layers, which contribute to its flexibility. The principal plasticizer is water, normally present at 7–12%. Gupchup and Zatz (12) provide an excellent review of the structural characteristics of human nail.

NAIL PLATE PERMEABILITY

In Vitro Measurements

The first systematic studies on nail plate permeability were carried out by Walters and colleagues in the late 1970s (13–16). These indicated marked differences between the permeability characteristics of the nail plate and epidermis which were attributed to the relative amounts of lipid and protein within the structures (13) and possible differences in the physicochemical nature of the respective phases. The nail plate was permeable to dilute aqueous solutions of a series of low MW homologous alcohols but permeation decreased as a function of increasing alkyl chain length up to octanol. Interestingly, the applied concentration of alcohols was a determinant of their penetration velocities, with pure liquid forms giving a five fold decrease in permeation (14). It was suggested that the nail plate possesses a highly "polar" penetration route that was capable of excluding permeants on the basis of their hydrophobicity. The existence of a minor "lipid" pathway through the nail plate, which could become rate-controlling for hydrophobic solutes, was suggested based on the significant decrease in permeation of hydrophobic n-decanol following nail plate delipidization (14).

Mertin and Lippold (17–19) extensively studied nail and hoof penetration in vitro. Hoof membrane was mainly used to examine permeation from different formulations. Permeability coefficients through both nail plate and hoof membranes did not increase with increasing oil-water partition coefficient (range from 7 to >51,000) or lipophilicity, indicating that these barriers behaved like hydrophilic gel membranes rather than lipophilic partition membranes (as in stratum corneum). Further studies with paracetamol and phenacetin showed that maximum flux was a function of drug solubility in water or in the swollen keratin. Mertin and Lippold were able to predict the maximum flux of ten antimycotics through the nail plate on the basis of their penetration rates through hoof membrane and their water solubilities. Their speculative extrapolation on permeation of amorolfine was in remarkably close agreement to the value obtained by Franz (20) using human nail plate. Bovine hoof membranes were also used by Monti et al. (5) to evaluate the effect of formulation on the transungual permeation of ciclopirox. Comparison of an experimental water-soluble lacquer (based on hydroxypropyl chitosan) with the marketed water-insoluble lacquer (Penlac) showed that, although steady-state permeation rates were similar, lag-times were considerably less for the experimental lacquer. This was tentatively attributed to a strong adhesion between hydroxypropyl chitosan and nail plate keratin. This group also used bovine hoof membrane to determine penetration of piroctone olamine into keratinous matrices (21). Although no transmembrane permeation was observed, following 30 hours exposure, approximately 11% of the drug penetrated into the hoof.

Several investigators have evaluated nail plate penetration of drugs following topical application in vitro (22,23) and in vivo (24–28). Kobayashi et al. (22) demonstrated that molecular size was the principal determinant of the rate and extent of permeation across nail plate. Furthermore, measurement of nail permeation of a series of *p*-hydroxybenzoic acid esters indicated, in broad agreement with earlier work of Walters et al. (14), that permeant lipophilicity was not an important determinant and that permeation decreased with increasing hydrophobicity. Very importantly, their studies also showed that, for the model permeant 5-fluorouracil, normal nail plate had similar permeation characteristics to infected nail plate, suggesting that normal plates can be used to predict drug distribution in diseased plates.

Recognizing the possibility of photodynamic therapy for onychomycosis (29,30), Donnelly et al. (6) investigated delivery of 5-aminolevulinic acid (ALA) to the nail from a bioadhesive-patch in vitro. After 72 hours approximately 90% of the applied drug had penetrated the nail, with an average flux of $2.54 \ 10^{-4} \ mg/cm^2 \ s^{-1}$. This was quite a remarkable rate of penetration and, given that ALA is a small highly polar molecule, further confirmation of the hydrophilic nature of the nail barrier. They concluded that it might be possible to use topical ALA PDT therapy as a viable alternative in the treatment of onychomycosis.

Hui et al. (31) developed a drilling technique for assessing drug delivery to the inner nail plate in vitro and used it to determine the effect of dimethyl sulfoxide (DMSO) on the penetration of urea, salicylic acid and ketoconazole. Nail plate composition suggests that it would be comparatively insensitive to the effects of stratum corneum penetration enhancers that produce their effects mainly by delipidization or fluidisation of intercellular lipids. The nail plate is incapable of absorbing much applied DMSO (32) and a decrease in absorption of methanol and hexanol applied with DMSO was noted by Walters et al. (16). On the other hand, an increase in nail plate content of econazole when applied in a formulation containing

DMSO was reported (33) and, following pretreatment with DMSO, an increase in the nail absorption of the anti-fungal amorolfine was demonstrated (20). Hui et al. (31) determined that DMSO was capable of enhancing the concentration of all three permeants in the ventral region of the nail plate but, paradoxically, reduced the concentration of ketoconazole and salicylic acid in the dorsal regions. The data for the effects of DMSO remain ambiguous.

Hui et al. (34) determined the effects of the lipophilic skin penetration enhancer 2-n-nonyl-1,3-dioxolane (SEPA) on the in vitro nail delivery of econazole and to evaluate the nail penetration of ciclopirox from three topical formulations (4). In the first study (34) lacquer formulations containing econazole with and without SEPA (18%) were applied twice daily for 14 days to human nail plates. The amounts of econazole in the inner part of the nail plate were 11.1 mcg/mg nail powder (with SEPA) and 1.78 mcg/mg (without SEPA). The amounts of econazole that had permeated through the nail plates were 48 mg (with SEPA) and 0.2 mg (without SEPA). In a separate study, radiolabeled SEPA was unsurprizingly found not to significantly penetrate the nail, and the mechanisms of penetration enhancement were presumed to be at the formulation/nail interface.

In the subsequent study over 14 days (4) Penlac lacquer (8% ciclopirox) was evaluated alongside the gels Loprox (0.77% ciclopirox) and an experimental formulation containing 2% ciclopirox. Ciclopirox delivery into and through the nail was greater from the marketed gel than from either the experimental gel or the nail lacquer. The amount of drug that penetrated into and through the nail was also greater from the marketed gel. It was concluded that the formulation played an important role in the delivery of ciclopirox. Notwithstanding the differences in the amount of ciclopirox delivered, all three formulations delivered sufficient drug to generate "in nail" concentrations far in excess of the minimum inhibitory concentrations (MICs) for most nail invasive dermatophytes and yeasts.

In our laboratory we have refined the nail drilling technique to allow determination of drug distribution in three layers of the nail plate (dorsal, intermediate, and ventral) and successfully adapted the technology as a rapid formulation-screening tool.

Quintanar-Guerrero et al. (35) evaluated the influence of keratolytic agents (papain, urea, and salicylic acid) on the permeability of three imidazole anti-mycotics (miconazole nitrate, ketoconazole, and itraconazole) using healthy human nails in vitro. In the absence of any enhancer the nail was relatively impermeable to these anti-mycotics. Furthermore, permeation of these anti-mycotics was not improved by pretreatment with salicylic acid alone (20% for 10 days), or by application of the drug in a 40% urea solution. The combined effects of papain (15% for 1 day) and salicylic acid (20% for 10 days) were capable of enhancing nail plate permeability.

In contrast, Mohorcic et al. (36), evaluating the use of keratinolytic enzymes to decrease barrier properties, found that keratinase acted on the intercellular regions and caused corneocytes on the dorsal surface to separate. Permeation studies using bovine hoof membranes showed that the enzyme doubled the flux and membrane-vehicle partition coefficient of the model penetrant, metformin, but had little effect on the diffusion coefficient. This suggests that the effect of the enzyme was confined to the outer surface layers of the hoof membrane.

IN VIVO MEASUREMENTS

The pharmacokinetics of sertaconazole, an imidazole antifungal drug, following topical application was evaluated in vivo (28). Sixteen healthy adults were treated with nail patches containing sertaconazole (3.63 mg), which were placed on a thumbnail of each subject. Patches were replaced weekly over six weeks. Nail clippings, used nail patches and blood samples were analyzed for sertaconazole. Concentrations $> 100\,\mu g/g$, exceeding the MICs for all relevant dermatophytes, were detected in all treated nail samples. Analysis of the residual patches indicated that 16–71% of the drug had penetrated into the nail. No sertaconazole was detected in plasma samples. It was concluded that nail patches should have beneficial therapeutic effects.

Ceschin-Roques et al. (24) assessed the bioavailability of 8% ciclopirox from a lacquer formulation. Nail lacquer was applied to the fingernails of healthy volunteers and the total amount of ciclopirox in the nail was $3.35\,\mu g/mg$ following 30 days treatment (sufficient to kill the fungal pathogens).

Similarly, van Hoogdalem et al. (26) evaluated the in vivo nail penetration of oxiconazole. Six healthy volunteers were treated with 1% w/v oxiconazole lotion applied to the nail twice daily for 6 weeks and nail clippings were collected every 2 weeks over an 8-week period. Maximum drug levels in the upper 0–50 µm layers varied between 120 and 1420 ng/mg. Total nail uptake was less than 0.2% of the topical dose. Co-delivery with acetylcysteine (15% w/v in the oxiconazole lotion), a compound that will disrupt keratin disulfide bonds, generated a statistically significant prolonged residence time of oxiconazole in the 51–100 µm nail layers. Peak drug levels in the upper 0–50 µm layer increased from 790 ng/mg to 1570 ng/ml. They concluded that the effect of acetylcysteine was related to increased binding of oxiconazole to nail constituents.

CLINICAL DATA SUPPORTING TOPICAL THERAPY OF NAIL DISEASES

For many years dermatologists believed that topical treatment for anything other than the most superficial infections of the nail plate was futile.

The nail plate was viewed as an impermeable barrier only to be breached via the blood supply to the germinative nail matrix and prolonged oral dosing with powerful anti-fungal agents was the order of the day. However, as our knowledge of the nail plate barrier has improved, our ability to rationally develop anti-fungal agents and delivery vehicles specifically for the topical treatment of nail diseases has increased. The dermatologists' armamentarium has been supplemented with nail lacquers and other formulations including those containing tioconazole, amorolfine, ciclopirox, clobetasol-17-propionate, and tazarotene. However, the true test of any therapeutic regimen is efficacy.

The conservative approach is to supplement oral therapy with topical treatment. Nakano et al. (9) performed a pilot study to assess the safety and efficacy of pulse therapy with oral terbinafine in 66 patients with onychomycosis. Each pulse consisted of oral terbinafine (500 mg/day) for 1 week followed by a 3-week interval. Topical 1% terbinafine cream was applied daily. Efficacy was assessed 1 year after treatment initiation. There was a complete cure in 51 patients (approximately 77%), marked improvement in five patients, improvement in five patients and slight improvement in one patient. Four patients showed no change. Although they concluded that terbinafine pulse therapy in combination with topical application of terbinafine cream was safe and effective, it was not possible to determine whether the topical applications improved the outcome. An earlier study (37) using a similar oral treatment regimen but with no supplemental topical therapy reported 74% cure rate, suggesting that topical application was of little additive benefit. However, it is important to appreciate that the application vehicle is a very important determinant for successful delivery of drug to the nail and that the cream used in the Nakano study was probably not optimized in this respect. Furthermore, the highly lipophilic nature of terbinafine suggests that it would not penetrate into the nail to any great extent.

A better indication of the usefulness of supplemental topical therapy can be obtained from the work of Rigopoulos et al. (38) who evaluated the combination of systemic and topical anti-fungals to improve the cure rates and reduce the duration of systemic treatment for onychomycoses. They used itraconazole pulse therapy combined with amorolfine and compared this with itraconazole alone in the treatment of nail Candida. Ninety patients with Candida fingernail were randomized into two treatment groups of 45. Group 1 received itraconazole pulse therapy for 2 months with amorolfine 5% solution nail lacquer application for 6 months, while group 2 received monotherapy with three pulses of itraconazole. Eighty-five patients, with a mean duration of onychomycosis of 11 months, were analysed. After three months of therapy, mycological cure was seen in 32 (74%) of 43 patients in group 1 and in 25 (60%) of 42 patients in group 2. Following 9 months therapy, a global cure was seen in 40 patients (93%) in group 1 and in 34 patients (81%) in group 2. Compared with oral itraconazole alone, the combination achieved greater mycological cure and increased total cure rate. Although statistical analysis showed no statistically significant difference ($p > 0.1$) between the two treatment groups, the combination of topical amorolfine and oral itraconazole exhibited considerable synergy.

Baran and Coquard (27) treated 13 onychomycotic patients, aged 25–78 years, with a solution of 1% fluconazole and 20% urea in an ethanol–water mixture, applied once daily. There was complete resolution of the condition in four cases and four patients demonstrated a 90% improvement. Of four patients with onychomycoses in both big toenails, two showed 50% improvement bilaterally and in the remaining two patients there was a 90% improvement in one nail and a 50% improvement in the other. Overall the response to local therapy was appreciable.

Gupta et al. (39) reviewed the efficacy and safety of 8% ciclopirox nail lacquer in the treatment of onychomycosis. In one study, 223 patients were randomized to treatment and in another, 237 subjects were randomized. Both studies were conducted in the United States. The active and placebo formulations were applied daily for 48 weeks and mycologic evaluation was performed every 12 weeks. Data from these pivotal trials demonstrated that ciclopirox nail lacquer was significantly more effective than placebo in the treatment of onychomycosis. At the end of the treatment period, the mycologic cure rate in the first study was 29% and 11% in the ciclopirox and vehicle groups, respectively, and in the second study the cure rate was 36% and 9%, respectively. In non-US studies, mycologic cure rates ranged from 47% to 86%, and the lacquer demonstrated a broad spectrum of activity showing efficacy against Candida species and some non-dermatophytes. The authors concluded that the nail lacquer provided a treatment choice with a favorable benefit-to-risk ratio. In subsequent studies, topical ciclopirox efficacy has been confirmed and, more recently, the efficacy of the lacquer in a case of infantile congenital candidal onychomycosis was reported to be excellent (40).

Not all nail diseases are fungal or bacterial infections. Psoriasis can affect the entire nail plate and is a common feature in psoriasis patients. Recently, a new lacquer formulation containing 8% clobetasol-17-propionate was evaluated for the efficacy and safety (7). Ten patients, with both nail bed and matrix psoriasis, were treated with the nail lacquer applied once daily for 21 days and subsequently twice weekly for 9 months. There was a reduction of all the nail alterations, including nail pain, within 4 weeks of initiating therapy and response was directly related to the length of treatment. The lacquer was a safe and effective treatment for nail bed and matrix psoriasis.

Tazarotene gel has also been evaluated as a therapy for nail psoriasis. In a double-blind, randomized, vehicle-controlled, parallel-group trial, 31 patients with fingernail psoriasis were randomized to receive tazarotene or vehicle gel, which was applied daily for up to 24 weeks to 2 target fingernails, one under occlusion and one unoccluded (41). Tazarotene treatment resulted in a significantly greater reduction in onycholysis (loosening of the nail plate-nail bed connection) in both occluded and non-occluded nails together with a significantly greater reduction in pitting in occluded nails. The gel was well tolerated.

CONCLUSION

The permeability characteristics of the human nail plate are well understood and topical formulations can be designed to optimize drug delivery into the nail. The formulations are well tolerated upon prolonged use. Upon clinical examination the topical formulations have been found to be reasonably effective as mono-therapies and have been shown to be synergistic with oral therapy. Treatment with topical agents has been described as cost effective (42) with topical amorolfine being the most effective monotherapy both in terms of efficacy and cost (43,44). Although present consensus is that dual therapy (oral and topical) affords the most effective treatment (45), further investigation into means to enhance penetration into and permeation across the nail plate will inevitably lead to more effective topical preparations.

REFERENCES

1. Hay R. Literature review. Onychomycosis. J Eur Acad Dermatol Venereol 2005; 19(Suppl. 1):1–7.
2. Elewski E. Onychomycosis: pathogenesis, diagnosis, and management. Clin Microbiol Rev 1998; 11(3):415–29.
3. Baran R, Gupta AK, Pierard GE. Pharmacotherapy of onychomycosis. Expert Opin Pharmacother 2005; 6(4):609–24.
4. Hui X, Wester RC, Barbadillo S, et al. Ciclopirox delivery into the human nail plate. J Pharm Sci 2004; 93(10):2545–8.
5. Monti D, Saccomani L, Chetoni P, et al. In vitro transungual permeation of ciclopirox from a hydroxypropyl chitosan-based, water-soluble nail lacquer. Drug Dev Ind Pharm 2005; 31(1):11–7.
6. Donnelly RF, McCarron PA, Lightowler JM, et al. Bioadhesive patch-based delivery of 5-aminolevulinic acid to the nail for photodynamic therapy of onychomycosis. J Contr Rel 2005; 103(2):381–92.
7. Sanchez Regana M, Martin Ezquerra G, Umbert Millet P, Llambi Mateos F. Treatment of nail psoriasis with 8% clobetasol nail lacquer: positive experience in 10 patients. J Eur Acad Dermatol Venereol 2005; 19(5):573–7.
8. Bristow IR, Baran R. Topical and oral combination therapy for toenail onychomycosis: an updated review. J Am Podiatr Med Assoc 2006; 96(2):116–9.
9. Nakano N, Hiruma M, Shiraki Y, et al. Combination of pulse therapy with terbinafine tablets and topical terbinafine cream for the treatment of dermatophyte onychomycosis: A pilot study. J Dermatol 2006; 33:753–8.

10. Runne U, Orfanos CE. The human nail—structure, growth and pathological changes. Curr Probl Dermatol 1981; 9:102–49.
11. Baden HP, Goldsmith LA, Fleming B. A comparative study of the physicochemical properties of human keratinized tissues. Biochim Biophys Acta 1973; 322:269–78.
12. Gupchup GV, Zatz JL. Structural characteristics and permeability properties of the human nail. J Cosmet Sci 1999; 50:363–85.
13. Walters KA, Flynn GL, Marvel JR. Physicochemical characterization of the human nail: I. Pressure sealed apparatus for measuring nail plate permeabilities. J Invest Dermatol 1981; 76:76–9.
14. Walters KA, Flynn GL, Marvel JR. Physicochemical characterization of the human nail: Permeation pattern for water and the homologous alcohols and differences with respect to the stratum corneum. J Pharm Pharmacol 1983; 35: 28–33.
15. Walters KA, Flynn GL, Marvel JR. Penetration of the human nail: the effects of vehicle pH on the permeation of miconazole. J Pharm Pharmacol 1985; 37: 498–9.
16. Walters KA, Flynn GL, Marvel JR. Physicochemical characterization of the human nail: solvent effects on the permeation of homologous alcohols. J Pharm Pharmacol 1985; 37:771–5.
17. Mertin D, Lippold BC. In vitro permeability of the human nail and of a keratin membrane from bovine hooves: Influence of the partition coefficient octanol/water and the water solubility of drugs on their permeability and maximum flux. J Pharm Pharmacol 1997; 49:30–4.
18. Mertin D, Lippold BC. In vitro permeability of the human nail and of a keratin membrane from bovine hooves: Penetration of chloramphenicol from lipophilic vehicles and a nail lacquer. J Pharm Pharmacol 1997; 49:241–5.
19. Mertin D, Lippold BC. In vitro permeability of the human nail and of a keratin membrane from bovine hooves: Prediction of the penetration rate of antimycotics through the nail plate and their efficacy. J Pharm Pharmacol 1997; 49: 866–72.
20. Franz TJ. Absorption of amorolfine through human nail. Dermatology 1992, 184(Suppl. 1):18–20.
21. Dubini F, Bellotti MG, Frangi A, et al. In vitro antimycotic activity and nail permeation models of a piroctone olamine (octopirox) containing transungual water soluble technology. Arzneimittelforsch 2005; 55(8):478–83.
22. Kobayashi Y, Komatsu T, Sumi M, et al. In vitro permeation of several drugs through the human nail plate: relationship between physicochemical properties and nail permeability of drugs. Eur J Pharm Sci 2004; 21:471–7.
23. Neubert RH, Gensbugel C, Jackel A, et al. Different physicochemical properties of antimycotic agents are relevant for penetration into and through human nails. Pharmazie 2006; 61(7):604–7.
24. Ceschin-Roques CG, Hanel H, Pruja-Bougaret SM, et al. Ciclopirox nail lacquer 8%: in vivo penetration into and through nails and in vitro effect on pig skin. Skin Pharmacol 1991; 4:89–94.
25. Schatz F, Brautigam M, Dobrowolski E, et al. Nail incorporation kinetics of terbinafine in onychomycosis patients. Clin Exp Dermatol 1995; 20:377–83.

26. van Hoogdalem EJ, van den Hoven WE, Terpstra IJ, et al. Nail penetration of the antifungal oxiconazole after repeated topical application in healthy volunteers, and the effect of acetylcysteine. Eur J Pharm Sci 1997; 5:119–27.

27. Baran R, Coquard F. Combination of fluconazole and urea in a nail lacquer for treating onychomycosis. J Dermatol Treat 2005; 16(1):52–5.

28. Susilo R, Korting HC, Greb W, et al. Nail penetration of sertaconazole with a sertaconazole-containing nail patch formulation. Am J Clin Dermatol 2006; 7(4):259–62.

29. Smijs TGM, Schuitmaker HJ. Photodynamic inactivation of the dermatophyte *Trichophyton rubrum*. Photochem Photobiol 2003; 77:556–60.

30. Kamp H, Tietz H-J, Lutz M, et al. Antifungal effect of 5-aminolevulinic acid PDT in *Trichophyton rubrum*. Mycoses 2005; 48:101–7.

31. Hui X, Shainhouse Z, Tanojo H et al. Enhanced human nail drug delivery: nail inner drug content assayed by new unique method. J Pharm Sci 2002; 91: 189–95.

32. Kligman AM. Topical pharmacology and toxicology of dimethyl sulfoxide. J Am Med Assoc 1965; 193:796–804.

33. Stuttgen G, Bauer E. Bioavailability, skin and nail penetration of topically applied antimycotics. Mycosen 1982; 25:74–80.

34. Hui X, Chan TCK, Barbadillo S, et al. Enhanced econazole penetration into human nail by 2-N-nonyl-1,3-dioxolane. J Pharm Sci 2003; 92(1):142–8.

35. Quintanar-Guerrero D, Ganem-Quintanar A, Tapis-Olgium P, et al. The effect of keratolytic agents on the permeability of three imidazole antimycotic drugs through the human nail. Drug Dev Ind Pharm 1998; 24:685–90.

36. Mohorcic M, Torkar A, Friedrich J, et al. An investigation into keratolytic enzymes to enhance ungual drug delivery. Int J Pharmaceut 2006; doi:10.1016/j.ijpharm.2006.09.042.

37. Alpsov E, Yilmaz E, Basaran E. Intermittent therapy with terbinafine for dermatophyte toe-onychomycosis: a new approach. J Dermatol 1996; 23(4): 259–62.

38. Rigopoulos D, Katoulis AC, Ionnides D, et al. A randomized trial of amorolfine 5% solution nail lacquer in association with itraconazole pulse therapy compared with itraconazole alone in the treatment of Candida fingernail onychomycosis. Br J Dermatol 2003; 149(1):151–6.

39. Gupta AK, Fleckman P, Baran R. Ciclopirox nail lacquer topical solution 8% in the treatment of toenail onychomycosis. J Am Acad Dermatol 2000; 43(Suppl. 4):S70–S80.

40. Sardana K, Garg VK, Manchanda V, et al. Congenital candidal onychomycoses: effective cure with ciclopirox olamine 8% nail lacquer. Br J Dermatol 2006; 154:573–5.

41. Scher RK, Stiller M, Zhu YI. Tazarotene 0.1% gel in the treatment of fingernail psoriasis: a double-blind, randomized, vehicle-controlled study. Cutis 2001; 68(5):355–8.

42. Gupta AK, Lynde CW, Barber K. Pharmacoeconomic assessment of ciclopirox topical solution, 8% oral terbinafine, and oral itraconazole for onychomycosis. J Cutan Med Surg 2006; 10(Suppl. 2):S54–S62.

43. Lecha M, Effendy I, Feuilhade de Chauvin M, et al. Treatment options— development of concensus guidelines. J Eur Acad Dermatol Venereol 2005; 19(Suppl. 1):25–33.
44. Marty JP, Lambert J, Jackel A, et al. Treatment costs of three nail lacquers used in onychomycosis. J Dermatol Treat 2005; 16:299–307.
45. Baran R, Kaoukhov A. Topical antifungals drugs for the treatment of onychomycosis: an overview of current strategies for monotherapy and combination therapy. J Eur Acad Dermatol Venereol 2005; 19:21–9.

29

Immediate Topical Drug Delivery Using Natural Nano-Injectors

Tamar Lotan

NanoCyte Inc., Jordan Valley, Israel

INTRODUCTION

The skin, the human body's largest organ, presents the most accessible avenue for drug delivery. Transdermal administration increases patient compliance and drug bioavailability, and reduces first-pass metabolism and side effects. Practical transdermal drug delivery is, however, limited due to the presence of the stratum corneum, the relatively impermeable outermost layer of the skin. This thin layer forms an effective barrier to the penetration of external molecules (1).

During the last several decades various approaches have been tried in an attempt to better penetrate the stratum corneum (2–4). These methods can be divided into two main groups: the chemical enhancer/passive approach and the physical energetic devices/active approach. The passive approach includes different types of formulations, including chemical enhancers, liposomes, ethosomes, or large reservoir patches (5). Practical limitations of these methods include their compatibility primarily to small-size lipophilic molecules, and their slow delivery rate necessitating prolonged, hours-long applications.

The physical approach primarily employs high energy devices such as needle-free injectors, low frequency ultrasound, iontophoresis, electroporation, microneedles, thermal methods, and others (6). These methods have the advantage of rapidly permeating the skin barrier. But, as these methods are device-dependent, they generally necessitate professional administration and suffer from higher costs and lower patient compliance.

In this chapter, we describe a naturally derived micro-device which can be applied as part of a topical formulation, but which can deliver drug as rapidly as a physical energetic device. These natural micro-devices can be isolated from one of the most ancient multicellular organisms on earth, the sea anemone. Sea anemone, hydra, coral, and jellyfish all belong to the Cnidaria phylum whose origin is dated to 700 million years ago. The micro-device is a sophisticated microcapsule containing a folded nano-injector that has a capability to penetrate the skin at 40,000 g in a fraction of a second (7). In the following sections these micro-devices are described and the implications for their use in active transdermal drug delivery are discussed.

CHARACTERIZATION OF THE NATURAL MICRO-DEVICE

Cnidarians have been known and described since ancient times and appear prominently in Greek mythology. The enormous power of the Hydra to renew its organs and the freezing effect of the Medusa (jellyfish) has been a topic of many storytellers, painters, and sculptors. In the modern world, these organisms were already identified and characterized by the time of the first microscopes. To date, more than 10,000 members of the Cnidaria phylum have been identified. A consistent characteristic of all these organisms is the presence of millions of specialized stinging cells which may comprise up to 47% of the organism (7). Although several species, such as some jellyfish, are toxic to humans, in nature the primary role of these cells is in the capture of prey or in defense (8).

Of primary interest for transdermal drug delivery are these stinging cells, which contain a highly complex microcapsule incorporating a unique nano-injection system (9). In order to adapt this nano-injection system for transdermal drug delivery, the microcapsules must be isolated and purified from the living cells without impairing their injection and penetration capability (10). The microcapsules can then be kept as a dry powder until use. To activate the nano-injection system the microcapsules need to be re-hydrated which thereby causes pressure to built-up within the microcapsules. The high rate of fluid inflow causes the nano-injectors to be ejected at high-speed from the microcapsule. The nano-injectors thereby penetrate the skin and deliver the drug to the subcutaneous tissue almost instantaneously.

To drive this process, high energy levels must develop within the microcapsule. This occurs due to a combination of the high tensile strength of the microcapsule wall, and to an internal matrix embedded within the microcapsule which serves as the "battery" of the process. The microcapsule's envelope and the nano-injector's walls are composed of fibrils of short collagen (11,12). The distribution of these fibrils along the walls of the microcapsule provides the high tensile strength which is nearly equal to steel.

This is necessary to withstand the high osmotic pressures which will develop within the microcapsule during activation (13,14).

The "battery" of the process is a condensed matrix of short chains of poly γ-glutamate and cations (15–17). When hydrated, the poly γ-glutamate aggregate dissociates causing the internal osmotic pressure within the microcapsule to increase to 150 atm. This high internal osmotic pressure generates additional high levels of drug solution to flow into the micro-capsule. The high internal pressure causes the nano-injector to be ejected out the microcapsule at extremely high speed, delivering its drug content to the skin (Fig. 1). Using a high-speed cinematography it has been shown that the nano-injector is released at a high acceleration of 40,000 g (18). The dis-charge process is completed in about 3 milliseconds and is considered to be one of the fastest events in cell biology.

Among the different Cnidaria species there are about 30 types of microcapsules, all of which act according to the above common principle but which differ in their size, shape and the length of the nano-injector (Fig. 2) (19). All the microcapsules contain highly packed nano-injectors whose lengths can reach up to 50 times of the capsule's dimensions. Nano-injectors vary from 50 to 800 μm in length but their diameters are very thin and in most of the cases they are less than 1 μm.

Although the nano-injector is ejected at high acceleration, contact between the microcapsules and the skin is necessary in order to obtain high

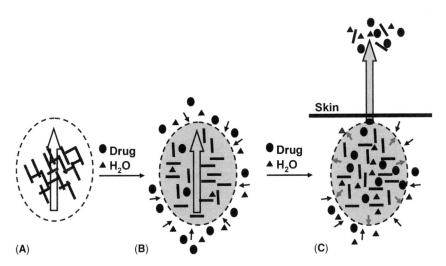

Figure 1   Microcapsule mode of operation: (**A**) the microcapsule at the inactive state; (**B**) after activation with a soluble drug the poly γ-glutamate matrix dissociates result-ing in increased flow of the drug solution into the microcapsule; (**C**) high pressure is built up within the microcapsule, accelerating the nano-injector into the skin. The drug is delivered through the nano-injector into the epidermal skin layer.

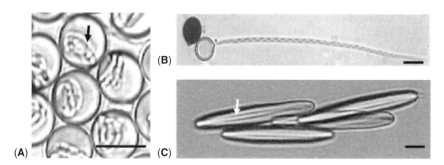

Figure 2 Different types of microcapsules: **(A)** round-shape microcapsules 8 µm in diameter. The arrow points to the folded nano-injector within the microcapsule; **(B)** a round-shaped microcapsule after discharge; **(C)** a rod-shaped microcapsule. The arrow points to the nano-injector within the microcapsule. Scale bar, 10 µm.

efficiency of drug delivery. Therefore any formulation containing the microcapsules must be spread evenly over the skin. The dry powder containing the microcapsules can be formulated as a suspension, gel, lotion or stick and it can also be attached to an adhesive patch. However, in order to keep the active potential of nano-injection, the formulation must be water-free.

When the nano-injectors are applied to the skin they are in the non-hydrated inactive state. Activation occurs by adding the drug in a solution, gel, or a lotion over the microcapsule layer thereby hydrating the microcapsules and triggering the injection process. As activation occurs almost immediately the entire process can be completed in less then 5 minutes.

DELIVERY OF HYDROPHILIC AND PEPTIDE COMPOUNDS TO THE SKIN

Hydrophilic compounds and large peptides are the most difficult substances to deliver transcutaneously. As the nano-injection system is highly compatible with hydrophilic compounds we initially tested the system using these molecules. We chose compounds for which immediate delivery would be beneficial, and for which topical application could increase patient compliance. In the following sections the delivery results of several compounds are presented.

5-Fluorouracil

5-Fluorouracil (5-FU) is a commonly used chemotherapeutic agent that affects both the DNA and RNA of dividing cells. It is used to treat skin conditions such as basal cell carcinoma, solar keratoses, psoriasis, and warts. 5-FU is available for topical application as a cream, but due to local toxicity it must be applied cautiously. NanoCyte microcapsules could limit skin exposure, as the drug is delivered almost immediately allowing the treated skin area to be rinsed free after only 5 minutes.

This was tested in vitro in a diffusion cell system on a full nude mice skin. The application consisted of first applying anhydrous gel containing the microcapsules over the skin followed by a 5% solution of 5-FU. The control application was similar except that the anhydrous gel did not contain the microcapsules. Five minutes after application the skin was thoroughly washed and samples were collected for up to 24 hours from the receiver compartment below the skin. Under these test conditions a significantly greater amount of drug ($80 \, \mu g/cm^2$) was delivered utilizing the microcapsules as compared to the controls (less than $10 \, \mu g/cm^2$) (Fig. 3).

Salicylate

Triethanolamine salicylate (salicylate) is intended for the temporary relief of arthritic or rheumatic pain. Salicylate-containing cream is used regularly to provide a continuous drug supply to the affected area. As the medication diffuses passively into the skin there often is a long delay (up to several hours) from the time of cream application to patient perceiving pain relief.

The nano-injection system provides immediate active delivery and thus may provide faster onset of pain relief. Thereafter, the passive cream could be applied for prolonged gradual drug delivery. The actual application can be done with one cream that can serve both for the initial activation of the NanoCyte system, and also for the prolonged delivery.

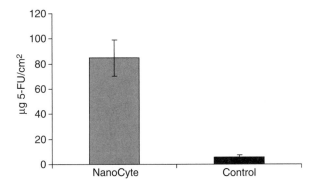

Figure 3   Immediate delivery of 5-FU to the skin. NanoCyte microcapsules were formulated in 2% hydroxypropyl cellulose in ethanol. The gel was applied on the skin and activated with 5% 5-FU solution. After 5 minutes, 5-FU was washed from the skin and samples were taken from the reservoir under the skin for up to 24 hours. The 5-FU delivery was compared to the same gel formulation without NanoCyte microcapsules, $n = 5$. The values are demonstrated as μg 5-FU/cm^2 of skin with its standard error of the mean. *Abbreviation*: 5-FU, 5-fluorouracil.

The amount of active compound delivered to the skin is dependant on the drug concentration. Using an in vitro diffusion cell system, a comparison between two drug concentrations was tested. The NanoCyte microcapsules were applied to the skin and were activated either in 5% or 10% salicylate solution. As a control, the same formulation was used but without the microcapsules and using the higher 10% salicylate concentration. The applied materials were washed from the skin after 5 minutes and the kinetics of the delivery was tested for 24 hours.

These results show a linear increase in delivery for 5% and 10 % salicylate of 60 and 120 μg/cm², respectively. In contrast, the control application of 10% salicylate without NanoCyte microcapsules resulted in a delivery of less than 10 μg/cm² (Fig. 4). The kinetics of the delivery through the skin layers demonstrates the potential for fast onset by the NanoCyte system. With the NanoCyte microcapsules about half of the salicylate is already delivered below the skin in the first 30 minutes following application, and most of the material (80%) is delivered in 3 hours. In contrast, only 63% of the drug is delivered by the control preparation after 5 hours and the actual amount delivered is 10 times less (Table 1).

Peptide

Transcutaneous delivery of peptides is an attractive alternative to needle injection. However, despite recent advances topical delivery of peptides has

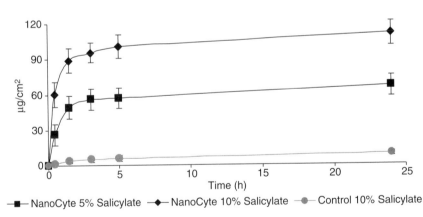

Figure 4 Delivery kinetics of salicylate: NanoCyte microcapsule gel (2% HPC in ethanol) was applied on the skin and activated with either a 5% or 10% salicylate solution. After 5 minutes, the solution was washed from the skin and samples were taken from the reservoir under the skin after 0.5, 1.5, 3, 5, and 24 hours. The salicylate delivery was compared to the same gel formulation without NanoCyte microcapsules, $n=4$. The values are demonstrated as μg salicylate/cm² of skin with its standard error of the mean.

Table 1 Percent Delivery of Salicylate after Application (Standard Error)

	0.5 hr	1.5 hr	3 hr	5 hr	24 hr
NanoCyte 5% salicylate	39(9.2)	74(9.6)	84(9)	86(8.5)	100(9)
NanoCyte 10% salicylate	54(10.8)	80(10.1)	86(8.5)	91(9.9)	100(10.3)
Control 10% salicylate	17(0.9)	43(1.9)	54(2.2)	63(2.5)	100(2.1)

met with limited success. As the NanoCyte system is based on nano-injection, similar to needle injection, we were interested to test the system's compatibility with peptides. A model peptide drug of 1100 Da that contains eight amino acids and which is proven to be highly stable was tested in vitro. The skin membrane was treated with NanoCyte microcapsules followed by the peptide solution. After 5 minutes the applications were washed from the skin leaving no residue. Three peptide concentrations were tested: 2.5%, 5%, and 10%. As a control the same formulation was used without NanoCyte microcapsules and using a 5% peptide solution. The delivered peptide was collected for 24 hours from the compartment under the skin.

The results demonstrate immediate delivery of the peptide in a concentration-dependent manner. Increasing the peptide concentration resulted in more peptide delivery of up to $100\,\mu g/cm^2$. As expected, negligible amounts were found following application of the control preparation absent the microcapsules (Fig. 5).

The possibility of delivering peptides to the skin in a topical manner opens new possibilities in the field of skin care and esthetics. The skin care arena is a growing market that is looking for new treatments based on cell biology. A growing portion of the new treatments are based on peptides like the SNAP 25 botox-like peptides and peptides that induce collagen and elastine synthesis. The NanoCyte topical system may provide a good delivery vehicle for these applications.

PENETRATION INTO KERATINOUS TISSUE

The above data demonstrate that the nano-injection system can immediately penetrate the stratum corneum, the tough outer layer of the skin. As these microcapsules are capable in nature of penetrating arthropod cuticle, we tested their potential to penetrate other hard tissues such as hairs, and nails. Figure 6 demonstrates the potential of the nano-injector system to penetrate a solid keratinous target. This may open the field for hair nourishment care as well as for nail treatments such as for onychomycosis. As the analytical study of the delivery profile is in process we do not yet have the results.

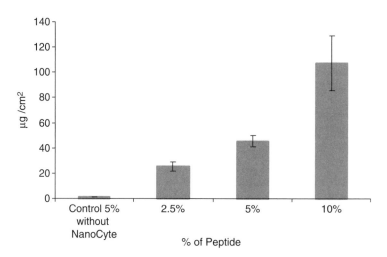

Figure 5 NanoCyte delivery of peptide is concentration-dependent: NanoCyte microcapsule gel was applied on the skin and activated with 2.5% ($n = 6$), 5% ($n = 21$) and 10% ($n = 8$) peptide. The control was composed of the same gel formulation with 5% peptide but without NanoCyte microcapsules ($n = 5$). After 5 minutes the application was washed out from the skin and samples were taken from the reservoir under the skin for up to 24 hours. The values are demonstrated as μg peptide/cm^2 of skin with its standard error of the mean.

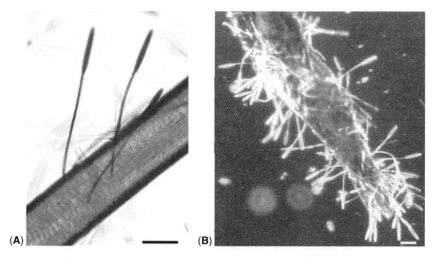

Figure 6 Penetration of hard keratinous tissues: **(A)** NanoCyte nano-injectors within a hair bundle; **(B)** NanoCyte nano-injectors penetration into nail plate. Scale bar, 50 μm.

SAFETY AND TOLERABILITY

The safety and tolerability of the nano-injection system was tested on 100 human volunteers using a single-patch primary dermal irritation study. An additional 30 volunteers were tested for sensitization using a repeat insult patch test consisting of 10 repetitive applications. The activation of the microcapsules in the safety studies was either with saline or buffer. In these studies there were no cases of contact irritation or sensitization suggesting the likelihood of safe utilization of this technique in humans.

During the application process the microcapsules are left on the skin while the short nano-injectors penetrate the stratum corneum. The application is relatively non- invasive as the penetration point is smaller than 1 µm and the nano-injector can penetrate only up to a depth of 50 µm. Nevertheless, we tested how long the nano-injector remains in place until it is cleared from the skin. This study was performed on four pigs, as they have skin similar to humans. On each pig up to 29 topical NanoCyte applications were performed and activation was done using saline. Half of the NanoCyte applications were gently wiped with medical gauze immediately following the application in order to determine if this mechanical treatment is sufficient to remove the microcapsules and nano-injectors from the skin. Tape stripping of the skin was preformed immediately after application (time 0) and at 2, 3, and 7 days after application. The skin samples collected by stripping were analyzed by immunohistochemistry.

The results demonstrated that after 2 days only traces of microcapsules and nano-injectors can be seen. Nevertheless, wiping the site immediately after application is sufficient to remove virtually all of the microcapsules and nano-injectors. This indicates that the capsules will readily dust off from the skin in actual use.

CONCLUSION

The NanoCyte delivery platform combines fast drug delivery with the high compliance of a topical application. The compatibility of the system with hydrophilic and peptide compounds is attractive as there is an unmet need to deliver these molecules across the skin. The power of the nano-injectors in penetrating hard surfaces as skin, hair, and nail offers a novel alternative for cosmeceutical and therapeutics applications.

REFERENCES

1. Trommer H, Neubert R. Overcoming the stratum corneum. The modulation of skin penetration. Skin Pharmacol Physiol 2006; 19:106–21.
2. Hadgraft J, Lane ME. Skin permeation: The years of enlightenment. Int J Pharm 2005; 305:2–12.

3. Barry BW. Breaching the skin's barrier to drugs. Nat Biotechnol 2004; 22:165–7.
4. Prausnitz MR, Mitragotri S, Langer R. Current status and future potential of transdermal drug delivery. Nat Rev Drug Discov 2004; 3:115–24.
5. Benson HAE. Transdermal drug delivery: Penetration enhancement techniques. Curr Drug Deliv 2005; 2:23–33.
6. Nanda A, Nanda S, Ghilzai N. Current developments using emerging transdermal technologies in physical enhancement methods. Curr Drug Deliv 2006; 3:233–42.
7. Tardent P. The cnidarian cnidocyte: A high-tech cellular weaponry. Bioessays 1995; 17:351–62.
8. Lotan A, Fishman L, Loya Y, Zlotkin E. Delivery of a nematocyst toxin. Nature 1995; 375:456.
9. Hessinger DA, Lenhoff HM. The Biology of Nematocysts, San Diego, CA: Academic Press, 1988.
10. Lotan T, Natural nano-injector as a vehicle for novel topical drug delivery. In: Bronaugh RL, Maibach HI, eds. Precutaneous Absorption Drugs-Cosmetics-Mechanisms-Methodology. Vol. 155. New York: Taylor & Francis, 2005: 521–8.
11. Kurz EM, Holstein TW, Petri BM, Engel J, David CN. Mini-collagens in hydra nematocytes. J Cell Biol 1991; 115:1159–69.
12. Engel U, Pertz O, Fauser C, Engel J, David CN, Holstein TW. A switch in disulfide linkage during minicollagen assembly in Hydra nematocysts. EMBO J 2001; 20:3063–73.
13. Holstein TW, Benoit M, Herder Gv, Wanner G, David CN, Gaub HE. Fibrous mini-collagens in hydra nematocysts. Science 1994; 265:402–4.
14. Ozbek S, Engel U, Engel J. A switch in disulfide linkage during minicollagen assembly in hydra nematocysts or how to assemble a 150-bar-resistant structure. J Struct Biol 2002; 137:11–4.
15. Lubbock R, Amos WB. Removal of bound calcium from nematocyst contents causes discharge. Nature 1981; 290:500–1.
16. Weber J. Ploy gamma-glutamic acids are the major constituents of nematocysts in hydra (hydrozoa, Cnidaria). J Biol Chem 1990; 265:9664–9.
17. Szczepanek S, Cikala M, David CN. Poly-gamma-glutamate synthesis during formation of nematocyst capsules in Hydra. J Cell Sci 2002; 115:745–51.
18. Holstein T, Tardent P. An ultrahigh-speed analysis of exocytosis: Nematocyst discharge. Science 1984; 223:830–33.
19. Kass-Simon G, Scappaticci AA. The behavioral and developmental physiology of nematocysts. Can J Zool 2002; 80:1772–94.

30

DOT Matrix® Technology

Juan A. Mantelle

Noven Pharmaceuticals, Inc., Miami, Florida, U.S.A.

BACKGROUND

Introduction

The concept of delivering drugs through the skin for systemic activity has been around throughout recorded history. Only during the last 30 years, however, has there been meaningful advancement in the area, fueled by the recognition of the potential benefits of transdermal drug delivery. Transdermal drug delivery systems (TDDS) either have been or are being developed in practically every known therapeutic category.

This chapter is focused on how the evolution of transdermal systems led to the development of DOT Matrix® technology by Noven Pharmaceuticals, Inc., and how the implementation of this technology has resulted in many firsts in TDDS technology. In order to properly explain the DOT Matrix story, the "state" of transdermals is presented as a series of decision-making processes where the many facets of product development are evaluated and the process is elucidated.

Why Transdermals?

Systemic drug delivery via TDDS presents several opportunities and benefits as compared to traditional oral delivery. As compared to pills, TDDS, or patches, offer the following advantages, among others:

1. avoidance of the first pass liver metabolism resulting in lower required doses;
2. easy discontinuation of dosing by simply removing the patch;

3. providing steady drug delivery and, consequently, steady blood levels for the dosing duration;
4. multiple-day dosing potential;
5. increased compliance;
6. control over the duration of dosing;
7. life cycle extension opportunities for older molecules at lower costs with lower risks.

Types of Transdermals—Evolutionary Steps

1. *Creams, ointments, plasters and salves*: As the first in the evolutionary process for systemic transdermal drug delivery, these types of TDDS have been around for centuries. Over the years, these types of TDDS have taken on many different configurations, from the simple grinding of plants and roots into a paste to more sophisticated and elegant emulsions, hydrogels, and ointments. Although efficacious when used properly, they have several drawbacks. First, they typically require large surface areas to achieve the therapeutic doses required due to their lack of occlusion. Secondly, dosing can be erratic since the patient must spread the preparation over the required surface area of the skin in order to achieve the target blood levels, in some cases over areas as large as $300 \, cm^2$.

2. *Reservoir systems*: Reservoir TDDS (Fig. 1) typically consist of a drug containing reservoir or gel held between an outer occlusive layer and a rate controlling membrane. On the other side of the membrane, there is

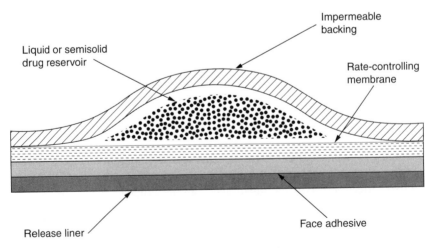

Figure 1   Reservoir transdermal system with face adhesive.

a pressure sensitive adhesive (PSA) which is, in turn, in contact with the disposable release liner.

This type of TDDS typically utilizes rubber-based PSAs as they are more permeable and inert to the drug and the vehicles utilized in the reservoir. In order to properly anchor the rate controlling membrane to the occlusive backing, a perimeter is present in the system that is not in direct contact with the reservoir components. As can be expected, this perimeter or border absorbs drug and vehicle until it equilibrates with storage time.

These systems constitute an advance in the transdermal evolutionary process in that their surface area, and consequently their delivery and dosing, is more reproducible and they require lesser surface areas due to their occlusive nature. The primary drawback to these systems has been the types of delivery vehicles (enhancers or solubilizers) used which have a tendency to be irritating. In addition, the adhesive properties can be compromised by these vehicle/drug combinations.

3. *Solid matrix systems*: Solid matrix systems (Fig. 2) are no longer available in the U.S. market but are worth mentioning due to their role in the evolutionary process. In 1980s, they were very prevalent in the nitroglycerin market. The principle behind these systems was to provide a "solid reservoir" with no need for a rate controlling membrane. The PSA could then be kept remote from the drug-containing solid matrix and thus prevent the deterioration of the adhesive properties with storage time.

Solid matrix systems, although an advancement in the evolutionary process in that they yielded reproducible dosing, encountered many problems since the solid matrix tended to ooze and detach from the occlusive backing. As such, their use slowly declined resulting in their removal from the market. However, they opened the door for use of acrylic PSAs and hence they played a significant role in the evolutionary process.

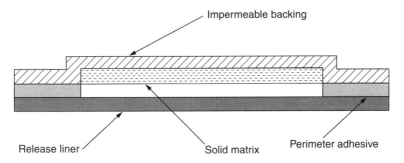

Figure 2 Solid matrix transdermal system with perimeter adhesive.

4. *Drug-in-adhesive systems*: Drug-in-adhesive (DIA) TDDS (Fig. 3) evolved almost by mistake although many would argue that it was an inevitable outcome. Some of the first commercial embodiments resulted from placing acrylic PSAs on the face of matrix systems and noticing their affinity for the drug and fluid vehicles in these solid matrices. Upon storage, almost all, if not all of the drug, was absorbed by these acrylics leaving the solid matrix practically devoid of drug and vehicles.

DIA systems are comprised of an occlusive backing, the drug and excipient containing PSA layer, and a disposable release liner. The PSA layer can be rubber based (e.g., polyisobutylene, silicone, natural rubber) or acrylic based.

DIAs constituted a significant advance in the evolutionary process in that the drug and vehicles are incorporated directly into the PSA and as such, for most designs there is no need for the perimeter or border. In addition, these units can be made on continuous motion machines like adhesive coaters. Dosing is reproducible, and the adhesives are designed with the drug and vehicles already incorporated so the adhesive properties typically do not deteriorate upon storage.

The primary drawback of these systems comes from the need to balance drug and vehicle loading/solubility with the adhesive properties. The compromise, almost invariably, is that the TDDS ends up being larger in order to accomplish the aforementioned balance (i.e., less drug and vehicle loading per unit area).

5. DOT Matrix (Fig. 4): The latest evolutionary step in TDDS was the development of the DOT Matrix system in the mid-1990s by Noven Pharmaceuticals, Inc. Structurally similar to the DIA systems that preceded it, in that it consists of an occlusive backing, a drug and vehicle-containing PSA layer and a disposable release liner, that is where the similarities end. DOT Matrix technology incorporates the learnings from all of its predecessors into a TDDS that solves the

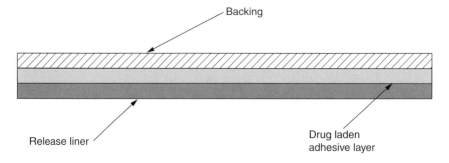

Figure 3 Drug-in-adhesive transdermal system.

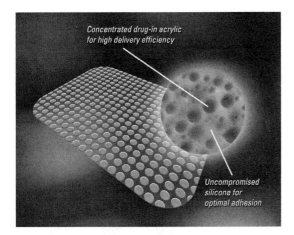

Figure 4 Circular image is the surface of the drug/adhesive layer of a DOT Matrix™ patch photographed with a scanning electron microscope.

patch design dilemma of achieving a Comfortable (non-irritating), Adherent, Reproducible and Small transdermal system (a combination of physician/end-user preferred properties referred to by the acronym CARS).

From the reservoir systems came the recognition that rubber based PSAs have very little, if any, affinity for the drugs or vehicles and are essentially nonreactive. From the DIA systems came the use of acrylic PSAs with their potential for drug and vehicle solvation. From experimentation came the recognition that these two types of PSAs (rubber based and acrylic) are essentially nonmiscible and as such can be utilized jointly to serve distinctly separate functions within the finished product. The rubber based PSA is utilized primarily for proper skin adhesion whereas the acrylic's PSA properties are allowed to be compromised in order to achieve maximum drug and vehicle loading. The resulting product is one with a delivery optimized thermodynamics matrix system, which, by design, delivers greater amounts of drug per unit area without the need for irritating chemical enhancers and provides the comfort and adhesion properties which today's consumers demand.

DEVELOPMENT OF TDDS SYSTEMS

Intellectual Property Considerations

Intellectual property (IP) in the area of TDDS has seen a proliferation in the number of U.S. patents as well as in the number of companies which are including the word "transdermal" in their patent specifications as well as the claims. Figure 5 shows that as recently as 1980 there was only one patent in

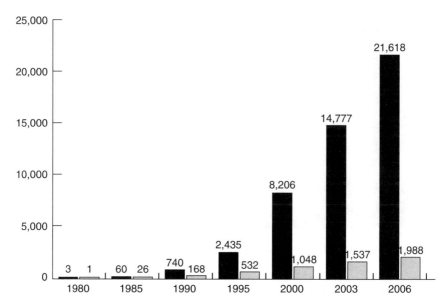

Figure 5   U.S. patents incorporating the word "transdermal" in the specification or claims.

the United States with the word transdermal in the claims while there were three which included it in the specification. By the middle of 2006, these numbers had grown to 1988 and 21,618, respectively.

For those planning to enter the field of the TDDS there are, as can be surmised from the above, many IP obstacles. Gone are the days when IP would be granted for general polymer classes with multiple drugs. Hence, some of the strategies being utilized now include:

1. "Picture" claims:
   a. narrow composition windows,
   b. new methods of manufacturing.
2. Expiring patents:
   a. making older technology new again by utilizing advances in PSA technology.
3. New chemical entities (NCEs):
   a. patenting these NCEs in TDDS.
4. Pharmacokinetic-based IP:
   a. IP based on the specific blood levels achieved and the duration of delivery.
5. Novel skin permeation enhancers:
   a. IP based on the discovery of new combinations of enhancers or surprising results with known chemical entities.

6. Novel polymeric systems/combinations:
   a. IP based on newly created PSA systems or surprising results from combinations of known systems.

Formulation Considerations

Overcoming the resistance of the stratum corneum to the passage of drug into the systemic circulation remains the primary barrier to TDDS development. As such, many different modalities can be utilized to achieve this, namely:

1. enhanced drug solubilization
2. chemical enhancement
3. mechanical enhancement
4. electrical enhancement
5. thermal enhancement

Enhanced drug solubilization traditionally has come from utilizing the base form of a given API. This approach is not without its own drawbacks since the base form is typically more unstable to atmospheric influences such as light, oxygen, and moisture. Another known option is the use of pro-drugs that are lipophilic as presented to the skin but are then converted to the parent molecule in the system (e.g., norethindrone acetate, which converts readily to norethindrone.) Enhanced drug solubilization is achieved in the DOT Matrix® TDDS by modifying the Hildebrand solubility parameter of the acrylic PSA to achieve saturation at a target level and thus maximize the thermodynamic driving force in the system. The net result of this approach has been the creation of the smallest 17-β estradiol product in the market (Vivelle-Dot™) (Table 1) as well as the first ever TDDS to deliver methylphenidate (Daytrana™) at a rate of $80 + \mu g/cm^2/hr$ (30 mg from a $37.5\,cm^2$ patch over 9 hours) (Table 2). This delivery rate is achieved without the need for irritating chemical enhancers.

Chemical enhancement consists of utilizing vehicles which either fluidize or bridge the stratum corneum. As such, most of these vehicles have been shown to be irritating to the skin so their use has been limited to a handful of molecules (e.g., ethanol, triacetin, low molecular weight alcohols, fatty acids, fatty acid esters, and fatty acid alcohols).

Mechanical enhancement of TDDS through the use of micro-needles, micro-protrusions, and other methods has been proposed for many years, but there are no commercial embodiments to date. The IP field in this area is growing as fast as or faster than that of passive TDDS since this approach appears to offer a methodology which bypasses the stratum corneum barrier by effectively creating a mechanical hole through it. Hollow as well as solid needles, micro-blades, drug-laden needles, etc. are just some of the proposed

Table 1 Based on Label Claim for 0.05 mg/day Dose

Product	Patch size	Estradiol content	% depletion
Vivelle-Dot	5.0 cm^2	0.8 mg	22.4
Vivelle	14.5 cm^2	4.3 mg	4.0
Climara[c]	12.5 cm^2	3.9 mg	9.0
Estraderm	18.0 cm^{2a}	4.0 mg	4.4
Mylan[c]	23.7 cm^{2b}	1.9 mg	18.0
Alora	18.0 cm^2	1.5 mg	11.6
Esclim	22.0 cm^2	10.0 mg	1.8

[a]Active area is cm^2.
[b]Active area is 15.5cm^2.
[c]7-day patch; others are 3.5-day.

embodiments which are in development today with the promise of larger molecules, including smaller peptides and proteins now being considered suitable candidates.

Alternative modes of mechanical enhancement have been developed which utilize heat, electrical current or radio frequency to create pores in the stratum corneum and hence reduce the barrier to hydrophilic drugs.

Table 2 Properties of Commercialized Transdermals

	Drug	Molecular weight	Daily TD dose	Smallest patch size (cm^2)	In-vivo permeation rate (g/cm^2/hr)
1.	Scopolamine	303.35	0.33 mg/day	2.5	5.5
2.	Nitroglycerin	227.09	1.6 mg/16 hr	5.0	20.0
3.	Clonidine	230.10	0.1 mg/day	3.5	1.19
4.	Estradiol	272.38	0.1 mg/day	10.0	.42
5.	NETA	340.45	0.14 mg/day	9.0	0.65
6.	Ethinyl Estradiol	296.40	0.02 mg/day	20.0	0.042
7.	Norelgestromin	327.47	0.15 mg/day	20.0	0.31
8.	Nicotine	162.23	7.0 mg/day	7.0	42.0
9.	Testosterone	288.42	2.5 mg/day	7.5	14.0
10.	Fentanyl	336.50	0.6 mg/day	10.0	2.5
11.	Lidocaine	234.34	21.33 mg/12 hr	140.0	12.0
12.	Oxybutynin	357.49	3.9 mg/day	39.0	4.16
13.	Methylphenidate	233.31	12.0 mg/12 hr	12.5	80.0
14.	Selegiline	187.28	6.0 mg/day	20	12.5
15.	Buprenorphine	467.64	0.12 mg/day	6.25	0.8

Although the way in which the pores are created is obviously different from the micro-needles or micro-blades, the result is similar in that the stratum corneum's permeability barrier is compromised to achieve the required drug permeation.

Electrical enhancement, otherwise referred to as iontophoresis, utilizes charged molecules with an electrical source to achieve permeation through the stratum corneum. Although these systems have been proposed for over 20 years, their commercial success has been limited by the bulkiness of the power source, costs, and the practicality of the systems for daily use. Once again, the hope is that these systems can be used to achieve therapeutic levels of larger molecules or higher doses.

Thermal enhancement is a more recent development wherein an external heat source is applied to the patch resulting permeation enhancement which can be tailored to provide a sharp peak, if needed, or simply a sustained, yet higher delivery rate.

Which Types of TDDS to Use and When?

With all of the available options for TDDS development, which option is best suited to a particular molecule? To follow are some general criteria which can help in the decision-making process when selection of a passive system is required.

1. Reservoir systems:
   a. volatile API—room temperature processing.
   b. expensive API—higher yields.
   c. difficult to solubilize API—reservoir can accommodate larger vehicle loading.
2. Traditional DIA systems:
   a. inexpensive API—need higher drug loading to achieve the target delivery rates;
   b. low doses/smaller molecules—where larger patch sizes are not problematic.
3. DOT Matrix® systems
   a. expensive API—highly efficient delivery via the customized polymeric systems;
   b. higher doses/larger molecules—higher thermodynamic driving force results in an enhanced ability to deliver these;
   c. volatile API—customized solvent system enables differential volatilization resulting in lesser drug loss during processing
   d. small size—for applications where a discreet patch is required
   e. customizable wear properties—wear properties can be optimized, via the selection and customization of the PSA system used.

THE DOT MATRIX EXPERIENCE

Adhesives

The DOT Matrix systems, by virtue of the blend of rubber based (silicone) PSAs with the acrylic PSAs affords the formulator several unique opportunities. The first and probably most remarkable feature is the fact that the acrylic PSA can be tailored, via modification of the reactive moiety, to achieve the desired solubility potential for the API while still maintaining the integrity of the polymeric system. Second, by altering the ratio of the two PSAs, one can also significantly alter the total delivery as well as the shape of the pharmacokinetic curve. Furthermore, by adjusting the functionality and molecular weight of these PSAs, stability and wear properties can be tailored to each API and intended wear time, respectively.

Efficiency

The binary adhesive system used in the DOT Matrix systems provides the formulator the ability to saturate the acrylic PSA without concern for its loss of PSA properties. As Table 1 illustrates, the attainment of higher drug concentrations permits a higher depletion rate for the given wear period, resulting in less drug being discarded at the end of the dosing period.

Firsts

DOT Matrix has, in the years since its creation provided the transdermal market with many firsts, namely:

1. the first two drug transdermal systems (CombiPatch®, Estalis®);
2. the first, and still only, 17-β Estradiol product to deliver 0.10 mg/day from a patch size of 10 cm² (Vivelle-Dot™, the smallest estrogen patch on the market);
3. the first and only TDDS to deliver more than 45 μg/cm²/hr of any drug (Daytrana™ delivers upwards of 80 μg/cm²/hr of methylphenidate).

CONCLUSION

Passive transdermal drug delivery is poised to become a more prevalent therapeutic choice as the technology has progressed to the point where larger molecules and larger doses in almost all therapeutic categories are in advanced development. With this added exposure to the general population comes the responsibility of the pharmaceutical companies to make these patches more esthetically appealing, flexible, and adhesive for the intended dose duration. The DOT Matrix system has already expanded this frontier and set the standard for passive transdermal drug delivery. The number of molecules that are contemplated in the various therapeutic categories for this system continues to expand as the PSA technology and consequent versatility has progressed to better suit the needs of the formulator. Acrylic PSAs with various reactant moieties in a wide range of concentrations have progressed the solubilization potential of these systems significantly and further advancement is occurring almost daily. Future developments will be more challenging, but the DOT Matrix systems are continuing to expand the horizon of APIs that can be delivered transdermally.

31

The PassPort™ System: A New Transdermal Patch for Water-Soluble Drugs, Proteins, and Carbohydrates

Alan Smith and Eric Tomlinson

Altea Therapeutics Corporation, Atlanta, Georgia, U.S.A.

The PassPort™ System is a novel transdermal technology developed by Altea Therapeutics Corporation that enables the delivery of water-soluble small drugs, peptides, proteins, carbohydrates, and nucleotides from a convenient and cost-effective transdermal patch.

Commercially available transdermal patches can only deliver small lipophilic molecules (< 500 Da) that can readily dissolve and diffuse through the lipid-rich intercellular matrix of the stratum corneum. In contrast, numerous clinical studies have demonstrated that the PassPort System can enable water-soluble small molecule and large macromolecular drugs to enter the skin through aqueous microchannels formed though the stratum corneum. The PassPort System uses focused microsecond pulses of thermal energy to ablate the stratum corneum and create multiple microchannels up to 50 μm in depth that just impinge into the viable epidermis. These microchannels fill with interstitial fluid through which water-soluble molecules permeate to reach the viable tissues of the skin. From there, molecules can have either local effect or, by entering the circulation via the microcapillaries or lymphatic system, systemic effect. The PassPort System is easy to use and patients report a painless application with no sensation of heat.

The PassPort System comprises a single-use disposable PassPort Patch and a re-useable handheld applicator. The PassPort Patch consists of a conventional transdermal patch drug reservoir attached to an array of metallic filaments (a "porator"). A patient clips a PassPort Patch to an applicator

(Fig. 1) and applies the porator to the skin surface. A single click of the activation button of the applicator causes the microchannels to be formed through the stratum corneum. The patient then removes the applicator from the skin surface, thereby automatically leaving the transdermal patch (but not the porator) on the skin. A simple fold-over step aligns the transdermal patch over the newly formed microchannels.

Pressing the activation button of the Applicator releases a single pulse of electrical energy to the porator, where the filaments convert the electrical energy into thermal energy. Rapid conduction of this thermal energy into tiny areas of the surface of the skin painlessly ablates the stratum corneum under each filament to create the microchannels.

The Applicator has built-in features that allow it to be programed to provide dosing control and monitoring. It can store the time and date of each application event which can be used to monitor prescription compliance and to prevent diversion. The applicator can be further programed with lock-out features to prevent drug misuse or abuse.

Altea Therapeutics has developed novel formulations for the PassPort System that result in rapid and sustained transdermal delivery of therapeutic amounts of highly water-soluble drugs including proteins, carbohydrates, nucleotides, and low-molecular weight molecules. These novel formulations lead to high utilization of drug during the dosing period. The technology and formulation attributes, together with low cost scaleable manufacturing processes, allow for an economically attractive cost of goods. Altea Therapeutics has demonstrated in clinical studies that using the PassPort System enables the efficient transdermal delivery of large amounts of drugs.

The intellectual property that surrounds the PassPort System includes both device and drug claims that protect the thermal ablation process as well as the novel controlled release aspect of the drug release from polymer film formulations. Altea Therapeutics is prosecuting 16 patent families that cover

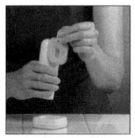 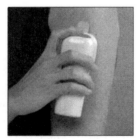 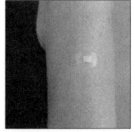

Clip patch to applicator   Apply to skin   Commence treatment

Figure 1   Use of the PassPort™ Transdermal Delivery System.

the use, composition, and manufacture of its technology. To date, 15 U.S. patents and 16 international patents have issued and numerous patent applications are pending in numerous countries and patent jurisdictions worldwide.

The PassPort System enables drug delivery through the skin by thermal ablation of microscopic areas of the stratum corneum to form an aqueous pathway into the viable tissues of the skin (1). Thermal ablation is accomplished by contacting an array of electrically resistive filaments to the skin surface and briefly heating the filaments by applying a short controlled pulse of electric current. Conditions can be adjusted to create microchannels typically in the range of 50–200 µm wide at the skin surface and 30–50 µm deep. The dimensions of the microchannels are controlled by several factors, including the temperature–time profile and the geometry of the filaments that contact the skin. Thermal ablation has also been investigated in clinical studies for the rapid extraction of interstitial fluid from the skin for glucose monitoring (2).

Studies using the PassPort System have shown the feasibility of delivering small water soluble drugs, exemplified by hydrophilic opioids morphine sulfate, fentanyl citrate, and hydromorphone hydrochloride (3) in human subjects, and large peptides, proteins, carbohydrates and nucleotides exemplified by insulin in animal (4) and human (5,6) studies, and preclinical animal studies that have shown the delivery of parathyroid hormone (7), interferon alpha (8), influenza HA, hepatitis B surface antigen (9), and DNA plasmid-based vaccines (10) (Fig. 2)

BASAL INSULIN TRANSDERMAL PATCH

Altea Therapeutics is developing a novel transdermal patch for the sustained and efficient delivery of basal levels of insulin for people suffering from diabetes. The anticipated differentiating features of the product include:

- reduced risks of hypoglycemia
- greater patient compliance than injectable basal insulin
- earlier adoption of insulin in diabetes management
- product storage at room temperature

There is a major unmet need for a pain-free, convenient, and cost-effective alternative to long-acting insulin injections as confirmed through physician market research. The basal insulin transdermal patch has the potential to capture a greater than US$ 2 billion share of the current worldwide basal insulin market and offers features and benefits that can expand the market due to an expected earlier introduction of basal insulin in diabetes management.

Altea Therapeutics is developing a 12-hour wear product for overnight delivery of basal insulin and a 24-hour wear product for daily delivery of

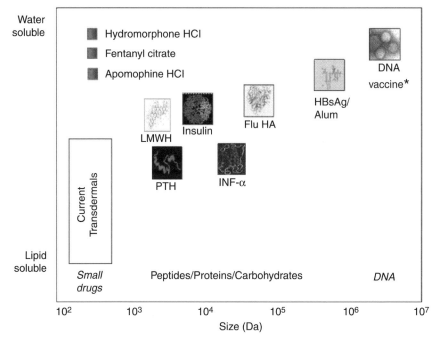

Figure 2 Transdermal delivery of water-soluble small drug salts and macromolecules using the PassPort™ System.

basal insulin. The company has achieved sustained and constant insulin delivery at therapeutic levels over a 24-hour application of a basal insulin transdermal patch in healthy subjects. Clinical data from a euglycemic glucose clamp study show efficient delivery of insulin and a pharmacodynamic effect of transdermal insulin comparable to subcutaneous injection of a long-acting insulin analog (Fig. 3). Steady-state pharmacodynamics as determined by the glucose infusion rates are reached at ~4 hours after patch application, and were maintained until the basal insulin transdermal patch was removed, whereupon they rapidly decrease (Fig. 3).

The basal insulin transdermal patch is designed to deliver 0.3 IU of biologically active insulin per hour per cm^2 and at a delivery efficiency of 20% relative to subcutaneous injection. Transdermal patches range in functional area from $2 \, cm^2$ to $8 \, cm^2$ and are designed to be stable at room temperature.

Steady basal levels are required for regulating glucose metabolism and achieving basal glycemic control. Clinicians increasingly appreciate the need for basal insulin in the management of diabetes, with products that provide and maintain basal insulin levels comprising the fastest-growing sector of the insulin market. The basal insulin transdermal patch will be the first non-injectable basal insulin product to provide equivalent or better glycemic control and equal or lower incidence of hypoglycemia than long-acting

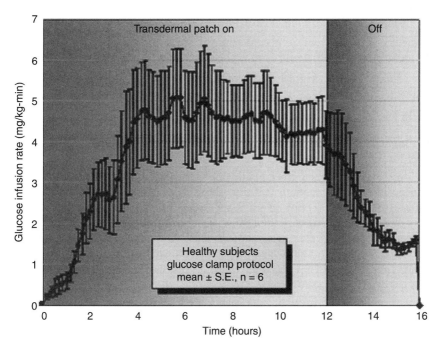

Figure 3 Glucose infusion rates in healthy subjects during a phase 1 clinical trial. The basal insulin transdermal patch was applied for 12 hours.

injectable insulin products, such as insulin glargine (Lantus®) and insulin detemir (Levemir®).

A recent assessment of the potential for a basal insulin transdermal patch revealed that 81% of primary care physicians and 77% of endocrinologists surveyed would switch their patients from basal insulin injections to a basal insulin transdermal patch (11). Furthermore, 71% of physicians stated they would use the product to introduce basal insulin earlier in their treatment regimen for type 2 diabetes. Worldwide, approximately 40 to 50 million people with type 2 diabetes and 10 million people with type 1 diabetes require basal insulin therapy. The worldwide market for all forms of insulin was over US$ 7 billion in 2005 and is estimated to be more than US$ 11 billion by 2011. The basal insulin market is the fastest growing insulin sector, generating over US$ 2.6 billion in worldwide sales in 2005.

FENTANYL CITRATE TRANSDERMAL PATCH

Altea Therapeutics is developing the first transdermal patch containing a potent opioid, fentanyl citrate that enables patients to achieve rapid and safe control of their pain. The differentiating features of the product include:

- fast onset of action and fast drug elimination
- rapid dose titration
- deterrents against abuse and misuse

The fentanyl citrate transdermal patch has the potential to create a new standard of care in opioid-based pain management. Market research with physician groups confirms the potential of the product due to its significantly improved safety, efficacy, and anti-abuse performance over existing products with market research estimates for annual sales of over US$ 1 billion. The fentanyl citrate transdermal patch is designed to provide rapid, steady and safe management of moderate to severe chronic pain. The transdermal patch is small, comfortable to wear and is intended for daily application.

Use of the highly water-soluble citrate salt form of fentanyl results in a pharmacokinetic profile that is similar to intravenous infusion of fentanyl citrate over 24 hours; namely: quick rise to steady state levels followed by rapid elimination after patch removal or cessation of infusion (Fig. 4). Such important attributes are unachievable with marketed fentanyl transdermal patches, including Duragesic, that use the base form of fentanyl.

The fentanyl citrate transdermal patch achieves efficient drug delivery during application, with little drug remaining in the transdermal patch after

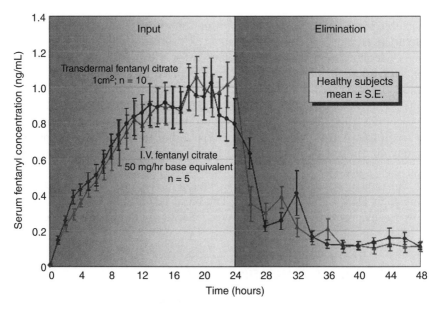

Figure 4 PassPort™ transdermal fentanyl citrate:comparison to intravenous infusion.

use. The transdermal patch is applied to the skin using a simple handheld Applicator that can be programed to include additional features including time and date stamping for each dose and dose lock-out features to prevent unscheduled dosing. Furthermore, there is no drug delivery unless the transdermal patch is applied with its applicator, and external heat sources such as heating pads are expected to have no significant effect on drug delivery. The four dose strengths of the fentanyl citrate transdermal patch match the approved doses of Duragesic (12.5, 25, 50, 100 μg/hr) but the fentanyl citrate transdermal patch will be about ten times smaller in functional area and have higher bioavailability.

Fentanyl transdermal patches have been used for over 15 years in the management of moderate to severe pain. Unfortunately, accidental misuse and abuse of this and other opioid products have resulted in dose-related deaths and serious side effects, overshadowing the important role opioids have in pain management. Currently marketed fentanyl patches contain the lipid-soluble base form of fentanyl and require 3 days wear per application. Following application of an initial patch, it takes between 24 and 72 hours to reach peak fentanyl serum concentrations and up to 2–3 applications of the three-day patch to achieve steady-state plasma drug concentrations. This slow rise to analgesic concentrations can lead to a patient wrongly applying a second patch during the first few days—leading to excessive skin accumulation of the fentanyl base that can lead to overdosing. Fentanyl base depots in the skin, resulting in slow elimination from the blood and making rapid discontinuation of therapy difficult in the event of an overdose. The pharmacokinetics of currently marketed fentanyl transdermal patches can also lead to difficulties in dose titration/patch change by the patient or the physician. Currently marketed fentanyl transdermal patches, used as directed by the label, lose efficacy sometime during the third day of therapy. Further, there is a potential for external heat sources, such as heating pads or electric blankets, to cause an increase in release of fentanyl base from the patch.

Despite these documented safety issues, currently marketed fentanyl transdermal patches, containing the base form of the drug, have achieved widespread use. This is primarily due to the potency of the fentanyl molecule and it's effectiveness in the management of moderate to severe pain coupled with the transdermal route of administration that eliminates the need for the patient to take immediate release pills every 4–6 hours.

According to a recent market research study, physicians believe that reduction of the abuse liability of currently available long-acting opioids is considered to be the most important need (12). Of the interviewed physicians, 82% were likely to prescribe the product. The global opioid market was approximately US$ 8.3 billion in 2005, with long-acting opioids accounting for more than half of that total at US$ 4.6 billion. The worldwide peak sales for Duragesic were US$ 2.4 billion.

REGULATORY CONSIDERATIONS

The PassPort System is a combination drug-device product with the primary mode of action being based on the drug. Therefore, in the United States, the product will require a New Drug Application (NDA) through the drug division (FDA-CDER) with the device division (FDA-CDRH) acting in a consulting role. For drugs already approved by other routes of administration, the systemic toxicology data for the reference listed drug will be referenced in the NDA submission as a 505(b)(2) application, and results of new studies focused on skin toxicology will be provided.

COMPETITIVE ADVANTAGE

Transdermal delivery using the PassPort System offers several potential benefits. Delivery through the skin bypasses metabolism in the gastrointestinal tract which typically results in the very low bioavailability of oral formulations of proteins and peptides. Transdermal patches are conventionally used to achieve steady serum levels of drug and avoid the "peak-valley" effect, however they are limited for use with small molecule lipophilic drugs. This is mainly due to the barrier function of the stratum corneum, the outer layer of dead skin cells, which is the rate-limiting step for transdermal transport. Various technologies have been used to overcome the barrier of the stratum corneum layer including the use of microfabricated needles, blades, or projections, iontophoresis, ultrasound, and electroporation. Challenges to commercialization of these technologies include pain/sensation, reproducibility, size, cost of goods, ease of use, and topical response. The design and development of the PassPort System has addressed these challenges and the technology is being optimized to meet the specific requirements for each therapeutic indication and drug.

REFERENCES

1. Eppstein J, Hatch M, Yang D. Microporation of human skin for drug delivery and monitoring applications, US Patent 5,885,211, March 23, 1999.
2. Smith A, Yang D, Delcher H, Eppstein J, Wilkes S. Fluorescein kinetics in interstitial fluid harvested from diabetic skin during fluorescein angiography: Implications for glucose monitoring, Diabet Technol Therapeut 1999; 1:21–7.
3. Smith AM, Gomez-Panzani E, Mills SE, Rainey G, Tolia G, Tagliaferri F, Spratlin V. 24-Hour Transdermal Delivery of Hydromorphone Hydrochloride, 25th Annual Scientific Meeting of the American Pain Society, San Antonio, Texas, May 2006.
4. Joshi DP, Chaturvedula A, Chang SL, Mills SE, Smith AM, Banga AK. Steady insulin infusion via micropores through the stratum corneum in hairless rats. AAPS Pharm Sci 2003; 5(4):S1:T3106.

5. Smith AM, Eppstein JA, Delcher HK, McRae MS, Woods TJ, Williams DJ, Hatch MR. Transdermal insulin infusion through thermally created micropores in humans. Diabetes 2001; 50(2):A132.
6. Smith AM, Woods TJ, Williams DJ, Delcher HK, Eppstein JA, McRae MS. Transdermal basal insulin delivery through micropores. Diabetes 2002; (51):A47.
7. Chang S-L, Smith AM, Mills SE, Joshi DP, Badkar AV, Banga AK. Transdermal delivery of human parathyroid hormone 1–34 by thermally created micropores and electrotransport. AAPS PharmSci 2001; 3(3).
8. Badkar AV, Smith AM, Eppstein JA, Banga AK. Transdermal Delivery of interferon Alpha-2b using microporation and iontophoresis in Hairless Rats. Pharmaceutical Research 2007; 24(7):1389–95.
9. Smith AM, Eppstein JA, Woods TJ, McRae MS, Allen DW, Hatch MR. Transdermal hepatitis B vaccine delivery through thermally created micropores in human subjects, Fourth Annual Conference of Vaccine Research, NIAID, Washington DC, April 25, 2001.
10. Bramson J, Dayball K, Evelegh C, Wan YH, Page D, Smith A. Enabling topical immunization via microporation: A novel method for pain-free and needle-free delivery of adenovirus-based vaccines. Gene Therapy 2003; 10: 251–60.
11. Conducted by Navigant Consulting on behalf of Altea Therapeutics.
12. Conducted by Pain Insights on behalf of Altea Therapeutics.

Part V: Nasal Technologies

——————————— **32** ———————————

Nasal Drug Delivery

Pradeep K. Karla, Deep Kwatra, Ripal Gaudana, and Ashim K. Mitra
University of Missouri-Kansas City, Kansas City, Missouri, U.S.A.

INTRODUCTION

The global drug delivery market was valued at US$ 426.9 billion in 2005 and is estimated to reach US$ 543.8 billion by 2010 (1). Nasal delivery commands the fourth position in market share, with US$ 3 billion in sales, following oral controlled release, pulmonary and parenteral delivery routes. Though the potential for growth in the oral sector is extensive, successful delivery of molecules like proteins and peptides need an alternative route to the parenteral route via a new delivery system (77). Verma et al. stated that "Products based on new drug delivery systems have significantly increased in recent years, and this growth is expected to continue in the near future. Many biopharmaceuticals present challenges to drug delivery scientists because of their unique nature and difficulty in delivery through conventional routes. Therefore, future research will focus on the delivery of these complex molecules through different routes, including intranasal and pulmonary routes" (28). The delivery of drugs non-invasively through the nasal route has been rapidly growing from just a specialized application field to a competent formulation option. It is not only convenient to the patient, but the route can also incorporate sustained, controlled, or instantaneous delivery of the drugs with better metabolism profiles and high target specificity. Apart from intranasal drug products that are indicated in the treatment of allergic rhinitis and minor local infections, it is feasible for a number of systemic drugs in a number of different therapeutic categories. Intranasal drug delivery is a popular way to treat respiratory ailments and administer drugs for sinus conditions, such as congestion and allergies.

As per Guo et al., "The nasal mucosa, although providing an extensive, highly vascularized surface of pseudostratified ciliated epithelium, secretes mucus that is subjected to mucociliary clearance" (85). Absorption is influenced by anatomical and physiological factors as well as by properties of the drug and the delivery system (75).

To optimize nasal administration, bioadhesive hydrogels, bioadhesive microspheres (dextran, albumin, and degradable starch), and liposomes have been extensively studied. Prescription drugs for pain management, migraine headaches, osteoporosis, etc., have benefited from the nasal route of administration. Companies are working on technologies and delivery devices that will overcome some of the challenges of delivering prescription drugs nasally, such as delivering the correct dosage, and ensuring higher absorption of drug in nasal mucosa. In this chapter, the nasal route and its applications are described in depth in relation to new drug delivery technologies currently in the market (76).

NASAL ANATOMY AND PHYSIOLOGY

Nasal Cavity

The exterior nose contains the nostrils and comprises of one-third of the nasal cavity. It is dual chambered ~ 5 cm high and ~ 10 cm long. Inside the cavities, the walls are lined with turbinates, which form the slit-like cavities that maintain the humidification and temperature regulation of inspired air. The total surface area of the nasal cavity in the human adult is ~ 150 cm^2 (77). The nose has three functional zones in the nasal cavity which include the vestibular, olfactory and respiratory areas and function as a protective barrier against foreign material. According to Turker et al., "The vestibular area serves as a baffle system filtering the airborne particles (2), the olfactory epithelium is capable of metabolizing drugs (3), and respiratory mucosa acts as a major site for absorption of drugs" (4,78). The nasal cavity also contains the nasal associated lymphoid tissue (NALT) which is mainly located in the nasopharynx. Numerous microvillus on the epithelial surface results in a large surface area available for drug absorption. A highly vascularized subepithelial layer, direct flow of venous blood from nose to systemic circulation which avoids loss of drug by first pass metabolism, a porous endothelial basement membrane, a high blood flow per cm^3 and olfactory nerves that are directly connected to brain all allows for efficient systemic and brain delivery of drugs.

Respiratory, Olfactory Epithelia, and Lymphoid Tissue

The anterior part of the nasal cavity is covered with squamous epithelium. It gradually changes into the respiratory epithelium that comprises pseudostratified columnar epithelium which is covered in microvilli. Four major types of cells; the ciliated and non ciliated columnar cells, goblet cells and basal cells constitute the pseudostratified columnar epithelium (Fig. 1).

Goblet cells are involved mainly in the secretion of mucus. The mucus layer covering the epithelial cells consists of a highly viscous upper layer and a lower layer of relatively low viscosity in which cilia can move. The mucus layer is propelled toward the throat with a half-time of clearance of about 15–20 minutes and is continuously renewed. The olfactory epithelium constitutes only about 5% of the total area of the nasal cavity in man, but is of considerable interest in drug delivery because it provides a direct pathway from this region of the nasal cavity to the brain (5).

The olfactory epithelium is a modified (pseudostratified) respiratory epithelium, comprising subtentacular cells that provide mechanical support by covering neuronal receptor cells and basal cells that are able to differentiate into neuronal receptor cells (57). Nasal epithelial cells (both respiratory and olfactory) are interconnected on the apical side of the membrane by narrow belt like structures that totally surround the cells (junctional complexes). These complexes, which comprise in series, the zona occludens,

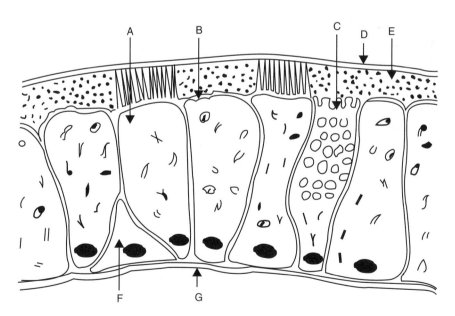

Figure 1   Cell types of the nasal epithelium showing ciliated cell (**A**), nonciliated cell (**B**), goblet cell (**C**), gel mucus layer (**D**), sol layer (**E**), basal cell (**F**), and basement membrane (**G**). *Source*: From Ref. 84 with permission.

the zona adherens, and the macula adherens, form a dynamic regulatable semi-permeable diffusion barrier between the epithelial cells (6). The zona occludens is also known as the tight junction. The normal diameter of the tight junctions in the nasal cavity is considered to be of the order of 3.9–8.4 Å (7,12).

The review by Illum states that "The zona occludens (tight junctional complex) consists of a variety of transmembrane proteins (e.g., occludins, claudins, junctional adhesion molecules) and cytosolic proteins (e.g., ZO-1, ZO-2, and ZO-3). Located in the cell membrane, the occludins project two loops into the intercellular space with the C- and N-termini remaining in the cytosol. Loops from two opposing transmembrane proteins interact (noncovalently) across the intercellular space. The C-terminal of the transmembrane proteins (e.g., occludin) then interacts with the N-terminal of the cytosolic proteins (e.g., ZO-1) which again connects via their C-terminals to the F-actin, thereby coupling the tight junction proteins to the cytoskeleton. The barrier properties and the assembly of the tight junctions are influenced by a range of signaling pathways. Generally, for many of these signaling pathways, the phosphorylation of the tight junction proteins or the displacement of the perijunctional actin-myosin ring is the final effect of modulation (7,8). Protein kinase C (PKC) is strongly involved in the complicated signal transduction process that regulates the tight junctions. Chitosan and their polycationic materials were shown to open tight junctions by a PKC activation mechanism" (9,12).

The NALT in humans is normally associated with Waldeyer's ring, i.e., the tubal, the palatine and lingual tonsils and the adenoids. The NALT contains specialized M-like cells similar to those present in the Payer's patches in the gut. However, in man, mucosal lymphoid tissue is also present immediately under the nasal mucosa, where one can find B and T lymphocyte follicles, macrophages, and dendritic cells (10,12). The cells are capable of taking up antigen and processing these for immune stimulation. It is generally recognized that soluble antigens can penetrate the whole of the nasal mucosa and reach the superficial cervical lymph nodes to produce mainly a systemic immune response. In contrast, particulates are mainly taken up by the M-cells in the NALT. These are processed and reach the posterior cervical lymph nodes where a predominant secretory immune response is evoked. However, one should note that in vitro studies in cell cultures or ex vivo studies in excised nasal tissue have shown that, under such circumstances particles can also be endocytosed into nasal epithelial cells (11). Illum et al. have hypothesized that from the lymph nodes there is a possibility that the particulates can escape and eventually reach the blood stream. Studies on uptake of particulates from the gut (via the M-cells) have shown that small particles (~ 50 nm) were taken up to a higher extent than larger particles (~ 500 nm and ~ 3 mm) although the overall amount was small, e.g., less than 3%. No further studies have been performed to evaluate the optimal size range for particle uptake by M-like cells in the NALT. Potentially, however, given the similarity of the cells, the size range for optimal uptake could be the same (12).

INTRANASAL DRUG ABSORPTION

Passage through the mucus and then the underlying cells is the initial step in intranasal drug absorption (13). Most of the enzyme activity in the nasal cavity occurs at the olfactory mucosa but still the activity per total weight of nasal mucosa is lower than in intestine (14). The mucus thus provides us with a paradigm wherein the longer the drug stays in the mucosa the more time it gets to get absorbed and gets more exposure to the catalytic enzymes. However, the physiological mucocilliary clearance reduces the residence time of the drug in the nasal cavity. Small, uncharged particles easily pass through and larger or charged particles are not able to pass. Mucin, the principal protein in the mucus, binds to solutes, hindering diffusion (68). The mucus undergoes static, hydrophobic and van der Waal interaction with the invading molecules. Structural changes in the mucus layer also occur due to environmental changes (i.e., pH, temperature, etc.), hindering molecular movement from the delivery site to the epithelium (13).

Several mechanisms have been proposed to describe the transport of drug molecules. According to a review in *Drug Delivery Technology* by Aurora, the following two mechanisms have been considered predominantly. According to the review, "The first mechanism involves an aqueous route of transport, which is also known as the paracellular route. This route is slow and passive. There is an inverse correlation between log intranasal absorption and the log molecular weight of water-soluble compounds. Poor bioavailability is generally observed for drugs with a molecular weight greater than ~ 1000 Da. Some small proteins and peptides are believed to be transferred through this route. The second mechanism involves transport through a lipoidal route that is also known as the transcellular process and is responsible for the transport of lipophilic drugs that show a rate dependency according to their lipophilicity. Drugs also cross cell membranes by an active transport route via carrier-mediated means or transport through the opening of tight junctions. For example, Chitosan, a natural biopolymer from shellfish, opens tight junctions between epithelial cells to facilitate drug transport" (15,69). Transcytosis by vesicle carriers is yet another mechanism of drug absorption utilized by certain drug molecules (16). A brief summary for various modes of transport of drug molecules across nasal epithelia is shown in Figure 2. The nasal cavity has proven to be a very effective route for drug absorption showing consistently good pharmacokinetic profiles. Experiments by Wermeling et al. (17) have shown that T_{max} and C_{max} values are higher for drugs delivered by the intranasal route than the intramuscular route, further proving the intranasal route as a

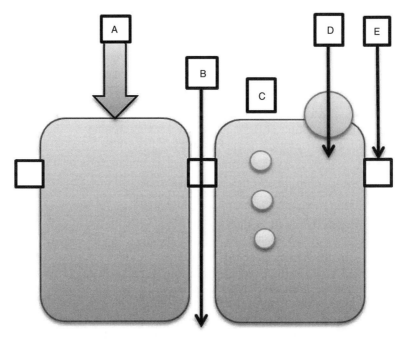

Figure 2 Drug transport pathways across the epithelium. Passive transcellular transport (**A**), paracellular transport (**B**), transcytosis (**C**), carrier-mediated transport (**D**), and intercellular tight junction (**E**).

potential route for drug delivery. However, nasopharyngeal irritation, eyes watering, and a bad taste were reported after intranasal doses and the results supported further development of the midazolam nasal spray that was tested. Various physico-chemical, anatomical, physiological and formulation parameters influencing intranasal drug absorption are represented in Figure 3 (17).

INTRANASAL DRUG FORMULATIONS

Many factors affect the efficiency and performance of an intranasal drug delivery system need to be considered in formulating an intranasal drug delivery system. Mucociliary clearance plays an integral role in removal of dust, allergens and bacteria in the nasal cavity which are entrapped on the mucus layer during inhalation (13). According to the review by Aurora, "The absorption of drugs is influenced by the residence (contact) time between the drug and the epithelial tissue. The mucociliary clearance is

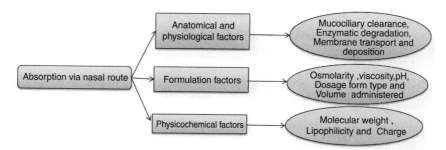

Figure 3 The physicochemical, anatomic, physiological, and formulation factors affecting the nasal absorption of drugs. *Source*: Adapted from Ref. 81.

inversely related to the residence time and therefore inversely proportional to the absorption of drugs administered" (69). But the mucociliary clearance cannot be prolonged for better absorption as it may disrupt the normal physiological functions. By using bioadhesive polymers, microspheres, chitosan, which increased the viscosity of the formulation, the residence time of drug in nasal cavity can be increased (69).

Many enzymes are present in the nasal mucosa which might affect the stability of drugs like proteases and amino-peptidase which may degrade drugs (especially proteins and peptides) on the mucosal surface (18). There are many immunoglobulin's present on the mucosal surface which may bind to the peptides and prevent their absorption due to increased molecular weight (15).

Drug concentration, dose and dose volume are three essential and mutually correlated parameters that may affect the efficiency of the nasal absorption. Their effect on drug absorption varies from drug to drug. Review by Aurora indicated that "Nasal absorption of L-Tyrosine was shown to increase with drug concentration in nasal perfusion experiments (19). However, in another study, aminopyrine was found to absorb at a constant rate as a function of concentration. In contrast, absorption of salicylic acid was found to decline with concentration. This decline is likely due to nasal mucosa damage by the permeant (20). The pH of a nasal formulation is important for the design of a intranasal formulation for the following reasons: (*i*) to avoid mucosal irritation; (*ii*) to maintain the drug in unionized form for absorption; (*iii*) to prevent growth of pathogenic bacteria in the nasal passage; (*iv*) for the stability of the excipients in the formulation such as preservatives; and (*v*) to maintain normal physiological ciliary movement. Lysozyme is found in nasal secretions, which is responsible for destroying certain bacteria at acidic pH (21). Under alkaline conditions, lysozyme is inactivated and the nasal tissue is susceptible to microbial infection. It is therefore advisable to keep the formulation at a pH of 4.5–6.5 keeping in mind the physicochemical properties of the drug as drugs are absorbed in the un-ionized form" (69).

Buffer capacity is a critical parameter in designing intranasal formulations. pH of nasal secretions can affect the amount of drug present in un-ionized form. Adequate formulation buffer capacity is thus needed to maintain the pH. Drug absorption can be also be affected by tonicity, by effecting shrinkage of epithelial cells and ceasing of ciliary activity.

Gelling agents are also an essential part of an intranasal formulation higher viscosity may increase the therapeutic effect (22). Hydroxypropyl cellulose as a drug carrier was effective in increasing the absorption of low molecular weight drugs but was not as effective for high molecular weight peptides (23).

The aqueous solubility of a drug is always a limitation for intranasal drug delivery or for that matter any form of drug formulation. Aurora has also mentioned that "Solubilizers such as conventional solvents or co-solvents for example glycols, small quantities of alcohol, transcutol (diethylene glycol monoethyl ether), medium chain glycerides and labrasol (saturated polyglycolyzed C_8–C_{10} glyceride) can be used to enhance the solubility of drugs. Other options include the use of surface active agents or cyclodextrins such as HP-β-Cyclodextrin that can serve as a biocompatible solubilizer and stabilizer in combination with lipophilic absorption enhancers. Most intranasal formulations are aqueous based and hence preservatives are needed to prevent microbial growth. Parabens, benzalkonium chloride, phenyl ethyl alcohol, EDTA, and benzoyl alcohol are some of the commonly used preservatives in intranasal formulations. Studies have shown that mercury-containing preservatives have a fast and irreversible effect on ciliary movement and should not be used in intranasal systems" (24,69). An extensive study has been conducted to develop preservative free intranasal delivery systems (25).

As application of drugs to the nasal cavity involves direct exposure to external air, use of antioxidants might help prevent the oxidation of drugs. Antioxidants that are commonly employed include tocopherol, sodium bisulfate, butylated hydroxytoulene, etc. Care should be taken to minimize the interactions between the execipient and the principle ingredient (19,69).

According to Aurora et al., "Many allergic and chronic diseases are often connected with crusts and drying of the mucous membrane. Certain preservatives/antioxidants are also likely to cause nasal irritation especially when used in higher quantities. Adequate nasal moisture is essential for preventing dehydration. Therefore, humectants can be added especially in gel-based intranasal products. Only humectants that avoid nasal irritation and are not likely to affect drug absorption should be used. Examples include glycerin, sorbitol and mannitol" (69).

The physicochemical properties of drugs play an important role in deciding the formulation characteristics. In his review, Aurora has mentioned that "The chemical form of a drug can be important in determining absorption. For example, conversion of the drug into a salt or ester form can alter its absorption (19). Studies on the effect of structural modification on absorption revealed that in situ nasal absorption of carboxylic acid esters of L-tyrosine was significantly greater than that of L-tyrosine. Polymorphism is known to affect the dissolution rate and solubility of drugs and thus their absorption through biological membranes" (69). So polymorphic stability and purity of drugs must be considered for intranasal formulations (20).

Molecular weight, particle size, solubility and dissolution rate are very important physiochemical properties effecting formulation characteristics. A linear inverse correlation exists between the absorption and molecular weight (up to ~300 Da) (69). As per Aurora, "absorption decreases significantly if the molecular weight is greater than ~1000 Da. It has been reported that particle sizes greater than 10 μm are deposited in the nasal cavity. Particles that are 2–10 μm can be retained in the lungs, while particles of less than 1 μm are exhaled. Drug solubility and dissolution rates are important factors in determining nasal absorption from powders and suspensions. The particles deposited in the nasal cavity need to be dissolved prior to absorption. If a drug remains as particles or is cleared away, no absorption occurs" (69).

The drugs administered to the intranasal route have been delivered through dosage forms such as nasal drops, sprays, powder insufflations, topical gels, nasal pledgets, emulsions and ointments. Sprays have been shown to have much better bioavailability as compared to powdered formulations. Conversely, powder formulations tend to provide better stability, less need for preservatives and offer the capability to administer drugs in larger doses.

Nasal Drops

Nasal drops are the simplest dosage form for nasal delivery. They are best suited for solutions. The main disadvantage of this system is dose inaccuracy. In nostrils, as compared to nasal sprays, nasal drops have been shown to deposit human serum albumin efficiently (26).

Nasal Sprays

In his review, Aurora has stated that "Both solution and suspension formulations can be formulated into nasal sprays. Due to the availability of metered dose pumps and actuators, a nasal spray can deliver an exact dose from 25 to 200 μL. The particle size and morphology (for suspensions) of the drug and viscosity of the formulation determine the choice of pump and actuator assembly" (69). These are the most common dosage forms where ever local effect is required (26).

Nasal Powders

This dosage form is the last resort if solution and suspension dosage forms are not possible (low stability). No preservative and superior stability of the formulation are advantages. As per review by Aurora "However, the suitability of the powder formulation is dependent on the solubility, particle size, aerodynamic properties and nasal irritancy of the active drug and/or excipients and a grittiness of the powder. Local application of drug is another advantage of this system but nasal mucosa irritancy and metered dose delivery are some of the challenges for formulation scientists and device manufacturers" (27,69).

Nasal Ointments

Nasal ointments or emulsions had been devised as an alternative to the nasal drops to address drug solubility and residence time issues. They suffer, however, from problems of dose inaccuracy and poor patient compliance. Ointments are limited to local drug delivery.

Nasal Gels

According to Aurora, "Nasal gels are high-viscosity thickened solutions or suspensions. Until the recent development of precise dosing devices, there was not much interest in this system. The advantages of a nasal gel include the reduction of post-nasal drip due to high viscosity, reduction of taste impact due to reduced swallowing, reduction of anterior leakage of the formulation, reduction of irritation by using soothing/emollient excipients and targeted delivery to mucosa for better absorption" (69). Nasal gels can be used for both systemic and local drug delivery. Vitamin B_{12} gel was developed recently as a prescription product (28).

Nasal Vaccine

Most of the pathogenic bacteria, viruses, and parasites enter human bodies through the mucosa. Air we inhale is filtered by the nose. Good immune response is difficult to attain with oral vaccination because of degradation and dilution in the stomach and intestines and thus the nasal delivery of vaccines has recently emerged as an excellent alternative to it (29,70).

The nose is easily accessible highly vascularized mucosal organ with large surface for absorption which can cause both mucosal and systemic immune responses. Suitability for mass-vaccination, needle-free vaccination and faster onset of strong immune response are the certain other major benefits of the nasal vaccination. Narrow nasal entrance, variable dosing with traditional delivery methods, complex geometry with narrow passages and mucociliary clearance are some of the major hurdles for nasal vaccination. Reformulation of vaccines and direct nose-to-brain transport when the brain is not the target organ also possess a concern for this delivery.

Microspheres

Microspheres of various polymers have been studied in vivo as nasal drug delivery systems. Microspheres of albumin, starch and DEAE-dextran absorbed water and formed a gel-like layer, which was cleared slowly from the nasal cavity (79). A degradable starch microsphere (DSM) is the most widely used microsphere system which has been shown to improve the absorption of insulin, gentamicin, human growth hormone, metoclopramide and desmopressin (30,31,78). The DSM was also shown to synergistically increase the effect of the absorption enhancers on the transport of the insulin across the nasal membrane. Illum et al. has introduced bioadhesive dextran microspheres for prolonging the residence time in the nasal cavity (32). They observed the slowest clearance for DEAE-dextran, where 60% of the delivered dose was still present at the deposition site after 3 hour. However, these microspheres were not successful in enhancing insulin absorption in rats.

Liposomes

Alpar et al. evaluated the potential adjuvant effect of liposomes on tetanus toxoid, to develop a non-parenteral immunization procedure (33). They found that tetanus toxoid entrapped in DSPC liposomes was stable also taken up intact in the gut. The permeability of liposome entrapping insulin through the nasal mucosa of rabbit has been studied and compared with the permeability of insulin solution with or without pre-treatment by sodium glycocholate (GC) (34,78). This comparison showed that the liposome had permeated more effectively after pre-treatment by GC. The loading and leakage characteristics of the desmopressin-containing liposomes and the effect of liposomes on the nasal mucosa permeation and were also investigated. The increase of permeability antidiuresis of desmopressin through the nasal mucosa occurred in the order positively charged liposomes > negatively charged liposomes > solution (35).

Gels

Chitin and chitosan have been widely exploited as vehicles in sustained nasal delivery systems. Nasal absorption of nifedipine from gel preparations resulted in rapid absorption and high C_{max} (26). The effect of polyacrylic acid gel on the nasal absorption of insulin and calcitonin was investigated in rats (36). According to Turker et al., "After nasal administration of insulin its absorption from 0.15 w/v polyacrylic acid gel is greater than with 1% w/v gel" (78). Zhou et al. have showed "The effects of putative bioadhesive polymer gels on slowing nasal mucociliary clearance in a rat model. The results showed that all the formulations decreased intranasal mucociliary clearance, thus increasing the residence time of the formulations in the nasal cavity" (80).

Nanoparticle Formulations

In the review by Illum et al., it has been stated that "Nanoparticle formulations can provide protection of drugs such as peptides and increase their longer residence time in the nasal cavity, of at least bioadhesive nanoparticles. This is the reason for the promotion of the uptake of the peptide over and above that of a simple drug solution or powder systems of the same material (37). In vitro evaluations have indicated that nanoparticles are taken up by the nasal tissue according to their size and surface characteristics but that the nanoparticles are not necessary transported to any great extent across the tissue. In vivo evaluations have suggested that particles can be taken up by M cells in the NALT and transported into the lymphatic system and hence to the blood stream. Nanoparticle systems seem to be well suited for the delivery of nasal vaccine. Nanoparticles containing (or coated with) antigenic materials can be transported to the lymphoid tissue by the M cells" (12). This approach will lower amounts of antigenic materials for vaccination. However, much work is needed to optimize such nanoparticle systems for vaccine delivery especially in terms of optimal particle size and surface characteristics.

Intranasal Gene Therapy

Intranasal gene therapy has caught attention as a noninvasive method for administering therapeutic genes. As stated by Han et al. in their review, "Intranasal administration of interleukin-12 genes has been studied as a method for treating osteosarcoma lung metastasis in mice" (38,41). Intranasal dosing of a plasmid DNA encoding transforming growth factor β1 was successfully developed to prevent the development of murine experimental colitis. This route has been also studied for administering cystic fibrosis transmembrane conductance regulator genes during treatment of patients with cystic fibrosis (39). Han et al. have also stated that "Intranasal administration of neurotrophic factors was found to offer some degree of brain targeting with minimal invasiveness" (81). Sniffing neuropeptide has been also exploited as a transnasal approach for targeting agents to the human brain (81). Recently, intranasal administration of nerve growth factor protein was shown to rescue recognition memory deficits in a transgenic mouse model (40). Another recent approach shows delivery of intranasally administered plasmid DNAs up to 14.1 kb in size, the brain, and their encoded genes could be expressed. Moreover, the authors have also supported mechanism for brain targeting of intranasally administered plasmid DNA via the olfactory bulb (41). These investigations will definitely form the basis for important therapeutic advances in the gene therapy of brain diseases by nasal route.

Preservative-Free Nasal Drug Delivery Systems

The main benefit in removing preservatives from formulations would be to reduce the potential for adverse effects on the nasal mucosa. According to Bommer et al., "Recently, the German health authorities (BfArM) issued a warning concerning the widely used popular preservative Benzalkonium-chloride" (71). According to Leskovsek et al. and Brouet et al., "The selection of the technology used in these specific devices, as well as the design of the protocols used to qualify the device, are key factors for success in the development of a non-preserved nasal spray product" (72,82). Brouet et al. also mentioned that "Multi-dose devices used in these products are specifically designed to protect the product to be dispensed and to prevent its microbial contamination. This can be achieved with the use of different technologies, which include the use of mechanical barriers, bacteriostatic agents, and filters. The choice of an appropriate protocol for microbial integrity testing is of great importance. Combinations of several of the tests are applied to verify the level of protection provided by the device" (25,82).

NOVEL NASAL DELIVERY SYSTEMS

Chitosan and Other Positively Charged Polymers

Recently, the polysaccharide material, chitosan has attracted a lot of interest as an intranasal delivery system that can efficiently deliver polar drugs (including peptides) to the systemic circulation and provide therapeutically relevant bioavailabilities. Resultant free amino groups enable the formation of positively charged chitosan salts with organic and inorganic acids. Chitosan glutamate is usually the pharmaceutically acceptable grade of chitosan for intranasal delivery. It has >80% acylation and high molecular weight (~250 kDa) (42).

A mixture of the chitosan-4-thiobutylamidine (TBA) conjugate, insulin and the permeation mediator reduced glutathione formulated into microparticles resulted in significant improvement in the delivery of peptide drugs. Also, in vivo evaluations of microparticles comprising chitosan-TBA have led to substantial higher potential for intranasal insulin administration than unmodified chitosan (43,44). Intranasal administration of chitosan-antigen nasal vaccines showed that the intranasal formulation induced significant serum IgG responses similar to and secretory IgA levels superior to what was induced by a parenteral administration of the vaccine (45). Chitosan powder was shown as the most effective formulation for intranasal delivery of insulin in the sheep model and chitosan nanoparticles did not improve the absorption enhancing effect of chitosan in solution or powder form (46). Illum et al. showed that in sheep model addition of chitosan to an intranasal formulation resulted in an increase in peak plasma insulin levels from 34 to 191 mIU/1 and a seven fold increase in area under the curve. Further these results were confirmed in human volunteers with 9–15% increase in nasal bioavailability as compared to a subcutaneous injection (47). Chitosan powder formulations have been shown to enable an efficient nasal absorption of goserelin in a sheep model where bioavailabilities of 20–40% were obtained dependent on the nature of the formulation (48). A thermosensitive hydrogel based on quaternized chitosan and poly(ethylene glycol) administered to the rat nasal cavity decreased the blood glucose concentration to 40–50% of initial blood glucose concentration for at least 4–5 hour after administration, and no apparent cytoxicity was observed after application (49). In a recent study on the effect of polymer type and intranasal delivery device on distribution and clearance of bioadhesive formulations from the olfactory region in man it was found that all of the bioadhesive formulations were able to reach the olfactory region in the nasal cavity of human volunteers when delivered using a simple nasal drop device. Charlton et al. in 2007 stated that "Furthermore, the formulations displayed a significantly increased residence time on the epithelial surface. This was in contrast to a non-bioadhesive control delivered with the same device. In contrast, a pectin formulation administered with a nasal spray system did not show an increase in residence time in the olfactory region. It was further shown that the reproducibility of olfactory delivery of a polymer formulation was significantly better intra- than inter-subject" (50).

Cyclodextrins

Earlier work by Marttin et al. indicated certain promise with the use of cyclodextrins in animal models (44). Co-administration of the peptide with protease inhibitors and absorption enhancers was shown to increase methionine enkephalin permeation (4- to 94-folds). The increase was proportional to nasal transepithelial resistance reduction and permeation of paracellular marker dye (51). Formulations containing 5% dimethyl-beta-cyclodextrin were shown to be most efficacious in enhancing absorption of low molecular weight heparins both in vivo and in vitro (52). In vivo studies by Tas et al. on metoclopramide HCl nasal formulation indicated that nasal bioavailability was higher with gel formulation as compared to solution and powder form (53). It can be concluded that cyclodextrins increase nasal bioavailability by acting on tight junctions and thus increasing paracellular drug transport.

Phospholipids and Lipids

In the early 1990s attempts to develop nasal insulin product by Novonordisk (Denmark) using the phospholipid didecanoyl-L-α-phosphatidyl choline (DDPC) as an absorption enhancer were discontinued due to insufficient metabolic profiles when compared to subcutaneous insulin delivery and low bioavailability in diabetic patients (54). A powder formulation comprising small starch microspheres (SSMS) and a powder formulation comprising SSMS and L-alpha-lysophosphatidylglycerol (enhancers) were found to increase nasal bioavailability of granulocyte-colony stimulating factor (55). As stated by Scheerlinck et al., "key barrier to producing effective nasal immunizations is the low efficiency of uptake of vaccines across the nasal mucosa. A cannulation system was used to examine antibody response induced by nasal immunization with an ISCOMATRIX influenza vaccine" (56). For the first time it was shown that following nasal vaccination, specific antibodies enter the circulation of primed animals via the draining lymphatics as a wave that peaks approximately 5–6 days after vaccination (56).

NOSE TO BRAIN DELIVERY

The reason for rapid euphoria generated by the inhalation of cocaine was concluded to be due to a pathway that exists directly from nose to brain which enables cocaine to concentrate in certain areas of brain. As stated by Illum et al., "Various studies in animal models have confirmed that the concentration of cocaine in the brain was higher after intranasal administration than after intravenous injection, thereby showing the existence of the pathway from nose to brain" (57,58,81). The nose to brain pathway can be of interest for delivery of polar drugs which are poorly permeable across the blood brain barrier. It was suggested that they might reach a target in the brain more effectively via the intranasal route as compared to other routes (57). It was shown in a mouse model that [^{3}H]-dopamine reached the olfactory lobe after intranasal administration and that at 4 hours after administration the concentration in this tissue after intranasal administration was 27-times higher than after intravenous injection (59,60). It should be noted that percent drug accumulated in the brain that is administered via the nasal route is relatively low (~1%). Experiments on man for studying the effect on brain potentials and investigating transport of drug into cerebrospinal fluid after intranasal and intravenous administration by sampling of CSF from spinal tap were performed earlier. A significant accumulation of insulin in CSF after a single administration of 40 IU and no increase in plasma level was observed (61). The olfactory region situated at the loft of the nasal cavity is the only site in human body where the nervous system is in direct contact with the surrounding environment (81). Drugs have been shown to reach the CNS from the nasal cavity by a direct transport across the olfactory region. Drug might cross the olfactory epithelium by either the transcellular or paracellular route. Illum et al. also stated, "Furthermore, the drug can be transported through the olfactory neuron cells by intracellular axonal transport primarily to the olfactory bulbs" (81). The intracellular axonal pathway is a slow pathway that can take hours to deliver drugs to the CNS, whereas the two other pathways enable drug transport to happen fast. Illum et al. suggested this as the last pathway that is often evident in the experimental settings. In diseases such as Parkinson's disease, Alzheimer's disease, etc., where direct and rapid action on the brain might be beneficial, nose to brain delivery might be of great interest. A recent study on rats to delineate relative accumulation of huperzine A after intranasal, intravenous and gastric administration indicated significant accumulation of drug in CSF when administered via the intranasal route (62). Also, intranasal delivery of peptides which degrade rapidly in the blood is being widely investigated, as peptide concentrations required for therapeutic action on the brain can be relatively low (63).

INTRANASAL DRUG DELIVERY TECHNOLOGIES

According to Dr. Bommer, "The term drug delivery can be explained by the keywords 'controlled release' and 'devices.' Controlled release mechanisms ensure that the patients system is exposed to a therapeutically viable dose of drug over a certain period of time. A device can govern a patient's comfort and efficiency of therapy" (71). Micro and macro-molecules given through the nasal route to treat various disease symptoms are on the market (Table 1). Most of the current intranasally administered drugs are liquid formulations and delivered with a metered pump spray. The delivery of drugs as a liquid is effective for most of the compounds (27). The need for delivering drugs to patients efficiently with fewer side effects has inspired pharmaceutical companies to actively develop new drug delivery systems. Pharmaceutical companies are currently in the process of developing multiple platform technologies for controlled release and delivery of large molecules (28).

Verma et al. indicated that, as opposed to earlier days when nasal drops were widely used, present nasal dosage forms mainly consist of "preparations containing dispersed or dissolved drugs placed in a container that is squeeze- or spray-activated. Alternatively, liquid solutions can be delivered using metered atomizing pumps or metered-dose pressurized nasal inhalers. Butorphanol (Stadol NS Nasal Spray, Bristol Myers Squibb Co., U.S.A.), calcitonin (Miacalcin Nasal Spray, Novartis), dihydroergotamine (Migranal Nasal Spray, Novartis, Inc.), sumatriptan (Imitrex Nasal Spray, Glaxo-SmithKline), and desmopressin (DDAVP Nasal Spray, Aventis Pharma, U.S.A.) are some of the drugs marketed in the form of a nasal spray. Cromolyn sodium (Nasalcrom Nasal Solution, Fisons Pharmaceuticals) is

Table 1 Compounds that Appear in Marketed Products that Are Administered Systemically via the Nasal Cavity to Treat Various Disease Conditions

Compound	Condition treated	Industry
Nicotine	Smoking	Pharmacia & Upjohn Inc.
Dihydrogotamine	Migraine	Novartis
Sumatriptan	Migraine	Glaxo SmithKline
Zolmitriptan	Migraine	AstraZeneca
Ergotamine	Migraine	Novartis
Calcitonin	Osteoporosis	Novartis
Butarphanol	Migraine	Bristol-Myers Squibb
Desmopressin	Reduce the flow of urine	Ferring, Norgine
Buserelin	Migraine	Aventis
Estradiol	Post menopausal symptoms	Servier

Source: From Ref. 28.

available in a solution form. Budesonide (Rhinocort Nasal Inhaler, Astra) and beclomethasone diproprionate (Rino Clenil, Chiesi Farmaceutici) are marketed in the form of metered-dose pressurized aerosols. Beclomethasone diproprionate is also available in the form of a metered-dose manual spray unit with trade names Beconase AQ marketed by Glaxo-SmithKline, and Vancenase AQ marketed by Schering Plough Corporation" (28). The intranasal route is being explored to deliver new drugs. As quoted in the article in *Medical News Today* the prescription antihistamine Astelin® (azelastine HCl) nasal spray is found to relieve the major symptoms of pollen allergy, including sneezing, runny nose, and congestion, within 15 minutes of application compared to placebo and maintained efficacy at all time points for 8 hours in a randomized, single dose, double-blind, placebo-controlled study (64). According to an article published in the Newswire Web site, "Four out of every 10 children suffer from severe nasal allergy symptoms that may affect their overall well-being. Clinical research suggests that fluticasone furoate (FFNS) nasal spray, a once-a-day allergy medicine under Food and Drug Administration review, effectively treats sneezing, runny nose, nasal itching, and nasal congestion in children 2–11 years of age with seasonal and year-round nasal allergies. Moreover, the investigational drug was found to have no effect on children's short-term growth. The data from two Phase III studies on 1100 children designed to evaluate how safe and effective FFNS was in children with either seasonal allergies, which are caused by pollen, or year-round allergies, which are caused by dust mites, mold, and animal dander. In both studies FFNS was found to be effective in reducing nasal symptoms, compared to placebo, and was generally well tolerated. In addition, researchers presented data from two studies that evaluated whether FFNS affected key safety measures in children, including short-term lower leg growth and a hormonal process known as hypo-thalamic-pituitary-adrenal axis function. Both studies demonstrated that treatment with FFNS did not affect these important indicators of growth and hormonal function" (65).

Though intranasal liquid delivery of drugs is effective a number of factors limit this approach (27). As per compilation by Dubin, "The various factors involved include solubility of the drug in the vehicle, limited capacity of the nasal cavity to hold liquid without drainage to the throat or from its anterior portion, and stability of the formulation" (83). Delivery of a powdered dosage form has numerous advantages compared to liquid administration. The powdered method can lead to localized deposition of drug on surface of mucosa. This avoids widespread coating of nasal cavity, which happens with liquid formulation. As the powder formulation is exposed to a smaller surface area for a limited period of time, it is expected to be better tolerated than liquid formulation (27). According to Verma et al., "administration of powders requires nasal insufflators that are either mechanically or respiration actuated. In mechanical devices, a rubber bulb is connected through the dose reservoir to a nasal adapter. Squeezing the rubber bulb provides a stream of air that is capable of emitting the loaded powder in the insufflator. Rinoflatore (Fisons, Italy), Miat Nasal Insufflator (Miat, Italy), and Puvlizer (Teijin, Japan) are some of the marketed insufflators for nasal administration of powders. Respiration-actuated devices are a nose-adapted version of dry powder inhalers. With both types of devices, the drug is loaded in a gelatin capsule that is pierced just before activation. The capsule is located between the air jet producer and the nose adapter, and the flowing air stream creates turbulence inside the capsule, which aerolizes and releases the powder from the capsule. Nasal gels also can be used to provide an enhanced bioavailability compared with oral delivery. EnerB (Nature's Bounty, Inc.), a vitamin B_{12} dietary supplement, is available in gel form" (28). As per explanation by Illum et al., "Bioadhesive delivery systems provide effective strategies to overcome barrier to effective absorption, namely the mucociliary clearance. One of these delivery systems is ChiSys™ (West Pharmaceutical Services, Inc.), which is a patented proprietary technology intended for intranasal delivery of drugs and vaccines. ChiSys is based on the use of chitosan, a cationic polysaccharide obtained from partial deacetylation of chitin, which originates from shells of crustaceans" (66,73). According to an article in the Delsite Web site, "A wide array of drugs are being tested as lead candidates to be delivered as nasal powders. DelSite Biotechnologies is developing an influenza nasal powder vaccine that incorporates inactivated whole virion antigen in the GelVac dry powder delivery system, a unique in situ gelling powder formulation. GelVac is a proprietary nasal powder vaccine delivery system based on the GelSite® polymer, the primary functional ingredient that confers its unique in situ gelling property. The GelVac system combines the advantages of dry powder formulations and nasal immunization, including room temperature stability, prolonged shelf life, and no need for preservatives, and induction of systemic and mucosal immune responses. Upon hydration by nasal fluid, the GelVac powder formulation changes from dry powder particles to wet gel particles, resulting in the formation of a gel that adheres to nasal mucus, thus maximizing antigen exposure through prolonged nasal residence time and sustained antigen release. This vaccine was indicated to provide distinct advantages in meeting the critical needs for influenza pandemic preparedness and epidemic control, including room temperature stability, broader protection, antigen sparing, ease of administration and induction of both mucosal and systemic immune responses. Preclinical studies have shown that GelVac powder vaccine is highly immunogenic in animal models, inducing a strong immune response and a strong protective effect following challenge infection. The powder vaccine was found to be stable at ambient temperature for over eighteen months. The Phase I human safety study showed that the GelVac powder without an antigen was safe and well tolerated in humans" (67,74).

CONCLUSION

Considering the potential benefits of intranasal drug delivery, novel approaches to this mode of delivery will be continuously explored. However, the long-term use of a drug delivery system will mainly depend on local toxicity. To meet the challenges of designing an effective nasal formulation with commercial success, one has to consider all aspects, from the anatomy and physiology of the nose to all the critical steps of product development. By increasing the residence time and absorption, one can potentially overcome the major barriers. Overall, intranasal route accompanied by novel drug delivery technologies can be highly efficient for the delivery of complex therapeutic molecules.

ACKNOWLEDGMENTS

The authors would like to acknowledge Dr. Pal for his advice and critical evaluation of the manuscript. The NIH grants 1RO1AI071199-01A2 and 5RO1AI071199-02 are acknowledged for the financial support.

REFERENCES

1. Datamonitor, Drug Delivery: Global Industry Guide. 2006:20.
2. Mygind N, Dahl R. Anatomy, physiology and function of the nasal cavities in health and disease. Adv Drug Deliv Rev 1998; 29:3–12.
3. Sarkar MA. Drug metabolism in the nasal mucosa. Pharm Res 1992; 9:1–9.

4. Brime B, Ballesteros MP, Frutos P. Preparation and in vitro characterization of gelatin microspheres containing Levodopa for nasal administration. J Microencap 2000; 6:777–84.

5. Illum L. Is nose-to-brain transport of drugs in man a reality? J Pharm Pharmacol 2004; 56:3–17.

6. Madara JL. Modulation of tight junctional permeability. Adv Drug Deliv Rev 2000; 41:251–3.

7. Ward PD, Tippin TK, Thakker DR. Enhancing paracellular permeability by modulating epithelial tight junctions. Pharm Sci Tech Today 2000; 3:346–58.

8. Tsukamoto T, Nigam SK. Role of tyrosine phosphorylationinthere assembly of occluding and other tight junction proteins. Am J Physiol 1999; 276: F737–50.

9. Smith JM, Dornish M, Wood EJ. Involvement of protein kinase C in chitosan glutamate-mediated tight junction disruption. Biomaterials 2005; 26:3269–76.

10. Frieke Kuper C, Koornstra PJ, Hameleers DMH, et al. The role of nasopharyngeal lymphoid tissue. Immunol Today 1992; 13:219–24.

11. Behrens I, Vila Pena AI, Alonso MJ, Kissel T. Comparative uptake studies of bioadhesive nanoparticles in human intestinal cell lines and rats: The effect of mucus on particle adsorption and transport. Pharm Res 2002; 19:1185–93.

12. Illum L. Nanoparticulate systems for nasal delivery of drugs: A real improvement over simple systems? J Pharm Sci 2007; 96:473–83.

13. Khanvilkar K, Donovan MD, Flanagan DR. Drug transfer through mucus. Adv Drug Deliv Rev 2001; 28:173–93.

14. Gervasi PG, Longo V, Naldi F, Panattoni G, Ursino F. Xenobiotic-metabolizing enzymes in human respiratory nasal mucosa. Biochem Pharmacol 1991; 41:177–84.

15. Hussain A, Hirai S, Bawarshi R. Nasal absorption of the natural contraceptive steroid in rats—progesterone absorption. J Pharm Sci 1981; 70:466–7 (Letter).

16. McMartin C, Hutchinson LEF, Hyde R, Peters GE. Analysis of structural requirements for the absorption of drugs and macromolecules from the nasal cavity. J Pharm Sci 1987; 76:535–40.

17. Wermeling DP, Record KA, Kelly TH, Archer SM, Clinch T, Rudy AC. Pharmacokinetics and pharmacodynamics of a new intranasal midazolam formulation in healthy volunteers. Anesth Analg 2006; 103:344–9.

18. Harris AS, Nilsson IM, Wagner ZG, Alkner U. Intranasal administration of peptides: Nasal deposition biological response and absorption of desmopressin. J Pharm Sci 1986; 75:1085–8.

19. Huang C, Kimura R, Nassar A, Hussain A. Mechanism of nasal drug absorption of drug II: Absorption of L-tyrosine and the effect of structural modification on its absorption. J Pharm Sci 1985; 74:1298–301.

20. Hirai S, Yashika T, Matsuzawa T, Mima H. Absorption of drugs from the nasal mucosa of rat. Int J Pharm 1981; 7:317–25.

21. Thompson R. Lysozyme and its relation to antibacterial properties of various tissues and secretions. Arch Pathol 1940; 30:1096.

22. Pennington AK, Ratcliffe JH, Wilson CG, Hardy JG. The influence of solution viscosity on nasal spray deposition and clearance. Int J Pharm 1988; 43:221–4.

23. Suzuki Y, Makino Y. Mucosal drug delivery using cellulose derivatives as a functional polymer. J Control Release 1999; 62:101–7.

24. Van de Donk HJM, Muller Plantema IP, Zuidema J, Merkus FWHM. The effects of preservatives on the ciliary beat frequency of chicken embryo tracheas. Rhinology 1980; 18:119–30.

25. Simon S, Grosjean B, Brouet G, Orange N, Pacaud H, Herry S. Evaluation of the ability of an air-filtering nasal spray device to prevent the contamination of preservative-free formulations. Paper presented at the annual meeting of the AAPS in Denver, Colorado, 2000.

26. Behl CR, Pimplaskar HK, Sileno J, deMeireles J, Romeo VD. Effects of physicochemical properties and other factors on systemic nasal drug delivery. Adv Drug Deliv Rev 1998; 29:89–116.

27. Lambert P. Nasal Drug Delivery: The Powder Advantage (Report). Drug Discovery Development and Delivery, 2002.

28. Verma RK, Garg S. Current status of drug delivery technologies and future directions. Pharm Tech On-line 2001; 25:1–14.

29. Davis SS. Nasal vaccines. Adv Drug Deliv Rev 2001; 51(1–3):21–42.

30. Illum L, Farraj NF, Davis SS, Johansen BR, O'Hagan DT. Investigation of the nasal absorption of biosynthetic human growth hormone in sheep—use of a bioadhesive microsphere delivery system. Int J Pharm 1990; 63:207–11.

31. Critichley H, Davis SS, Farraj NF, Illum L. Nasal absorption of desmopressin in rats and sheep. Effect of a bioadhesive microsphere delivery system. J Pharm Pharmacol 1993; 46:651–6.

32. Illum L, Jorgensen H, Bisgaard H, Krogsgaard O, Rossing N. Bioadhesive microspheres as a potential nasal drug delivery system. Int J Pharm 1987; 39:189–99.

33. Alpar HO, Bowen JC, Brown MRW. Effectiveness of liposomes as adjuvants of orally and nasally administered tetanus toxoid. Int J Pharm 1992; 88: 335–44.

34. Maitani Y, Asano S, Takahashi S, Nakagaki M, Nagai T. Permeability of insulin entrapped in liposome through the nasal mucosa of rabbits. Chem Pharm Bull 1992; 40:1569–72.

35. Law SL, Huang K J, Chou HY. Preparation of desmopressin-containing liposomes for intranasal delivery. J Control Release 2001; 70:375–82.

36. Morimoto K, Morisaka K, Kamada A. Enhancement of nasal absorption of insulin and calcitonin using polyacrylic acid gel. J Pharm Pharmacol 1985; 37:134–6.

37. Illum L. Nanoparticulate systems for nasal delivery of drugs: A real improvement over simple systems? J Pharm Sci 2007; 96(3):473–83.

38. Jia SF, Worth LL, Densmore CL, Xu B, Zhou Z, Kleinerman ES. Eradication of osteosarcoma lung metastases following intranasal interleukin-12P gene therapy using a nonviral polyethylenimine vector. Cancer Gene Ther 2002; 9:260–6.

39. Hyde SC, Southern KW, Gileadi U, et al. Repeat administration of DNA/liposomes to the nasal epithelium of patients with cystic fibrosis. Gene Ther 2000; 7:1156–65.

40. De Rosa R, Garcia AA, Braschi C, et al. Intranasal administration of nerve growth factor (NGF) rescues recognition memory deficits in AD11 anti-NGF transgenic mice. Proc Natl Acad Sci USA 2005; 102:3811–6.

41. Han IK, Kim MY, Byun HM, et al. Enhanced brain targeting efficiency of intranasally administered plasmid DNA: An alternative route for brain gene therapy. J Mol Med 2007; 85(1):75–83.

42. Illum L. Nasal drug delivery—possibilities, problems and solutions. J Control Release 2003; 87:187–98.

43. Krauland AH, Guggi D, Bernkop-Schnurch A. Thiolated chitosan microparticles: A vehicle for nasal peptide drug delivery. Int J Pharm 2006; 307:270–7.

44. Marttin E, Verhoef JC, Merkus FW. Efficacy, safety and mechanism of cyclodextrins as absorption enhancers in nasal delivery of peptide and protein drugs. J Drug Target 1998; 6:17–36.

45. Illum L, Jabbal-Gill I, Hinchcliffe M, Fisher AN, Davis SS. Chitosan as a novel nasal delivery system for vaccines. Adv Drug Deliv Rev 2001; 51:81–96.

46. Dyer AM, Hinchcliffe M, Watts P, et al. Nasal delivery of insulin using novel chitosan based formulations: A comparative study in two animal models between simple chitosan formulations and chitosan nanoparticles. Pharm Res 2002; 19:998–1008.

47. Illum L, Farraj NF, Davis SS. Chitosan as a novel nasal delivery system for peptides drugs. Pharm Res 1994; 11:1186–9.

48. Illum L, Watts P, Fisher AN, Jabbal-Gill I, Davis SS. Novel chitosan based delivery systems for nasal administration of a LHRH-analogue. STP Pharm 2000; 10:89–94.

49. Wu J, Wei W, Wang LY, Su ZG, Ma GH. A thermosensitive hydrogel based on quaternized chitosan and poly(ethylene glycol) for nasal drug delivery system. Biomaterials 2007; 28:2220–32.

50. Charlton S, Jones NS, Davis SS, Illum L. Distribution and clearance of bioadhesive formulations from the olfactory region in man: Effect of polymer type and nasal delivery device. Eur J Pharm Sci 2007; 30:295–302.

51. Agu RU, Vu Dang H, Jorissen M, Kinget R, Verbeke N. Metabolism and absorption enhancement of methionine enkephalin in human nasal epithelium. Peptides 2004; 25:563–9.

52. Yang T, Hussain A, Paulson J, Abbruscato TJ, Ahsan F. Cyclodextrins in nasal delivery of low-molecular-weight heparins: In vivo and in vitro studies. Pharm Res 2004; 21:1127–36.

53. Tas C, Ozkan CK, Savaser A, Ozkan Y, Tasdemir U, Altunay H. Nasal absorption of metoclopramide from different Carbopol 981 based formulations: In vitro, ex vivo and in vivo evaluation. Eur J Pharm Biopharm 2006; 64:246–54.

54. Hilsted J, Madsbad S, Hvidberg A, Rasmussen MH. Intranasal insulin therapy: The clinical realities. Diabetologia 1995; 38:680–4.

55. Gill IJ, Fisher AN, Farraj N, Pitt CG, Davis SS, Illum L. Intranasal absorption of granulocyte-colony stimulating factor (G-CSF) from powder formulations, in sheep. Eur J Pharm Sci 1998; 6:1–10.

56. Scheerlinck JP, Gekas S, Yen HH, et al. Local immune responses following nasal delivery of an adjuvanted influenza vaccine. Vaccine 2006; 24:3929–36.

57. Illum L. Transport of drugs from the nasal cavity to the central nervous system. Eur J Pharm Sci 2000; 11:1–18.
58. Chow H, Chen Z, Matsuura GT. Direct transport of cocaine from the nasal cavity to the brain following intranasal cocaine administration in rats. J Pharm Sci 1999; 88:754–8.
59. Dahlin M, Bergman U, Jansson B, Bjork E, Brittebo E. Transfer of dopamine in the olfactory pathway following nasal administration in mice. Pharm Res 2000; 17:737–42.
60. Dahlin M, Jansson B, Bjork E. Levels of dopamine in blood and brain following nasal administration to rats. Eur J Pharm Sci 2001; 14:75–80.
61. Fehm HL. Manipulating neuropeptidergic pathways in humans: A novel approach to neuropharmacology. Eur J Pharmacol 2000; 405:43–54.
62. Yue P, Tao T, Zhao Y, Ren J, Chai X. Huperzine A in rat plasma and CSF following intranasal administration. Int J Pharm Dec 28, 2006 (Epub ahead of print).
63. Banks WA. The CNS as a target for peptides and peptide-based drugs. Expert Opin Drug Deliv 2006; 3:707–12.
64. http://www.medicalnewstoday.com/medicalnews.php?newsid = 63850
65. http://www.medicalnewstoday.com/medicalnews.php?newsid = 64068
66. Muzzarelli RAA. Chitin. In: Muzzarelli RAA, ed. Natural Chelating Polymers: Alginic Acid, Chitin, and Chitosan. Pergamon Press, New York, 1973: 83–252.
67. Yates KM, Ni Y. GelVac™ nasal powder: A new approach to vaccine delivery. BIO 2005 Annual International Convention, June 2005.
68. Wermeling DP, Miller JL, Rudy AC. Systematic intranasal drug delivery: Concepts and applications. Drug Deliv Tech 2002; 2(1):56–61.
69. Aurora J. Development of nasal delivery systems: A review. Drug Deliv Tech 2002; 2(7):70–3.
70. http://www.optinose.no/publications
71. http://www.drugdeliverytech.com/cgi-bin/articles.cgi?idArticle=386
72. Bommer R, Kern J, Hennes K, Zwisler W, Preservative-free nasal drug delivery systems. Med Device Technol 2004; 15(9):14–8.
73. Leskovsek NV. Don't hold your breath: FDA's phase-out of chlorofluorocarbon metered-dose inhalers will take years. Drug Delivery Technology; http://www.drugdeliverytech.com/cgi-bin/articles.cgi?idArticle=184
74. Illum L, Dodane V, Iqbal K. Chitosan Technology to Enhance the Effectiveness of Nasal Drug Delivery. Drug Delivery Technology; http://www.drugdeliverytech.com/cgi-bin/articles.cgi?idArticle=31
75. http://www.delsite.com/
76. Simón CA, Bartomeu RM, Pérez RA, Baena FA. Intranasal opioids for acute pain. Rev Esp Anestesiol Reanim 2006; 53(10):643–52.
77. http://www.devicelink.com/pmpn/archive/04/05/002.html
78. Türker S, Onur E, Özer Y. Nasal route and drug delivery systems. Pharm World Sci 2004; 26(3):137–42; http://www.touchbriefings.com/pdf/17/pt031_t_west_pharma.pdf
79. Morath LP. Microspheres as nasal drug delivery systems. Adv Drug Deliv Rev 1998; 29(1–2):185–94.

80. Mengping Z, Donovan MD. Intranasal mucociliary clearance of putative bioadhesive polymer gels. Int J Pharm 1996; 135:(1–2):17.

81. Illum L. Nasal drug delivery: New developments and strategies. Drug Discov Today 2002; 7(23):1184–9.

82. Brouet G, Grosjean B. Development of preservative-free nasal spray products. Drug Delivery Technology; http://www.drugdeliverytech.com/cgi-bin/articles.cgi?idArticle=179

83. Dubin C. Nothing to sneeze At. Excerpt from PFQ Magazine 2002; http://www.optinose.no/publications/files/20030129181011_PFQ_nasal_reprint.pdf

84. Ugwokea MI, Aguc RU, Verbekeb N, Kinget R. Nasal mucoadhesive drug delivery: Background, applications, trends and future perspectives. Adv Drug Deliv Rev 2005; 57(11):1640–65.

85. Guo C, Doub WH. The influence of actuation parameters on in vitro testing of nasal spray products. J PharmSci 2006; 95(9):2029–40.

33

Controlled Particle Dispersion®: A Twenty-First-Century Nasal Drug Delivery Platform

Marc Giroux

Kurve Technology, Inc., Bothell, Washington, D.C., U.S.A.

Peter Hwang

Stanford Sinus Center, Stanford University School of Medicine, Stanford, California, U.S.A.

Ajay Prasad

University of Delaware, Newark, Delaware, U.S.A.

INTRODUCTION

The idea of using the nasal cavity for drug delivery is centuries old. The devices used for nasal drug delivery were as antiquated and varied as the pharmaceutical compounds delivered. From the original snuff box to nose drops, from pressurized metered dose inhalers (pMDIs) to today's aqueous spray bottles—nasal drug delivery has never reached its full potential due to the limited efficacy that resulted from the poor design, and inadequate deliverability of the devices.

It is only in recent years that research has allowed a better understanding of the environment of the nasal cavity, which in turn determined the limiting factors in successfully introducing a formulation for maximum effect and efficacy.

Recent studies focus on the physics and fluid dynamics of the changes in the nasal cavity parameters during an inhalation with respect to the drug administered. Understanding these physical characteristics is the key to designing a device that acts upon this environment, thus overcoming the limiting obstacles that have stood in the way of successful nasal drug delivery. These obstacles include complex physical geometry, inhalation air flows, narrow pathways, individual anatomy, and variable anatomy within a single patient as well as from patient to patient.

Kurve Technology Bothell, WA, U.S.A. conducted and participated in research defining the success parameters for nasal drug delivery that helps to identify and overcome longstanding obstacles. The result is a technology platform—Controlled Particle Dispersion® (CPD)—capable of delivering formulations throughout out the entire nasal cavity, to the olfactory region and into the paranasal sinuses. CPD—used in the Kurve Technology's ViaNase™ and ViaNase ID™ devices—can also target specific areas of the nasal cavity to a limited extent.

Based on CPD, the ViaNase device family can optimize deposition around a given formulation, maximizing efficacy for each given treatment. The success of the technology platform opens treatment options across topical, systemic, and nose-to-brain areas, many of which were unattainable prior to the development of this platform.

This chapter clarifies the following:

- obstacles to nasal delivery found in the nasal cavity and the solutions needed to overcome these problems;
- how these solutions level the playing field across variable patient anatomy to serve broad patient populations across the many disease states targeted for nasal drug administration;
- how the ViaNase device can be optimized around a particular formulation to achieve the greatest efficacy possible; and
- fields of use for the technology platform.

THE PLAYING FIELD—THE NASAL CAVITY ENVIRONMENT

Complex Geometry

Figure 1 displays the complex geometry of the human nasal cavity. The narrow, black pathways are the air passages a droplet must traverse in order to deliver throughout the nasal cavity. The gray areas are highly vascularized mucosa covering the complex structure of the turbinates and septum. These highly vascularized mucosal surfaces are the target of the delivered drug.

A drug is introduced into this environment at the very bottom of the nasal cavity through a nostril opening. Current technologies (spray bottles, pMDIs) introduce formulations into this environment using very large droplets, traveling in one dimension and at great velocity as shown in Figure 2. The task of getting a droplet to travel through these complex

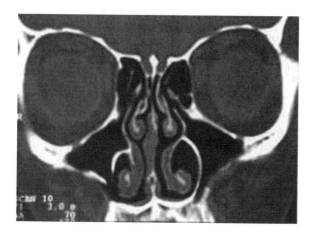

Figure 1 Frontal MRI slice of the nasal cavity.

airways is extremely difficult and it is impossible with current technologies such as spray bottles.

Nasal Cavity Airflow Patterns

Transportation and deposition of droplets within the nasal cavity are closely dependent on the existing airflow patterns. Figure 3 illustrates the inspired air profile that is the dominant airflow pattern in the cavity. Inspired air

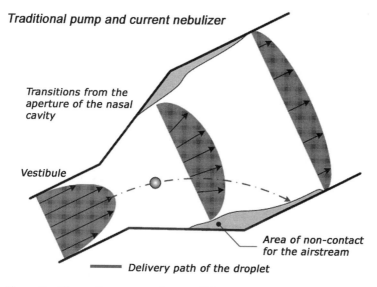

Figure 2 Linear flow pattern in a traditional spray pump.

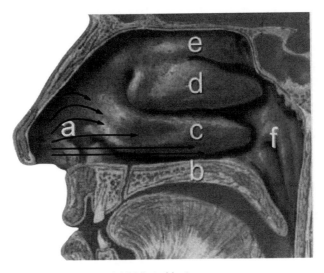

a: Nasal vestibule   d: Middle turbinate
b: Palate   e: Superior turbinate
c: Inferior turbinate   f: Nasopharynx

Figure 3   Nasal cavity anatomy and airflow patterns.

patterns largely determine where and how drug deposition in the nasal cavity occurs.

Several factors make it difficult to deliver drugs to these regions. Relatively low flow amounts are observed in the olfactory region (< 10% of the inspired air) and in the nasal meatuses. This is predominately due to the small cross-sectional area of these regions, relative to the total cross-sectional area of the entire nasal cavity.

In a study examining airflow patterns in the nasal cavity, the greatest airflow velocities were observed between the top of the palate and under the inferior turbinate (1). Velocities and flows decrease in the upper regions of the nasal cavity. The inferior airway has a relatively small cross-sectional area, compared to the anterior portion of the cavity, which increases the velocity of the inspired air. This causes airflow to move in a predominantly streamwise direction, i.e., a direction aligned with the primary flow direction along the axis of the inferior airway. However, it is desirable to disrupt the axial streamlined trajectories of inhaled particles flowing along the inferior airway.

An ideal delivery method creates an environment in which spatial extent is capable of altering the airstream created by the inspired air in order for droplets to deposit beyond this stream. This airflow stream is the greatest obstacle to the delivery of medications into the upper posterior of the nasal cavity, which allows access to the olfactory region and paranasal sinuses. Disruption of this airstream must occur in order to attain the desired result of effective nasal drug delivery. If a delivery technology does not disrupt the airflow streams, it will not deliver any more effectively than current technologies.

Current technologies offer nothing in the way of disrupting either air flow patterns or a means of diffusing throughout the narrow, complex air passages. In actuality, they create and disperse droplets in a linear, or one-dimensional flow, pattern directly away from the valve emitting the droplet. With the heavy droplet moving straight ahead it will deposit on the first obstacle it reaches. In the environment illustrated in Figure 1, this will happen almost immediately, where upon the droplet will be instantly subjected to gravitational settling and clearance to the stomach resulting in as much as 90% of all droplets sprayed into the nasal cavity being swallowed.

Controlled Particle Dispersion

CPD technology addresses the limitations associated with current technologies by controlling droplet size and delivery trajectories. The correct droplet size assures the droplets are delivered to the nasal cavity. Two limits defining the optimal droplet size include upper limit of size (mean diameter) set by the aerodynamic properties of droplet and a lower limit value minimizing peripheral deposition to the lungs.

CPD affects delivery path by generating a vortical flow which gives droplets the environment needed to disrupt the inherent air flow streams and penetrate into the entire nasal cavity (Fig. 4). Consequently, the airflow acquires two components: the primary flow which is still directed along the axial direction, and a secondary component which imparts a circular spin. The net result is that the flow streamlines trace spiral or helical paths as they navigate the nasal passage. The vortex accelerates droplets in an upward direction at the same time centrifuging the droplets to the outer edge of the vortex, i.e., to the walls of the nasal cavity. The centrifugal acceleration imparted to the droplets is proportional to the radial location of the droplet from the center of the vortex and the square of the angular velocity (speed with which it is being spun about the vortex axis). Because the droplets are typically 1000 times denser than air, they are ejected outwards (i.e., they are centrifuged away from the vortex core). The vortex sorts the droplets by size. The larger droplets move to the outer wall first, allowing the smaller droplets to move upwards.

This disrupts the existing airflow patterns in the nasal cavity causing the smaller droplets to move upwards and into the middle and superior airways. In studies of air patterns in the nasal cavity, standing eddies have been noted in the superior airway (1). The objective of CPD is to reach these upper regions to take advantage of these existing air patterns which prolong droplet residence time in the cavity.

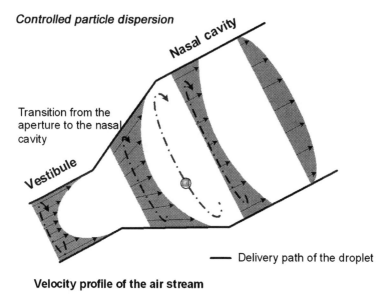

Figure 4 Vortical droplet flow created by CPD. *Abbreviation*: CPD, controlled particle dispersion.

CPD also uses the inspired airstream to enhance deposition. A comparison of spray bottle and CPD deposition patterns is shown in Figure 5. The inspired airstream enters the device through the nose piece. The airstream is aligned with the vortex axis and the flow acceleration along the nasal passage causing a stretching of the vortex (Fig. 6). Stretching the vortex increases its strength since vorticity is inversely proportional to its cross-sectional area. Incorporation of inspired air into the device design becomes a useful variable in the performance of the device as it can alter the air pattern in the nasal cavity and enhance the centrifugal forces generated by the vortex.

Droplet Size

In addition to airflow patterns, deposition is dependent on the diameter of the droplet delivered to the nasal cavity. Large droplets found in spray pumps tend to fall out of the airstream immediately because the liquid comprising the droplets has a density approximately 1000 times larger than the airflow on which the droplets ride. Consequently, large droplets fall out of the airflow either due to gravitational settling or because they possess far too much inertia to negotiate the bends within the nasal passage and are removed from the flow by inertial impaction. Aerodynamically controlling droplets this large is exceedingly difficult.

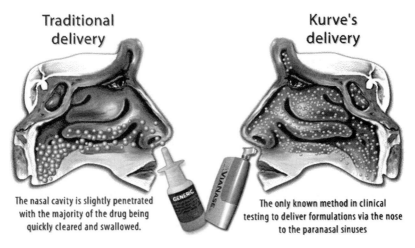

Traditional delivery

The nasal cavity is slightly penetrated with the majority of the drug being quickly cleared and swallowed.

Kurve's delivery

The only known method in clinical testing to deliver formulations via the nose to the paranasal sinuses

Figure 5 Deposition pattern comparison.

The ideal droplet size is smaller than that produced by a typical spray pump, but large enough to disrupt the air flow patterns and not be respirable to the lungs. The CPD technology platform produces droplet ranges from 3 to 100 μm and can target the dv50 in 1-μm increments. Due to the necessity of aerodynamically controlling the droplets, the CPD technology platform operates between 10 and 30 μm.

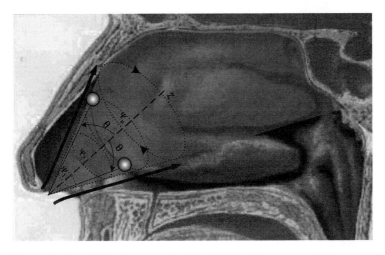

Figure 6 Vortical pattern produced by CPD. *Abbreviation*: CPD, controlled particle dispersion.

Droplet Velocity

The droplet velocity is inversely proportional to its residence time within the nasal passage. All factors being equal, a droplet with a smaller velocity has a higher probability of remaining in the airway longer but must follow the trajectory and pathway of the airstream.

Droplet Delivery Trajectories

Redirecting along cross-stream trajectories greatly improves particle residence time and penetration within the intranasal passages. If the flow is primarily in the axial direction of the inferior airway, the droplets will simply be pulled along the flow streamlines and quickly exit the intranasal passages. The ability to disrupt the primary "stream-wise" flow and impart a significant flow component in the cross-stream direction (i.e., a direction perpendicular to the primary or axial direction) is critical to dispersing droplets over the greatest possible area within the nasal passages.

VIANASE ID: A REPEAT USE, TWO-PART ELECTRONIC ATOMIZER

The ViaNase ID device with the CPD technology platform is a two-part system (Fig. 7). The first part of this two-part system is a base unit containing the electronics, compressor and the drug pedigree tracking equipment.

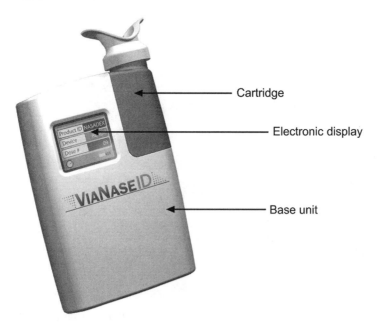

Figure 7 Kurve Technology's ViaNase ID™ device.

The second part is the cartridge into which the drug is introduced and which contains the CPD platform intellectual property. This cartridge is optimized around a particular formulation in order to produce the droplet size specified by the pharmaceutical partner and through which the ideal deposition area inside the nasal cavity is targeted. Each application of the ViaNase devices has a unique cartridge designed and optimized for delivery of the specific formulation.

FLEXIBILITY OF THE CPD PLATFORM

The CPD platform contains six critical-to-function design parameters that can be adjusted to create the optimal delivery environment for a given formulation. Manipulation of these design parameters allows CPD to function within an extremely wide range of fluid characteristics as well as maintain the ability to target specific areas of deposition within the nasal cavity. The design parameters are as follows:

- compressor flow
- droplet generator
- droplet separator
- cone geometry
- particle dispersion chamber–turbulent (vortical) flow
- nose piece interface

Within these six design parameters are nearly 3000 different configurations of the delivery cartridge, which allow adjustment for fluid characteristics and deposition targets. In addition, within each individual variable is a range of adjustments that further widen the breadth of the CPD platform.

The sophisticated technology of the CPD platform allows it to create droplets from virtually any liquid regardless of viscosity or surface tension. This includes solutions and suspensions as well as combinations of the two. The droplet generator is also significantly less harsh on the molecule itself than other technologies and can deliver intact large and small molecules, delicate proteins and peptides, and live vaccines. All of the formulations tested to date have been performed by independent laboratories and all have maintained purity throughout the testing cycles.

CRITICAL FACTORS IN DEVELOPMENT

Once the droplets have been generated it is necessary to control the droplets that exit the cartridge. This is done by sorting the undesirable droplets and recirculating them back through the droplet generator to be re-atomized.

Sorting of the droplets begins with the Droplet Separator™— the design of this feature determines how many of the droplets get sorted out of the airstream. Cone geometry also plays a role in droplet sorting and is used in conjunction with the Droplet Separator. These two features also play a key role in selecting the atomization rate and exit velocity in order to tailor the flow depending on the desired deposition inside the nasal cavity.

Turbulent flow is controlled by either passive and/or active means. One-way valves that allow inhalation air to be introduced along the axial flow of the exiting droplets create passive flow and add an extra 7 lpm to the exiting droplet flow. The device itself delivers 2.5 lpm to the user, allowing the energy from the additional 7 lpm to be used to assist in the creation of the turbulent, or vortical, flow. In the active system, air is fed from the compressor to the cartridge exit via cannulas which direct the droplets into their turbulent (vortical) flow. Both systems add inhalation air to the axial flow; only the active system provides direction of droplets via cannulas. These systems can be designed to deliver into both nostrils simultaneously or into one nostril at a time.

All six critical-to-function design features play a role in which droplets exit the device and where in the nasal cavity the highest concentration of droplets occurs. With nearly 3000 different variables, as well as individual ranges within those variables, the CPD platform can deliver virtually any liquid regardless of the formulation characteristics.

Pharmaceutical firms first develop molecules and test for efficacy prior to a search for a delivery mechanism. Device design flexibility is a crucial capability that can spell success or failure in the delivery of a particular molecule. Since nebulizers and spray bottles are quite limited in the viscosities delivered (4–5 cp), a formulation that is successfully delivered by spray bottle at 4 cp, may be a failure at 35 cp. Surface tensions and combination products further complicate this formulation life cycle issue.

From a financial perspective, reformulating a high viscosity drug adds significant and costly development time when it is even possible. This means money invested with no return as well as an increased time to market. Every month spent accommodating limited-scope devices is lost revenue with a drug on the market. In addition, excipients such as preservatives, mucoadhesives, and thixotropic additives can, in many instances, be limited or eliminated reducing formulation complexity, development time, and FDA hurdles. When partnered with a platform as sophisticated as CPD, fewer dollars are spent in development, gaining more time on the market under patent earning a quicker and larger return on investment.

The flexibility of CPD may allow a project to progress rather than being shelved for lack of a device since delivery is not often factored into development until a viable molecule has passed a certain amount of testing.

INTELLIGENT NASAL DRUG DELIVERY

Today's drug delivery tracking systems are designed to validate prescription drugs from manufacturer to retailer, with the intent of reducing fraud. Intent falls far short of the goal. Drug counterfeiting and fraud within the pharmaceutical industry's supply chain ranges from conservative estimates of $30 billion to more than $50 billion in annual losses to corporations, according to market studies by the World Health Organization and the U.S. Food and Drug Administration. According to a 2005 report released by the Center for Medicines in the Public Interest, counterfeit drug sales could reach $75 billion by 2010 (2).

Obviously, the industry and regulatory agencies around the world desire stronger systems that validate the product throughout the supply chain and perhaps even down to the patient level to avoid drug abuse/misuse. Attempting to curb drug counterfeiting, the pharmaceutical industry, with the support of the FDA, is developing a pedigree system that will track prescription drugs from manufacture to retail pharmacies using a variety of technologies including radio frequency identification (RFID). However, the envisioned systems end at the retail pharmacy. Drug delivery systems that validate the pedigree of the drug at the device and patient levels—steps that could significantly curtail the use of counterfeit drugs and the misuse of correctly prescribed drugs—are also necessary. Formulators welcome improved nasal delivery devices that promote and support patient compliance. Traditional spray bottles, while convenient, lack such advanced features as dose counters, lockouts, and timers that curb counterfeiting as well as improve patient acceptance and compliance.

Intelligent Nasal Delivery Systems

Intelligent nasal drug delivery technologies—based on the CPD technology platform—can offer dose counting, timers, and reminders while curtailing the use of counterfeit drugs, decreasing the misuse of correctly prescribed drugs, and improve patient compliance. ViaNase ID has active built-in electronics that can become a vital part of the pedigree system and can go a long way to curbing abuse/misuse at the patient level, adding that final step to the monitoring chain at the patient.

The ViaNase ID is powered by a main power switch that brings power to the device while leaving it in a locked position and therefore inoperable. An RFID tagged package, ampoule or bottle is brought to the device which has a built-in reader that recognizes the RFID tag (Fig. 8). This tag not only determines whether the machine will operate but how it will operate to some extent. In addition to unlocking the device, it can communicate with the rest of the electronics and set droplet generation parameters. For example, the RFID reader can communicate with internal electronics to run a

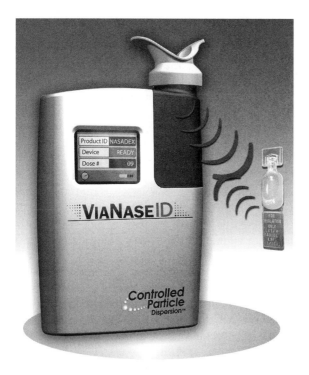

Figure 8 ViaNase ID reads an RFID tag on a drug ampoule. *Abbreviation*: RFID, radio frequency identification.

preprogrammed set of parameters that includes atomization rate and/or droplet size when it reads a particular tag.

Locking Out Counterfeits

Pedigree confirmation technology identifies or confirms such specific drug information as product name, total number of doses in the prescription, and expiration date by reading a coding technology placed on the drug packaging or unit dose ampoule. If a counterfeit drug has been improperly tagged, the device recognizes it as a counterfeit and remains locked. An added feature is tag destruction. Once a dose has been delivered the tag can no longer be used to unlock the device. The reader recognizes it as a "used dose" and remains locked to prevent abuse/misuse.

As an example, take the case of a controlled substance for breakthrough cancer pain. If the prescription calls for a dose to be delivered every four hours, the device times the interval between doses and will not unlock until the prescribed amount of time has passed. Also, it recognizes the tag and controls power to the compressor that plays a role in droplet size and atomization rate. The abuse of pain drugs is well known and the patient cannot unlock the device to dose more often than prescribed.

Improved Patient Compliance

Dose reminders and information via an electronic display can be extremely effective in increasing patient compliance numbers.

Intelligent nasal drug delivery devices can enhance patient compliance in the following ways:

- setting specific dose time in minutes per day or number of doses per day
- setting the total number of doses per prescription
- sounding an alarm when the dose is required
- sounding an alarm when cleaning is required

Monitoring Compliance

With intelligent drug delivery technology, such information as drug identification numbers, drug type, prescription order number, time/date of doses, total amount of drug delivered, and operating parameter records can be saved to a data storage card or downloaded to a PC or PDA. This information is useful for physicians, pharmacies, and clinical trial coordinators.

Traditional nasal delivery devices such as spray pumps do not meet the pharmaceutical industry's new requirements for pedigree confirmation, data transfer, and improved patient acceptance. Formulators, spending hundreds of millions of dollars developing new compounds, can consider intelligent nasal delivery systems to increase the odds of patient and physician acceptance, and thus commercial success.

DRUG–DEVICE COMBINATIONS

Emerging developments in the pharmaceutical field and combination drug–device products are setting the groundwork for increased licensing and collaboration between pharmaceutical and medical device companies.

Combining drugs and devices enhances the quality of treatment by increasing efficacy and reducing side effects. Such drug–device combination products augment a device's efficacy and/or safety, to deliver the drug locally. Consider the following data from the FDA:

- Approximately 10% increase in drug–device, drug–biologic, and device–biologic application submission since 2005 with no forecasted decrease.
- A total market for drug–device combinations worldwide valued at $5.4 billion in 2004 and expected to rise at an average annual growth rate of 13.6% to $11.5 billion by 2010 (3).

- Nasal drug delivery device combinations could be analogous to drug-eluting stents, which continue to show a 12% average annual growth. This will result in the market doubling to around $8 billion by the year 2010 (3). The United States presently dominates the market for drug– device combination products, due to wide acceptance of drug-eluting stents.
- The newly created Office of Combination Products was established to streamline the processing of complex drug–device products.

ELIMINATING FIXED DOSE COMBINATIONS

While not new to the medical community, combination drug products have long been tagged with a negative connotation. Physicians' objections to combining drugs limit the ability to prescribe specific doses and therapeutic combinations to fit a patient's particular needs. With CPD and the capability to design cartridges around non-fixed dose combinations (non-FDC), prescribers' concerns with having a lack of dose ranges for a given drug are addressed. CPD also addresses the medical community's concerns of compliance and reduce safety concerns.

The main obstacle to non-FDC development though involves product formulation and manufacturing issues. If the process is too expensive and the market too small, manufacturing a wide range of doses is impractical.

With CPDs intelligent delivery technology, non-FDC products can diffuse the impact of generic competition, revitalize established brands, fill gaps in product pipelines, and enhance patient compliance. This is true for a drug–device combination as well as a combination drug therapy additionally combined with the device. A drug combination can be defined as a product comprised of two or more regulated components that are physically, chemically, or otherwise mixed as a single entity, or two or more products packaged together. They are combined with a device to complete the therapy. For example, drugs such as a corticosteroid and an antibiotic can be combined into a straight drug/device combination with a single drug or a combination of all three. In each instance, the combination results in an improved overall product which provides patients with efficacious treatments and improves patient compliance.

DRUG–DEVICE PRODUCTS EVOLVING RAPIDLY

Drug–device combination products have evolved rapidly and are on the threshold of even greater change. Future products will require increasing collaboration and cooperation between the various medical and device regulatory systems—an important step in allowing these products to develop while ensuring the safety of patients. This is beneficial from many standpoints in that the pharmaceutical company can get patent extensions and product lifecycle management improvements while the patient gets better efficacy, simpler treatments, and a single product therapy.

The ViaNase devices lend themselves ideally to this scenario in their sophistication and versatility. The payer reimburses only one prescription when patient compliance and condition improves. The outlook for combination products has become quite positive as they clearly show improved efficacy in a single treatment. The formulators have a tougher job with combination products because they have to ensure that the two drugs are compatible in delivery and storage—subject to FDA scrutiny. However, CPD offers life cycle extension for the life of the Kurve patents as well as being able to lock out all direct competitors, generics and counterfeit compounds.

GENERIC VERSUS BRAND NAME

Large pharmaceutical companies—with few potential blockbuster drugs on the horizon—are aggressively protecting their patented drugs in the market. Tough competition also lies ahead for the generic industry as firms fear being shut out of the marketplace. The opportunity for CPD thus is two-fold: life cycle extension by preserving the brand, or generic product brand pricing by partnering with device manufacturers to lock out competitors. Presently, generic medicines account for 53% of all prescriptions dispensed in the United States and are used to fill more than one billion prescriptions every year (4).

INDUSTRY APPLICATIONS OF CPD

CPD has broad applications across topical treatments and systemic treatments, and, more recently, nose-to-brain therapies that utilize the olfactory and/or trigeminal pathway to directly access the brain for central nervous system (CNS) disorders.

TOPICAL TREATMENTS

Disorders directly affecting the nasal mucosa itself affect a large population of patients. Chronic rhinosinusitis affects 74 million people in the United States and the European Union. Americans spend $5.8 billion each year on health care costs related to rhinosinusitis (5). At least 35.9 million people in the United States have seasonal allergic rhinitis with an estimated equal number in the European Union (6). The influenza virus infects an estimated 17–50 million people in the United States each flu season (7). In addition, adults average 2–4 colds per year and children suffer 6–10 colds per year (8).

Sinusitis currently has no approved topical treatments of any kind making it one of the largest untreated chronic diseases in the United States.

CPD can reach the ostia of the paranasal sinuses and, in some patients, penetrate into these sinuses, enabling a topical treatment for sinusitis for the first time. Symptoms such as congestion and rhinorrea for cold and flu can be relieved using CPD as well.

The same principle applies to rhinitis. For a topical treatment, the drug should be applied directly on the affected mucosa. Since a spray bottle cannot deliver beyond the nasal vestibule, it does not deliver compounds to all of the affected mucosa, resulting in a less than efficacious therapy with significant compliance issues.

SYSTEMIC TREATMENTS

Systemic treatments via the nasal cavity are an exciting and growing area for nasal drug delivery. There are currently over 100 drugs in development for nasal drug delivery and the lion's share are for systemic delivery. The highly vascularized mucosa is ideal for many therapies that currently require an injection or for protein and peptide treatments that cannot survive the first-pass metabolism.

For the drugs that are mucosally available, efficacy can be maintained as well as rapid onset of action and absorption. Success is dependent on the device being able to access as much of this vascularized mucosa as possible—a feat current technologies are incapable of achieving. Efficacious systemic treatments through the nasal mucosa demand a device that is more effective at reaching beyond the nasal vestibule and does not quickly clear the compound out of the nasal cavity. CPD both reaches beyond the nasal vestibule and limits peripheral deposition to the lungs and stomach enabling many of these therapies to succeed.

NOSE-TO-BRAIN TREATMENTS

Nose-to-brain drug delivery is widely debated. Gaining definitive proof that the pathway exists through the olfactory region and/or the trigeminal nerve is difficult. In order to research this route of administration, among the first requirements is the delivery of a formulation to the target site, i.e., the olfactory region. Since a nasal spray bottle does not penetrate beyond the nasal vestibule, it is not a valid choice for administration.

Kurve's ViaNase device with CPD has shown clear evidence of reaching the olfactory region. Participation in a clinical study with the University of Washington and the Veterans Administration Hospital of Puget Sound showed statistically relevant symptom improvement in Alzheimer's patients (9). Based on the positive results of the first clinical study, a larger study has been funded by the U.S. National Institutes of Health.

Kurve currently has several nose-to-brain studies underway with pharmaceutical companies for central nervous system (CNS) disorders and is moving ahead with development and refinement of device design parameters for these formulations.

CONCLUSION

Through careful research and insight, Kurve Technology has thoroughly studied the physics and fluid dynamics of the environment of the nasal cavity to develop a versatile, sophisticated technology platform. CPD's breakthrough in deposition and efficacy alone enables the creation of the next generation of nasal drug delivery devices for nose-to-brain, topical and systemic therapy areas. The need for intelligent delivery and counterfeit controlling devices is also foreseen.

REFERENCES

1. Kelly JT, Prasad AK, Wexler S. Detailed flow patterns in the nasal cavity. J Appl Physiol 2000; 89:323–7.
2. Center for Medicines in the Public Interest Report, September 2005, www.cmpi.org
3. DeSorbo MA. Thinking inside the box: the world of drug delivery. Pharm Form Qual 2005; December.
4. www.gphaonline.org
5. www.niaid.nih.gov/factsheets/sinusitis.htm
6. www.aaaai.org/media/resources/media_kit/allergy_statistics.stm
7. www.medimmune.com/products/flumist/index.asp
8. www.niaid.nih.gov/healthscience/healthtopics/colds/overview.htm
9. Craft S. Therapeutic effects of daily intranasal insulin in early Alzheimer's disease. In: Proceedings of the International Conference on Alzheimer's Disease and Related Disorders. Madrid, Sept 2006.

34

DirectHaler™ Nasal: Innovative Device and Delivery Method

Troels Keldmann

DirectHaler A/S, Copenhagen, Denmark

INTRODUCTION

DirectHaler™ A/S has invented and developed a novel nasal delivery device and nasal delivery principle. The innovation takes advantage of the patient's anatomy with the aim to improve nasal delivery effectiveness and convenience. The integrated nasal device and delivery method enable nasal delivery of very fine particles, without the risk of pulmonary deposition. The nasal device has successfully been used in clinical trials, and has confirmed patient acceptability.

The single-use, disposable DirectHaler™ Nasal device is for both single and bi-dose delivery, in a pre-metered, pre-filled dose format. The device offers effective, accurate, repeatable and hygienic dosing, and is intuitively easy-to-use. Further, the straightforward device design possesses unequalled cost-effective manufacturability.

DIRECTHALER™ NASAL IS BOTH DELIVERY-METHOD AND DEVICE INNOVATION

When air is being blown out of the mouth against a resistance, then the airway passage between the oral and nasal cavities automatically closes. The same reflex is activated when a person blows up a balloon; none of the air escapes through the nose. This anatomical feature is activated when the patient uses DirectHaler Nasal for blowing their nasal dry powder dose into the nostril. Hereby the dose is captured in the nasal cavity, where it is

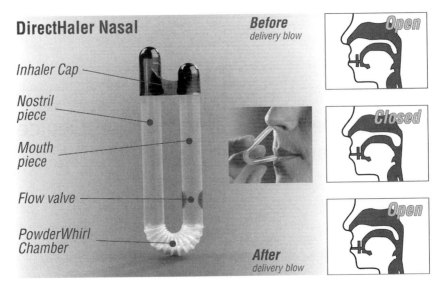

Figure 1   DirectHaler™ Nasal: Device and delivery method innovation.

intended to act or to be absorbed into the systemic circulation. After completion of the dose delivery blow, the nasal/oral connection returns to its normal open state (Fig. 1).

The delivery method holds potential to become the dominant delivery principle in nasal drug delivery. DirectHaler is the first drug delivery company to take advantage of this device-dependent reflex for enhancing nasal drug delivery. The increased interest in this principle for enhanced nasal delivery has recently led other companies to seek exploitation of the same delivery principle. However, DirectHaler has broadly issued device and delivery method patents for this area. Patents are issued in 44 countries, with priority dates going back to 1997.

REMOVING DISADVANTAGES OF CURRENTLY AVAILABLE SYSTEMS

A range of nasally delivered products have been on the market in recent decades. These products belong to therapeutic areas such as allergic rhinitis treatment, migraine relief, hormone replacement therapy (HRT) and common cold relief. These products have applied nasal delivery systems based primarily on four different formulation/device technology types: liquid nasal drops, liquid nasal spray, pressurized metered dose inhaler (hydrofluoroalkane, HFA; chlorofluorocarbon, CFC), and Dry Powder Inhalers/Insufflators. Performance and characteristics of these nasal delivery systems have been studied widely (Table 1), and a range of disadvantages have been

Table 1   DirectHaler™ Nasal Overcomes Disadvantages of Currently Marketed Nasal Delivery Device Systems

Disadvantages reported on current nasal delivery systems (Refs.)	Solved by DirectHaler Nasal
Risk of liquid dose dripping out from nostril after dose delivery (1)	Dry powder formulations adhere to the nasal mucousa
Risk of liquid dose being swallowed immediately after delivery—giving limited absorption time and unpleasant taste (2)	No risk of immediate swallowing Reduction of taste sensation
Complicated device priming procedure before first use, and if many days pass between uses (3,4,5)	Primeless
Risk of small delivered dose for the last actuations as container begins to empty; no dose counter, patient has to keep records to ensure the product is discarded before the dose size becomes insufficient (3,4,5)	Pre-metered, pro-filled unit dose/bi-dose device system. No risk of reduced dose
Acceptability problems for liquid formulations with preservatives, for chronic use (6)	No preservatives
Multi-dose containers include risk of contamination, necessitating preservatives in formulation and frequent device cleaning (6,7)	Hygienic single-use, disposable. No contamination risk
Unpleasant "cold-blow" and "hard-blow" of medication from pMDI (8)	Tempered & pleasant blow
Risk of pulmonary dose deposition for "snorting-in" DPI devices (9)	No risk of pulmonary deposition

Abbreviations: DPI, dry powder inhaler; pMDI, pressurized metered dose inhaler.

identified. The DirectHaler Nasal device and delivery method can solve or significantly reduce these disadvantages.

The liquid nasal spray/drop type is currently the most widely used nasal delivery system. A number of issues have been reported on this type:

- risk of liquid dose dripping out from nostril after dose delivery (1);
- risk of liquid dose being swallowed immediately after delivery—giving limited absorption time and unpleasant taste (2);
- complicated device priming before first use, and when many days between uses (3–5);
- risk of small delivered dose for "last doses"; no dose counter, patient has to keep records to discard the product before the dose size is insufficient (3–5);

- acceptability problems for liquid formulations with preservatives, for chronic use (6);
- multi-dose containers include risk of contamination, necessitating preservatives in formulation and frequent device cleaning (6,7).

Dry powder formulations can offer important advantages to liquid formulations: enabling higher drug pay-load per dose delivered, prolonging absorption time in nasal cavity, reducing temperature sensibility during product distribution/storage. Further, DirectHaler Nasal device eliminates priming, cleaning, risk of contamination and thereby eliminates the need for preservatives.

The pressurized metered dose inhaler (pMDI) technology has also been applied for nasal delivery. However, patient acceptability has not been impressive:

- unpleasant "cold-blow" (from the cooling effect of the propellant) and "hard-blow" (from the forceful and high velocity of dose plume) from pMDI (8).

In contrast, the patient contributes to the blow energy when utilizing DirectHaler Nasal. Therefore, the nasal dose blow is conveniently tempered for high patient acceptability.

Dry powder nasal formulations have historically been used mostly for locally acting drugs for rhinitis treatment by dry powder delivery devices. Among these, are pulmonary dry powder inhalers with a "nostril piece" instead of a "mouthpiece." Such devices are activated by the patients "snorting in" the medication. The lungs are generating the airflow, and therefore unfortunately the lungs will be the delivery place for part of the drug dose.

- Risk of "snorting in" powder dose being partly deposited in the lungs (9).

The DirectHaler Nasal device and method automatically activates the anatomical reflex, which closes the airway passage between the nasal cavity and oral cavity. This activated reflex removes the risk of pulmonary deposition of drug particles.

In summary, DirectHaler Nasal provides a novel opportunity for overcoming the above recognized problems of currently marketed nasal delivery device concepts (Table 1).

FACILITATING PURSUIT OF NEW HORIZONS FOR NASAL DELIVERY

New opportunities in nasal delivery include pursuit of an eventual possibility for "nose to brain" delivery, requiring dose particle deposition in the olfactory region. However, currently marketed nasal products seek to deliver particle sizes above 20–30 μm in order to prevent risk for deposition in the lower airways. Such large particle sizes are also preventing pursuit of more advanced nasal delivery to the olfactory region. Therefore, a key point in pursuing such new opportunities requires dose particles in the size range below $< 5\,\mu m$. A new nasal delivery method is therefore needed to prevent deposition of fine particle nasal dose in the lower airways. DirectHaler Nasal and its delivery method offer such characteristics.

PROVEN TECHNOLOGY APPLIED IN PULMONARY DELIVERY

The research and development (R&D) behind DirectHaler Nasal was initiated on the basis of experiences achieved in our R&D on dry powder inhalation technology for pulmonary delivery. With DirectHaler Nasal the ambition was to develop a disposable dry powder delivery device offering effective, accurate and repeatable dosing that is compact and easy-to-use. Our ambition was also to make it possible for pharmaceutical companies to manage manufacturing, filling, and packing of the devices. The innovative result of our nasal R&D is patent protected worldwide.

The nasal device comprises an engineered curved and bendable inhaler tube with a "mouth-to-nose" optimized corrugated flexible bend, and a double cap that seals each end of the inhaler tube. As DirectHaler Nasal is intended for nasal delivery of dry-powder formulations, it takes advantage of the PowderWhirl chamber for dispersion, and powder entrainment. The PowderWhirl chamber was originally developed for pulmonary delivery applications, where powder dispersion and gradual entrainment to the airflow is important.

Three principles governing airflow and powder dispersion are applied in the design (Fig. 2), so that DirectHaler Nasal delivers the complete dose gradually over one inhalation as a well-dispersed powder:

First, the air intake is designed for generating and feeding in turbulent air to the PowderWhirl chamber. Second, the corrugations of the PowderWhirl chamber are designed to generate turbulent whirls. These recirculation zones contribute to powder dispersion. Finally, the turbulent airflow forces the powder up on the inner walls of the corrugations. From here, it is gradually entrained into the inhaled air stream until the device is completely empty.

EASY-TO-USE IMPLIES EASE-TO-INSTRUCT/CHECK

DirectHaler Nasal is intuitively easy to use, which will minimize the instruction task and ease any checking of the patient's technique. The pre-metered and prefilled powder dose in the DirectHaler Nasal is always visible due to device transparency. This allows the patient to have visual contact with the dose—ensuring confirmed "dose ready" before delivery and "dose taken"

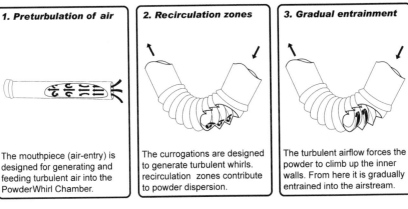

1. Preturbulation of air	**2. Recirculation zones**	**3. Gradual entrainment**
The mouthpiece (air-entry) is designed for generating and feeding turbulent air into the PowderWhirl Chamber.	The currogations are designed to generate turbulent whirls. recirculation zones contribute to powder dispersion.	The turbulent airflow forces the powder to climb up the inner walls. From here it is gradually entrained into the airstream.

Figure 2 Three powder dispersion principles are applied simultaneously in DirectHaler™ Nasal.

after delivery. The compact device dimensions ensure portability and discretion in using the device.

To use DirectHaler Nasal, the cap is taken off, leaving both ends of the tube open and the dose resting at the bottom of the "U." Holding and pressing the mouthpiece between the thumb and forefinger, the patient inserts, due to the flexible bend, the nostril piece into a nostril and the mouthpiece into their mouth. They then blow into the mouthpiece and thereafter completely release the finger pressure on the tube (Fig. 3). The blow of the patient closes the airway passage between the nasal and oral cavities, and then disperses the powder dose and transports it via the nostril piece to the nasal mucosa.

ACCOMMODATING SENSITIVE POWDERS AND SPECIAL APPLICATIONS

Active substances and their formulations often have variable sensitivities to moisture, light, temperature and mechanical impact. Some therapeutic applications require delivery of two doses; one to each nostril. To accommodate such potential requirements, we have developed additional types of device caps. Examples are shown in Figure 4, along with the original cap. Such new caps enable bi-dose storage, and dose encapsulation, along with customized device appearance—both designed for optimal ease of use.

1. Type 1 (left side): the powder dose is sealed inside the cap with a foil strip, which is easily torn off for dose loading to the PowderWhirl chamber, before removing the cap and delivering the dose.

2. Type 2 (center): the isolated dose inside the cap is loaded by pressing the two cap parts together until a "click" is heard.

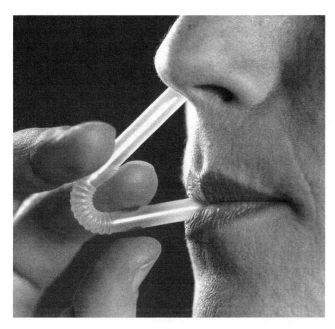

Figure 3   Applying DirectHaler™ Nasal.

HOW CAN THE DEVICE APPEAR SO STRAIGHTFORWARD?

The high degree of function-integration in only two device components (with a total weight of 0.6 g) has been achieved by an R&D philosophy focusing on identifying the essential device functionality requirements, and on sophisticated engineering.

The analysis of nasal delivery device concepts shows that these possess a range of mechanism that make the devices complicated to use and/or expensive to manufacture. As a new and innovative device concept, the DirectHaler Nasal device eliminates the need for a number of the "common device" mechanisms. This has allowed us to focus on new principles for nasal delivery.

Figure 5 shows our identification of the most essential functional elements for a powder based nasal device technology. Moving from left to right in the diagram means moving from overall aim to the detailed functional elements.

UNIQUE DEVICE MANUFACTURABILITY

DirectHaler Nasal is straightforward and cost effective to manufacture, fill, and assemble using high-speed standard mass production technology. The device tube is manufactured using extrusion and roll forming and the device

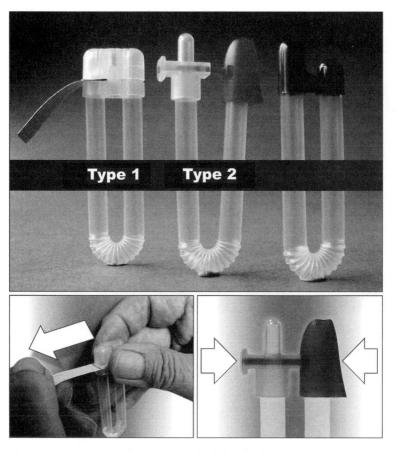

Figure 4   Different device cap types for DirectHaler™.

cap by injection moulding. The device's initial design was partly inspired by the design of a standard drug capsule. Thus, powder dose filling is carried out using modified high-speed capsule filling equipment supplied by MG2 (Fig. 6), ensuring high-precision pre-metered doses.

The overall extremely straightforward DirectHaler manufacturing process—rare in the inhaler market—adds flexibility when it comes to choosing a device supply strategy.

One option is to adopt an overall "turn-key" drug delivery business concept, including complete manufacturing, filling, and packing lines that are placed locally for regional supply of the finished product. Another option is for pharmaceutical companies to take advantage of the straightforward and efficient production process, which allows them to manage device manufacturing, filling, and packing in house, without the usual contract manufacturing and filling link in the supply chain.

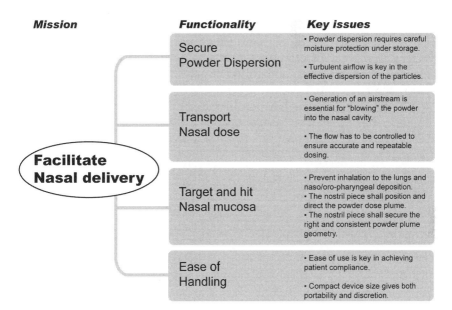

Mission	Functionality	Key issues
	Secure Powder Dispersion	• Powder dispersion requires careful moisture protection under storage. • Turbulent airflow is key in the effective dispersion of the particles.
Facilitate Nasal delivery	Transport Nasal dose	• Generation of an airstream is essential for "blowing" the powder into the nasal cavity. • The flow has to be controlled to ensure accurate and repeatable dosing.
	Target and hit Nasal mucosa	• Prevent inhalation to the lungs and naso/oro-pharyngeal deposition. • The nostril piece shall position and direct the powder dose plume. • The nostril piece shall secure the right and consistent powder plume geometry.
	Ease of Handling	• Ease of use is key in achieving patient compliance. • Compact device size gives both portability and discretion.

Figure 5 Defining the key device functionality for facilitating nasal delivery.

BUILDING FURTHER ON THE ADVANTAGES OF NASAL DELIVERY

The manufacturing simplicity and compactness of the DirectHaler Nasal opens new opportunities to address future needs for combination therapy.

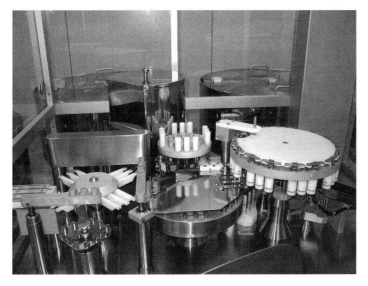

Figure 6 Equipment for integrated filling and assembly of DirectHaler™ Nasal.

The DirectHaler device can be considered as the basic "building block" in any combination therapy or dosing sequencing involving nasal delivery. This means that the DirectHaler device could be the "nasal component" in a combination therapy consisting of for instance: One nasal dose + one oral dose in the same blister pack (Fig. 7).

Such innovative combination therapy options for use of two delivery routes at the same time would enable design of delivery systems for achieving, for example:

- local action (nasal) + systemic action (oral);
- rapid onset of action (nasal) + delayed and sustained release (oral).

ENABLING TARGETING OF THE COMPLETE RESPIRATORY SYSTEM

The "building block" characteristic of DirectHaler Nasal can be exploited further, as this characteristic is shared with our pulmonary device technology: DirectHaler Pulmonary.

Dosing to the complete respiratory system has previously only been possible by special nebulizers with face masks, and limited portability. Such highly specialized equipment is expensive, complicated, and mainly suitable for stationary use.

The DirectHaler technologies eliminate these limitations, and open a completely new option for drug delivery to the whole respiratory system with dry powder formulations: DirectHaler Pulmonary and DirectHaler Nasal are the first unit-dose devices which can be clicked together as one device (Fig. 8). Enabling specific dosing to the nasal and pulmonary airways, and thereby targeting the complete airway system. Such targeting can

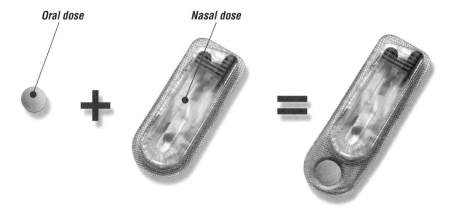

Figure 7 Combining an oral dose with DirectHaler™ Nasal.

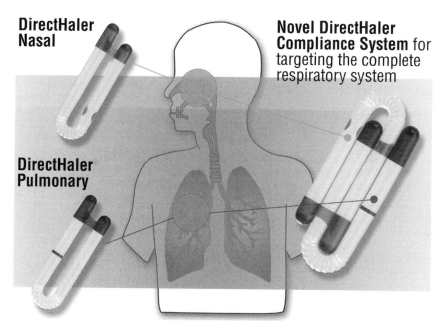

Figure 8 DirectHaler^TM combination unit for pulmonary and nasal delivery.

be highly relevant in treatment of respiratory diseases, and in prevention/ treatment of respiratory infections (also in relation to biodefence).

As the two devices are packed together and applied separately, it allows utilizing of separate formulation technologies for reaching nasal airways and for the pulmonary airways. This is important, as nasal delivery and pulmonary delivery has their own requirements for powder formulation characteristics.

CONCLUSION

The DirectHaler Nasal technology offers advanced nasal delivery characteristics in a straightforward, patent protected, and cost effective device embodiment. The DirectHaler Nasal device removes disadvantages of currently available nasal delivery technologies, and enables pursuit of new therapeutic approaches exploiting the nasal route of administration.

REFERENCES

1. Novartis, Miacalcin, product leaflet, http://www.miacalcin.com
2. GSK, Imigran/Imitrex, product leaflet, http://www.migrainehelp

3. AstraZeneca, Rhinocort, product leaflet, http://www.astrazeneca-us.com/pi/Rhinocort_Aqua.pdf
4. Schering-Plough, Nasonex, product leaflet. http://www.nasonex.com/framework/skins/default_ default/pdf/patients_instructions.pdf.
5. GSK, Flonase, product leaflet, http://www.flonase.com/use/howto.html
6. Devillers G. Exploring a pharmaceutical market niche and trends: Nasal spray drug delivery. New trends and unmet needs. Drug Deliv Technol 2003; 3(3):1–4.
7. Brook I. Bacterial contamination of saline spray/drop solution in patients with respiratory tract infection. Am J Infect Control 2002; 30:246–7.
8. Geller DE. New liquid aerosol generation devices: Systems that force pressurized liquids through nozzles. Respiratory Care. 2002; 47(12):1392–405.
9. Thorsson L, Newman SP, Weisz A, Trofast E, Moren F. Nasal distribution of budesonide inhaled via a powder inhaler. Rhinology 1993; 31(1):7–10.

Part VI: Vaginal Technologies

35

Intravaginal Drug Delivery Technologies

A. David Woolfson

School of Pharmacy, Queen's University Belfast, Medical Biology Centre, Belfast, Northern Ireland, U.K.

HISTORICAL

For thousands of years, women have been administering a wide range of substances to the vagina, primarily for contraception or for the treatment of infection. The Kahun papyrus, an ancient Egyptian treatise on gynecology, mentions such contraceptive methods as the use of a vaginal suppository containing crocodile dung mixed with honey and sodium carbonate. In the papyrus of Ebers, another ancient Egyptian document on medicine, the recommended method was to insert into the vagina acacia tips containing gum arabic which, when dissolved in water, liberated lactic acid. This latter preparation is not dissimilar in concept to modern day intravaginal administration of lactic acid pessaries in order to restore or maintain the natural, slightly acidic pH of the vagina. More alarmingly, in the nineteenth century, abortion, suicide, and homicide attempts using vaginally administered arsenic and other poisons were not uncommon. Thus, it has long been realized that exogenous chemicals, when administered intravaginally, could find their way into the systemic circulation. However, this belief was not formalized until the publication of the seminal study by Macht (1) in 1918, which described the absorption of alkaloids, inorganic salts, esters, and antiseptics through the vagina, thus demonstrating for the first time the potential for systemic drug delivery via this route.

INFLUENCE OF VAGINAL ANATOMY AND PHYSIOLOGY ON DRUG DELIVERY

Anatomical and physiological considerations have a direct influence on the design of intravaginal drug delivery systems. The functions of the human vagina, a portion of the female reproductive system, are connected with conception and birth, and its physiology changes with the female life cycle, in addition to variations occurring during the monthly cycle (2,3). From the drug delivery viewpoint, therefore, the vagina is a potential space that contains a non-constant environment. Thus, the design of intravaginal drug delivery systems must take account of the anatomy and physiology of the vagina.

The vagina is a highly expandable, slightly S-shaped fibromuscular collapsible tube situated between the rectum, which lies posterior to it, and the urethra and bladder, which lie anterior to it (Fig. 1). It extends from the lower part of the uterine cervix to the external part of the vulva known as the labia minor (4). The vault of the vagina is divided into four areas relative to the cervix (5). These are the posterior fornix, which is capacious, the anterior fornix, which is shallow, and two lateral fornices. The anterior wall of the vagina averages 6–7 cm in length, whereas the posterior wall is slightly longer (approximately 7.5–8.5 cm) due to the intrusion of the cervix below the vault.

The walls of the vagina are composed of four distinctive layers, the stratified mucosa, submucosa, muscularis, and the tunica adventitia (6). The stratified mucosa, which offers the main barrier to drug absorption, consists of an epithelium and an underlying lamina propria, with the thickness of the epithelium varying by 200–300 mm as a result of changes in estrogen levels during the menstrual cycle. Therefore, the degree of estrogenization of vaginal epithelium has important consequences for drug permeation through the tissue.

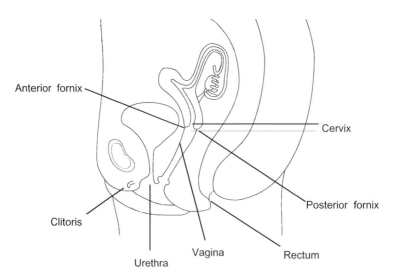

Figure 1   Vaginal anatomy in relation to drug delivery.

The cellular structure of vaginal epithelium consists of five distinct cytological layers, the basal, parabasal, intermediate, transitional, and superficial layers (7). The basal cells, typically cuboidal in shape and characterized by the presence of microvilli on the surface of the cell membrane (8) are responsible for the continuous production of squamous cells. Parabasal cells are polygonal in shape and differ slightly from the basal cells in having a substantially greater amount of surface microvilli. The cells of the intermediate layer are of the largest cell type and also exhibit microvilli. The transitional cells that follow may show noticeable signs of involution characterized by the reduction of microvilli and intercellular junctions (8). The superficial layer, as the name suggests, are the cells of the outermost layer, squamous in shape and normally devoid of keratin (9). These cells store considerable amounts of glycogen, which is released into the vaginal lumen when the surface cells are exfoliated (10).

All layers of the epithelium consist of living cells that renew continuously as they are stimulated by hormonal action and intracellular communication. The constant loss and renewal of cells is characteristic of epithelial membranes. Epithelial cells are very closely packed and are joined together by junctional complexes (11). Thus, there is no room for blood vessels between adjacent epithelial cells. The epithelium must therefore receive nourishment from the underlying connective tissue, which has large intercellular spaces that can accommodate blood vessels and nerves. Epithelial membranes are attached to the underlying connective tissue by the basement lamina, consisting primarily of proteins and polysaccharides.

Vaginal epithelium is in constant contact with vaginal fluid, formed primarily from transudate which passes through the vaginal wall from the blood vessels. It is mixed with vulval secretions from sebaceous and sweat glands, with minor contributions from Bartholin's and Skene's glands (4). Vaginal fluid may also contain several enzymes, enzyme inhibitors, proteins, carbohydrates, amino acids, alcohols, hydroxy-ketones, and aromatic compounds (12).

Vaginal fluid is normally mixed with cervical mucus and sloughed cells from the vaginal epithelia to the extent that this mucus, produced by glandular units within the cervical canal, is the major component of the fluid. The amount, composition, and physical characteristics of cervical mucus change with the menstrual cycle (13), are making its production estrogen dependent. At the time of ovulation, the amount of cervical secretions further increases, resulting in an increase in the overall volume of vaginal fluid. Consequently, there is an increase in fibrosity, pH, and mucin content and a decrease in the viscosity, cellularity, and albumin concentration (12), with potential effects on drug delivery. Thus, since vaginal fluid is aqueous in nature, it follows that any drug intended for systemic absorption via the vaginal epithelium will require a degree of aqueous solubility.

For drugs that have ionizable functional groups, vaginal pH, in particular, may exert a significant effect on absorption. The vaginal fluid in healthy mature women has a typical pH of between 4 and 5 (5). The pH value is maintained by the commensal micro-organism *Lactobacillus acidophilus,* which produces lactic acid from glycogen contained in the sloughed mature cells of the vaginal mucosa. The acidic nature of the vaginal fluid is of importance since it offers natural resistance to the colonization of pyrogenic organisms.

Normally, vaginal pH is low in infancy and gradually increases as the concentration of maternal hormones in the infant's body recedes, reaching a pH of 7 where it remains until puberty (13). The pH of vaginal fluid in the adult rises during menstruation, but it may also increase after periods of frequent acts of coitus as both vaginal transudate, formed during coitus, and ejaculate are alkaline. Physiologically, the anterior fornix of vagina has the lowest pH, which gradually rises toward the vestibule (2). Intravaginal pH may also be affected by the presence of cervical mucus, which has a pH in the range 6.5–9 (14), and by the amount of lubricating vaginal secretions. These changes could influence the release profile from intravaginal drug delivery devices by, e.g., altering the ratio of charged to uncharged (lipophilic) species of a weakly basic drug, and thus its solubility in vaginal fluid, together with its permeability through the predominantly lipophilic epithelial barrier.

Drug transport across vaginal epithelium may also be affected by enzymatic activity associated with vaginal fluid. For example, enzymatic degradation of polypeptides may lead to low vaginal absorption of these drugs (15). The basal layer of the vaginal epithelium has a high activity of enzymes found in the citric acid cycle, in fatty acid metabolism, and in 17-ketosteroidogenesis, e.g., succinic dehydrogenase, diaphorase, acid phosphatase, b-glucuronidase, and phosphoamidase (16). The outer cell layers of the vagina contain b-glucuronidase, acid phosphatase, and smaller quantities of a-naphthylesterase, diaphorase, phosphoamidase, and succinic dehydrogenase. Basal cell layers contain b-glucuronidase, succinic dehydrogenase, diaphorase, small amounts of acid phosphatase, and a-naphthylesterase. Levels of alkaline phosphatase, lactate dehydrogenase, aminopeptidase, and esterase activity are all high in the follicular phase of the menstrual cycle, but fall immediately prior to ovulation (16). The presence of infective diseases can, of course, affect the levels and types of enzymes found in vaginal fluid (17).

Vaginal epithelium has a rich blood supply originating primarily from the internal iliac artery but, in some cases, may come from the first part of the uterine artery (9). One aspect of the vascularity of vaginal tissue that has recently attracted attention is the concept of a "first uterine pass effect" or direct preferential vagina-to-uterus transport. Evidence of higher than expected uterine tissue concentrations after vaginal administration of progesterone (18) has been advanced as one possible consequence of this effect. A "counter current" flow of absorbed permeant between venous and arterial systems supplying the vagina has been postulated as a possible mechanism for this event. It has been suggested that the "first uterine pass effect" may allow targeted drug delivery to the uterus via the vaginal route, thereby maximizing the desired effects while minimising the potential for adverse systemic effects. However, the concept remains unproven and may yet engender further controversy.

The vaginal environment is a dynamic and closely interrelated mix of facultative and obligate anaerobic microbes, mainly *Lactobacillus*, *Bacteroides*, and *Staphylococcus* species, with new strains constantly being introduced (19). These microorganisms possess enzymes that enable them to survive and replicate under a given vaginal environment. It is well established that only those microorganisms that can replicate and compete for nutrients in the vagina can become established as part of the natural vaginal flora (3). Medication has been found to have a direct influence on the vaginal microflora. The selective eradication of certain microorganisms by administration of antibiotics may result in the colonization of the vagina by opportunistic pathogens. Sjoberg and co-workers (20) investigated the effects of phenoxymethylpenicillin on normal vaginal flora in six subjects. Gram-negative strains developed in 4 of the 6 women and, in one of the subjects, *Lactobacilli* species had disappeared completely, to be replaced by *Escherichia coli*.

Several research groups have investigated the possible effects of intravaginal drug delivery devices on the normal vaginal microflora (21,22). For example, intrauterine devices (IUD) have been known to cause local mechanical irritation of the vagina, thus resulting in an increased number of leukocytes and increased mucus secretion on the site of irritation. As a consequence of this, vaginal pH increases, favouring the proliferation of non-acidophilic pathogens (3). A higher prevalence of anaerobes in IUD users compared with non-IUD users has been reported (23). In contrast, however, other studies found no significant changes in vaginal flora between users and non-users of contraceptive elastomeric intravaginal rings (24,25).

INTRAVAGINAL DRUG ABSORPTION

Systemic drug absorption across the vaginal epithelium membrane involves drug release from the delivery system, drug dissolution in vaginal fluid and membrane penetration. Local intravaginal drug treatment follows drug release, dissolution, and delivery throughout the vaginal space. The significant absorption capability of the vagina for exogenous substances, including drugs, is now well recognized. Originally regarded as relatively passive and impermeable to foreign agents, the intravaginal absorption of numerous compounds has now been noted. The emphasis in human clinical trials has been primarily on the systemic delivery of contraceptives (26) and, more recently, on estrogenic and progestogenic compounds for hormone replacement therapy (27). Currently, there is substantial interest in the intravaginal delivery of therapeutic peptides and proteins (15).

A significant advantage of intravaginal drug delivery is that the route avoids hepatic first-pass metabolism. For example, intravaginal delivery of estrogenic compounds, which are subject to extensive first-pass metabolism, requires a significantly lower dose than the oral route in order to achieve the required serum concentration of circulating steroid.

The absorption of drugs or other exogenous substances from the vagina depends on the condition of the epithelial membrane, the nature of the delivery system and on physicochemical factors relating to the penetrant, including molecular weight and size, lipophilicity, ionization state. The local pharmacological action of the drug, thickness of the vaginal wall, presence of cervical mucous, and the presence of specific cytoplasmic receptors may also be important. Drug absorption is also modified by changes in the thickness of the vaginal wall influenced by the ovarian cycle or by pregnancy and by post-menopausal changes in vaginal epithelium and intravaginal pH.

The pathways for drug diffusion across vaginal epithelium are essentially similar to other epithelial tissues (15) and are well represented by the "fluid mosaic model" as a lipid continuum interspersed with aqueous pores, the latter forming an aqueous "shunt" route (28). The lipid continuum predominates in vaginal drug absorption.

The permeability coefficient of a drug across a vaginal epithelial barrier membrane may be considered as the product of the amount of drug penetrating the membrane per unit time per unit area drug (flux) and the membrane thickness, divided by the drug concentration in the delivery vehicle. For drugs with a high vaginal membrane permeability coefficient, absorption is mainly controlled by permeability across the hydrodynamic diffusion layer formed by vaginal fluid sandwiched between the vaginal epithelial membrane and the delivery device (29). For drugs with a low vaginal membrane permeability, vaginal absorption is mainly controlled by permeability across the vaginal epithelium (29). Consequently, in vaginal drug delivery, for systemic drug absorption to occur, the penetrant substance must have sufficient lipophilicity to diffuse through the lipid continuum of the membrane, but also require some degree of aqueous solubility to ensure dissolution in vaginal fluid. This is sometimes a difficult compromise to achieve.

The sequence of events that occurs in intravaginal drug delivery depends, in part, on the nature of the delivery system that is employed, i.e., whether it is solid or semi-solid, swellable or erodible, soluble or insoluble, immediate or controlled release. For the purposes of illustration, Flynn et al. (30) have described the sequence of events that occur when a solid polymeric reservoir device is used as the delivery system for a hydrophobic drug, such as a steroidal hormone. The drug is initially present as a homogeneous distribution of fine particles within the core of the device, with a small proportion in solution within the polymer system. Drug in solution diffuses through the polymeric sheath, followed by partitioning and diffusion through the vaginal fluid forming the hydrodynamic layer sandwiched between the device and vaginal wall. The drug then passively diffuses along a concentration gradient, primarily through the lipid continuum of vaginal mucosal epithelium (the transcellular route). In practice, the concentration gradient established with a matrix system is actually a series of such gradients, comprising that between the device and depletion zone boundaries, the gradient across the hydrodynamic layer and that across the epithelial membrane, between the mucosal and serosal sides (30).

The bioavailability of an intravaginally administered drug can be modified by the use of chemical penetration enhancers, typically acting on epithelial tight junctions to provide an alternative intercellular penetration route that may be particularly significant in the vaginal absorption of higher molecular weight species, such as therapeutic peptides and proteins. The overall permeability of vaginal epithelium to penetrant species is greater than the rectal, buccal or transdermal routes, but less than the nasal and pulmonary routes (31).

DESIGNING AN INTRAVAGINAL DRUG DELIVERY SYSTEM: KEY CONSIDERATIONS

There are a wide range of delivery systems applicable to intravaginal drug delivery, very few of which are specifically designed for the vaginal route. General delivery platforms that may be used intravaginally include creams, foams, pessaries, gels, tablets, and particulate systems. Some of these incorporate the use of one or more mucoadhesive polymeric components (32,33). The best examples of specifically designed intravaginal delivery systems generally involve solid polymeric systems, typically either elastomers (34) or hydrogels. The choice of optimum delivery system for the intravaginal route depends on a consideration of the following considerations.

- The choice between local or systemic delivery may determine, e.g., the use of a traditional dosage form, such as a semi-solid cream or gel, or a system that promotes increased intravaginal residence with an increased possibility of absorption across vaginal epithelium.
- Site-specific application may be preferable or it may be required that the drug is distributed rapidly throughout the vaginal space. The latter approach may be best suited to, e.g., intravaginal administration of an antimicrobial agent. Site-specific delivery will require the use of a self-locating system, typically a mucoadhesive formulation, although an intravaginal ring, due to its elastomeric nature, will remain located high in the

vaginal space. Conversely, for rapid distribution throughout the space, semi-solid or fast-dissolving solid systems will be required. For semi-solids, flow properties and viscoelastic character will be critical determinants of their ability to spread rapidly from their point of application.

- Intravaginal drug release may be required to be immediate or modified (sustained or controlled release). Drug release by the intravaginal route is most commonly immediate but a viscoelastic semi-solid can be designed to offer some increase in duration of delivery, as can solid hydrogels or intravaginal tablets. For controlled, zero order release sustained over prolonged periods (days, extending to months), solid polymeric systems may be most suitable, provided they are compatible with the physicochemical nature of the drug to be delivered. Intravaginal applications of controlled release relate to systemic drug delivery applications, typically for potent drugs such as steroid sex hormones and, perhaps, peptides or peptidomimetic agents.
- For systemic drug delivery by the intravaginal route, the physicochemical and pharmacological nature of the penetrant are of paramount importance. The drug to be delivered should be considered in relation to its polarity and partition characteristics, molecular weight and size, both in respect of epithelial penetration, release into vaginal fluid and performance in either water-based or more hydrophobic delivery systems.
- Vaginal delivery may not be universally acceptable in all cultures, and within cultures the preference for systems that can be self-inserted and removed, or considerations relating to leakage, will vary considerably.
- From an industrial perspective, a cost-benefit analysis is an important factor in deciding upon the choice of delivery system. Capital costs, e.g., are considerably higher for specifically designed intravaginal systems than for those capable of manufacture on generic equipment, such as semi-solids and intravaginal tablets. These costs must be considered in relation to the commercial value of the active component(s) and the likely benefits in relation to the disease state.

INTRAVAGINAL DELIVERY OF HIV MICROBICIDES AND VACCINES

There are presently an estimated 40 million people carrying HIV, with around 25 million of these being in sub-Saharan Africa (35). The majority (around 90%) of new HIV infections in this region, which remains blighted by the AIDS pandemic, occur via heterosexual vaginal intercourse (35,36). In the continued absence of a vaccine against HIV, and for a variety of cultural reasons, there is a clear and urgent need for a female-controlled approach to prevention of vaginal infection by HIV (37). Microbicides are agents, or formulations thereof, that reduce the transmission of HIV during sexual intercourse (38,39). Whilst first-generation microbicides were intended to offer a physical barrier to viral infectivity, the focus is now primarily on specific chemical agents that may block viral entry or attachment to vaginal epithelia, or interfere with one or more modes of viral reproduction. Although a vaginal microbicide may potentially act at any stage of the HIV infectivity cycle, it is preferable to disrupt the cycle as early as possible so as to minimize the risk of systemic infection (40). Vaginal microbicides have further stimulated research into the development of vaginal delivery systems, particularly those that can provide continuous release of a microbicidal agent (41,42).

Mucosal vaccination is a potential administration route for eliciting antigen-specific mucosal and systemic immunogenicity. Conventional immunisation strategies rely on immunological memory, whereby an appropriate immune response is generated upon subsequent post-vaccination exposure to the infectious agent (43). However, it is not at all clear if retroviruses, and particularly lentiviruses such as HIV, can ever be eliminated once the host is infected. Hence, vaccine design may have to break with tradition and assume that sterilizing immunity at the portal of viral entry will be required. Thus immunological memory may not be enough to protect against HIV, but may require maintenance of constant and elevated level of local specific immune effector function. In practice, this may mean the delivery of HIV viral antigen to vaginal epithelium, possibly in a repeated or continuous mode (44). Thus, in the future development of an effective HIV vaccine, vaginal delivery technologies (45) may have a key role to play.

INTRAVAGINAL DRUG DELIVERY TECHNOLOGIES

Intravaginal drug delivery systems can be thought of as being adapted from semi-solid topical systems (usually, by design of a vaginal applicator device) or designed specifically for intravaginal use. Existing delivery platforms are summarized in Table 1. Intravaginal drug delivery may be intended for a local effect, such as barrier contraceptive methods, the prevention/treatment of infection or estronization of vaginal epithelium. It may also be intended to provide controlled, sustained systemic delivery of a range of possible therapeutic agents, including steroid sex hormones for contraception or estrogen/hormone replacement therapy (46). One exciting area for development is the use of the vaginal route for non-parenteral delivery of peptide and protein drugs, with the assistance of appropriate penetration enhancement strategies (47).

Conventional solutions, semi-solids (ointments, creams, and some gels), tablets, and pessaries all suffer from problems of retention and spreadability when used intravaginally. Semi-solids, in particular, are perceived as messy in use and prone to leakage. Conventional systems often do not offer sufficient flexibility in design, in respect of controlling the drug release rate and sustaining

Table 1 Intravaginal Drug Delivery Technologies

Delivery platform	Physicochemical aspects
Gels/hydrogels	Rapid drug release from conventional gels Most suitable for relatively polar drugs Usually designed as mucoadhesive systems Viscoelastic rheology may enhance intravaginal residence time
Tablets	Unlike oral solid dosage forms, limited applications for controlled release—most suitable for immediate release applications May be formulated with mucoadhesive polymers
Pessaries/suppositories	Rapid drug release Can accommodate drugs in solution or suspension
Particulate systems (naoparticles, microspheres, etc.)	Controlled release possible via matrix, reservoir, swelling or erodible mechanisms Bioadhesive polymers may improve retention May enhance intravaginal drug distribution May offer protection for labile drugs Can be combined with other systems such as gels, where the gel acts as a carrier
Intravaginal rings	Suitable for highly lipophilic drugs, such as steroids, but may be modified for delivery of a wider range of actives Processing temperature may not be suitable for thermolabile actives Variety of release profiles, including zero order release, possible through alteration of ring design

release over periods extending from days to, perhaps, months. Thus, specific intravaginal drug delivery designs are continuing to evolve. These are largely based on non-specific mucoadhesive hydrogel systems, cytoadhesive targeted systems, solid hydrogels or intravaginal elastomeric rings. Penetration enhancement may be a necessary feature of certain delivery systems, particularly where the penetrant is a biomolecular species (48), although certain absorption enhancers may induce histological damage. Where such damage is irreversible, an enhancement strategy will clearly be unacceptable.

Bio(Muco)Adhesive Semi-Solids

Bioadhesive polymers can control the rate of drug release from, and extend the residence time of, intravaginal delivery systems. Vaginal epithelium, although it is not strictly a mucosal epithelium since it does not possess secretory goblet cells, is, in practice, coated with cervical mucus from vaginal fluid. Thus, the term mucoadhesive is preferable in this case. Mucoadhesive formulations may contain one or more therapeutic agents, or they may primarily be designed as moisturisers to control vaginal dryness.

Mucoadhesive hydrogels are weakly crosslinked polymers which are able to swell in contact with water and to spread onto the surface of mucus (49). Their ability to achieve an intimate contact with an absorbing membrane, to localize drug delivery systems at a certain place and to extend residence time are the main factors in their use in intravaginal drug delivery (50).

Mucoadhesion can be understood as a two-step process, in which the first adsorptive contact is governed by surface energy effects and a spreading process. In the latter phase, the diffusion of polymer chains across the polymer-mucus interface may enhance the final bond (51). Water plays an important role in mucoadhesion, the invading water molecules liberating polymer chains from their twisted and entangled state and, thus, exposing reactive sites that can bond to tissue macromolecules. The adhesion of dried hydrogels to moist tissue can be quite substantial, with water uptake from the tissue surface facilitating surface dehydration and exposing surface depressions that may act as anchoring locations (52). Thus, the majority of hydrogels applied for intravaginal use are based on mucoadhesive polymers, including poly(acrylic acid)s and polycationic materials such as chitosan. However, other hydrogels systems are also being investigated. For example, Zulfiqar et al. have prepared and characterized a range of polyurethane hydrogel networks for potential vaginal application based on poly(ethylene glycol) and hexamethylene diisocyanate using 1,1,1-tris(hydroxymethyl) ethane as the cross-linking agent. Intravaginal implantation of the hydrogel into rats produced no pathological changes in the tissue (53).

Spreading and retention, and consequent "messiness," of semi-solid vaginal mucoadhesive systems, such as gels, is a major issue in intravaginal drug delivery. Brown et al. reported a scintigraphic evaluation of vaginal dosage forms in post-menopausal women (54). The vaginal spreading and clearance of a radiolabelled pessary formulation and a commercial poly-carbophil gel was assessed in six healthy, post-menopausal female volunteers over a six hour period by gamma scintigraphy. In five out of the six subjects studied, clearance of the two formulations exhibited very little intra-subject variation. However, there was considerable inter-subject variability in clearance. Importantly, there was no evidence to suggest that either of the formulations dispersed material beyond the cervix, into the uterus, in any of the subjects studied. The authors concluded that the lack of significant retention of these products in most of the volunteers had obvious implications for the delivery of therapeutic agents.

The drawbacks associated with mucoadhesive gel systems has prompted further developments in advanced semi-solid vaginal delivery systems. Such systems may be based on the use of thermogelling polymers such as Pluronic F127 (55), on polymer modifcations to provide enhanced rheological performance (56) or by the addition of a controlled release functionality through the use of particulate carriers within the mucoadhesive gel (57–59). Mucoadhesive hydrogel films (60) offer another interesting alternative, but often present manufacturing difficulties due to the need to remove relatively large quantities of water from polymeric hydrogels.

Vaginal Pessaries or Suppositories

Vaginal pessaries or suppositories (the terms often being used interchangeably) containing such substances as natural gums, fatty acids, alum, and rock salts were originally used in ancient Egyptian times as contraceptives. One of the earliest technical papers describing a suppository-based vaginal device was published in 1947 by Rock et al. (61). The paper described the administration and adsorption of penicillin from a cocoa butter base in non-pregnant women with vaginitis, near-term pregnant women, and women recently post partum. Appreciable serum levels were measured in both the vaginitis and postpartum groups, but not in the near-term group, the latter presumably due to changes in the vaginal epithelial tissue. The results also clearly demonstrated variations in absorption resulting from the menstrual cycle. These suppository/pessary systems are now most commonly used to administer drugs to promote cervical ripening prior to child-birth, and for local drug delivery to the vagina. An interesting recent application is the use of a suppository formulation containing a lyophilized *Lactobacillus* species intended to restore the natural vaginal flora to a healthy state, thus stimulating local anti-infective properties (62).

Solid Polymeric Carriers

Solid polymeric carriers represent perhaps the only class of specifically designed intravaginal drug delivery systems and comprise either solid hydrogels or elastomeric intravaginal rings (63). The former category relies on shape to remain in place within the vaginal space, whereas the intravaginal ring relies on its elastomeric properties, thus exerting a slight tension on the vaginal walls. Such systems are non-messy and can be used to generate a variety of controlled delivery profiles over periods ranging from several days to several months. The elastomeric system requires predominantly hydrophobic drugs or modifications to the polymer or formulation (or both) in order to cope with hydrophilic actives. By contrast, hydrogel systems, which are typically highly biocompatible, are more suitable for hydrophilic actives but perform poorly in the delivery of more hydrophobic agents.

Carriers for Intravaginal delivery of Peptide and Protein Drugs

Peptide and protein drugs suffer from low bioavailability when administered orally, and thus commonly require parenteral administration. However, intravaginal delivery may offer an exciting and viable alternative for certain drugs in this category associated with female health issues (15). Richardson et al. demonstrated that vaginal absorption of insulin in sheep from either insulin solutions or a bioadhesive microsphere delivery systems is significantly enhanced by the addition of lysophosphatidylcholine (LPC) (48). While the vaginal absorption of insulin from solution was minimal, the addition of LPC resulted in a rapid rise in plasma insulin and a pronounced fall in plasma glucose levels. The absolute bioavailability of the peptide from the latter solution was 13%. The hypoglycaemic response to vaginally administered insulin was also improved using the microsphere delivery system, compared to insulin solution alone, and was further enhanced by LPC. Vaginal absorption of insulin from each formulation appeared to be influenced by the estrous cycle and was thought to correlate with changes in vaginal histology. Niosomes prepared from sorbitan monoesters have also been shown effectively deliver insulin vaginally in a rat model (64).

The ability to deliver macromolecular species intravaginally suggests the possibility of using vaginal epithelium as a portal for vaccine administration. Such work remains in the early stages, but some promising results have been reported in animal studies. Thus, starch microspheres containing LPC have also been assessed in sheep for vaginal delivery of a 40 kDa glycoprotein fragment from influenza virus haemagglutinin (TOPS) (65). Three groups of sheep received intravaginal immunisation with either a TOPS solution, TOPS/LPC as a powder formulation, and TOPS and LPC in solution, while a fourth group received intramuscular immunisation with TOPS adsorbed to an aluminium hydroxide gel. At day 45, the serum IgG and the vaginal wash IgA antibody responses induced by TOPS-DSM/LPC powder formulation were significantly greater than those induced by intravaginal immunisation with the TOPS solution. However, the highest levels of antibodies in serum and vaginal wash samples were induced by intramuscular immunisation with TOPS/aluminium oxide gel formulation. Intravaginal immunization with TOPS and LPC did not result in the induction of enhanced levels of antibodies in serum or vaginal wash.

Calcitonin is a polypeptide hormone used to treat postmenopausal osteoporosis and Paget's disease of the bone and in the management of malignant hypercalcaemia. The preparation, characterization and clinical evaluation in rats of calcitonin-containing vaginal delivery systems based on hyaluronic acid esters (HYAFF) microspheres have been reported (66,67). HYAFF biopolymers are derived from chemically-modified hyaluronic acid and are considered to be mucoadhesive (68). HYAFF microspheres are typically prepared by a solvent evaporation method (47). Spherical microspheres containing salmon calcitonin (sCT) and having a diameter of about 10 mm in diameter were prepared by a solvent extraction method solution. The efficiency of incorporation was high, with approximately 80–90% of the peptide recovered by extraction from the microspheres, while assessment of the biological activity of the peptide confirmed that the pharmacological activity of sCT was unaffected by the microsphere preparation process. The microspheres produced enhanced hypocalcaemic responses in rats compared with a simple sCT solution (22 vs. 12%, respectively), but maximal effect also occurred more rapidly after administration (130 vs. 195 minutes, respectively). Microscopic examination of the rat vaginal epithelium clearly showed the presence of numerous microspheres in the vaginal lumen and closely attached to the epithelial tissue. In a related experiment, where technetium-labelled microspheres were administered to the vagina of a sheep that had been treated with a radio-labelled gel, the distribution, spreading and clearance of the microspheres were determined using gamma-scintigraphy. The results demonstrated the bioadhesive properties of the HYAFF microspheres under in vivo conditions and suggest that the microspheres were solely confined to the vaginal tract.

FUTURE PROSPECTS FOR INTRAVAGINAL DRUG DELIVERY

Intravaginal drug delivery is increasingly of interest to the drug delivery community. Delivery systems for this route can broadly be subdivided into those that are adaptations of technologies used for other routes, such as semi-solids or vaginal 'tablets' that may incorporate mucoadhesive polymers or particulate carriers, and those systems specifically designed for vaginal application. In the latter category, some technologies have long been known, e.g., the use of pessaries. Perhaps of greater interest are more recent developments utilising solid polymeric carriers that can offer sustained and/or controlled delivery of a range of actives for both local and systemic administration. Partuclate controlled-release systems, formulated in a mucoadhesive carrier, are also of increasing interest, possibly combined with emerging semi-solid formulations displaying high performance rheological characteristics. Thus, future developments are likely to centre on specifically-developed high performance intravaginal products for female health, in combination with novel strategies for the intravaginal delivery of macromolecular actives. Thus, intravaginal delivery of biomolecules such as therapeutic peptides and proteins will be of significant interest. The non-viral delivery of DNA across vaginal epithelium may also attract attention, given the relatively low absorption barrier of this tissue. The ability to deliver biomolecules by a non-parenteral route remains the great challenge in drug delivery. The delivery of biomolecular actives that have implications for female health is therefore likely to provide one of the main drives for the further development of novel intravaginal drug delivery technologies. However, the greatest incentive for the development of advanced vaginal drug delivery systems is likely to be the need for continuous delivery of vaginal microbicides and possible vaginal immunisation strategies in the continued fight against the HIV/AIDS pandemic.

REFERENCES

1. Macht DI. The absorption of drugs and poisons through the vagina. J Pharmacol Path 1918; 10:509–22.
2. Kistner RW. Physiology of the vagina. In: Hafez ESE, Evans TN, eds. Human Reproductive Medicine: The Human Vagina. Vol. 2, New York: North-Holland, 1978:109–20.
3. Paavonen J. Physiology and ecology of the vagina. Scand J Infect Dis Suppl. 1983; 40:31–5.
4. Deshpande AA, Rhodes CT, Danish M. Intravaginal drug delivery. Drug Dev Ind Pharm 1992; 18:1225–79.
5. Tindall VR. Jeffcoate's Principles of Gynaecology. London: Butterworths, 1987.
6. Gartner LP, Hiatt JL. Color Atlas of Histology. Baltimore: Williams and Wilkins, 1994.
7. Burgos MH, De Vargas-Linares CE. Ultrastructure of the vaginal mucosa. In: Hafez ESE, Evans TN, eds. Human Reproductive Medicine: The Human Vagina. Vol. 2, New York: North-Holland, 1978:63–93.
8. Yu K, Chien YW. Vaginal delivery and absorption of drugs. In: Swarbrick J, Boylan JC, eds. Encyclopedia of Pharmaceutical Technology. New York: Marcel Dekker, 1995:153–85.
9. Leeson TS, Leeson CR, Pap AA. Textbook of Histology. Philadelphia: Saunders, 1988.
10. Telford IR. Bridgman CF. Introduction to Functional Histology. Grand Rapids: Harper Collins, 1995.
11. Fox SI. Human Physiology. 6th ed. Boston: McGraw-Hill, 1999.
12. Wagner G, Levin RJ. Vaginal fluid. In: Hafez ESE, Evans TN, eds. Human Reproductive Medicine: The Human Vagina. Vol. 2, New York: North-Holland, 1978:121–37.
13. Washington N, Wilson CG. Physiological factors affecting drug delivery and availability, In: Swarbrick J, Boylan JC, eds. Encyclopedia of Pharmaceutical Technology. New York: Marcel Dekker, 1995:137–69.
14. Masters WH, Johnson VE. Human Sexual Response. Boston: Little, Brown, 1966.
15. Richardson JL, Illum L. Routes of delivery—Case studies. The vaginal route of peptide and protein drug delivery. Adv Drug Del Rev 1992; 8:341–66.
16. Wendell Smith CP, Wilson PM. The vulva, vagina and urethra and the musculature of the pelvic floor. In: Philipp E, Setchell M, Ginsburg J, eds. Scientific Foundations of Obstetrics and Gynaecology. London: Butterworth Heinemann, 1991:84–5.
17. Draper DL, Landers DV, Krohn MA, Hillier SL, Wiesenfeld HC, Heine RP. Levels of vaginal secretory leukocyte protease inhibitor are decreased in women with lower reproductive tract infections. Am J Obstet Gynecol 2000; 183:1243–8.

18. Weber AM, Walters MD, Schover LR, Mitchinson AV. Vaginal anatomy and sexual function. Obstet Gynecol 1995; 86:946–9.
19. Jaszczak S, Hafez ESE. Human Reproduction, Conception and Contraception 2nd ed. Philadelphia: Harper and Row, 1980.
20. Sjoberg I, Grahn E, Hakansson S, Holm SE. Influence of phenoxymethyl pencillin on the vaginal ecosystem. Gynecol Obstet Invest 1992; 33:42–6.
21. Curtis EM, Pine L. Actinomyces in the vaginas of women with and without intrauterine contraceptive devices. Am J Obstet Gynecol 1981; 140:880–4.
22. Welch JS. Quantitative and qualitative effects of douche preparations on vaginal microflora. Obstet Gynecol 1993; 81:320–1.
23. Goldacre MJ, Watt B, Loudon N, Vessey MP. Vaginal microbial flora in normal young women. Brit Med J 1979; 1:1450–9.
24. Roy S, Wilkins J, Mishell DR. The effect of a contraceptive vaginal ring and oral contraceptives on the vaginal flora. Contraception 1981; 24:481–91.
25. Schwan A, Ahren T, Victor A. Effects of contraceptive vaginal ring treatment on vaginal bacteriology and cytology. Contraception 1983; 28:341–7.
26. Roy S, Mishell DR. Vaginal ring clinical studies: Update. In: Zatuchni GI, Goldsmith A, Shelton JD, Sciarra JJ eds. Long-Acting Contraceptive Delivery Systems. Philadelphia: Harper and Row, 1983:581–94.
27. Nash HA, Brache V, Alvarez-Sanchez F, Jackanicz TM, Harmon TM. Estradiol delivery by vaginal rings: potential for hormone replacement therapy. Maturitas 1997; 26:27–33.
28. Singer SJ, Nicolson GL. The fluid mosaic model of the structure of cell membranes. Science 1972; 175:720–2.
29. Chien YW. Novel Drug Delivery Systems. 2nd ed. New York: Marcel Dekker, 1992.
30. Flynn GL, Ho NFH, Hwang S, et al. Interfacing matrix release and membrane absorption–analysis of steroid absorption from a vaginal device in rabbit doe. In: Paul DR, Harris FW, eds. Controlled Release Polymeric Formulations. Washington, DC: American Chemical Society, 1976: 87.
31. Sayani AP, Chien YW, Systemic delivery of peptides and proteins across absorptive mucosae. Crit Rev Ther Drug Carrier Syst 1996; 13:85–184.
32. Gursoy A, Bayhan A. Testing of drug release from bioadhesive vaginal tablets. Drug Dev Ind Pharm 1992; 18:203–21.
33. Gursoy A, Sohtorik I, Uyanik N, Peppas NA. Bioadhesive controlled release systems for vaginal delivery. STP Pharm Sci 1989; 5:886–92.
34. Jackanicz TM. Vaginal ring steroid-releasing systems, In: Zatuchni GI, Sobrero AJ, Speidel JJ, Sciarra J, eds. Vaginal Contraception: New Developments. Philadelphia: Harper and Row, 1979:201–12.
35. UNAIDS/WHO AIDS Epidemic Update: December 2006. http://www.unaids.org/en/HIV_data/epi2006/default.asp (Accessed 8 January 2007)
36. Royce RA, Sena A, Cates W, Cohen MS. Current concepts: Sexual transmission of HIV. N Engl J Med 1997; 336:1072–8.
37. Wang YC, Lee CH. Characterization of a female controlled drug delivery system for microbicides. Contraception 2002; 66:281–7.
38. Shattock RJ, Solomon S. Microbicides—aids to safer sex. Lancet 2004; 363: 1002–3.

39. Shattock RJ, Moore JP. Inhibiting sexual transmission of HIV-1 480 infection. Nat Rev Microbiol 2003; 1:25–34.
40. Malcolm RK, Woolfson AD, Toner C, Lowry D. Vaginal microbicides for the prevention of HIV transmission. Biotech Gen Eng Rev 2004; 21:81–121.
41. Woolfson AD, Malcolm RK, Morrow RJ, Toner CF, McCullagh SD. Intravaginal ring delivery of the reverse transcriptase inhibitor TMC 120 as an HIV microbicide. Int J Pharm 2006; 325:82–9.
42. Geonotti AR, Katz DF. Dynamics of HIV neutralization by a microbicide formulation layer: Biophysical fundamentals and transport theory. Biophys J 2006; 91:2121–30.
43. Krambovitis E, Spandidos DA. HIV-1 infection: Is it time to reconsider our concepts? Int J Mol Med 2006; 18:3–8.
44. Veazey RS, Shattock RJ, Pope, Kirijan JC, Jones J, Hu Q, Ketas T, et al. Prevention of virus transmission to macaque monkeys by a vaginally applied monoclonal antibody to HIV-1 gp120. Nature Med 2003; 9:343–6,.
45. Saltzman WM, Sherwood JK, Adams DR, Haller P. Long-term vaginal antibody delivery: delivery systems and biodistribution. Biotech Bioeng 2000; 67:253–64.
46. Woolfson AD, Elliott GRE, Gilligan CA, Passmore CM. Design of an intravaginal ring for the controlled delivery of 17beta-estradiol as its 3-acetate ester. J Cont Rel 1999; 61:319–28.
47. Lee VHL. Enzymatic barriers to peptide and protein absorption. Crit Rev Ther Drug Carr Sys 1988; 5:69–98.
48. Richardson JL, Farraj NF, Illum L. Enhanced vaginal absorption of insulin in sheep using lysophosphatidylcholine and a bioadhesive microsphere system. Int J Pharm 1992; 88:319–25.
49. Duchêne D, Touchard F, Peppas NA. Pharmaceutical and medical aspects of bioadhesive systems for drug administration. Drug Dev Ind Pharm 1988; 14:283–318.
50. Brannonpeppas L. Novel vaginal drug-release applications. Adv Drug Del Rev 1993; 11:169–77.
51. Lehr CM, Bouwstra JA, Boddé HE, Junginger HE. A surface energy analysis of mucoadhesion: Contact angle measurements on polycarbophil and pig intestinal mucosa in physiologically relevant fluids. Pharm Res 1992; 9:70–5.
52. Longer MA, Robinson JR. Fundamental aspects of bioadhesion. Pharm Int 1986; 7:114–7.
53. Zulfiqar M, Quddos A, Zulfiqar S. Polyurethane networks based on poly (ethylene oxide). J Appl Polymer Sci 1993; 49:2055–60.
54. Brown J, Hooper G, Kenyon CJ, et al. Spreading and retention of vaginal formulations in post-menopausal women as assessed by gamma scintigraphy. Pharm Res 1997; 14:1073–8.
55. Bilensoy E, Rouf MA, Vural I, Sen M, Hincal AA. Mucoadhesive, thermosensitive, prolonged-release vaginal gel for clotrimazole: Beta-cyclodextrin complex. AAPS Pharmscitech 2006; 7:38.
56. Valenta C, Kast CE, Harich I, Bernkop-Schnurch A. Development and in vitro evaluation of a mucoadhesive vaginal delivery system for progesterone. J Cont Rel 2001; 77:323–32.

57. Ning MY, Guo YZ, Pan HZ, Chen XL. Preparation, in vitro and in vivo evaluation of liposomal/niosomal gel delivery systems for clotrimazole. Drug Dev Ind Pharm 2005; 31:375–83.
58. Pavelic Z, Skalko-Basnet N, Filipovic-Grcic J, Martinac A, Jalsenjak I. Development and in vitro evaluation of a liposomal vaginal delivery system for acyclovir. J Cont Rel 2005; 106(18):34–43.
59. Pavelic Z, Skalko-Basnet N, Schubert R. Liposomal gels for vaginal drug delivery. Int J Pharm 2001; 219:139–49.
60. Yoo FJW, Dharmala K, Lee CH. The physicodynamic properties of mucoadhesive polymeric films developed as female controlled drug delivery system. Int J Pharm 2006; 309:139–45.
61. Rock J, Barker RH, Bacon WB. Vaginal Absorption of Penicillin. Science 1947; 105:13–5.
62. Kale VV, Trivedi RV, Wate SP, Bhusari KP. Development and evaluation of a suppository formulation containing Lactobacillus and its application in vaginal diseases. Nat Prod Mol Ther Ann NY Acad Sci 2005; 1056:359–65.
63. Malcolm RK, Woolfson AD, Russell JA, Tallon P, McAuley L, Craig DQM. Influence of silicone elastomer solubility and diffusivity on the in-vitro release of drugs from intravaginal rings. J Cont Rel 2003; 90:217–25.
64. Ning MY, Guo YZ, Pan HZ, Yu HM, Gu ZW. Niosomes with sorbitan monoester as a carrier for vaginal delivery of insul in: Studies in rats. Drug Del 2005; 12:399–407.
65. O'Hagan DT, Rafferty D, Wharton S, Illum L. Intravaginal immunization in sheep using a bioadhesive microsphere antigen delivery system. Vaccine 1993; 11:660–4.
66. Richardson JL, Ramires PA, Miglietta MR, et al. Novel vaginal delivery systems for calcitonin. 1. Evaluation of HYAFF calcitonin microspheres in rats. Int J Pharm 1995; 115:9–15.
67. Rochira M, Miglietta MR, Richardson JL, Ferrari L, Beccaro M, Benedetti ML. Novel vaginal delivery systems for calcitonin. 2. Preparation and characterization of HYAFF(R) microspheres containing calcitonin. Int J Pharm 1996; 144:19–26.
68. Sanzgiri YD, Topp EM, Benedetti L, Stella VJ. Evaluation of mucoadhesive properties of hyluronic acid benzyl esters. Int J Pharm 1994; 107:91–7.

36

Vaginal Rings for Controlled-Release Drug Delivery

R. Karl Malcolm

School of Pharmacy, Queen's University Belfast, Medical Biology Centre, Belfast, Northern Ireland, U.K.

INTRODUCTION

The concept of controlled drug delivery to the human vagina using vaginal rings was first described in a 1970 patent application (1) and a series of subsequent publications (2,3) following the discovery that a range of molecules, including steroids, could be released from silicone elastomer in a controlled and predictable manner (4). Consequently, the major early focus for vaginal ring technology was the development of steroid-releasing rings for contraception, a reflection of the concern over burgeoning global population in the developing world and the need to improve family health by controlling conception rates. However, a number of development issues, largely concerned with the choice and safety of the progestin, seriously hindered contraceptive ring development to the extent that the first vaginal ring to reach the market in 1992 was, in fact, Pfizer's estrogen replacement therapy product Estring®, providing continuous and controlled delivery over 3 months of 17β-estradiol for local treatment of menopausal symptoms (Fig. 1, Table 1). Two other rings have since reached the market; Organon's contraceptive product Nuvaring®, simultaneously delivering the steroids etonogestrel and ethinylestradiol over 21 days, and Warner Chilcott's Femring™ (Menoring® in the U.K.), which provides continuous controlled administration of an estradiol prodrug, 17β-estradiol-3-acetate, over 3 months (Fig. 1, Table 1). In this chapter, a brief introduction to vaginal ring technology is provided, followed by a review of the scientific

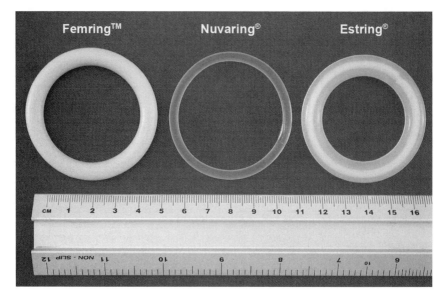

Figure 1 Photograph showing the marketed vaginal rings.

literature relating to each of the three current commercial ring products. Finally, the potential future clinical applications of vaginal ring technology are considered.

VAGINAL RINGS

Vaginal rings are flexible, torus-shaped, elastomeric, or thermoplastic devices that provide long-term, controlled delivery of substances to the vagina for either local or systemic effect. They are easily inserted by the woman herself, and are positioned in the upper third of the vagina, generally adjacent to the cervix. Although the exact location of ring placement is not critical for clinical efficacy, it may have implications for comfort in some women. Ring removal is also easily performed by the woman.

    The simplest design of vaginal ring contains solid drug homogeneously dispersed throughout the polymeric matrix (so-called homogeneous or matrix rings), such that drug release rates are proportional to both the drug loading and the surface area of the device. Drug release from these systems is via a matrix permeation mechanism, involving dissolution of the solid drug in the polymer followed by diffusion of the solubilized molecules through the polymer network. Drug near the surface of a matrix ring is released first, creating a drug-depleted layer, which other solubilized molecules in the inner layers of the ring must diffuse through in order to be released. As time progresses, the surface area of this inward-moving

Table 1 Description of Marketed Vaginal Rings

Vaginal ring product Name/Company/ Dimensions/ Duration of use	Active(s) Chemical formula/ Molecular weight/ Release rate	Chemical Structure of Active
Estring® Pfizer 55.0, 9.0 mm 90 days	Estradiol $C_{18}H_{24}O_2$ MW: 272.39 0.0075 mg/day	
Nuvaring® Organon 54.0, 4.0 mm 3 weeks	Etonogestrel $C_{22}H_{28}O_2$ MW: 324.46 0.120 mg/day	
	Ethinyl estradiol $C_{20}H_{24}O_2$ MW: 296.40 0.015 mg/day	
Femring® Warner Chilcott 56.0, 7.6 mm 3 months	Estradiol-3-acetate $C_{20}H_{26}O_3$ MW: 314.41 0.05 / 0.10 mg/day	

depletion boundary decreases with simultaneous increase in the thickness of the drug-depleted zone. Therefore, the daily amount of drug released decreases with time as the drug close to the surface of the ring becomes exhausted and the diffusional pathway for the remaining drug increases, while the corresponding cumulative drug release versus root time plot is linear.

The "sandwich" and "core" vaginal ring designs (also known as "shell" and "reservoir," were developed to provide constant daily release rates throughout the duration of application, resulting in linear cumulative release versus time profiles, and conforming to zero-order release kinetics. The sandwich design consists of a narrow drug-loaded polymer layer located below the surface of the ring and positioned between a non-medicated central core and a non-medicated outer membrane. The position of the drug core close to the surface ensures efficient delivery of drugs having poor polymer diffusion characteristics, while also minimizing costs owing to relatively low drug loadings. Core-type rings contain the drug(s) within one or more central core which is encapsulated by a drug-free outer polymer membrane. Several individual, small drug-loaded cores of various lengths may be incorporated into the same core ring, thereby allowing multiple drug administration at pre-determined and independent release rates. The release rates of both core and sandwich ring designs may be further modified by changing the thickness of the rate-controlling outer membrane.

The range of materials that may be used for the manufacture of vaginal rings is limited by the requirements for biocompatibility, flexibility and high drug permeability. Commercial ring products are made from either silicone (polydimethylsiloxane) elastomer or polyethylene vinyl acetate (PEVA) copolymers, the former being a chemically cross-linked polymer system and the latter a thermoplastic polymer. Silicone elastomer rings are generally made by elevated-temperature reaction injection molding of room-temperature vulcanized silicone elastomers, while PEVA rings are manufactured by high-temperature co-extrusion of two different grades of the polymer.

ESTRING®

Estring is a reservoir-type vaginal ring designed for localized delivery of estradiol to reduce postmenopausal urogenital symptoms (Fig. 1, Table 1). First marketed in Sweden in 1992, it comprises a silicone elastomer (Silastic®) core loaded with estradiol hemihydrate (2 mg) surrounded by a nonmedicated Silastic polymer membrane, and permits constant release of estradiol at a rate of approximately 7.5 µg/day for 90 days, after which the ring is removed and replaced. Prior to the development of Estring, a number of different matrix (or "homogeneous") and reservoir (or "core")-type vaginal rings had been investigated for estrogen replacement therapy. However, reservoir-type rings, containing an estradiol-loaded core surrounded by a non-medicated polymer sheath, offered the advantage of providing constant low daily doses and stable plasma concentrations over extended time periods (5). Early clinical studies in postmenopausal women demonstrated a high maturation value in the vaginal mucosa, a very significant improvement in vaginal atrophy, and the restoration of vaginal pH to levels normally seen in fertile women (< 5.5) (6,7). Moreover, a strong preference for the ring over other forms of estrogen administration has commonly been reported, and no major side-effects or endometrial proliferation have been observed during treatment (6–9).

Estrogens are known to have a favorable effect on serum lipid profiles, lowering low density lipoprotein cholesterol (HDL) and elevating high density HDL. Given that the menopause is an estrogen deficient state, the possibility that estrogen replacement therapy may have a positive effect on abnormal lipid profiles exists, and ultimately on the incidence of coronary heart disease. Naessen et al. have reported that the ultra-low doses of estradiol administered during Estring use, primarily intended for local effect, may in fact, improve serum lipid profile in elderly women with a pattern and magnitude similar to that reported after conventional estrogen doses or first-generation lipid-lowering agents (10). In a subsequent study in 2002, Estring administration was shown not to significantly change endometrial thickness or uterine diameter in elderly women, indicating that there may be a "therapeutic window" for systemic effects of ultra-low doses of estradiol in elderly women without any apparent increase in endometrial thickness (8).

In addition to its ability to alleviate postmenopausal urogenital symptoms, Estring has also been shown useful in prolonging the time to next recurrence among postmenopausal women with recurrent urinary tract infection and to decrease the number of recurrences per year (11).

A review of the use of Estring for estrogen replacement therapy in postmenopausal women has also been published (12).

NUVARING®

Nuvaring is a non-biodegradable, flexible, transparent, colorless contraceptive vaginal ring (Fig. 1, Table 1), developed by Organon, Inc. and first marketed in 2002. It contains two active compounds, the progestin etonogestrel (11.7 mg), and the estrogen ethinyl estradiol (2.7 mg), located within a central polyethylene-co-vinyl acetate (28% w/w vinyl acetate) core as a supersaturated eutectic mixture (13), and surrounded by a non-medicated polyethylene-co-vinyl acetate (9% w/w vinyl acetate) sheath layer. The slow permeation of the steroid molecules through the low vinyl acetate content nonmedicated sheath provides for controlled release, resulting in mean daily release rates of 120 µg etonogestrel and 15 µg of ethinyl estradiol over a 3-week period of use. The ring is designed to be used continuously for 3 weeks, and then removed for 1 week, before being replaced with a new ring.

Numerous clinical studies have been reported describing various aspects of Nuvaring use, including a large number of clinical studies comparing Nuvaring with combined oral contraceptives (COC) (14–40). In summary, Nuvaring offers similar efficacy and tolerability to COC (14,22,24,25,37), better cycle control (15,19,22,25,38), and very high levels of compliance (14,16,24,37,38) and user acceptability/satisfaction (14,16, 32,38–40). The most frequently reported adverse events associated with Nuvaring use are headache, leukorrhea and vaginitis, as well as a number of ring-related local effects, such as discomfort during intercourse, foreign body sensation, and occasional ring expulsion. However, much fewer of the estrogen-related events common with COC, such as nausea and breast tenderness, are reported (14,16). Also, no clinically relevant changes in blood biochemistry, hematology, blood pressure, heart rate, body weight, physical examination, cervical cytology, or endometrial histology have been associated with long-term Nuvaring use (18,37). Extended use regimens to alter bleeding schedules have also been investigated (22). Co-usage of Nuvaring with tampons (33) and other orally or vaginally administered medicines (23,34,35) has been shown not to significantly influence etonogestrel and ethinyl estradiol serum levels.

The anatomical positioning of Nuvaring, which is not critical for its contraceptive efficacy, has been assessed using three-dimensional magnetic resonance imaging demonstrating that the ring resides adjacent to the cervix, and in most situations the entire cervix rests inside the ring (21). Furthermore, the otherwise circular form of the ring is compressed laterally in vivo to form a gentle oval shape. Scanning electron microscopy has been used to evaluate the surface of Nuvaring both before and after use in a volunteer with normal vaginal flora and has shown that no penetration of bacteria into the bulk of the ring or general surface modification takes place over a 28-day period of use (41).

FEMRING®

Femring (Fig. 1, Table 1) is a reservoir-type vaginal ring device (56.0 mm outer diameter, 7.6 mm cross-sectional diameter) developed by Warner Chilcott which provides controlled release of the estradiol prodrug 17β-estradiol-3-acetate (Fig. 2) for the treatment of vasomotor symptoms and vulvovaginal atrophy associated with the menopause. The ring comprises a centralized silicone elastomer core (2.0 mm cross-sectional diameter) in which the solid active agent is dispersed, which is encapsulated within a non-medicated silicone elastomer rate-controlling outer sheath. The length of the active core within the ring is varied to provide two Femring products having

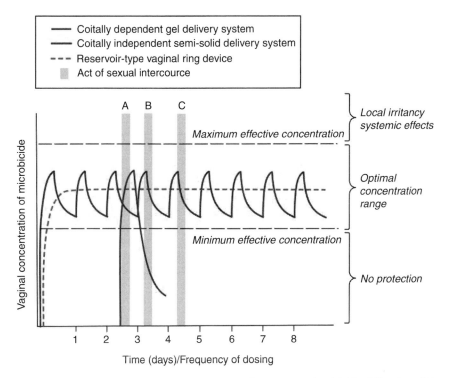

Figure 2 Projected vaginal concentrations of an HIV microbicide following: (**A**) vaginal administration of a coitally dependent gel delivery system prior to intercourse, (**B**) daily vaginal administration of a coitally independent semi-solid delivery system, and (**C**) single application of a reservoir-type vaginal ring device.

different daily release rates. Femring 0.05 mg/day has a central core that contains 12.4 mg of estradiol acetate, and releases at a rate equivalent to 0.05 mg of estradiol per day for 3 months; Femring 0.10 mg/day has a central core that contains 24.8 mg of estradiol acetate, and releases at a rate equivalent to 0.10 mg of estradiol per day for 3 months. After release from the rings, the estradiol acetate is rapidly hydrolyzed to estradiol, producing mean serum estradiol concentration of 40.6 and 76 pg/mL, respectively, corresponding to apparent in vivo estradiol delivery rates of 0.052 and 0.097 mg/day.

The initial concept behind Femring (i.e., a silicone elastomer vaginal ring providing systemic levels of estradiol suitable for estrogen replacement therapy [ERT]) was first described by Woolfson et al., who investigated the release characteristics of a range of estradiol prodrug derivatives from reservoir-type silicone rings (42). The best in vitro release rates under sink conditions, in combination with substantial aqueous solubilities as indicated by the release rates into saline, were observed for the acetate and propionate esters. A combination of drug release characteristics, short plasma half-life and a toxicologically acceptable hydrolysis product indicated that 17β-estradiol-3-acetate was the prodrug of choice for ring delivery of ERT. In vivo, an IVR device releasing 100 μg/day of estradiol as its 3-acetate ester maintained over 84 days a circulating plasma concentration in the region of 300 pmol/L, within the clinically desirable range for ERT. Subsequent large-scale trials in postmenopausal women have demonstrated a significant improvement in climacteric and vasomotor symptoms with Femring compared with placebo oral tablet or placebo ring (43–45) and significantly increased bone mineral density for Femring compared with Estring (46). Patient evaluations of Femring tolerability and acceptability were excellent, and comparable with those of oral estrogen therapy (43,44).

FUTURE APPLICATIONS FOR VAGINAL RINGS

In addition to their use in contraception and HRT, vaginal rings are also being developed for other clinical applications, including vaginal administration of HIV microbicides. These are chemical substances that, when formulated appropriately and applied to the vagina before intercourse with an infected partner, have the potential to either prevent or reduce HIV transmission via a range of different mechanisms. Although no effective microbicide products are currently available, there is a push to have a first-generation HIV microbicide on the market within the next 5 years. The vast majority of lead microbicide candidates currently being evaluated in human clinical are formulated as coitally dependent semi-solid vaginal gels, designed to be administered a short time prior to every act of intercourse. However, it is recognized that such gel formulations will require high levels of user compliance to be effective, and that optimal protection from infection might best be afforded by the of coitally independent microbicide formulations providing sustained or controlled release. The rationale for this approach is presented in Figure 2. A single application of a coitally-dependent microbicide gel formulation administered immediately prior to intercourse would provide protective vaginal microbicide concentrations for only a limited duration—protection would be afforded for sex act A, but not for acts B or C. A highly retentive, sustained release, coitally independent, semi-solid microbicide formulation administered once daily could provide protection against all three sex acts by maintaining the vaginal microbicide concentrations within the optimal concentration range. Alternatively, application of a single controlled release microbicide formulation such as a vaginal ring device, could theoretically provide continuous pre-programmed release of the microbicide over very long periods of time, such that microbicide levels were constantly maintained within the optimal concentration range.

Current vaginal ring designs are permeation-controlled delivery systems, requiring the active agent to first dissolve in and then diffuse through the polymeric matrix that constitutes the ring. Consequently, existing vaginal ring products have been limited exclusively to the release of small molecular weight hydrophobic actives, as exemplified by the steroid molecules of Estring, Nuvaring, and Femring. However, a number of potential HIV microbicides have been shown to be released from silicone elastomer vaginal rings at rates theoretically capable of providing long-term protection in vivo, including the surface-active agent nonoxynol-9 (47,48), and the non-nucleoside reverse transcriptase inhibitors TMC120 (49–51) and UC781 (51). A comprehensive discussion of the issues relating to the potential use of vaginal rings for the controlled release of HIV microbicides has been published recently (51). In particular, the high user acceptability of vaginal rings seen with commercial products, coupled with their ability to provide controlled and continuous release of vaginal HIV microbicides over long periods of time suggest that they may have a significant role to play in helping to reduce the rates of heterosexually transmitted HIV. Importantly, multi-active vaginal rings releasing more than one microbicidal agent could readily be developed to provide enhanced HIV protection via a combination of mechanisms or to meet the needs of women also requiring fertility control.

REFERENCES

1. Duncan GW. Medicated devices and methods. US Patent 3,545,439, 1970.
2. Mishell DR, Talas M, Parlow AF, Moyer DL. Contraception by means of a silastic vaginal ring impregnated with medroxyprogesterone acetate. Am J Obstet Gynecol 1970; 107:100–7.
3. Mishell DR, Lumkin ME. Contraceptive effect of varying doses of progestogen in Silastic vaginal rings. Fert Steril 1970; 21:99–103.
4. Dziuk PJ, Cook B. Passage of steroids through silicone rubber. Endocrinology 1966; 78:208–11.
5. Schmidt G, Andersson SB, Nordle O, Johansson CJ, Gunnarsson PO. Release of 17-beta-estradiol from a vaginal ring in postmenopausal women–pharmacokinetic evaluation. Gynecol Obstet Invest 1994; 38:253–60.
6. Henriksson L, Stjernquist M, Boquist L, Cedergren I, Selinus I. A one-year multicenter study of efficacy and safety of a continuous, low-dose, estradiol-releasing vaginal ring (Estring) in postmenopausal women with symptoms and signs of urogenital aging. Am J Obstet Gynecol 1996; 174:85–92.
7. Barentsen R, vandeWeijer PHM, Schram JHN. Continuous low dose estradiol released from a vaginal ring versus estriol vaginal cream for urogenital atrophy. Eur J Obstet Gynecol Reprod Biol 1997; 71:73–80.
8. Naessen T, Rodriguez-Macias K. Endometrial thickness and uterine diameter not affected by ultralow doses of 17 beta-estradiol in elderly women. Am J Obstet Gynecol 2002; 186:944–7.

9.   Weisberg E, Ayton R, Darling G, et al. Endometrial and vaginal effects of low-dose estradiol delivered by vaginal ring or vaginal tablet. Climacteric 2005; 8(1): 83–92.

10. Naessen T, Rodriguez-Macias K, Lithell H. Serum lipid profile improved by ultra-low doses of 17 beta-estradiol in elderly women. J Clin Endocrin Metab 2001; 86:2757–62.

11. Eriksen BC. A randomized, open, parallel-group study on the preventive effect of an estradiol-releasing vaginal ring (Estring) on recurrent urinary tract infections in postmenopausal women. Am J Obstet Gynecol 1999; 180: 1072–9.

12. Sarkar NN. Low-dose intravaginal estradiol delivery using a silastic vaginal ring for estrogen replacement therapy in postmenopausal women: a review. Eur J Contracept Reprod Health Care 2003; 8:217–24.

13. van Laarhoven JAH, Vromans H. Influence of supersaturation on the release properties of a controlled release device based on EVA copolymers. J Cont Rel 2003; 87:210–3.

14. Ahrendt HJ, Nisand I, Bastianelli C, et al. Efficacy, acceptability and tolerability of the combined contraceptive ring, NuvaRing, compared with an oral contraceptive containing 30 mug of ethinyl estradiol and 3 mg of drospirenone. Contraception 2006; 74:451–7.

15. Milsom I, Lete I, Bjertnaes A, et al. Effects on cycle control and bodyweight of the combined contraceptive ring, NuvaRing, versus an oral contraceptive containing 30 mug ethinyl estradiol and 3 mg drospirenone. Human Reprod 2006; 21:2304–11.

16. Roumen FJME, ten Berg MMTO, Hoomans EHM. The combined contraceptive vaginal ring (NuvaRing (R): First experience in daily clinical practice in The Netherlands. Eur J Contracept Reprod Health Care 2006; 11:14–22.

17. Roumen FJME, Dieben TOM. Comparison of uterine concentrations of ethinyl estradiol and etonogestrel after use of a contraceptive vaginal ring and an oral contraceptive. Fertil Steril 2006; 85:57–62.

18. Bulten J, Grefte J, Siebers B, Dieben T. The combined contraceptive vaginal ring (NuvaRing) and endometrial histology. Contraception 2005; 72(5): 362–5.

19. Sarkar NN. The combined contraceptive vaginal device (NuvaRing (R): A comprehensive review. Eur J Contracept Reprod Health Care 2005; 10:73–8.

20. van den Heuvel MW, van Bragt AJM, Alnabawy AKM, Kaptein MCJ. Comparison of ethinylestradiol pharmacokinetics in three hormonal contraceptive formulations: the vaginal ring, the transdermal patch and an oral contraceptive. Contraception 2005; 72:168–74.

21. Barnhart KT, Timbers K, Pretorius ES, Lin K, Shaunik A. In vivo assessment of NuvaRing (R) placement. Contraception 2005; 72:196–9.

22. Miller L, Verhoeven CHJ, in't Hout J. Extended regimens of the contraceptive vaginal ring—A randomized trial. Obstet Gynecol 2005; 106(3):473–82.

23. Dogterom P, van den Heuvel MW, Thomsen T. Absence of pharmacokinetic interactions of the combined contraceptive vaginal ring NuvaRing (R) with oral amoxicillin or doxycycline in two randomised trials. Clin Pharmacokin 2005; 44:429–38.

24. Oddsson K, Leifels-Fischer B, de Melo NR, et al. Efficacy and safety of a contraceptive vaginal ring (NuvaRing) compared with a combined oral contraceptive: a 1-year randomized trial. Contraception 2005; 71:176–82.

25. Oddsson K, Leifels-Fischer B, Wiel-Masson D, et al. Superior cycle control with a contraceptive vaginal ring compared with an oral contraceptive containing 30 mu g ethinylestradiol and 150 mug levonorgestrel: a randomized trial. Human Reprod 2005; 20:557–62.

26. Duijkers I, Killick S, Bigrigg A, Dieben TOM. A comparative study on the effects of a contraceptive vaginal ring NuvaRing(R) and an oral contraceptive on carbohydrate metabolism and adrenal and thyroid function. Eur J Contracept Reprod Health Care 2004; 9:131–40.

27. Duijkers IJM, Klipping C, Verhoeven CHJ, Dieben TOM. Ovarian function with the contraceptive vaginal ring or an oral contraceptive: a randomized study. Human Reprod 2004; 19:2668–73.

28. Duijkers IJM, Verhoeven CHJ, Dieben TOM, Klipping C. Follicular growth during contraceptive pill or vaginal ring treatment depends on the day of ovulation in the pretreatment cycle. Human Reprod 2004; 19:2674–79.

29. Baker E. Incidence of vaginitis with the etonogestrel/ethinyl estradiol vaginal ring. J Reprod Med 2004; 49:699–9.

30. Magnusdottir EM, Bjarnadottir RI, Onundarson PT, et al. The contraceptive vaginal ring (NuvaRing®) and hemostasis: a comparative study. Contraception 2004; 69:461–7.

31. Tuppurainen M, Klimscheffskij R, Venhola M, Dieben TOM. The combined contraceptive vaginal ring (NuvaRing®) and lipid metabolism: a comparative study. Contraception 2004; 69:389–94.

32. Novak A, de la Loge C, Abetz, L. Development and validation of an acceptability and satisfaction questionnaire for a contraceptive vaginal ring, NuvaRing®. Pharmacoeconomics 2004; 22:245–56.

33. Verhoeven CHJ, Dieben TOM. The combined contraceptive vaginal ring, NuvaRing®, and tampon co-usage. Contraception 2004; 69:197–9.

34. Verhoeven CHJ, van den Heuvel MW, Mulders TMT, Dieben TOM. The contraceptive vaginal ring, NuvaRing®, and antimycotic co-medication. Contraception 2004; 69:129–32.

35. Haring T, Mulders TMT. The combined contraceptive ring NuvaRing® and spermicide co-medication. Contraception 2003; 67:271–2.

36. Killick S. Complete and robust ovulation inhibition with NuvaRing. Eur J Contracept Reprod Health Care 2002; 7(Suppl. 2):13–8.

37. Roumen F. Contraceptive efficacy and tolerability with a novel combined contraceptive vaginal ring, NuvaRing. Eur J Contracept Reprod Health Care 2002; 7(Suppl. 2):19–9.

38. Vree M. Lower hormone dosage with improved cycle control. Eur J Contracept Reprod Health Care 2002; 7(Suppl. 2):25–5.

39. Szarewski A. High acceptability and satisfaction with NuvaRing use. Eur J Contracept Reprod Health Care 2002; 7(Suppl. 2):31–1.

40. Novak A, de la Loge C, Abetz L, van der Meulen EA. The combined contraceptive vaginal ring, NuvaRing®: an international study of user acceptability. Contraception 2003; 67:187–94.

41. Miller L, MacFarlane SA, Materi HL. A scanning electron microscopic study of the contraceptive vaginal ring. Contraception 2005; 71:65–7.
42. Woolfson AD, Elliott GR, Gilligan CA, Passmore CM. Design of an intravaginal ring for the controlled delivery of 17 beta-estradiol as its 3-acetate ester. J Cont Rel 1999; 61:319–28.
43. Buckler H, Al-Azzawi F. UK VR Multicentre Trial Grp. The effect of a novel vaginal ring delivering oestradiol acetate on climacteric symptoms in postmenopausal women. Brit J Obstet Gynecol 2003; 110:753–9.
44. Al-Azzawi F, Buckler HM. United Kingdom Vaginal Ring Invest. Comparison of a novel vaginal ring delivering estradiol acetate versus oral estradiol for relief of vasomotor menopausal symptoms. Climacteric 2003; 6:118–27.
45. Speroff L. Efficacy and tolerability of a novel estradiol vaginal ring for relief of menopausal symptoms, Obstet Gynecol 2003; 102:823–34.
46. Al-Azzawi F, Lees B, Thompson J, Stevenson JC. Bone mineral density in postmenopausal women treated with a vaginal ring delivering systemic doses of estradiol acetate. Menopause 2005; 12:331–9.
47. Malcolm K, Woolfson D, Russell J, Andrews C. In vitro release of nonoxynol-9 from silicone matrix intravaginal rings. J Cont Rel 2003; 91:355–64.
48. Malcolm K, Woolfson D. Blocking the heterosexual transmission of HIV: Intravaginal Rings for the controlled delivery of topical microbicides. Drug Del Syst Sci 2001; 1:117–21.
49. Malcolm RK, Woolfson AD, Toner CF, Morrow RJ, McCullagh SD. Long-term, controlled release of the HIV microbicide TMC120 from silicone elastomer vaginal rings. J Antimicrob Chemother 2005; 56:954–6.
50. Woolfson AD, Malcolm RK, Morrow RJ, Toner C. Intravaginal ring delivery of the reverse transcriptase inhibitor TMC 120 as an HIV microbicide. Int J Pharm 2006; 325:82–9.
51. Woolfson AD, Malcolm RK, Morrow RJ, Toner CF, McCullagh SD. Potential use of vaginal rings for prevention of heterosexual transmission of HIV: a controlled-release strategy for HIV microbicides. Am J Drug Delivery 2006; 4: 7–20.

37

Phospholipids as Carriers for Vaginal Drug Delivery

Mathew Leigh

PHARES Drug Delivery AG, Muttenz, Switzerland

INTRODUCTION

Vaginal drug delivery systems are traditionally used to deliver contraceptives and to treat vaginal infections or inflammatory conditions. Recent advances have also advocated this route for systemic applications, notably for administration of peptides, proteins, vaccines, and antimicrobial agents. Physicochemical properties of drugs such as molecular weight, lipophilicity, ionization, molecular size, chemical nature, and local action can all influence drug absorption and permeability (1). Drugs should ideally be in molecular dispersion prior to absorption and should be able to penetrate the cervical mucus. In addition, the formulation should be sufficiently bioadhesive to prevent removal of the dosage form by gravity and vaginal secretions. Vaginal epithelium has displayed variable permeability to drugs of different physicochemical properties, with small lipophilic drugs tending to be more readily absorbed than hydrophilic macromolecules.

Optimized vaginal delivery systems should provide the opportunity for controlled and prolonged release of drugs. Mucocutaneous drug delivery systems can be designed to maximize the efficacy of the active and minimize the cost. While a number of systems have been developed (e.g., containing permeability/stability enhancing and bioadhesive agents), phospholipids offer considerable benefits as vectors for vaginal drug delivery.

PHOSPHOLIPIDS

Phospholipids are a functionally versatile class of compounds, ubiquitously distributed in human, animal, plant, and microorganism cells. They are important elements in the structure of biological membranes acting essentially as the "solvent matrix." They have found widespread use within cosmetic, agro-food, and pharmaceutical applications. Phospholipids are traditionally used as emulsifiers in many pharmaceutical products and are key components in liposome formulations, which are generally associated with high cost, niche applications.

The term phospholipid refers to a lipid containing phosphoric acid as a mono- or diester. Two types of phospholipids exist, glycerophospholipids (phosphodiglycerides) or sphingophospholipids, together with their corresponding hydrolysis products. The glycerophospholipids are the most abundant and possess a hydrophilic head group containing phosphorus and one other chemical subgroup (e.g., choline, ethanolamine, inositol, serine). The head is attached to a to a glycerol backbone, which in turn is linked to the hydrophobic fatty acids.

Phospholipids are extremely well tolerated from a physiological stance. Their highly favorable toxicity profile has prompted widespread inclusion in many formulations. They are natural substances which occur in foods and are accepted as toxicologically safe. For oral use, lecithin (primarily a mixture of phospholipids) is GRAS listed ("generally recognized as safe") by the U.S. Food and Drug Administration (FDA) and is included in many drug monographs. Lecithin is also listed in the FDA Inactive Ingredients Guide (inhalations, IM and IV injections, oral capsules, suspensions, and tablets, rectal, topical, and vaginal preparations). Phospholipids are included in non-parenteral and parenteral medicines licensed in the European Union.

LIPOSOMES

Liposomes are vesicular structures widely utilized in topical delivery systems and are versatile vectors for drug delivery. While research is fairly limited, liposomes have been used in vaginal therapy with promising results (2–7). Liposomes have the potential to associate amphipathic or lipophilic drugs and can be modified to impart controlled release properties. However, pre-formed liposomes are not ideal delivery vectors and have a number of attendant problems. The major drawbacks are limited drug loading and poor storage stability. It is difficult to attain effective drug loading within the liposomes and drug molecules often leak from the structures. Energy intensive manufacturing techniques such as extrusion, high pressure homogenization, and solvent evaporation methods are also time-consuming and expensive. Not surprisingly, this tends to promote development of high cost niche products.

PRO-LIPOSOMES

The pro-liposome approach was developed as a straightforward, reproducible, and reliable manufacturing technique for large-scale production of liposome dispersions (8,9). Today, it is one of the most cost effective and widely used methods for producing commercial liposome products. This technology is based upon the intrinsic property of hydrated membrane lipids to form vesicles on contact with water. A typical formulation consists of suitable fractions of phospholipids with an active, which may be lipophilic or amphipathic. The formulation does not, however, contain sufficient water to allow liposome formation under stored conditions. Liposomes are only formed when the formulation comes into contact with a moist aqueous environment such as found in the body's skin or mucosal surfaces. It is designed particularly for the molecular dispersion and delivery of water-insoluble materials, where association efficiencies approaching 100% can be achieved. Pro-liposomes have been employed as a basis for a number of site specific drug delivery approaches.

SUPRAVAIL® MUCOCUTANEOUS DELIVERY

Background

SupraVail® is the name given to the platform technology for delivering poorly water soluble drugs as molecular associates to maximize bioavailability. These associates are formed from lipid complexes that may be liquids, semi-solids, or solids. The complexes can be incorporated into various dosage forms for different routes of administration. SupraVail dosage forms have the intrinsic capacity to form lipid aggregates where the drug is in molecular association. Depending upon the type of phospholipids selected, these structures may be vesicles, micelles, or mixed micelles. The particular SupraVail technology for topical and mucosal applications is a semi-solid pro-liposome gel. These formulations utilize fractionated phospholipids to form vesicular structures in vivo, triggered by the aqueous environment found on mucosal surfaces. These have a high potential to associate with both lipophilic and hydrophilic compounds. The type of phospholipid fraction used for mucocutaneous application will depend on the physicochemical properties of the drug and also on the required characteristics for the formulation. The key to SupraVail delivery is, first, to disperse the drug in a monomolecular state within phospholipid bilayers. Second, in the presence of excess water the bilayers readily convert into discrete vesicular structures. The important feature in this process is that the drug should remain associated with the vesicles even after conversion. While the phospholipid and drug form the basis of the formulation, a number of excipients can be readily incorporated to optimize the product characteristics.

SupraVail® Vaginal Gels

A gel presentation is particularly suitable for vaginal administration. It is non-greasy, esthetically appealing and offers the potential for improved drug retention. In SupraVail gels, the phospholipid adopts a liquid crystalline matrix and forms a bilayered translucent gel. Lipophilic drugs readily associate with the phospholipid molecules. The SupraVail gel is particularly suitable for incorporation of lipophilic drugs and thus act as excellent carriers for anti-fungal and steroid compounds. On contact with the mucosal surface, the bi-layered gel formulation converts readily in vivo to vesicular structures.

A typical SupraVail formulation will consist of three essential components: phospholipids, hydrophilic media, and active compound. Other excipients, such as polymers to improve bioadhesion and stabilizers, e.g., buffers and antioxidants, may also be added if necessary.

Figure 1 shows a freeze fracture of a bilayered gel and Figure 2 shows a freeze fracture of a liposome dispersion formed from a pro-liposome gel after contact with water.

Selection of Drugs to Treat Local Vaginal Infections

Vaginal delivery systems are frequently required to treat local fungal infections, particularly candidiasis. The low aqueous solubility of antifungal

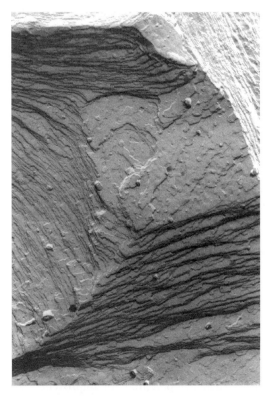

Figure 1   Freeze fracture of a bilayered gel.

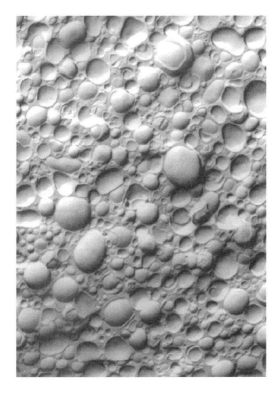

Figure 2 Freeze fracture of a liposome dispersion formed from a pro-liposome gel after contact with water.

drugs such as amphotericin, miconazole, clotrimazole, and nystatin make them ideal compounds for delivery using the SupraVail approach.

Candidiasis

The term *candidiasis* is the most common fungal infection affecting humans, and was originally ascribed to infections due to a single yeast species, *Candida albicans*. It has now been expanded to encompass a range of yeast species of the genus *Candida*. While systemic candidiasis occur, the most common candidiasis infections are superficial lesions especially of the mucous surfaces of the vagina or mouth.

Therapy for Vaginal Fungal Infections

Vaginal candidiasis is primarily treated with antifungal cream or pessaries inserted high into the vagina (including during menstruation). Vulvitis and superficial sites of infection can be readily treated with appropriate creams. The drugs of choice include the imidazole drugs (clotrimazole, eco-nazole, fenticonazole, isoconazole, and miconazole) and nystatin. The poor aqueous solubility of the antifungal agents in these conventional formulations means that they are not in a molecular state and consequently have reduced drug concentration at the active sites.

DEVELOPMENT OF A SUPRAVAIL AMPHOTERICIN B GEL

Development

A SupraVail gel can be employed in topical drug delivery for treating mucosal fungal infections. While preliminary studies have centred on amphotericin B, it also presents as an ideal formulation strategy for antifungal agents such as miconazole, clotrimazole, and nystatin. It consists of selected fractions of phospholipid dispersed in an anhydrous hydrophilic medium, wherein the drug is partitioned between the hydrophobic membrane lipid bilayer formed in the gel and the hydrophilic solvent phase. It confers many unique features for drug delivery to mucosal surfaces, notably:

- It is a highly efficient lipophilic carrier, utilizing natural lipid to molecularly disperse the drug. Phospholipids have natural affinity for biological membranes and are generally nontoxic and nonirritant.
- The drug is in molecular dispersion in the bilayers offering improved drug activity.
- The vehicle is nontoxic and contains pharmaceutically acceptable excipients.
- Difficulties associated with liposomal preparations, e.g., stability and loading, are circumvented because the pro-liposomes only convert to vesicular structures (liposomes) in vivo, i.e., on the mucosa.
- The product has a low initial microbiological burden and does not encourage microbial growth (preservative free).
- SupraVail formulations can be produced economically and reliably on a large scale.
- The product is economically viable (i.e., in similar price range as current topical antifungal therapies).

Formulation Issues and Product Stability

Key factors in obtaining a satisfactory pro-liposome amphotericin B gel suitable for direct application to the vaginal mucosa should take into consideration the following factors:

- stability and packaging
- drug concentration
- manufacturing method
- excipients
- antifungal activity
- release profile

Stability and Packaging

The stability of the drug and phospholipid components can be maximized through the selection of an appropriate hydrophilic base. Accelerated and real-time stability studies were undertaken in a variety of tube and pump packs. Both accelerated and real-time stability data predicted a shelf life of 24 months at 25°C/60% relative humidity.

Drug Concentration

The amphotericin B concentration was 1% w/w. More than 95% of the drug resides in the lipid bilayers, effectively protecting the drug from degradation during storage, compared to the unprotected form.

Manufacturing Method

The pilot manufacturing method for producing 5 kg of the gels utilized a conventional high-shear mixer. The process may be readily scaled up for larger production batches.

Excipients

A number of studies were performed to assess the effects of modifying the standard pro-liposome gel. These included addition of antibacterial agents, antioxidants, chelating agents, and complexing agents. None of these agents (at the concentrations used) were found to alter the degradation or encapsulation profiles for the drug in the pro-liposome gel. The gel passes the relevant European Pharmacopoeia microbial challenge test and was deemed to have sufficient antimicrobial activity without need for preservatives.

Antifungal Activity

The pro-liposomal amphotericin B gels demonstrated a superior antifungal activity than equivalent concentrations of drug in aqueous suspension. These findings were substantiated by growth inhibition both in solid media (cup-plate diffusion assay) and in liquid media. A comparison of the activity of amphotericin B in a SupraVail formulation against a commercially marketed product is shown in Figure 3. The data shows that higher antifungal properties were obtained with the phospholipid preparation.

Release Profile

The release of the drug can be controlled by altering the composition of the formulations. The release of three amphotericin B gels was determined at 37°C. It can be seen from Figure 4 that the amphotericin B can either be released immediately or more gradually, where about 40% diffuses out after 2 hours.

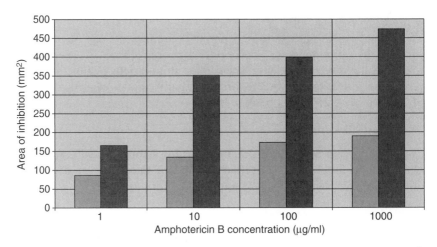

Figure 3 Comparison of antifungal activity of amphotericin B in SupraVail®
against commercially marketed suspension.

DEVELOPMENT OF ALTERNATIVE ANTI-FUNGAL DRUGS IN A SUPRAVAIL® GEL

While amphotericin B was selected as a test model drug, development pro-
grammes have also been instigated for a number of other drugs, namely clotrimazole, miconazole, and nystatin. In addition to the excellent association
(Table 1) and stability profiles (6 months accelerated stability data), these
prototype formulations also have supporting microbiological efficacy data.

REGULATORY ISSUES

While the SupraVail gel must comply with the normal demands for a standard mucocutaneous gel preparation, no specific regulatory issues arise. The
phospholipids used for the SupraVail gels are of exceptionally high specification and exceed the general pharmacopoeial requirements for lecithin.
drug master files are also available for selected fractions. While it may be
necessary to perform a tolerability study for the final product (active in association with all excipients), it is believed that there would be no requirement
to undertake extensive toxicological profiling of the individual formulation
components.

COMPETITIVE ADVANTAGE

The formulation components are readily available in bulk quantities at
competitive prices and would readily lend themselves to mass marketing of
competitively priced products. In addition, the manufacturing process

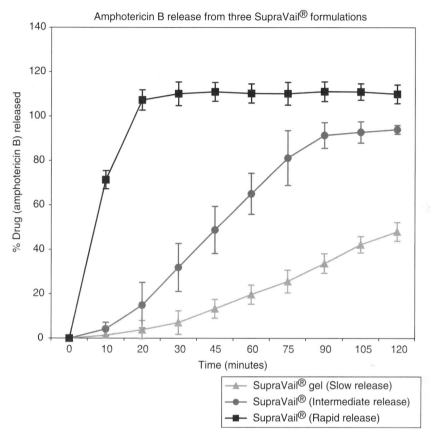

Figure 4 Release profile of amphotercin B from three SupraVail® gel formulations.

involves standard mixing equipment and facilitates production of large scale batches economically and reliably.

There is a potential to reduce drug dosage in these formulations. Enhanced bioavailability and drug activity have been demonstrated by presenting the drug to membranes in molecular dispersion. These formulations are also nontoxic and nonirritant and do not require the inclusion

Table 1 Association of Drug after Conversion

Formulation	Percentage association after conversion
1% Amphotericin B	99.2
1% Miconazole	97.7
1% Clotrimazole	97.3

of preservatives. The gel formulations can be packaged in a number of presentations (e.g., pumps, tubes, jars).

The SupraVail gel is highly versatile and is suitable for inclusion of a number of drug compounds. While initial research has focused on the hydrophobic antifungal agents, it could be readily adapted for delivery of other actives (e.g., steroids, peptides, vaccines, and antimicrobial agents).

FUTURE DIRECTIONS

There is considerable promise for development and expansion of the innovative SupraVail platform technology, particularly for poorly soluble compounds. The dual-vector nature of phospholipids facilitates incorporation of both hydrophobic and hydrophilic drugs. Gels, foams, and creams can be developed and individually tailored for specific actives. The phospholipid(s) can be carefully selected and blended with actives/excipients to confer superior stability, efficacy and patient acceptability profiles.

REFERENCES

1. Richardson JL, Illum L. Routes of delivery–Case studies. The vaginal route of peptide and protein drug delivery. Adv Drug Deliv Rev 1992; 8:341–66.
2. Kobrinskii GD, Mel'nikov VR, Kulakov VN, L'vov ND, Bolotin IM, Barinskii IF. Treatment of experimental genital herpes, with liposomal interferon. Biomed Sci 1991; 2:29–32.
3. Jain SK, Singh R, Jain VV. Mucoadhesive liposomes bearing metronidazole for controlled and localised vaginal delivery. Proc Int Symp Control Release Mater 1996; 23:701–2.
4. Jain SK, Singh R, Sahu B. Development of a liposome based contraceptive system for intravaginal administration of progesterone. Drug Dev Ind Pharm 1997; 23:827–30.
5. Foldvari M, Moreland A. Clinical observations with topical liposome-encapsulated interferon alpha for the treatment of genital papilloma virus infections. J Liposome Res 1997; 7:115–26.
6. Pavelic Z, Skalko-Basnet N, Jalsenjak I. Liposomes containing drugs for treatment of vaginal infections. Eur J Pharm Sci 1999; 8:345–51.
7. Pavelic Z, Skalko-Basnet N, Jalsenjak I. Liposomal gel with chlorampenicol: Characterisation and *in vitro* release. Acta Pharm 2004; 54:319–30.
8. Williams P. Liposomes and the pro-liposome method. SOEFW J 1992; 6:377–8.
9. Perrett S, Golding M, Williams P. A simple method for the preparation of liposomes for pharmaceutical applications: Characterization of the liposomes. J Pharm Pharmacol 1991; 43:154–61.

38

SITE RELEASE®, Vaginal Bioadhesive System

Jennifer Gudeman, Daniel J. Thompson, and R. Saul Levinson
KV Pharmaceutical Company, St. Louis, Missouri, U.S.A.

INTRODUCTION

In women's health care, the utilization of intravaginal creams for both bacterial and fungal infections, as well as other unique localized female health conditions, is commonplace. In fact, it is estimated that the treatment of vaginitis accounts for more than 10 million physician office visits per year, and represents the most common reason for patient visits to an OB-GYN physician (1). However, vaginal cream products have historically been fraught with the following inherent problems: product leakage and irritation, multiple days dosing, supine application, and soon. All these factors contribute to poor compliance, and potentially disrupt achievement of therapeutic efficacy. Although improvements in vaginal cream dosing regimens have occurred, i.e., from 7-day dosing regimens to 3-day dosing creams, the method to achieve this is frequently an increase in the concentration of drug delivered per application (2). As many side effects of medications are dose related, this "improvement" represents additional challenges to successful therapy. Additionally, traditional vaginal administration of medication is often messy, and typically requires nighttime dosing to decrease the accompanying product leakage.

While there are disadvantages to traditional vaginal drug therapy, there are also significant advantages with this route of administration as compared to oral treatment, such as decreased systemic exposure of medication, direct application at the site of infection, and the likelihood of a faster onset of action (3). Thus, the ideal vaginal delivery system should target the positive attributes of traditional vaginal delivery while mitigating

521

the recognized shortcomings of vaginal drug delivery (4). SITE RELEASE®
was designed with these goals in mind.

Improvements in pharmaceutical dosage forms and drug delivery
systems that result in less frequent and more tolerable dosing regimens are
well received by both the patient and the physician alike. Increasing patient
convenience through product design enhancement can lead to improved
drug regimen compliance resulting in a high degree of therapeutic efficacy.
By focusing on the needs of the patient and the clinician, and addressing the
negatives of conventional vaginal creams and ointments, the unique bioadhesive drug delivery system SITE RELEASE was developed.

DESCRIPTION OF TECHNOLOGY

SITE RELEASE is a unique vaginal delivery system that is composed of a
high internal phase ratio, water-in-oil emulsion. A typical high internal phase
emulsion is composed of 70–90% internal phase by volume. Previously, these
high internal phase emulsions were thought to be inherently unstable (5).
The internal phase of the emulsion acts as the carrier of an active drug. The
drug-laden internal dispersed phase globules serve a dual purpose for both
the sequestering and the controlled release of the active agent (Fig. 1). The
high internal phase ratio emulsion containing dispersed phase globules

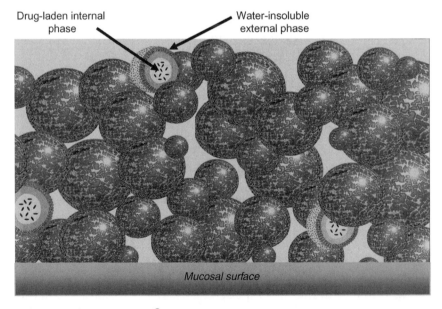

Figure 1   SITE RELEASE® system is a biphasic system containing a drug-laden
internal phase and a water-insoluble external phase. The system is bioadhesive to
mucosal surfaces.

develops a high affinity for surfaces, especially mucosal tissues. After introduction of the drug containing emulsion to mucosal tissue, a thin bioadhesive film of contiguous drug-laden internal phase globules forms on the mucosal surface. This tenacious, bioadhesive film acts as a drug delivery platform providing for a controlled release of the active drug.

Importantly, the process of bioadhesion is not affected by the presence of moisture; the drug delivery film actually forms on wet tissue. Furthermore, the drug delivery platform forms a single dose, remains intact and functional for more than 4 days; conversely, conventional non-bioadhesive creams and ointments remain only for a few hours after a single application (6,7). By incorporating bioadhesion and the controlled release of an active drug, SITE RELEASE can meter the release of active drug over several days, with a single dose application.

Currently, SITE RELEASE has been applied commercially in two vaginal medications: Gynazole-1® (2% butoconazole nitrate), indicated to treat vulvovaginal candidiasis (VVC) and Clindesse® (2% clindamycin phosphate), indicated to treat bacterial vaginosis (BV). The SITE RELEASE formulation is composed of generally recognized as safe materials and includes as major components an aqueous phase, a hydrophobic or oily phase, and appropriate emulsifiers, preservatives, and other excipients. For the patient, each product has several distinct advantages attributed to the SITE RELEASE delivery system:

- minimization of product leakage that often occurs with conventional vaginal creams and ointments (5),
- the desirable approved option of administering the medication day or night,
- a single application of an anti-infective medication that achieves therapeutic equivalency to multi-day conventional creams (8),
- continuous exposure to active drug resulting in a more rapid relief of irritating symptoms (7),
- low dose of active pharmaceutical ingredient.

PHARMACOLOGICAL CONSIDERATIONS

A basic tenet of pharmacology is that an increased dose often yields increased adverse effects. In the case of topical vaginal preparations, such as the creams and ointments used to treat VVC, an increase in the amount of drug exposed to the living tissues can be expected to cause a greater incidence of adverse effects, such as irritation, burning, and discomfort. In contrast, a single dose of Gynazole-1 and Clindesse accomplishes a therapeutic response equivalent to the response seen with multiple dose products because of the bioadhesive and controlled release properties of SITE RELEASE. Furthermore, a dramatic "dose sparing" effect, because of the controlled release of the active agent, is realized: Gynazole-1 contains only 100 mg of active drug, 2% butoconazole nitrate (a total of 5 g of cream); likewise, Clindesse employs the same 2% concentration of clindamycin phosphate (100 mg per 5 g of cream). Comparing this to the amount of drug delivered over 3 days with the conventional butoconazole nitrate product, a total of 15 g of formulated product is introduced intravaginally to deliver a total of 300 mg of butoconazole nitrate. Similarly, a traditional clindamycin-based vaginal medication (Cleocin-7®) delivers 700 mg of medication during the treatment period (9).

CLINICAL EVALUATION AND REGULATORY STATUS

In vitro analysis of the controlled-release formulation of butoconazole nitrate revealed a slow and steady sustained release of the active ingredient throughout a 7-day period while shaken in a pH 4.3 acetate buffer designed to simulate vaginal fluid, as shown in Figure 2 (6). In contrast, a conventional vaginal cream containing the same active ingredient, butoconazole nitrate, rapidly disintegrated and began to release its active drug immediately. This conventional vaginal cream released 100% of its active drug (butoconazole nitrate) within the first several hours (Fig. 2). The data illustrate the dramatic disparity in the delivery of active drug dependent on the emulsion system used.

The bioadhesive properties of SITE RELEASE have been clinically demonstrated in two separate studies. Weinstein et al. studied the vaginal retention time of both Gynazole-1, using the SITE RELEASE system and of a standard vaginal cream containing butoconazole nitrate 2%. Sixteen healthy females were treated intravaginally with either the standard

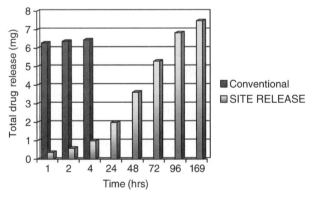

Figure 2   Release of butoconazole nitrate from the Gynazole-1® SITE RELEASE® formulation vs. a standard cream formulation containing the same active ingredient.

cream or the controlled-release Gynazole-1 and monitored daily over 7 days. The amount of cream excreted and captured in feminine minipads was monitored for 7 days. Analysis of the data demonstrated a median vaginal retention time of approximately 2.5 days for the standard cream. The median vaginal retention time of Gynazole-1 treated patients was 4.2 days ($P = 0.0024$) (6). These data demonstrate that Gynazole-1 remained intact in the vagina 63% longer than a standard formulation with the same active ingredient, butoconazole nitrate. The bioadhesive properties of the SITE RELEASE system enable Gynazole-1 to deliver a therapeutic effect over several days with a single application.

In another study, 44 healthy volunteers were enrolled in a parallel double-blind design to determine the vaginal retention time of a formulated antifungal in the SITE RELEASE emulsion against a comparable antifungal in a standard commercial formulation. Women were given a single application of one of the two formulations. Subjects were provided sanitary pads during the course of the 48-hour multi-point analysis. The returned sanitary pads were assayed using HPLC methodology for detectable drug content. The SITE RELEASE formulation containing active drug yielded approximately 50% of the product leakage found with the standard cream formulation (Fig. 3) (4). Hence, the inherent design of the SITE RELEASE system to be bioadherent to mucosal surfaces, leads to a significant reduction in product leakage from the vaginal cavity. The minimization of product leakage from the vagina can contribute to improved patient compliance and successful therapeutic efficacy.

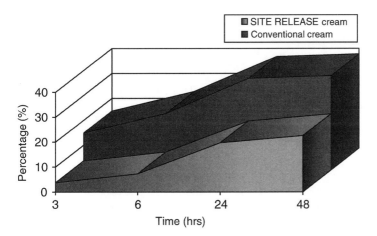

Figure 3 Percentage of accumulated cream in sanitary napkins following vaginal application of equivalent doses captured at different controlled times (3, 6, 24, and 48 hours). $N = 28$ healthy volunteers. At all times, the differences are statistically significant ($P < 0.05$).

From a therapeutic standpoint, the bioadhesive properties of Gynazole-1 in the SITE RELEASE system enable one-time product dosing. Brown et al. confirmed the efficacy of both Gynazole-1 and miconazole 7 when studied in 205 infected patients (8). All 205 patients were confirmed by both clinical and KOH smear to have vulvovaginal candidiasis. The clinical cure rates at 7–10 days post-therapy initiation were comparable between Gynazole-1 and miconazole 7 at 92% and 96%, respectively (Table 1). No statistical difference in the clinical cure rates between the two therapies was observed. Similarly, 30 days after treatment completion, clinical cure rates were 88% and 86% for Gynazole-1 and miconazole 7, respectively (Table 1). The microbiologic cure rates were also comparable between therapies at both the initial follow-up and 30-day follow-up visits. The data demonstrate that therapeutic equivalency can be achieved with the SITE RELEASE emulsion when compared to a standard cream dosed over 7 days. Similarly, a randomized controlled trial of 253 women with BV demonstrated that a single dose of Clindesse was comparable in efficacy to 7 daily doses of vaginal clindamycin 2% cream (10). According to the standard Amsel criteria (a compilation of four signs and symptoms including vaginal odor, discharge, pH, and presence of clue cells), single dose of Clindesse provided an equivalent clinical cure to that of 7 daily doses of traditional vaginal clindamycin 2% cream.

From this same study, the resolution of each of the primary individual symptoms of BV can also be examined: "whiff test" for vaginal odor, percentage clue cells, discharge, and vaginal pH (Fig. 3). Again, all data gathered demonstrated that a single dose of clindamycin, given via the SITE RELEASE delivery system as Clindesse, resulted in equivalent efficacy as 7 doses of vaginal clindamycin 2% cream.

Table 1 Efficacy of Gynazole-1[®], Single-Day Treatment versus Miconazole, 7-day Treatment

	Treatment groups		
Cure rate (%)	Gynazole-1[®]	Miconazole 7	*P**
First clinical follow-up: no. of patients treated/cured	101/93(92)	104/100(96)	0.24
Second clinical follow-up: no. of patients treated/cured	84/74(88)	93/80(86)	0.92
First microbiologic follow-up: no. of patients treated/cured	98/85(87)	101/93(92)	0.75
Second microbiologic follow-up: no. of patients treated/cured	77/57(74)	87/67(77)	0.24

Beyond greatly enhanced convenience, patients will likely have increased compliance with a therapeutic regimen that requires fewer doses (11). In the aforementioned study, women enrolled in the Clindesse study arm were found to be 95.4% compliant with the whole single-dose treatment duration (10). Conversely, women randomized to the 7-day treatment of clindamycin had a decrease in compliance correlated to increasing doses of therapy. By day 3 of therapy, compliance with 7-day clindamycin was 89.1%, a statistically significant decrease in compliance compared to the 95.4% found with 1-dose of Clindesse. Compliance with clindamycin-7 continued to decrease, and was determined to be 65.3% on day 7 of therapy. Furthermore, the data were obtained via a clinical study, under circumstances where compliance is expected to be higher than "real-life" use when patients may abandon therapy after a few days worth of treatment.

The SITE RELEASE system enables a drug-containing emulsion to remain adhered topically for a prolonged duration. Increased duration of topical adherence means a longer, continuous exposure to the therapeutic activity of the active drug contained within the emulsion. Interestingly, this longer duration of vaginal retention, and slower release of medication, result in decreased systemic exposure when compared to traditional intravaginal creams, which often exhibit a "bolus" type of effect. In a single-center, open-label, cross-over study (12) of 20 participants, subjects were randomized to receive a single dose of Clindesse, or traditional vaginal clindamycin cream (each containing 100 mg clindamycin phosphate). After a 2-week washout period, participants received a single dose of the other medication. Area-under-the-curve (AUC) from time zero to the last detectable concentration (AUC_{0-t}) was significantly lower with Clindesse compared to the traditional clindamycin 2% multi-dose cream: 98.61 ng vs. 794.21 ng × h/mL, respectively. Likewise, C_{max} was also lower for Clindesse compared to the traditional multi-dose vaginal clindamycin cream: 3.18 ng/mL vs. 42.27 ng/mL (p < 0.001 between formulations). Overall, Clindesse™ demonstrated approximately 12% bioavailability compared to that of a standard intravaginal clindamycin cream. Importantly, although this was a single-dose study, the same standard clindamycin cream is typically dosed daily (100 mg QD) for 7 days. Thus, the marked decrease in systemic exposure of medication with Clindesse compared to a single dose of conventional cream, would further be amplified with the use of such cream in its conventional (seven dose) manner. Moreover, this sustained release property also appears to confer a more rapid onset of action and faster amelioration of irritating symptoms. Brown et al. reported that Gynazole-1 resulted in significant relief in severe/very severe symptoms associated with VVC as early as 1 day post-drug application. This statistically significant difference was compared (8) to the relief demonstrated with a conventional cream dosed daily for seven consecutive days (Fig. 4). Thus, not only can SITE RELEASE reduce product leakage and dosing requirements, but its

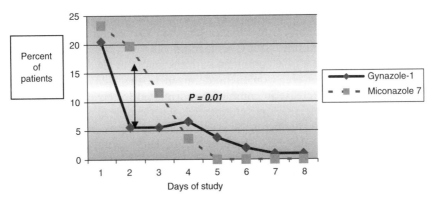

Figure 4 Proportion of patients with severe/very severe symptoms of VVC after single application of Gynazole-1® and during seven daily applications of Miconazole 7 vaginal cream. *Abbreviation*: VVC, vulvovaginal candidiasis.

bioadherence can facilitate a continuous exposure to active drug, which may result in a more rapid therapeutic effect. Of more than 25,000 women surveyed whom had used Gynazole-1, greater than three-quarters cited "fast relief" as the most important attribute in a product when treating a yeast infection (7). In addition to Gynazole-1 demonstrating faster symptomatic relief compared to miconazole-7, Gynazole-1 has also been demonstrated elsewhere to have a significantly faster onset of action compared to oral fluconazole (13). From the aforementioned survey, women report a very high level of satisfaction with Gynazole-1: 97% of women report that they would use Gynazole-1 again.

CONCLUSION

As evidenced by efficacy data, a single dose bioadhesive topical cream formulation of either butoconazole nitrate or clindamycin phosphate is as efficacious as multiple dose conventional creams in the treatment of VVC or BV, respectively. The bioadhesive technology employed in both Gynazole-1 and Clindesse is SITE RELEASE, a patented high internal phase emulsion delivery system. This dual phase emulsion system represents an improvement over standard commercialized creams, by means of improving the convenience and duration of drug delivery while maintaining therapeutic effectiveness and even simultaneously reducing the dose of medication. The bioadherence of the SITE RELEASE system is confirmed in the clinical setting by both a significant reduction in product leakage and faster time to relief when compared to a conventional cream applied to the vaginal cavity. The SITE RELEASE system design meets an increasing need in the management of women's health care by offering a delivery system designed to contribute to improved patient compliance for two very common gynecologic infections.

In addition, the SITE RELEASE delivery system represents a potential opportunity for the incorporation of various drug moieties to treat other disease states.

REFERENCES

1. Schwebke JR. Gynecologic consequences of bacterial vaginosis. Obstet Gynecol Clin N Am 2003; 30:685–94.
2. Anon. Vaginal Antifungal Monograph. Drug Facts and Comparisons. St. Louis:Wolters Kluwer Health, 2005.
3. Ferris DG, Litaker MS, Woodwards L, Mathis D, Hendrich J. Treatment of bacterial vaginosis: a comparison of oral metronidazole, metronidazole vaginal gel, and clindamycin vaginal cream. J Fam Pract 1995; 41(5):443–9.
4. Merabet J, Thompson D, Levinson RS. Advancing vaginal drug delivery. Expert Opin Drug Delivery 2005; 2:769–77.
5. United States Patent 5,266,329 and United States Patent 4,551,148.
6. Weinstein L, Henzl MR, Tsina IW. Vaginal retention of 2% butoconazole nitrate cream: comparison of a standard and a sustained-release preparation. Clin Ther 1994; 16:930–4.
7. Data on file, KV Pharmaceutical, St. Louis, MO. 2008.
8. Brown D, Henzl MR, Kaufman RH and the Gynazole-1 Study Group. Butoconazole nitrate 2% for vulvovaginal candidiasis: new single-dose vaginal cream formulation vs. seven-day treatment with miconazole nitrate. J Repr Med 1999; 44:933–8.
9. Cleocin-7 Vaginal Cream Package Insert. Pfizer Pharmaceutical. New York, NY. 2005.
10. Faro S, Skokos CK. The efficacy and safety of a single dose of Clindesse™ vaginal cream versus a seven-dose regimen of Cleocin-7® vaginal cream in patients with bacterial vaginosis. Infect Dis Obstet Gynecol 2005; 13:155–60.
11. Richter A, Anton SE, Koch P, Dennett SL. The impact of reducing dose frequency on health outcomes. Clin Ther 2003; 25:2307–35.
12. Levinson RS, Mitan SJ, Steinmetz JI, Gattermeir DJ, Schumacher RJ, Joffrion JL. An open-label, two-period, crossover study of the systemic bioavailability in healthy women of clindamycin phosphate from two vaginal cream formulations. Clin Ther 2005; 27:1894–900.
13. Seidman LS, Skokos CK. An evaluation of butoconazole nitrate 2% Site Release® vaginal cream (Gynazole-1®) compared to fluconazole 150 mg tablets (Diflucan®) in the time to relief of symptoms in patients with vulvovaginal candidiasis. Infect Dis Obsttet Gynecol 2005; 13:197–206.

39

Clindamycin Vaginal Insert

Janet A. Halliday and Steve Robertson

Controlled Therapeutics (Scotland) Limited, East Kilbride, Lanarkshire, U.K.

INTRODUCTION

Controlled Therapeutics (Scotland) Ltd. (CTS), a wholly owned subsidiary of Cytokine PharmaSciences, Inc., has developed the C-Vad™ vaginal insert for the treatment of bacterial vaginosis. This product uses a unique, patent-protected, vaginal delivery system to administer a drug with confirmed efficacy in an effective and convenient manner. The retrievable pessary is covered by granted international patents. The polymer-clindamycin hydrochloride combination is the subject of a U.S. patent application.

Bacterial vaginosis (BV) is the most common cause of abnormal vaginal discharge in women of childbearing age and accounts for up to 10 million physician office visits in the United States each year. Although there are other vaginal treatment options, these give a 30-day cure rate of less than 50% (1), have a high relapse rate and require up to 7 days dosing. The available creams and ovules complete their drug release within a few hours after insertion and leak from the vagina, losing drug product, staining undergarments, and becoming uncomfortable to the patient. Oral treatments are effective, but their associated unpleasant GI effects and interference with alcohol metabolism make them undesirable as a treatment option.

Due to its continuous, controlled release of clindamycin directly to the vagina, the C-Vad insert is expected to improve efficacy over currently available treatments, reduce treatment duration to 1 day, and provide patients with a cleaner, neater approach to successful cure. Improved initial efficacy may also reduce the current 70% relapse rate for BV.

INTELLECTUAL PROPERTY

The patented, removable vaginal pessary is the same delivery system used in the licensed medicinal product, known as both Cervidil® and Propess® is a vaginal insert containing dinoprostone for cervical ripening. This product has been marketed worldwide for more than 10 years and has been successfully used in more than 3 million births. In addition to the retrievable pessary patent, C-Vad is protected by extensive know-how surrounding the design, loading, and manufacture of controlled-release hydrogel polymers.

BACKGROUND

Bacterial vaginosis is the result of an imbalance of vaginal flora caused by a reduction of the normal lactobacillary bacteria, and a heavy overgrowth of mixed anaerobic flora, including *Gardnerella vaginalis*, *Mycoplasma hominis*, and *Mobiluncus* species. The cause of the change of the vaginal flora is unknown. The reported prevalence of BV is between 8% and 23% of U.S. women of childbearing age (1). For the up to 8 million women so affected, BV is the most common cause of vaginal symptoms leading them to seek medical care (1,2). In addition to its unpleasant nature, this infection has also been associated with premature birth and maternal and neonatal infections. BV also increases susceptibility to other infections, such as HIV, and may be a contributory factor in pelvic inflammatory disease.

Existing vaginal treatments deliver their product rapidly, allow the drug product to escape from the vagina, and must be repeated for up to 7 days and result in an initial cure in only 60–70% of cases (1). Clindesse® launched in 2005 had a 33% therapeutic cure rate in its phase III study (3). BV recurs in up to 29% of women using existing therapies at 1 month and in 50–70% by 3 months (2). Oral treatments are associated with GI upset, often severe, and interfere with alcohol metabolism.

Existing Therapies

Various preparations are available for the treatment of BV, with both systemic and vaginal therapeutic approaches. The active ingredient in these preparations is either metronidazole in the form of generic tablets, Flagyl® tablets, Metrogel®, generic gel or clindamycin phosphate Cleocin® cream, Dalacin® in the European Union, Cleocin® ovules or Clindesse™ bioadhesive gel launched in the United States in 2005.

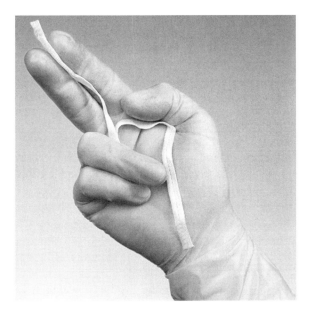

Figure 1 C-Vad™ vaginal insert, a controlled-release hydrogel insert containing clindamycin hydrochloride for the treatment of bacterial vaginosis.

DESCRIPTION OF TECHNOLOGY

Physical Properties and Formulation

The C-Vad vaginal insert has three components: the polymer, the active drug, and the retrieval tape. The non-biodegradable hydrogel polymer insert is 30 mm long, 10 mm wide and 1.5 mm thick and contains clindamycin hydrochloride dispersed throughout its matrix. The hydrogel polymer is contained within an inert, polyester, woven retrieval tape. The tape itself has no physiological activity but allows simple withdrawal of the product is designed to be non-wicking (Fig. 1) and is provided with a custom designed applicator (Fig. 2).

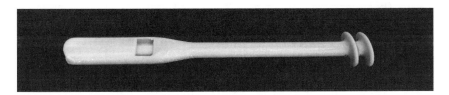

Figure 2 Custom designed applicator.

Scale Up and Manufacturing

CTS' purpose-built, state-of-the-art facility is dedicated to the production of drug delivery products based upon these unique hydrogel polymers. At the scale required for phase III studies and market launch the existing processes can meet the volumes. Once market penetration rises then an alternative process will be introduced. A continuous process to manufacture the polymer is in development for implementation in 2009.

The hydrogel technology is based on a polyurethane polymer composed of polyethylene glycol, chain extended with an isocyanate and cross-linked with a triol (4). By adjusting the thickness, crystallinity, and solvent uptake properties the polymer controls the release of drug over a period of many hours. In vitro release rates at different thicknesses are shown in Figure 3.

CLINICAL RESULTS

Clindamycin phosphate was initially utilized in the product because it is most commonly used for vaginal preparations. Studies performed on the precursor clindamycin phosphate insert, however, showed that the product had inadequate shelf life. Substitution of the hydrochloride salt for the phosphate has demonstrated acceptable stability in further studies and this formulation has therefore been chosen for further clinical development.

The C-Vad vaginal insert has been designed to release drug in a sustained and controlled manner for 24 hours. Once in place, the polymer

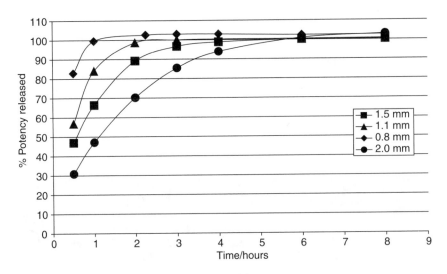

Figure 3 In vitro release rate at various thicknesses.

absorbs water, causing it to hydrate. This action creates a concentration gradient that releases the active ingredient and bathes the surrounding tissues with clindamycin. In addition to the expected superior efficacy from this direct and prolonged effect, this method is also expected to have fewer side effects due to lower systemic exposure than oral and ovule preparations. Moreover, there is no leakage from the product, a benefit that should improve patient acceptability and compliance.

In Vivo Studies

A Phase I clinical study of a precursor vaginal insert containing clindamycin phosphate was carried out. The product was identical to the current formulation except for the substitution of phosphate in place of the hydrochloride salt. This study tested two dosage strengths in two polymer thicknesses (50 mg/0.8 mm and 100 mg/1.5 mm) in non-pregnant, healthy women to determine the pharmacokinetics and release profile of the vaginal inserts. Used inserts were collected and analyzed for drug residue to allow the determination of the drug-release profile.

The product has a PK profile with a systemic exposure similar to marketed vaginal ovule and cream BV products, indicating that C-Vad should perform at least as well as these preparations. Vaginal lavage samples also established that clindamycin was present at therapeutic levels for up to 72 hours after a single, 24-hour use of C-Vad. Measurable amounts of clindamycin were determined in lavage samples from volunteers up to 48 and 72 hours post insertion for a 50- and 100-mg clindamycin vaginal insert (CVI). These levels are well above the 0.125 and 0.5 μg/ml MIC levels for *Gardnerella* and *Bacteroides*, respectively. A concentration of ≥900 μg/ml was found 48 hours after insertion. This approximates to 7000 and 2000 times the reported MIC for *Gardnerella* and *Bacteroides*, respectively (5,6). Concentrations of 133 μg/ml clindamycin were measured at 96 hours for the 100 mg sample described above (Table 1).

Table 1 Clindamycin Concentrations in Lavage Samples after Dosing with 50 or 100 mg CVI

Dose lavage time point (hr)	50-mg CVI Mean concentration (μg/mL)	100-mg CVI Mean concentration (μg/mL)
25	3400	7111
48	1200	4267
72	1067	333
96	89	134

Abbreviation: CVI, clindamycin vaginal insert.

The release profile showed medication was released at a consistent rate for the entire 24-hour application. The inserts are several times smaller than the average tampon routinely used during a woman's menses, and were well tolerated.

REGULATORY PLAN

The company proposes to market the product initially in the United States. Clindamycin hydrochloride, is already marketed in an IV dosage form. The vaginal delivery system is well known to regulatory authorities since it is the same system approved around the world in Cervidil® and Propess®. Clindamycin is widely used to treat bacterial vaginosis and is supported by a large body of medical literature.

The inserts will be manufactured by CTS at its GMP facility in East Kilbride, near Glasgow, Scotland.

FUTURE ACTIVITIES

The goal is to achieve rapid marketing approvals in the United States and Europe. The next step will be a Phase II, placebo-controlled clinical trial to demonstrate the efficacy and safety of C-Vad. Based on literature data that confirm vaginal clindamycin is effective in the treatment of BV, we expect that C-Vad will have a cure rate equivalent or superior to marketed 3–7 day products. This proof-of-concept study will be quickly rolled over into a single phase III study.

POTENTIAL MARKET

The U.S. market for intravaginal BV products is presently more than $130 million per year (IMS, 2004). The market in Europe is slightly smaller, principally due to lower pricing. CPSI expects that C-Vad will generate sales of $35–50 million annually in the United States alone.

REFERENCES

1. Marrazzo JM. Evolving issues in understanding and treating bacterial vaginosis. Expert Rev Anti-Infective Ther 2004; 2:913–22.
2. Hanson JM, McGregor JA, Hillier SL, et al. Metronidazole for bacterial vaginosis. A comparison of vaginal gel vs. oral therapy. J Reproduct Med 2000; 45: 889–96.
3. Clindesse package label, revised 02/05.
4. Graham NB. In: Peppas NP, ed. Hydrogels in Medicine and Pharmacy. Vol. 2. Boca Raton, FL: CRC Press, 1987: 95–113.

5. Joesoef MR, Schmid GP, Hillier SL. Bacterial Vaginosis: Review of treatment options and potential clinical indications of therapy. Clin Infect Dis 1999; 28(Suppl. 1):S57–65.
6. Martindale, The Extra Pharmacopoeia 33rd ed. P. 188. The Pharmaceutical Press. London.

40

Bioresponsive Vaginal Delivery Systems

Patrick F. Kiser

Department of Bioengineering, University of Utah, Salt Lake City, Utah, U.S.A.

INTRODUCTION

Bioresponsive polymers (also known as "smart," "intelligent," bio-interactive or stimulus-sensitive polymers) respond to small external signals with large changes in their polymer conformation or properties to affect changes in their performance (Fig. 1) (1–3). A wide variety of uses have been envisioned for these types of polymer constructs. Polymer constructs have been engineered to act as actuators, valves, responsive surfaces, diagnostics, and drug delivery systems (4). In drug delivery applications, four major physiological signals have been utilized to trigger a physical change in the polymer construct or the release of entrapped drug: temperature changes (5), pH changes (6), and soluble molecules or enzymes. Utilizing these signals, drug delivery systems have been devised that target diverse therapeutic areas, with anticancer (7), diabetes (8,9), and pH sensitive coatings (10) being the most ubiquitous.

Two of the most common classes of bioresponsive polymers that have been studied are the temperature responsive polymers and pH responsive polymers. Many polymers in water exhibit temperature responsive behavior or a lower critical solution temperature (LCST) inwater. In this case, the polymer is in a soluble state (sol) at a temperature below the LCST, and when warmed to the LCST it undergoes a phase transition, becoming insoluble. When a semisolid gel is formed when the polymer precipitables, this is known as a temperature induced sol to gel phase transition. One common composition of temperature sensitive polymers are domains or moieties that exhibit both hydophobicity and hydrophilicity, and the balance between these domains can be adjusted to change the LCST (1).

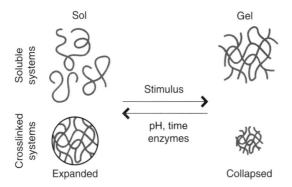

Figure 1 Bioresponsive polymer systems undergo phase transitions in response to external stimuli. These phase transitions can result in the reversible dissolution/gelation of a polymer or reversible volume changes as a polymer becomes hydrated and dehydrated.

Changes in the association of these domains with each other and with solvent result in the LCST behavior. Mechanistically, the temperature change causes desorportion of bound water from the soluble polymer chains, inducing the hydrophobic domains of the soluble polymer to associate into extended insoluble networks (11). In this class, the two most common polymeric compositions studied are based on triblock copolymers of poly (ethylene oxide)-poly(propylene oxide)-poly(ethylene oxide) also known as poloxamers, and polymers containing poly(N-isopropyl acrylamide) (poly (NIPAAm)).

The behaviors of pH sensitive systems are modulated through ionic interactions (12,13). Typically, these materials are structured form crosslinked hydrogel networks which undergo reversible osmotic swelling and contraction due to the presence of fixed ionizable groups attached to the polymer network (13,14). The increase in the network pore size with swelling can be used to increase diffusion of entrained soluble compounds within the hydrogel network, thereby triggering drug release with swelling. Finally, Hofmann (15) and others (16) have pioneered the development of a number of "dual" response systems that are sensitive to both temperature and pH.

Vaginal drug delivery using bioresponsive polymers has received relatively little attention in comparison to other areas of bioresponsive drug delivery. This is likely because sustained drug delivery (17–20) has been the major goal in vaginally applied therapeutics, and there is a lack of physiologically relevant signals from the diseases that are normally targeted with vaginal drug delivery systems. Yet there are several rationales to apply bioresponsive polymers to vaginal delivery. Many semi-solid vaginal delivery systems suffer from lack of retention of the dosage form in the vagina. When a woman is standing, the vaginal cavity is oriented at a 45° angle inferior, and the combined effect of squeezing and gravity induced flows (21–23), along with the production of vaginal exudate, tends to promote leakage of the dosage form from the vaginal cavity. Therefore, a system that could be triggered by a temperature change upon application to gel in situ may assist in retention of the dosage form, thereby increasing the dose duration (24–26). Bioadhesive or mucoadhesive systems that aim to accomplish the same effect have been recently reviewed (27).

A number of physiological signals other than temperature exist in the vaginal milieu, and these could be used to signal a polymer phase transition for delivery systems designed to target contraception and the prevention of male to female transmission of sexually acquired diseases. One of the most interesting signals is the seminal fluid itself, because semen is the carrier for the target of both contraceptive and anti-STD agents. By taking advantage of molecules endogenous to semen and not endogenous to the vaginal lumen, one might be able to accomplish site specific triggered drug delivery within the vaginal lumen using bioresponsive polymer systems.

Two signals contained within seminal fluid that are currently being explored as triggers for drug release are proteases (28), e.g., human kallikrein III also known as prostrate specific antigen, present at high concentration in semen (29–31), and pH changes due to the presence of semen in the vagina (32–34). A healthy vaginal lumen is acidic (pH 4–5), and acidic vaginal exudate has a low buffering capacity (35). Seminal fluid, on the other hand, has a significantly higher pH (7.5–8.5) and is relatively highly buffered (36). Therefore the presence of seminal fluid induces a large change in the vaginal pH after coitus. In addition, an increase in vaginal pH also results from various types of infections, including trichomoniasis vaginitis and bacterial vaginosis (37). Utilizing these signals we have designed several bioresponsive polymers that use the presence of seminal fluid as a trigger for release of pharmaceutical actives from the vaginal gel and into semen.

DESCRIPTION OF THE TECHNOLOGY

There are only a few examples of published bioresponsive delivery systems that have been studied for vaginal delivery and/or the prevention of STDs (Table 1). Bergeron et al. have pioneered the use of thermosensitive polymers (in this case poloxamers) for the prevention of STDs (24,38,39). The rationale is that at ambient temperature a low viscosity sol during application allows the fluid to flow via capillary action into the vaginal rugae, coat the genital tissue and provide improved biodistribution. Furthermore as discussed above, when the thermosensitive polymer passes through its LCST and gels in situ, the increased viscosity should aid in retention and extended duration of active agents in the vaginal lumen. They have demonstrated that their poloxamer formulation is effective for treating herpetic lesions in a murine model (24). Currently, this thermosensitive polymer in

Table 1   Composition, Application of Published Bioresponsive Vaginal
Delivery Systems

Composition[a]	Sensitivity	Therapeutic area	References
Poloxamer	Temp.	Topical antiviral	24,38,53,54
Poloxamer-g-poly(acrylic acid)	Temp.	Vaginal delivery	41,42,55–57
Poloxamer with poly carbophil	Temp.	Vaginal candidiasis	25
p(NiPAm-co-AA-BMA)	Temp.	pH Topical antiviral	26
In situ crosslinking system	pH	Topical antiviral	48

[a]All of these materials are semisolid gels.
Abbreviations: AA, acrylic acid; BMA, n-butyl methacrylate.

combination with the surfactant sodium lauryl sulfate, is in phase I/II
clinical trials as an anti-HIV microbicide (40). Ron et al. have devised
bioadhesive thermosensitive block copolymers, based on poloxamers functionalized with poly(acrylic acid) blocks, that have been envisioned for use
as bioadhesive vaginal delivery vehicles (11,41–43). Chang et al. have made
syringable mixtures of poloxamers and polycarbophils for sustained delivery
of clotrimazole against vaginal candidiasis (25). More recently, we have
devised a dual temperature and pH responsive delivery system (Fig. 2) based
on random copolymers of NIPAAm and acrylic acid (AA) as a semen
triggered vehicle for delivery of polymer therapeutics against STDs and in
particular HIV (26).

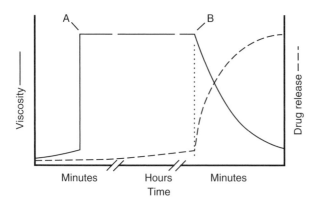

Figure 2   Theoretical behavior of a semen-triggered vaginal delivery system. The
dosage form would undergo an in situ gelling reaction when applied and go through
a large viscosity change (**A**). The drug would be retained in the vaginal lumen for an
extended period of time. In the presence of semen (**B**) the system would rapidly
release the entrained drug to inactivate pathogens that might be present in the seminal fluid.

The design aim of this dual temperature and pH bioresponsive vehicle was to produce a polymer system that could efficiently deploy and coat genital tissue; could gel in situ to retain the vehicle after deployment; and that could release entrapped macromolecular antiviral agents into semen when the polymer comes in contact with seminal fluid (Fig. 3). Therefore, a thermosensitive polymer was chosen to accomplish the first two processes. The rationale driving the use of pH triggered release was to deliver a therapeutic concentration of the antiviral agents into the potentially infected seminal fluid at a maximum rate, thereby inactivating infectious viral particles before they could defuse or come in contact with cells which may be infected by the STD (Fig. 3C). To accomplish this, we designed a random terpolymer of NIPAAm, n-butyl methacrylate (BMA) and AA, poly (NiPAAm-co-BMA-co-AA) (Fig. 4) (3,44). At vaginal pH (~4.5) the AA groups are largely protonated, thereby providing a polymer that has thermosensitive properties similar to poly(NiPAAm). However, when the polymer is exposed to seminal fluid the pH change in the vaginal lumen causes the AA groups to become ionized. This increased charge density and increased degree of hydration in the polymer disrupts the gel phase and forces the polymer construct to undergo a gel to sol phase transition (Fig. 3). Thus the delivery system can be applied to the vagina as a liquid, and it will become a gel in situ at acidic vaginal pH to form a potentially well distributed coating layer on the genital tissues (Figs. 2 and 3A,3B). Later, when the delivery system comes in contact with semen it would undergo a sol to gel phase transition and release the entrained macromolecular active agents into semen and inactivate the STDs carried therein (Figs. 2 and 3C).

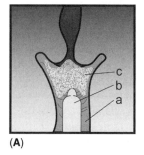 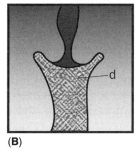 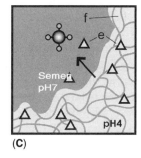

(A) (B) (C)

Figure 3 Diagram of how a prototype temperature-sensitive and pH-sensitive formulation undergoes in situ gelling, retention, and semen-triggered release. The gel would be applied as a liquid to the vaginal lumen in an applicator (**A**) and it would spread over susceptible tissue. After a brief time the gel warms to body temperature and (**B**) gels in situ. When semen comes in contact with gel (**C**), the pH change from acidic vaginal/formulation pH to near neutral pH induces a gel to sol phase transition and the entrained drug is released from the vehicle.

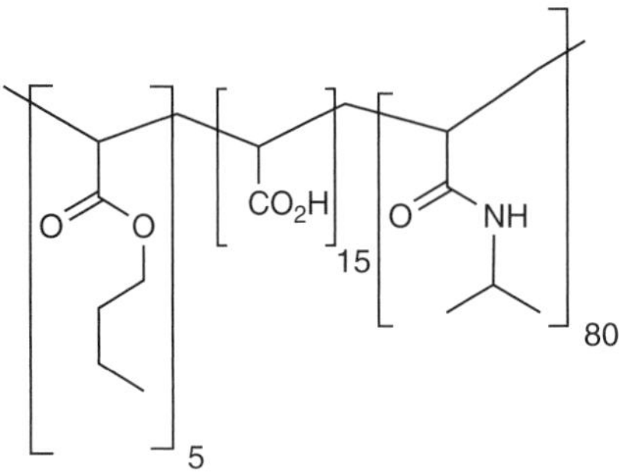

Figure 4 Chemical structure and composition of the copolymer selected with N-isopropyl acrylamide, AA and butyl methacrylate. The NIPAAm monomer provides the temperature sensitivity, and the AA moieties provide the pH sensitivity. *Abbreviation*: AA, acrylic acid.

RESEARCH AND DEVELOPMENT

Antiviral delivery systems are targeted largely to users in the developing world where resources are scarce, and therefore it is important that the active agents and the delivery system components are able to be produced at low cost. The copolymer system (Fig. 4) that was developed (26) was synthesized in such a way that it could be made inexpensively in bulk, using standard single step free radical or emulsion-based polymerization technology. It is envisioned that the polymers and active pharmaceutical ingredients would be co-formulated in the polymer system below the LCST. The liquid polymer could then be packaged in a blister pack or syringe like applicator for use.

Feasibility studies were conducted with this delivery system as it relates to vaginal delivery of macromolecular and small molecule antiviral agents (26). After synthesizing a library of copolymers and studying their pH and temperature gelling behaviors, a copolymer with the composition of NIPAm 80 mol%, AA 15 mol% and BMA 5 mol% was selected that had properties which appeared to be suitable for vaginal delivery (Fig. 4). These polymers were then formulated so that they were isotonic with blood plasma and at the acidic pH of the vagina using pH 4.2 acetate buffer. The rheological behavior was studied as a function of temperature and polymer concentration. Polymer concentration was adjusted to 70 mg/mL at pH 4.2 to set the LCST for this composition just below body temperature. With a polymer number average molecular weight of approximately 1100 kDa a system was obtained which underwent a thirty fold increase in complex viscosity moving from 25°C to 37°C (Fig. 5A). To investigate the ability of the formulated pH and thermosensitive copolymer to resist erosion in the presence of simulated vaginal fluid and simulated seminal fluid, thin layers of the polymer were made and the resistance to erosion under agitation was evaluated (45). In the presence of simulated vaginal fluid the copolymer eroded significantly less then current marketed vaginal formulations. As

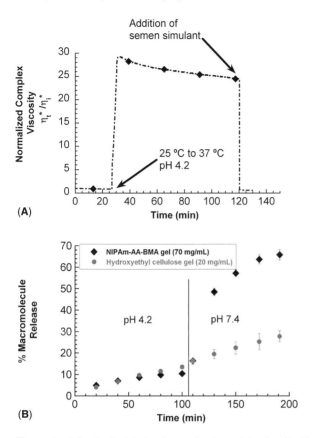

Figure 5 Rheological behavior and release kinetics for the 80:15:5 NiPAAm, AA and BMA temperature and pH responsive delivery system. (**A**) Plot of complex viscosity normalized to the initial complex viscosity ($n^* = 1.206$ Pa s). A 70 mg/mL solution of the polymer was made in 100 mM pH 4.2 acetate buffer containing sorbitol to adjust the osmolality to 310 mOsm/kg. The sample was loaded on the TA-550 rheometer plate and complex viscosity was measured in four steps (*i*) at 25°C for 25 minutes, (*ii*) during a temperature ramp from 25°C to 37°C in 3.4 minutes, (*iii*) at 37°C for 1.5 hr, then in the presence of 1:1 mixture of seminal fluid. (**B**) For the release study, a gel sample loaded with FITC-Dextran (Mn = kD) was equilibrated with vaginal fluid simulant at 37°C for 105 minutes prior to addition of seminal fluid simulant. The amount of the entrained macromolecular model released was monitored by fluorescence in the receptor chamber above the gel. *Abbreviations*: AA, acrylic acid; BMA, n-butyl methacrylate. *Source*: From Ref. 26.

expected and indicated by our rheological examinations of the material at seminal pH (Fig. 5A), the terpolymer eroded rapidly in the presence of the seminal fluid simulant. This simulates the behavior of the material after being exposed to semen during intercourse.

In a series of in vitro release studies of entrapped macromolecular agents it was observed that the dissolution of the polymer gel resulted in a burst release of entrapped agent by significantly reducing the diffusion constant of the entrapped agent upon going through the gel to sol phase transition (Fig. 5B). This rapid dissolution of the gel layer after exposure to semen and subsequent rapid drug release are critical to the desired performance of this delivery system. A relatively small amount of macromolecular agent was released from the system when it was in the gel state. Cytocompatibility of intravaginal delivery systems meant to prevent the transmission of sexually acquired diseases is a critical early measure of the safety of the delivery system. Studies using the standard FDA protocol for cytocompatibility in the L929 fibroblast cell line showed the 80:15:5 NiPAAm:AA:BMA copolymer to be less cytotoxic than the well tolerated and commercially used Carbopol polymers.

REGULATORY ISSUES

Currently, there are no approved female-initiated products on the market which prevent sexually transmitted diseases. Additionally, there are no delivery systems for any indication on the market that display both pH sensitivity and temperature sensitivity. Therefore, the entire product class of bioresponsive vaginal formulations represents a new frontier in vaginal drug delivery. Another consideration relative to the development of any anti-STD products is that a large fraction of the users—particularly in the case of prophylactic anti-HIV therapeutics—live in the developing world. Clinical trials designed to show preventative efficacy present a significant cost barrier due to their size requirements and associated costs of conducting this type of clinical trial in developing countries, where scientific and clinical infrastructures are still being established (46). Secondly, all novel functional drug delivery systems made from new polymers require the generation of a drug master file. Particularly in the area of anti-HIV delivery systems where commercial interest is limited, due to the lack of developed markets, the cost of generating the drug master file is inhibitory in the further development of these systems. Furthermore, functional vehicles like the ones described above would be classified as a combination product according to FDA definitions under 21 CFR 3. The request for designation of the combination product requires that a description be provided to the FDA of all known modes of action, and scientific basis for the most important therapeutic action of the product. It could be difficult to generate in vivo data that elucidates the relative importance of the various modes of action for these types of functional delivery systems. Generation of these data will likely involve complex imaging modalities to ascertain in situ gelling, tissue distribution, prevention of viral transport, and retention and delivery of antiviral agents into tissue and into semen. These issues along with a lack of appropriate animal models present a difficult challenge in the face of regulatory requirements.

Finally, for the widespread deployment of this type of delivery system, a number of practical and clinical hurdles need to be overcome to satisfy regulatory requirements. These include potential manufacturing and formulation difficulties with a polymeric material that can phase separate during processing or at elevated temperatures during storage. And finally, as topical anti-STD agents complete phase III clinical trials and are registered, next generation bioresponsive vaginal delivery systems will have to be shown in a clinical trial to be as effective as or an improvement over approved products (46).

TECHNOLOGY POSITION/COMPETITIVE ADVANTAGE

Currently, there are 5 anti-STD microbicides in phase IIb/III clinical trials and a large number of others in earlier stages (46). All of the vehicles in phase III are simple semisolid gels that have largely not been optimized for deployment or drug release characteristics. Therefore, the use of a thermosensitive polymer system could provide a significant improvement in the deployment of the drug delivery system in the vaginal lumen and potentially improved patient adherence because of the low application volume that might be achieved with this of gel. Furthermore, the use of site and compartment specific delivery systems operate under an assumption that local delivery of drug into a biological compartment (in this case compartment of semen) should provide a improved pharmacological effect in comparison to current formulations. If the rate of delivery of the antiviral agent into semen is maximized by removing the diffusion barrier of the gel, then the maximum rate of mixing with seminal fluid will occur, providing the greatest pharmacological effect in the shortest possible time. Furthermore, systems like the dual sensitive polymers describe above could compliment the long duration intravaginal ring systems being developed to deliver antiretroviral drugs into genital tissue for 30 days or more (47). A semisolid gel that remains active for 24 hours could be used by the subset of the user population that does not require long duration protection, thus providing a number of choices for users depending on their individual needs.

FUTURE DIRECTIONS

There are a number of specific directions in which semen-triggered bioresponsive materials may be used in vaginal delivery of antiviral agents and contraceptives. We are interested in non-thermosensitive polymer systems that can be made to undergo a sol to gel phase transition within the vaginal lumen (48) and particle systems that are degradable by enzymes in semen (26). In addition, polymers which provide a barrier to viral diffusion could act as a first level of protection in the early events of sexual transmission of infectious agents (49). To realize the potential of this technology will require the advancement of new animal models (in particular primate models) and imaging modalities (50) that allow us to study the deployment and activity of bioresponsive delivery vehicles like those described in this chapter. Furthermore, since semen-triggered delivery is largely relevant to agents that can act in the vaginal lumen, particularly in the anti-HIV area, there are a few agents that will act within this compartment on HIV directly. Therefore, in order to fulfill the potential of this mechanism of action, further discovery efforts will have to be completed on classes of compounds that can inactivate HIV in seminal fluid. Finally, the area of user acceptability is an extremely important and largely overlooked aspect of development of these kinds of products (51,52). It is unknown how women from diverse cultural backgrounds will respond to materials that change properties within their vaginas. Studies that address these issues will need to be completed as part of the overall preclinical program.

REFERENCES

1. Hoffman AS. Intelligent polymers in medicine and biotechnology. Artif Organs 1995; 19:458–67.
2. Hoffman AS. Environmentally sensitive polymers and hydrogels. MRS Bulletin 1991; September:42–6.
3. Hoffman AS, Afrassiabi A, Dong LC. Thermally reversible hydrogels: II. Delivery and selective removal of substances from aqueous solutions. J Control Release 1986; 4:213–22.
4. Galaev IY, Mattiasson B. 'Smart' polymers and what they could do in biotechnology and medicine. Trends Biotech 1999; 17:335–40.
5. Jeong B, Kim SW, Bae YH. Thermosensitive sol–gel reversible hydrogels. Adv Drug Deliv Rev 2002; 54:37–51.
6. Kiser PF, Wilson G, Needham D. A synthetic mimic of the secretory granule for drug delivery. Nature 1998; 394:459–62.
7. Duncan R. The dawning era of polymer therapeutics. Nature Rev Drug Discov 2003; 2:347–60.
8. Matsumoto R, Yoshida R, Kataoka K. Glucose-responsive polymer gel bearing phenylborate derivative as a glucose-sensing moiety operating at the physiological pH. Biomacromolecules 2004; 5:1038–45.
9. Lowman AM, Morishita M,Kajita M, Nagai T, Peppas NA. Oral delivery of insulin using pH-responsive complexation gels. J Pharm Sci 1999; 88:933–7.
10. Patel M, Patel B, Patel R, Patel J, Bharadia P, Patel M. Carbopol: A versatile polymer. Drug Deliv Tech 2006; 6:32–4.
11. Orkisz MJ, Bromberg L, Pike R, Lupton EC, Ron ES. Rheological properties of reverse thermogelling poly(acrylic acid)-g-(oxyethylene-b-oxypropylene-b-oxyethylene) polymers (smart hydrogel). Book ofAbstracts, 213th ACS National Meeting, San Francisco, April 13–7, PMSE-169; 1997.

12. Hoffman AS. Hydrogels for biomedical applications. Adv Drug Deliv Rev 2002; 43:3–12.
13. De SK, Aluru NR, Johnson B, Crone WC, Beebe DJ, Moore J. Equilibrium swelling and kinetics of pH-responsive hydrogels: models, experiments, and simulations. Journal of Microelectromechanical Systems 11:544–55.
14. Eichenbaum GM, Kiser PF, Simon SA, Needham D pH and ion-triggered volume response of anionic hydrogel microspheres. Macromolecules 1998; 31:5084–93.
15. Chen GH, Hoffman AS. Graft-copolymers that exhibit temperature-induced phase-transitions over a wide range of pH. Nature 1995; 373:49–52.
16. Suh JM, Bae SJ, Jeong B. Thermogelling multiblock poloxamer aqueous solutions with closed-loop sol-gel-sol transitions upon increasing pH. Adv Mater 2005; 17:118–20.
17. Brannon-Peppas L. Novel vaginal drug release applications. Adv Drug Deliv Rev 1993; 11:169–77.
18. Okada H, Hillery AM. Vaginal drug delivery. In: Hillery AM, Lloyd AW, Swarbrick J, eds. Drug Delivery and Targeting for Pharmacists and Pharmaeutical Scientists. London: Taylor & Francis, 2001; 301–28.
19. Hussain A, Ahsan F. The vagina as a route for systemic drug delivery. J Control Release 2005; 103:301–13.
20. Merabet J, Thompson D, Levinson RS. Advancing vaginal drug delivery. Expert Opin Drug Deliv 2005; 2:769–77.
21. Kieweg SL, Geonnotti AR, Katz DF. Gravity-induced coating flows of vaginal gel formulations: In vitro experimental analysis. J Pharmal Sci 2004; 93:2941–52.
22. Kieweg SL, Katz DF. Squeezing flows of vaginal gel formulations relevant to microbicide drug delivery. J Biomech Eng 2006; 128:540–53.
23. Kieweg SL, Katz DF. Interpreting properties of microbicide drug delivery gels: Analyzing deployment kinetics due to squeezing. J Pharm Sci 2007; 96: 835–50.
24. Piret J, Gagne N, Perron S. Thermoreversible gel as a candidate barrier to prevent the transmission of HIV-1 and herpes simplex virus type 2. Sex Transm Dis 2001; 28:484–91.
25. Chang JY, Oh YK, Kong HS. Prolonged antifungal effects of clotrimazole-containing mucoadhesive thermosensitive gels on vaginitis. J Control Release 2002; 82:39–50.
26. Gupta KM, Barnes SR, Tangaro RA. Temperature and pH sensitive hydrogels: An approach towards smart semen-triggered vaginal microbicidal vehicles. J Pharm Sci 2007; 96:670–81.
27. Valenta C. The use of mucoadhesive polymers in vaginal delivery. Adv Drug Deliv Rev 2005; 57:1692–712.
28. Lee CW, Aliyar AW, Gupta KM, Kiser PF. Triggering microbicide release by enzymes in semen. Abstract. Microbicides 2006, Cape Town, South Africa, 2006.
29. Lilja H. Biology of prostate-specific antigen. Urology 2003; 62:27–33.
30. Balk SP, Ko YJ, Bubley GJ. Biology of prostate-specific antigen. J Clin Oncol 2003; 21(2):383–91.

31. Lilja H. A kallikrien-like serine protease in prostrate fluid cleaves the predominant seminal vesicle protein. J Clin Invest 1985; 76:1899–903.
32. Masters WH, Johnson VE, Reproductive Biology Research Foundation (U.S.). Human Sexual Response. 1st ed. Boston: Little Brown, 1966.
33. Fox CA, Meldrum SJ, Watson BW. Continuous measurement by radiotelemetry of vaginal pH during human coitus. J Reprod Fertil 1973; 33:69–75.
34. Tevi-Benissan C, Belec L, Levy M, et al. In vivo semen-associated pH neutralization of cervicovaginal secretions. Clin Diagn Lab Immunol 1997; 4:367–74.
35. Owen DH, Katz DF. A vaginal fluid simulant. Contraception 199; 59:91–5.
36. Owen DH, Katz DF. A review of the physical and chemical properties of human semen and the formulation of a semen simulant. J Androl 2005; 26:459–69.
37. Sagawa T, Negishi H, Kishida T, Yamada H, Fujimoto S. Vaginal and cervical pH in bacterial vaginosis and cervicitis during pregnancy. Hokkaido Igaku Zasshi 1995; 70:839–46.
38. Roy S, Gourde P, Piret J, et al. Thermoreversible gel formulations containing sodium lauryl sulfate or n-lauroylsarcosine as potential topical microbicides against sexually transmitted diseases. Antimicrob Agents Chemother 2001; 45: 1671–81.
39. Piret J, Lamontagne J, Bestman-Smith J, et al. In vitro and in vivo evaluations of sodium lauryl sulfate and dextran sulfate as microbicides against herpes simplex and human immunodeficiency viruses. J Clin Microbiol 2000; 38:110–9.
40. US National Institutes of Health. US Clinical Trials database: Safety, Tolerance and Acceptability Trial of the Invisible Condom® in Healthy Women, 2005.
41. Bromberg L. Novel family of thermogelling materials via C-C bonding between poly(acrylic acid) and poly(ethylene oxide)-b-poly(propylene oxide)-b-poly (ethylene oxide). J Phys Chem B 1998; 102:1956–63.
42. Bromberg LE, Ron ES. Temperature-responsive gels and thermogelling polymer matrices for protein and peptide delivery. Adva Drug Deliv Rev 1998; 31:197–221.
43. Ron ES, Roos EJ, Staples AK, Bromberg LE, Schiller ME. Interpenetrating polymer networks for sustained dermal delivery. In: Proceedings of the International Symposium on Controlled Release of Bioactive Materials, 1996; 128–9.
44. Young-Hee Kim YHB, Sung Wan K. pH/Temperature-sensitive polymers for macromolecular drug loading and release. J Control Release 1994; 28:143–52.
45. Geonnotti AR, Peters JJ, Katz DF. Erosion of microbicide formulation coating layers: Effects of contact and shearing with vaginal fluid or semen. J Pharm Sci 2005; 94:1705–12.
46. Ramjee G, Shattock R, Delany S, McGowan I, Morar N, Gottemoeller M. Microbicides 2006 conference. AIDS ResTherapy 2006; 3:25.
47. Woolfson AD, Malcolm RK, Toner CF, et al. Potential use of vaginal rings for prevention of heterosexual transmission of HIV: a controlled-release strategy for HIV microbicides. Am J Drug Deliv 2006; 4:7–20.

48. Roberts MC, Hanson MC, Massey AP, Karren EA, Kiser PF. Dynamically restructuring hydrogel networks formed with reversible covalent crosslinks. Adv Mater 2007, 19:2503–7.

49. Geonnotti AR, Katz DF. Dynamics of HIV neutralization by a microbicide formulation layer: biophysical fundamentals and transport theory. Biophys J 2006; 91:2121–30.

50. Henderson MH, Couchman GM, Walmer DK, et al.. Optical imaging and analysis of human vaginal coating by drug delivery gels. Contraception 2007; 75:142–51.

51. Morrow K, Rosen R, Richter L, et al. The acceptability of an investigational vaginal microbicide, PRO 2000 Gel, among women in a phase I clinical trial. J Women's Health 2002; 12:655–66.

52. Hardy E, Jimenez AL, de Padua KS, Zaneveld LJ. Women's preferences for vaginal antimicrobial contraceptives. III. Choice of a formulation, applicator, and packaging. Contraception 1998; 58:245–9.

53. Gagne N, Cormier H, Omar RF, et al. Protective effect of a thermoreversible gel against the toxicity of nonoxynol-9. Sex Transm Dis 1999; 26:177–83.

54. Haineault C, Gourde P, Perron S, et al. Thermoreversible gel formulation containing sodium lauryl sulfate as a potential contraceptive device. Biol Reprod 2003; 69:687–94.

55. Bromberg LE. Enhanced nasal retention of hydrophobically modified poly-electrolytes. J Pharm Pharmac 2001; 53:109–14.

56. Orkisz MJ, Bromberg L, Pike R, Lupton EC, Ron ES. Rheological properties of reverse thermogelling poly(acrylic acid)-g-(oxyethylene-b-oxypropylene-b-oxyethylene) polymers (Smart Hydrogel(TM)). Abstr Pap Am Chem S 1997; 213:169–PMSE.

57. Qiu Y, Park K. Environment-sensitive hydrogels for drug delivery. Advanced Drug Deliv Rev 2001; 53:321–39.

41

Pulmonary Delivery of Drugs by Inhalation

Paul B. Myrdal and B. Steven Angersbach

College of Pharmacy, University of Arizona, Tucson, Arizona, U.S.A.

INTRODUCTION

Therapy via inhalation has traditionally targeted the localized treatment of lung disease. The potential to administer drugs with limited oral bioavailability, as well as the means to achieve both local and systemic exposure has subsequently made inhalation delivery a rational modality for the development of therapies for a wide range of diseases. The aim of this section is to provide an overview of the contemporary technologies and strategies for pulmonary drug delivery. General chapters discussing small molecular weight molecules (Hickey and Mansour) and protein powders for inhalation (Chan) are complemented by those highlighting current and future trends in approved systems, such as nebulizers (Knoch and Finlay), and metered-dose inhalers (Ashurst). Additionally, specific advanced technologies for pulmonary delivery are discussed in the chapters by Cipolla and Johansson (Aradigm), Wachtel and Moser (Boehringer Ingelheim), Leone-Bay and Grant (MannKind), Clark and Weers (Nektar Therapeutics), and Nikander and Denyer (Respironics).

PRINCIPLES

The potential for inhalation dosing to afford both local and systemic activity of drugs continues to make this an attractive area of research. In addition to the classic treatments for asthma and lung disease, accomplished through topical delivery of small molecules, the large surface area of the peripheral lung and highly permeable alveolar cell layer offer access to the systemic blood and lymphatic circulation. The behavior of inhaled particles in the respiratory tract is dependent on the properties of the particles themselves, as well as the inspiratory characteristics of the patient (1,2).

Suitability of particles for inhalation delivery depends on the aerodynamic diameter of the particles, which is determined by size, shape and density. Studies have indicated that aerosol particles < 6 μm in diameter have the ability to bypass the central airways and deposit in the peripheral lung region, if they are subjected to low rates of inspiration (1–3). In order for a larger fraction of particles to reach the peripheral lung, however, a diameter range of two to three microns is ideal (4). The deposition of these particles is through sedimentation, whereas the Brownian diffusion can be appreciable for smaller particles (< 1 μm) and particles > 6 μm have a higher probability of impaction in the upper airways and oropharyngeal cavity. Particles may also increase or decrease in size due to hygroscopic effects. It has been shown that high relative humidity can exert a nearly instantaneous effect on particle diameter and distribution characteristics (5,6).

The dependency on patient coordination for successful administration of drugs via inhalation is a classic complication. Conventional therapy requires the patient to inhale suitably sized particles early in inspiration, continuing to inhale deeply at a low and even rate. Deposition has been shown to be enhanced by a modest period of breath holding following inspiration (7). Increased rates of inhalation correspondingly increase the fraction of particles experiencing oropharyngeal impaction, and variability among patients is quite high (8). Additionally, obstruction of the airways, such as that due to disease, lead to increased localized deposition of inhaled particles (9).

CONVENTIONAL DELIVERY METHODS

Therapy via inhalation has traditionally targeted the localized treatment of lung disease. Indeed, the metered-dose inhaler has been the primary pulmonary delivery system for over 50 years, while the earliest patents for nebulizers date back to the late nineteenth century. The potential to administer drugs with limited oral bioavailability, or to reduce systemic exposure, or as the means to achieve both local and/or systemic activity, has subsequently made inhalation delivery a logical target for the development of therapies for a wide range of diseases. An overview of the common pulmonary delivery technologies follows.

Pressurized Metered-Dose Inhalers

The pressurized metered-dose inhaler (MDI) remains the most prevalent pulmonary delivery system (see Chapter 49). MDIs are applicable to the delivery of both solution and suspension based drug formulations and their small size and the vast base of knowledge regarding their mechanics and formulation behavior have no doubt contributed to their continuing popularity. Conventional MDIs have been formulated as chlorofluorocarbon (CFC) propellant based devices. As noted in the first edition, however, due to their adverse effects on the atmospheric ozone, CFCs are being phased out, thus necessitating the use of alternative propellants or propellant systems.

Due to physicochemical differences from CFCs, including, but not limited to, solubility of active drug entities and aerosol behavior, reformulation of existing MDI products continues to receive extensive research. The compatibility and behavior of excipients in the alternative propellants may also be different from that in conventional CFC based MDIs. Furthermore, changes in formulation have, in some cases, required the use of alternative materials for components of the device itself (10).

Since the publication of the first edition of this book, in addition to the continued research surrounding the phasing out of CFCs, much work has also been directed towards the development of formulations which afford once daily dosing, as well as the opportunity to deliver agents previously limited to other (e.g., oral) routes. Longstanding and well-known issues with MDIs, such as the requisite patient coordination of actuation and inspiration and relatively low lung deposition are being addressed both through the use of add on devices, such as holding chambers, and through reengineering of the device itself (11–14). Additionally, new methods to address these issues, as well as some previously given less attention such as the development of dose counting devices incorporated in the MDI, are the subjects of current research (see Chapter 49).

Dry Powder Inhalers

Initial development of the conventional dry powder inhaler (DPI) as an alternative to MDIs began in the 1960s and 1970s and today, they are the second most common type of inhalation device (15,16). DPIs are classified as either, "passive," in which the patient, through breathing, produces the energy necessary to deliver the medication from the powder bed to the lung or, "active," in which the energy necessary to aerosolize the powder is provided by such means as compressed air or a battery. The year 2006 saw the first FDA approval of a DPI employing an active dispersion device. Although the mechanism employed in the active DPIs reduces the dependence on patient coordination to achieve inhaler actuation and particle size distribution, distribution of those particles in the lung is still suggested to be dependent on the patient's inspiratory flow rate and volume of inspiration (17,18).

DPIs have been utilized to administer drugs for both local and systemic purposes and are capable of delivering both small molecular weight and macromolecules (19). An advantage of conventional DPIs, when compared to MDIs, is the elimination of the need for synchronization of aerosol generation and patient inspiration (10). Development of the device itself may, however, be considered to be more involved than that of MDIs, as many DPIs are developed for use with a specific formulation. In contrast, aerosol generation via MDI is typically accomplished through a more generic "device," with the differences existing in the formulation itself. Differences in formulation, metering system, and dispersion mechanism all play a crucial role in the design of a DPI and it is important to note that formulations which may work in one device will not necessarily work in another device (10,19).

Traditionally, formulation methods have involved initial precipitation or crystallization from solution or spray drying, followed by milling to achieve the desired respirable particle size (19). In recent years, supercritical fluid technology for the preparation of particles has been an area of active research and recent advances have expanded the applicability of SCF technology to include such species as biopolymers and biomacromolecules, as well as small molecular drugs (see Chapter 44) (20–22). Advances in approved products employing DPI technology include several which allow less frequent dosing than conventional MDIs, due to their longer duration of action (19).

Historical as well as new challenges posed by technological advances exist for the development of DPIs. There is currently only one FDA approved excipient for dry powder products (23). Alternate materials which allow for controlled delivery and are suited for pulmonary administration are desirable; they do, however, necessitate thorough toxicological studies. Additionally, dissolution testing of modified-release technology and improved ability to predict DPI performance are the subjects of ongoing research (see Chapter 44).

Issues also remain for the formulation of protein powders for inhalation. Specifically, biochemical stability of proteins may be compromised during the production process. Typically, stabilization utilizing excipients such as carbohydrates have been employed. Conventional excipients may, however, not be ideal for use with all proteins and the investigation of alternatives is an area of active research. Furthermore, powder dispersibility is also required, but has typically been confounded by the formulation techniques employed to achieve biochemical stability. Methods to address these challenges are under development (see Chapter 47).

Nebulizers

Nebulizers, the third common pulmonary delivery technology currently in use, have found applicability in administering some types of drugs not available for use with MDIs or DPIs, as well as for those patients who may not be able to achieve adequate therapy with the more common systems. Indeed, for children, administration via nebulizer may be the only practical way to achieve efficacy. Furthermore, nebulizers are able to achieve the delivery of high doses of drug to the lung and typically allow a range of adjustments, making them applicable to a wide field of formulations. Conventional nebulizers are typically either of the jet or ultrasonic type, with the former being commercially dominant, and are suitable for administration of aqueous, as well as solvent:water solutions and suspensions, for water insoluble drugs (10).

Recent regulatory shifts have altered the nature of nebulizer and formulation development and approval. As discussed in the first edition of this book, FDA regulations which came into effect in the United States in 2002 require that all inhalation solutions for nebulization be sterile. This has increased the prevalence of single use nebulization solution containers, as they may be formulated without the addition of preservatives (10). Furthermore, the recognition of drug and nebulizer interactions, as well as differences in lung deposition achieved from device to device, has led to the approval of specific drug formulation nebulizer combinations. This shift of paradigm promises improvement of both efficacy and safety and products based on this philosophy continue to be developed (see Chapters 45 and 46).

Technology advances also are touching the nebulizer market. As is commonly known, the conventional nebulizer is not as easily transportable as are MDIs or DPIs and treatment times tend to be of significantly greater length. However, recent advances in piezoelectric and electromechanical systems have allowed great reductions in size and a corresponding increase in portability. These systems show promise to allow production of small portable nebulizers. Further, the development of technology which allows timing of aerosol delivery to the patient's inspiration affords improvement in the resultant lung deposition and decrease in waste of aerosol to the environment. The ability for healthcare professionals to better monitor patient usage data is also being incorporated into the newest generation of commercially available nebulizers, through the incorporation of a cradle and software which facilitates the download of data from the device (24) (see Chapters 45 and 46).

CONTEMPORARY APPROACHES TO CONVENTIONAL DELIVERY

The dominant delivery technologies for pulmonary administration of drugs continue to be the MDIs and DPIs. Traditional forms of these devices have been adequate for the dosing of medications with a large therapeutic index. The trend toward administration of an increasing array of drugs, however, has necessitated an increase in efficiency and a decrease in variability (10). Historical causes of variance, such as the dependence of efficacy on the synchronization of actuation and patient inspiration remain an issue of the traditional designs. New methods of reducing or eliminating this dependency are now successfully addressing this problem, while novel formulations enhance the absorption of poorly soluble drugs. Issues of patient compliance are being addressed through the inclusion of dose counting devices (see Chapter 49), as well as computerized patient data monitoring (see Chapter 45).

The 1987 Montreal protocol calls for an initial limit to the use of CFC propellants and an end to their utilization in the United States by 2009 (25,26). The ongoing phasing out of CFCs, as well as the desire to achieve systemic delivery, via pulmonary administration, of agents which may be unsuitable for oral delivery, such as gene medications, proteins and peptides, has contributed to the intensive research currently underway (10,27). The limited number of excipients approved for use in inhaled products, however, has posed challenges for formulation and reformulation alike (19). New methods of analysis, however, have facilitated improved testing of propellant systems in the MDI device (28–30). Despite the acknowledged challenges, the potential to achieve locally high therapeutic doses, while avoiding systemic exposure of drugs with undesirable side effect profiles has further added to the interest in pulmonary drug delivery.

Efficient delivery of drugs via the pulmonary route and decreased waste to the environment is of concern due to not only the cost associated with the medications, in particular some of the newer biologics, but also to minimize exposure of caregivers. Specific efforts to address these issues are underway and mean lung deposition via the newest generation of nebulizers has been reported to exceed 60%, with exhaled fractions of 1% or less; these compare favorably to conventional nebulizers, with typical waste during exhalation exceeding 50% (31–33). Similar deposition has also been accomplished with inhalers incorporating Soft Mist™ technology (see Chapters 45 and 48). Clinical data have shown plasma concentrations in the systemic circulation greater than 90% of the emitted dose for model species, using a novel electromechanical inhalation drug delivery system (34,35) (see Chapter 43). Similar improvements to the delivery of drugs have been made in other areas, as well.

The large surface area of the peripheral lung, offering the potential for systemic absorption of drugs, coupled with the ability to design formulations for localized therapy, has made the pulmonary delivery of medications an area of intensive research. Additionally, agents that may be unsuited for alternative dosing regimens, such as those with low oral bioavailability, or providing undesirable side effect profiles when administered systemically, have the potential to be successfully administered via inhalation. For some treatments, traditional administration techniques may be suboptimal with regard to patient convenience and compliance and the ability to offer such alternatives as needle free delivery is highly attractive.

Recent advances in delivery systems include the development of propellant free devices incorporating alternate aerosolization mechanisms (see Chapter 48), as well as those which employ both an electromechanical device and complementary dosage form, helping to optimize efficiency, reduce variability, and enhance stability upon long-term storage of the active drug substance (see Chapter 43). Improvement in the design of nebulizer systems, affording the ability to monitor and coordinate aerosol delivery to the breathing pattern of the patient has resulted in enhanced lung deposition, decreased waste to the environment upon exhalation and improved patient compliance (see Chapter 45). Specific technologies designed to more closely replicate the endogenous release of substances such as insulin, illustrate the potential for pulmonary delivery to not only replace traditional methods of administration for currently approved drugs, but to improve upon their action via this delivery method (see Chapter 51). Other techniques involve the advanced engineering of the process technology or the formulation itself, and a decreasing dependence on the device to produce efficient deposition (see Chapter 50). The FDA approval of Exubera®, a macromolecule DPI product for the administration of insulin in 2006 has paved the way for advances in pulmonary delivery on many fronts. Indeed, clinical trials are ongoing for multiple drugs employing this technology platform (see Chapters 44 and 50). Indeed, while many medications currently under investigation for pulmonary delivery are commonly commercially available employing other delivery methods, this route of administration is garnering increasing attention for its potential to facilitate the delivery of antigens, genes, and nucleic acids (19).

MODIFIED RELEASE APPROACHES TO DELIVERY

The therapeutic possibilities of administering medications for both local and systemic activity via the lung are greatly enhanced by the potential for the development of controlled release formulations. Although currently marketed HFA-MDI based products rely on the pharmacokinetic properties and biological response of the active drug substance (i.e., half-life, receptor binding) to afford once daily dosing, the development of controlled release formulations is an area of active and intense research. One such approach involves the use of oligolactic acid, a novel excipient which is biodegradable and biocompatible, to achieve sustained release (see Chapter 49). Furthermore, controlled-release formulations which have shown early stage positive results in other treatment modalities are presently undergoing testing in pulmonary delivery applications. A theme of these formulations is the use of biocompatible and biodegradable excipients.

One of the noted challenges of developing controlled-release formulations for pulmonary administration is the different residence time of these formulations, depending on where in the lung they are deposited. Specifically, different clearance mechanisms are present in different parts of the respiratory tract, thereby resulting in varying duration of effective drug levels (36). This characteristic may, however, also be used to therapeutic advantage, through the rational selection and design of formulations for sustained release. Another consideration which must be taken into account is the need to avoid undesirable buildup of excipients in the lung, caused by slow clearance of these carrier species. A clear understanding of the kinetics involved and the clearance mechanisms at work is necessary to allow proper design of the formulation.

CONCLUSIONS

The ability to administer agents for both local and systemic activity has continued to stimulate keen interest in pulmonary drug delivery. We have seen formulation and device technology advances, resulting in increased efficiency of delivery, decreased waste, and the ability to better replicate endogenous release of critical biochemicals. The dependence on patient coordination and technique to achieve efficacy has also been minimized by the latest developments.

Two philosophical approaches are evident from the newest devices and formulations. The first is the development of unique drug–device combinations, which are optimized through specificity; the second is the development of device technology platforms, which may be tailored for the administration of a wide array of drugs. Both of these approaches have merit and it is proposed that, indeed, they may have a complementary relationship in the therapy of the patient. Finally, the ongoing development of controlled-release formulations affords great potential for both patient convenience and more consistent therapeutic drug levels.

REFERENCES

1. Gonda I. Targeting by deposition. In: Hickey AJ, ed. Pharmaceutical Inhalation Aerosol Technology. New York: Marcel Dekker, 1992: 61–82.
2. Gonda I. Physico-chemical principles in aerosol delivery. In: Crommelin DJA, Middha KK, eds. Topics in Pharmaceutical Sciences 1991. Stuttgart: Medpharm Scientific Publishers, 1992: 95–115.
3. Gonda I. Particle deposition in the human respiratory tract. In: Crystal RG, West JB. The Lung: Scientific Foundations, 2nd ed. Philadelphia: Lippincott-Raven, 1997: 2289–94.
4. Stahlhofen W, Gebhart J, Heyder J. Experimental determination of the regional deposition of aerosol particles in the respiratory tract. Amer Ind Hyg Assoc J 1980; 41:385–98.
5. Fuchs NA. Evaporation and Droplet Growth in Gaseous Media. Oxford: Pergamon Press, 1962: 1–37.
6. Chew NYK, Chan HK. Effect of humidity on the dispersion of dry powders. In: Dalby RN, Byron PR, Farr SJ, eds. Respiratory Drug Delivery VII. Raleigh: Serentec Press, 2000: 615–7.

7. Palmes ED, Altschuler B, Nelson N. Deposition of aerosols in the human respiratory tract during breath holding. In: Davies CN, ed. Inhaled Particles and Vapours II. New York: Pergamon Press, 1967: 339–49.

8. Morrow PE, Yu CP. Models of aerosol behavior in airways. In: Moren F, Newhouse MT, Dolovich MB, eds. Aerosols in Medicine. Amsterdam: Elsevier, 1985: 149–91.

9. Christensen WD, Swift DL. Aerosol deposition and flow limitation in a compliant tube. J Appl Physiol 1986; 60: 630–7.

10. Gonda I, Schuster J. Pulmonary delivery of drugs by inhalation. In: eds. Modified Release Drug Delivery Technology, 1st ed. New York: Marcel Dekker, 2003: 807–15.

11. Dalby RN, Tiano SL, Hickey AJ. Medical devices for the delivery of therapeutic aerosols to the lung. In: Hickey AJ, ed. Inhalation Aerosols: Physical and Biological Basis for Therapy. New York: Marcel Dekker, 1996: 441–73.

12. June DS, Schultz RK, Miller NC. A conceptual model for the development of pressurized metered-dose hydrofluoroalkane-based inhalation aerosols. Pharm Tech 1994; October: 40–52.

13. Pritchard JN, Genova P. Adapting the pMDI to deliver novel drugs: insulin and beyond. In: Dalby RN, Byron PR, Peart J, et al., eds. Respiratory Drug Delivery X. River Grove : Davis Healthcare International Publishing, 2006:133–41.

14. Lewis DA, Meakin BJ, Bramhilla G. New actuators versus old: reasons and results for actuator modifications for HFA solution MDIs. In: Dalby RN, Byron PR, Peart J, et al., eds. Respiratory Drug Delivery X. River Grove: Davis Healthcare International Publishing, 2006: 101–10.

15. Fisons Corporation. Intal (cromolyn sodium) a monograph. Rubin LD. Bedford, Massachusetts: s.n., 1973: 173.

16. Ganderton D, Kassem NM. Dry powder inhalers. In: Ganderton D, Jones T, eds. Advances in Pharmaceutical Sciences. London: Academic Press, 1992: 165–91.

17. Farr SJ, Rowe AM, Rubsamen R, et al. Aerosol deposition in the human lung following administration from a microprocessor controlled pressurized metered dose inhaler. Thorax 1995; 50: 639–44.

18. Hill M, Vaughan L, Dolovich M. Dose targeting for dry powder inhalers. In: Dalby RN, Byron PR, Farr SJ, eds. Respiratory Drug Delivery V. Buffalo Grove: Interpharm Press, 1996: 197–208.

19. Hickey AJ, Mansour HM. Formulation challenges of powders for the delivery of small molecular weight molecules as aerosols. In: Rathbone M, Hadgraft J, Roberts M, Lane M, eds. Modified Release Drug Delivery Technology, 2nd ed. New York: Informa Healthcare, 2007.

20. Chow AHL, Tong HHY, Chattopadhyay P, et al. Particle engineering for pulmonary drug delivery. Pharm Res 2007; 24(3): 411–37.

21. Chan HK. Dry powder aerosol delivery systems: current and future research directions. J Aerosol Med 2006; 19(1): 21–7.

22. Van Oort MM, Sacchetti M. Spray-drying and supercritical fluid particle generation techniques. In: Hickey AJ, ed. Inhalation Aerosols: Physical and Biological Basis for Therapy, 2nd ed. New York: Informa Healthcare U.S.A., Inc., 2007: 307–46.

23. U.S. FDA. Guidance for Industry: Metered Dose Inhaler (MDI) and Dry Powder Inhaler (DPI) Drug Products. Washington D.C.: U.S. FDA CDR, 1998.

24. Prince I, Denyer J, Nikander K. I-neb Insight: a new tool for monitoring inhaled medication use. In: Dalby RN, Byron PR, Farr SJ, et al., eds. Respiratory Drug Delivery X. Boca Raton: Davis Healthcare International Publishing, 2006: 769–72.

25. Montreal protocol on substances that deplete the ozone layers. Montreal Protocol 1987.

26. U.S. Food and Drug Administration. Use of ozone-depleting substances; removal of essential use designation, 2005.

27. Gonda I. The ascent of pulmonary drug delivery. J Pharm Sci 2000; 89: 940–5.

28. Gupta A. Myrdal PB. A novel method for the determination of solubility in aerosol propellants. J Pharm Sci 2004; 93(10): 2411–9.

29. Gupta A, Myrdal PB. Comparison of two methods to determine solubility of compounds in aerosol propellants. Int J Pharm Sci 2005; 292: 201–9.

30. Myrdal PB, Stein SW, Mogalian E, Hoye W, Gupta, A. Comparison of the TSI model 3306 impactor inlet with the Andersen Cascade Impactor: solution metered dose inhalers. Drug Dev Ind Pharm 2004; 30(8): 858–68.

31. Nikander K. Adaptive aerosol delivery: the principles. Eur Respir Rev 1997; 7: 385–7.

32. Denyer J, Nikander K, Smith NJ. Adaptive Aerosol Delivery (AAD) technology. Expert Opin Drug Deliv 2004; 1: 165–76.

33. Nikander K, Denyer J. Adaptive Aerosol Delivery (AAD) technology. In: Rathbone M, Hadgraft J, Roberts M, Lane M, eds. Modified Release Drug Delivery Technology, 2nd ed. New York: Informa Healthcare, 2007: Pages.

34. Ward ME, Woodhouse A, Mather LE. Morphine pharmacokinetics after pulmonary administration from a novel aerosol delivery system. Clin Pharmacol Ther 1997; 62: 596–609.

35. Dershwitz M, Walsh J, Morishige R. Pharmacokinetics and pharmacodynamics of inhaled versus intravenous morphine in healthy volunteers. Anesthesiology 2000; 93: 619–28.

36. Gonda I. Drugs administered directly into the respiratory tract: modeling of the duration of effective drug levels. J Pharm Sci 1998; 77: 340–6.

42

AERx®Pulmonary Drug Delivery Systems

David C. Cipolla and Eric Johansson

Aradigm Corporation, Hayward, California, U.S.A.

INTRODUCTION

Delivery of aerosolized drugs to the lungs presents significant opportunities, both for the topical treatment of lung disease; e.g., cystic fibrosis, asthma, Chronic Obstructive Pulmonary Disease, pulmonary hypertension, and lung cancer, and for the noninvasive delivery of systemically active compounds; e.g., insulin, apomorphine, and parathyroid hormone. Unlike other noninvasive methodologies, such as transdermal techniques, delivery via the lung takes advantage of a physiological "portal of entry" to the systemic circulation (1).

A number of constraints need to be satisfied in order to achieve efficient and reproducible delivery systems that comply with regulatory demands, are reasonably "patient-friendly" and are economically viable. Aradigm Corporation has been developing a family of pulmonary delivery systems (2) with these constraints in mind. To avoid the oropharynx and more central airways, particle diameters less than approximately 3.5 μm must be generated (3). Particle sizes can be affected by hygroscopic growth (4,5), and high relative humidity can cause significant increase in particle diameter on time scales similar to transit times for aerosols through the oropharynx and bronchial airways (6). Efficient deposition with a minimum amount of exhaled aerosol requires particles larger than approximately 1 μm (7), while regional deposition of aerosols is also affected by inhalation flow rate (8). Additionally, the U.S. Food and Drug Administration has mandated that liquid aerosol delivery systems utilize sterile dosage forms (9). This monograph describes a platform of unit dose liquid aerosol delivery technologies, the AERx® electromechanical system (2,10), and the AERx Essence® all-mechanical system (11,12).

THE AERx® SYSTEM

The AERx Essence aerosol drug delivery system was developed to efficiently deliver topical and systemically active compounds to the lung in a convenient manner while reducing variability through features ensuring proper user technique (12). A single use, disposable dosage form, the AERx Strip®, ensures sterility and robust aerosol generation. This dosage form is placed into the durable, reusable device for delivery. An early version of a single dose disposable system called AERx Ease® has also been described (13).

THE AERx STRIP® DOSAGE FORM

The AERx dosage form (Fig. 1) is a multi-layer laminate designed to both ensure the stability of the pharmaceutical compound on storage, and also to facilitate the robust generation of the aerosol (14). The formulation is packaged in a blister layer consisting of polymer components that ensure stability of the pharmaceutical compound and also provide a barrier to the loss of water during storage. This feature is particularly important for products designed to be stored and used at room temperature. An AERx product under development for its potential to treat asthma, hydroxy-chloroquine, was shown to have acceptable stability out to twelve months at

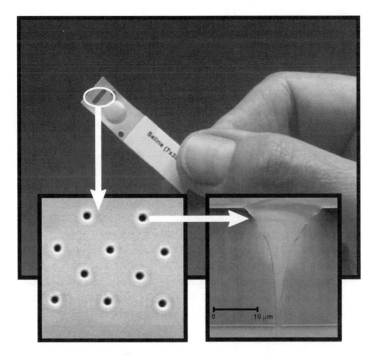

Figure 1 The AERx® dosage form, nozzle array, and cross-section image.

controlled room temperature (15) and this has now been extended to 24 months with less than a 5% increase in drug concentration due to loss of water. A foil overwrap could be used to provide even greater stability, if desired.

The AERx Strips dosage forms can accommodate a variety of formulations and excipients. Although aqueous-based formulations are generally preferred, for drugs which are unstable in water or poorly water soluble, e.g., testosterone, cosolvents such as ethanol have been used to improve their solubility (16). The AERx device has also been shown to reproducibly generate aerosols of optimized nanosuspension formulations with only a slight reduction in aerosol performance (17).

After the formulation is dispensed into the blister, a multi-layer laminate is heat sealed to the top of the blister. This laminate, in addition to providing the same storage and stability functions as the blister layer, also contains a single use disposable nozzle array. This nozzle array consists of hundreds of approximately one μm diameter (or smaller) holes laser micromachined into a polymer film (Fig. 1).

Prior to filling, the formulation is filtered to remove particulates. This, combined with the single use nature of the nozzle array, ensures that the aerosol generation process is not affected by nozzle blockage from particulates or dried formulation. The patient uses a pristine nozzle with every dose.

THE AERx® FAMILY OF DEVICES

Aradigm developed a family of devices for use with the AERx Strip dosage form. The first generation device, currently being used for the delivery of insulin, is a battery-powered, hand-held, electromechanical device designed for extremely precise systemic drug delivery. The device incorporates many features designed to eliminate possible causes of dosing irreproducibility. In order to eliminate variability due to uncontrolled inhalation rate, the device prompts, and trains the subject to inhale at the optimal rate by presenting multi-colored, flashing, and steady light emitting diodes. In addition to monitoring the inhalation flow rate, the device calculates an inhaled volume, and will only trigger the generation of aerosol if the inhalation rate is in the best range during a predetermined time early in the inspiration, a technique that has been previously shown to optimize lung deposition (18). When the patient achieves this optimum flow/volume "window," an electronically controlled motor actuates a piston, which pressurizes the formulation blister in the dosage form. When the formulation is pressurized, the heat seal peels open in a controlled region, and the formulation flows from the blister through the nozzle array, forming an aerosol. This aerosol is then entrained in the patient's inhalation air, and is delivered to the lungs.

In order to generate an optimal aerosol size distribution across the range of expected in use ambient conditions, the device provides an air temperature controlling module (19). This module is electrically preheated prior to the drug delivery event. During inspiration, the inhalation air is drawn through the module, thereby warming the air. Because the air is warmed, the aerosol generation always occurs in conditions of low relative humidity, reducing the possibility of hygroscopic growth (20).

There are many additional features that can be incorporated into this AERx platform, depending on the requirements of the therapy. For asthma and other lung diseases, an integrated instrument has been developed to measure indicators of lung function such as peak flow or FEV_1 (21). Compliance to critical dosing regimens can be ascertained with onboard memory that records the time and date of dosing event, along with other relevant dosing information. Applications such as pain management that require a greater number of doses followed by a predetermined lockout period can be accommodated. Use by a non-patient can be prevented with a patient identification feature which disables the device until a special patient ID bracelet is placed in contact with the device.

One particularly unique feature of this AERx platform is the ability to titrate fractional doses from a single dosage form (22). This is accomplished by controlling the stroke of the piston, and retracting it when the desired dose is achieved. This feature is valuable when the dose delivered needs to be tightly controlled, and varies in time or between patients. An example is the control of diabetes with insulin (23). The required dose can vary with such factors as measured blood glucose level, expected food intake, and body weight. Unlike any other aerosol drug delivery system, this feature allows the AERx system to deliver controlled fractions of the dosage form contents in accurate ten percent increments (20).

Aradigm also developed an all-mechanical, second-generation device platform called AERx Essence (Fig. 2). This device is intended for both systemic and precision topical delivery applications. While this device does not offer all of the features of the electromechanical AERx devices, key advances have allowed this design to offer very similar aerosol performance in a light, palm-size device (24). This mechanical AERx Essence device incorporates features to synchronize the delivery to the start of inhalation and then controls the flow rate during inhalation. The device is also designed to operate at half the flow rate of the first generation system; i.e., 30 LPM, making it well suited for younger patient populations. Preliminary in vitro performance of the AERx Essence platform has been shown to be reproducible with emitted aerosol from an individual device averaging $60.0 \pm 2.1\%$ (Fig. 3, $n = 40$ strips) and $58.8 \pm 2.8\%$ across four devices ($n = 40$ strips, 10 per device, data not shown). The fine particle fraction less than $4.95\,\mu m$ is 90% (data not shown), resulting in a predicted fine particle dose (ED × FPF) of approximately 54%. We anticipate that high efficiency and reproducibility will also be manifested in human clinical trials, as the key parameters affecting respiratory tract deposition—particle size,

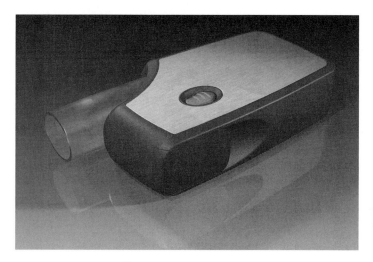

Figure 2 The AERx® Essence device.

actuation of delivery at a predetermined part of inspiration, and inspiratory flow rate, are well controlled.

CLINICAL DATA

The electromechanical AERx system has been tested in the clinic with a wide variety of small molecule (15,16,25), protein and peptide drugs (26–30), gene

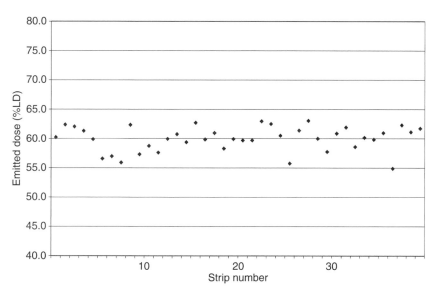

Figure 3 In vitro emitted dose performance of AERx® Essence.

vectors (31), and diagnostic agents (32,33). Pharmacokinetic studies with morphine sulfate (34,35) are illustrative of the potential capabilities of the technology. Peak plasma concentrations are achieved in less than 1 minute following inhalation, and greater than 90% of the morphine emitted from the device appears in the systemic circulation. Plasma concentration profiles are indistinguishable from intravenous injection (20).

Another well studied application of the AERx system is the delivery of human insulin for the management of diabetes (36,37). Clinical data show that glycaemic control similar to subcutaneous injection is achievable. However, minimum glycaemic levels are achieved in approximately 1 hour, versus approximately 2 hours for a subcutaneous injection. This rapid response is more similar to the gluco-dynamics in non-diabetics, and will allow insulin dosing at meal time, as opposed to dosing 30–60 minutes prior to meals, as is presently required with injections. Additionally, depth of inhalation has been shown to have a significant effect on insulin bioavailability (38), suggesting the need for breath control such as that demonstrated with the AERx system (20). An early prototype of AERx Essence was evaluated in gamma scintigraphic studies and demonstrated lung deposition consistent with the predicted fine particle dose (24).

CONCLUSIONS

Delivery of drugs by aerosol inhalation presents a significant opportunity for rapid, reproducible, noninvasive therapy. The AERx platform of devices takes advantage of this opportunity by optimizing aerosol characteristics, patient compliance with the correct breathing pattern, and by removing sensitivity to ambient conditions in the electromechanical versions of the devices. Clinical data with the AERx technology have shown that inhalation therapy is capable of reproducing, or in some cases improving upon, pharmacokinetics is following injections.

REFERENCES

1. Taylor G. The absorption and metabolism of xenobiotics in the lung. Adv Drug Deliv Rev 1990; 5:37–61.
2. Schuster J, Rubsamen R, Lloyd P, et al. The AERx™ aerosol delivery system. Pharm Res 1997; 14:354–7.
3. Task Group on Lung Dynamics, Deposition and retention models for internal dosimetry of the human respiratory tract. Health Phys 1996; 12:173–207.
4. Phipps PR, Gonda I, Anderson SD, et al. Regional deposition of saline aerosols of different tonicities in normal and asthmatic subjects. Eur Resp J 1994; 7:1474–82.
5. Ferron G, Kreyling W, Haider J. Inhalation of salt aerosol particles-II. Growth and deposition in the human respiratory tract. J Aerosol Sci 1987; 19:611–31.

6. Fuchs NA. Evaporation and Droplet Growth in Gaseous Media. Oxford: Pergamon Press,. 1962: 1–37.

7. Byron P. Prediction of drug residence times in regions of the human respiratory tract following aerosol inhalation. J Pharm Sci 1986; 75:433–8.

8. Hinds WC. Aerosol Technology. New York: Wiley, 1982: 211–31.

9. Draft Guidance for Industry, Nasal Spray and Inhalation Solution, Suspension, and Spray Drug Products, Chemistry, Manufacturing and Controls Documentation. U.S. Department of Health and Human Services, Food and Drug Administration, Center for Drug Evaluation and Research. 1999:8.

10. Schuster J, Farr SJ, Cipolla DC, et al. Design and performance validation of a highly efficient and reproducible compact aerosol delivery system: AERx™, In: Dalby RN, Byron PR, Farr SJ. eds. Respiratory Drug Delivery VI. Buffalo Grove: Interpharm Press. 1998: 83–90.

11. Schuster J, et al. New AERx In-Vivo Results. ISAM 13th Congress, Interlaken 2001.

12. Noymer P, Schuster J, Holst P, et al. AERx Essence: Efficiency and breath control without electronics. In: Dalby RN, Byron PR, Peart J, Suman JD, Farr SJ. eds. Respiratory Drug Delivery VI. Red Grove: Davis Healthcare International Publishing, 2004: 255–62.

13. Schuster J, Ament B, Walsh M, et al. Development of a novel single dose inhaler. In: Dalby RN, Byron PR, Peart J, Suman JD, Farr SJ, eds. Respiratory Drug Delivery X, River Grove: Davis Healthcare International Publishing, 2006: 417–20.

14. Farr SJ, Schuster J, Lloyd J, et al. AERx–development of a novel liquid aerosol delivery system: Concept to clinic. In: Dalby RN, Byron PR, Farr SJ. eds. Respiratory Drug Delivery V. Buffalo Grove: Interpharm Press, 1996: 175–85.

15. Dayton F, Owen S, Cipolla D, et al. Development of an inhaled hydroxy-chloroquine sulfate product using the AERx system to treat asthma. In: Dalby RN, Byron PR, Peart J, Suman JD, Farr SJ, eds. Respiratory Drug Delivery X, River Grove: Davis Healthcare International Publishing, 2006: 429–32.

16. Davison SL, Thipphawong J, Blanchard J, et al. Pulsed testosterone therapy: Pharmacokinetics and safety of inhaled testosterone in postmenopausal women. In: Programs & Abstracts, 84th Annual Meeting of the Endocrine Society. The Endocrine Society Poster no. P3–43. 2002: 504.

17. Shekunov B, Chattopadhyay P, Yim D, et al. AERx aerosol properties of drug-lipid nanosuspensions produced using supercritical fluid extraction of emulsions (SFEE) In: Dalby RN, Byron PR, Peart J, Suman JD, Farr SJ, eds. Respiratory Drug Delivery X. River Grove: Davis Healthcare International Publishing, 2006: 609–12.

18. Farr SJ, Rowe A, Rubsamen R, et al. Aerosol deposition in the human lung following administration from a microprocessor controlled pressurized metered dose inhaler. Thorax 1995; 50:639–44.

19. Schuster J, McKinley G, Lloyd P, et al. Developing systems for aerosol drug delivery that are independent of ambient conditions. Abstracts of the Aerosol Societies Drug Delivery to the Lungs X. London, 1999: 147–50.

20. Schuster J, Farr SJ. The AERx Pulmonary Drug Delivery System. In: Rathbone M, Hadgraft J, Roberts M, Lane M, eds. Modified Release Drug Delivery Technology. Informa Healthcare, 2002.
21. Gonda I, Schuster J, Rubsamen R, et al. Inhalation delivery systems with compliance and disease management capabilities, J Control Rel 1998; 53:269–74.
22. Schuster J, Hasegawa D. Dose titration with the AERx® system. Abstracts of the Aerosol Societies Drug Delivery to the Lungs XI. London. 2000:68–71.
23. Lasker RD. The diabetes control and complications trial, implications for policy and practice. New Eng J Med 1993; 329:1035–6.
24. Farr SJ, Schuster JA, Holst P, et al. Utilizing mechanical and nano-technology approaches to optimize bolus liquid aerosol delivery from AERx. Abstracts of the ISAM 15th Congress, Perth, Australia. J Aerosol Med 2005; 18:1, 88.
25. Mather LE, Woodhouse A, Elizabeth Ward M, et al. Pulmonary administration of aerosolised fentanyl: Pharmacokinetic analysis of systemic delivery, Brit J Clin Pharmacol 1998; 46:37–43.
26. Mudumba S, Khossravi M, Yim D, et al. Delivery of rhDNase by the AERx® pulmonary delivery system, In: Dalby RN, Byron PR, Farr SJ, Peart J, eds. Respiratory Drug Delivery VII. Buffalo Grove: Interpharm Press, 2000: 329–31.
27. Cipolla D, Boyd B, Evans R, et al. Bolus administration of INS365: Studying the feasibility of delivering high dose drugs using the AERx® pulmonary delivery system. In: Dalby RN, Byron PR, Farr SJ, Peart J, eds. Respiratory Drug Delivery VII. Buffalo Grove: Interpharm Press, 2000: 231–9.
28. Cipolla D, Farr SJ, Gonda I, et al. Pulmonary delivery and systemic absorption of a therapeutic protein using the AERx® system. J Aerosol Med 1997; 10:254.
29. Blanchard JD, Cipolla D, Liu K, et al. Lung deposition of interferon gamma-1b following inhalation via AERx® System and Respirgard II™ nebulizer. Am J Resp Crit Care Med 2003; 167(7):A373.
30. Sangwan S, Agosti JM, Bauer LA, et al. Aerosolized protein delivery in asthma: Gamma camera analysis of regional deposition and perfusion. J Aerosol Med 2001; 14(2):185–95.
31. Sorgi F, Gagne L, Sharif S, et al. Aerosol gene delivery using the AERx™ delivery system. Proc Int Symp Control Rel Bioact Mater 1998; 25:184–5.
32. Chan H, Daviskas E, Eberl S, et al. Deposition of aqueous aerosol of technetium-99 m diethylene triamine penta-acetic acid generated and delivered by a novel system, AERx®, in healthy subjects. Eur J Nucl Med 1999; 26:320–4.
33. Robinson M, Glass D, Bailey D, et al. Evaluation of a new aerosol delivery device, AERx™ for ventilation scans in patients with chronic obstructive airways disease, COAD. Resp Crit Care Med 1997; 155:A596.
34. Ward ME, Woodhouse A, Mather LE, et al. Morphine pharmacokinetics after pulmonary administration from a novel aerosol delivery system. Clin Pharmacol Ther 1997; 62:596–609.
35. Dershwitz M, Walsh J, Morishige R, et al. Pharmacokinetics and pharmacodynamics of inhaled versus intravenous morphine in healthy volunteers. Anesthesiology 2000; 93:619–28.

36. Farr S, McElduff A, Mather L, et al. Pulmonary insulin administration using the AERx® system: physiological and physicochemical factors influencing insulin effectiveness in healthy fasting subjects. Diabetes Tech Ther 2000; 2:185–97.
37. Clauson P, Balent B, Briunner G, et al. PK-PD of four different doses of pulmonary insulin delivered with the AERx® diabetes management system. In: Dalby RN, Byron PR, Farr SJ, Peart J, eds. Respiratory Drug Delivery VII. Buffalo Grove: Interpharm Press, 2000: 155–61.
38. Farr SJ, Gonda I, Licko V. Physicochemical and physiological factors influencing the effectiveness of inhaled insulin. In: Dalby RN, Byron PR, Farr SJ, eds. Respiratory Drug Delivery VI. Buffalo Grove: Interpharm Press, 1998: 25–33.

43

Formulation Challenges of Powders for the Delivery of Small Molecular Weight Molecules as Aerosols

Anthony J. Hickey and Heidi M. Mansour

School of Pharmacy, Division of Molecular Pharmaceutics, University of North Carolina-Chapel Hill, Kerr Hall-Dispersed Systems Laboratory, Chapel Hill, North Carolina, U.S.A.

INTRODUCTION

Those interested in the treatment of asthma have championed the use of dry powder inhalers (DPI) to deliver small molecular weight drug substances. One advantage of a DPI is that, unlike a pressurized metered dosed inhaler (pMDI), therapeutic administration requires minimal patient coordination to achieve inhaler actuation and drug delivery. Second, the use of a spacer is unnecessary with DPI delivery systems. Additionally, the propellant after-taste that patients often detect following pMDI inhalation is not present with DPI systems. The major therapeutic categories of compound delivered in this manner have been β_2-adrenergic agonists, corticosteroids, and other anti-inflammatories (mast cell stabilizers and leukotriene analogs) (1). The general structures of the major therapeutic categories of drug are shown in Figure 1 (2). Most of these drugs have molecular weights less than 1 kDa. Macromolecular drug delivery to the lungs has been defined to include molecules >5 kDa, with a window of opportunity for transport through the lung between 5 and 20 kDa (3). The transition from small molecular weight to large molecular weight may arbitrarily be designated to occur between 1 and 5 kDa.

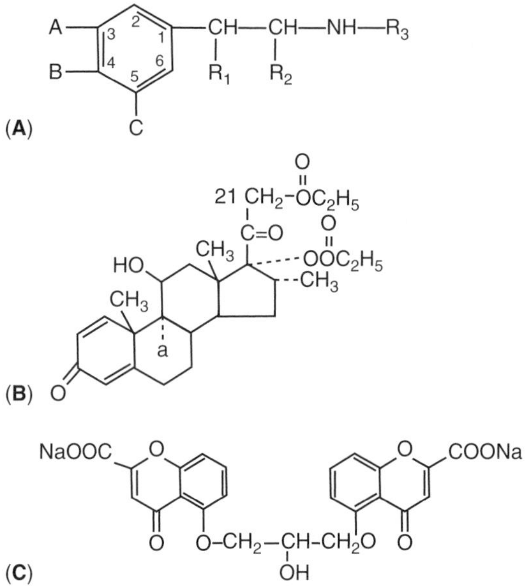

(A)

(B)

(C)

Figure 1 Chemical structures of **(A)** β-adrenergic agonist; **(B)** representative glucocorticoid (beclomethasone dipropionate); **(C)** disodium cromoglycate.

DPIs have been employed to deliver small molecular weight molecules and macromolecules for local and systemic absorption. In 2006, the first FDA-approved macromolecule (recombinant human insulin) DPI product, Exubera®, was introduced to the market. Its approval represents many firsts and milestones in pulmonary inhalation aerosol delivery. First, it does not employ large diluent particles and is, therefore, a carrier-free DPI drug delivery system that delivers a macromolecule in engineered particles in the solid-state for systemic absorption. Second, it represents the first and only FDA-approved DPI using an active dispersion device. Thus, the powder's dispersion is not dependent on the patient's inspiratory flow. While it lacks a traditional lactose carrier, it is important to recognize that the formulation contains excipients that do reach the lung. The solid-state amorphous insulin (α-helical protein conformation) formulation contains 60% insulin in a buffered sugar matrix (4). These excipients (sodium citrate dihydrate, mannitol, glycine, and sodium hydroxide) (5) are necessary for physical and chemical stability of the amorphous protein, enhance systemic absorption, and include buffers, salts, and mannitol.

The aim of this chapter is to discuss small molecular weight molecules. It is important to acknowledge that the scientific and particle engineering principles can be extended to small molecular weight molecules delivered for both systemic and local action. For the purpose of this review, comments will be restricted to molecules below 1 kDa and, within this range, biological molecules such as peptides and sugars will not be considered.

PATENT INFORMATION/STATUS

A number of small molecular weight compounds are available in the United States as dry powder products including disodium cromoglycate (Rhone-Poulenc Rorer), albuterol, fluticasone, salmeterol, Relenza (zanamivir, GlaxoWellcome), tiotropium, and budesonide (Astra-Zeneca). Other compounds are available elsewhere in the world, such as fenoterol (Boehringer Ingelheim) and terbutaline (Astra-Zeneca). Most of these drugs conform to the categories outlined earlier.

Since the publication of the First Edition, scientific and technological advances have been made and DPI pharmaceutical products approved. All of these new DPI products contain small molecular weight drugs and utilize passive devices which depend on a patient's peak inspiratory flow rate. Tables 1 and 2 list various common types of DPI devices and marketed DPI

Table 1 The Various Types of Common DPI Devices

Inhaler device name	Device manufacturer	Device power type
Unit dose (a capsule/ a blister with powder)		
Pulmonary Inhaler®	Nektar	Active device
Aerolizer®	Schering Plough	Passive device
Aerosolizer®	Novartis	Passive device
Cyclohaler®	Plastiope	Passive device
Handihaler®	Boehringer Ingelheim	Passive device
Inhalator®	Boehringer Inhelheim	Passive device
Rotahaler®	GlaxoSmithKline	Passive device
Spinhaler®	Aventis	Passive device
Multiple unit dose (multiple capsules or multiple blisters with powder)		
Accuhaler®	GlaxoSmithKline	Passive device
Diskhaler®	GlaxoSmithKline	Passive device
Diskus®	GlaxoSmithKline	Passive device
Eclipse®	Aventis	Passive device
Inhalator-M ® (Aerohaler®)	Boehringer Ingelheim	Passive device
Rotadisk®	GlaxoSmithKline	Passive device
Multidose (powder reservoir)		
Certihaler®	SkyePharma	Passive device
Clickhaler®	ML Labs	Passive device
Easyhaler®	Orion	Passive device
Novolizer®	ASTA Medica	Passive device
Pulvinal®	Chiesi	Passive device
Turbuhaler®	AstraZeneca	Passive device

Table 2   Currently Marketed DPI Products

DPI product name (manufacturer)	Pulmonary drug(s)	Carrier/excipients
Unit dose (a capsule/ a blister with powder)		
Exubera® (Pfizer marketed/Nektar innovation)	Amorphous rh-insulin (recombinant human)	Sodium citrate dihydrate, mannitol, glycine, and sodium hydroxide (no lactose monohydrate carrier)
Foradil Aerolizer® (Schering Plough)	Formoterol fumarate	Lactose monohydrate carrier
Spiriva Handihaler® (Boehringer Ingelheim)	Tiotropium bromide monohydrate	Lactose monohydrate carrier
Multiple unit dose (multiple capsules or multiple blisters with powder)		
Advair Diskus® (GlaxoSmithKline)	Fluticasone propionate/ Salmeterol	Lactose monohydrate carrier
Flovent Diskus® (GlaxoSmithKline)	Fluticasone dipropionate	Lactose monohydrate carrier
Flovent Rotadisk® (GlaxoSmithKline)	Fluticasone dipropionate	Lactose monohydrate carrier
Flovent Rotadisk® (GlaxoSmithKline)	Fluticasone propionate	Lactose monohydrate carrier
Relenza Rotadisk® (GlaxoSmithKline)	Zanamivir	Lactose monohydrate carrier
Serevent Diskus® (GlaxoSmithKline)	Salmeterol xinafoate	Lactose monohydrate carrier
Multidose (powder reservoir)		
Pulmicort Turbuhaler® (AstraZeneca)	Budesonide	No lactose monohydrate carrier

products, respectively (6,7). Interestingly, all of the approved DPI products are generally well, accepted by patients and have a significantly longer duration of action resulting in once-daily (e.g., Spiriva®) or twice-daily (e.g., Advair®) dosing (as opposed to 4–6 times daily with their MDI counterparts).

Over the past several years there have been many patents on DPI design and a smaller number on formulation strategies issued in the United States, Europe, and Japan (www.patents.ibm.com). Most of the formulation and processing patents have dealt with macromolecules. A much smaller number of patents have covered the delivery of small molecular weight molecules.

Patents based on physicochemical properties such as aerodynamic performance (8), surface roughness of carrier particles (9) or controlled release properties (10) have been filed. Compositional patents on the use of salt (11), surfactants (12), complexation (13) and microcapsules (14) are also notable. Particle engineering and novel devices have been employed in recent DPI research and investigated for future applications (7,15–24).

HISTORICAL PERSPECTIVE

Modern DPI development was initiated in the 1960s and 1970s (25,26). However, it could be argued that the principles of powder dispersion that launched this technology had been in existence for many years. The principles employed in devices such as the Wright's dust feed (27) and fluidized bed aerosol generator (27) can be linked closely to inhaler designs (24).

The properties of fine particles have been studied in depth. The fundamental forces of interaction (28), methods of manipulation (29), and processing steps (30) have been described in detail. The performance of dry powders has also been scrutinized. The focus of these studies has been the measurement of powder properties such as flow and dispersion (31). Electrostatic properties (32–35) have been evaluated as both static bulk (36–38) and aerodynamic features (35,39–41) in DPIs.

The key elements of DPI systems are the formulation, the metering system, and the dispersion mechanism. Formulation approaches have historically involved precipitation or crystallization either from solution or upon spraying from a nozzle. Additional processing may have been required in the form of attrition milling to reduce the particle size to that suitable for delivery to the lungs.

Crystallization remains a major method of manufacture of particles. The two key features of crystals are their molecular, or lattice, arrangement, which can be described in terms of seven crystal systems (42,43). These crystal systems can be divided into 32 classes based on rotational symmetry or 230 space filling categories based on Miller indices and Bravais lattices (44). The size and shape of crystals is also dictated by the crystal habit (45–50). The crystal habit is derived from the nature of particle growth. Growth, or the incorporation of molecules into the lattice system, may occur in each of the three spatial dimensions. However, growth may be inhibited in any of these directions, which will give rise to different sizes and shapes of crystal. Notably, for cubic crystals this can result in large cubes (growth in all dimensions), plates (growth in two dimensions), and rods or fibers (growth in one dimension).

It should be recognized that partially ordered/disordered phases are generally important in solid-state pharmaceuticals and in DPI particles, in particular. These partially ordered/disordered phases may be process-induced or intelligently designed into the particle for enhanced favorable performance and therapeutic properties (e.g., enhanced solubility and bio-availability). These phases include nanocrystals (non-amorphous state lacking long-range order), liquid crystals, plastic crystals, and amorphous phases. The phase has been demonstrated to affect pulmonary absorption (51). The current interest in formulation and inhalation aerosol character-ization lies in adopting strategies leading to DPI performance prediction. There is a great need for DPI performance prediction based on a strategy of physical characterization of the static and dynamic properties of DPIs (35,45,52).

Three categories of metering system may be identified including unit (single) dose, multiple unit dose, and reservoir systems. Single dose and multiple unit dose metering systems are somewhat inconvenient for chronic disease therapies where several doses/day are required. However, these systems offer protection for the drug from ambient environmental con-ditions. Reservoir systems are more convenient for long-term therapy but pose potential stability concerns due to the repeated sampling from the drug reservoir, which allows contact with the environment. Moisture ingress is the most significant potential disadvantage of such a system, which may be accompanied by microbial growth and changes in aggregation state due to capillary forces.

NEED FOR THE TECHNOLOGY

There have been many stimuli to the continuous development of DPIs over the last 40 years. Initially, the desire to have a handheld bolus dose delivery system that did not use propellants for commercial reasons led to powder systems. There are also a small number of patients who respond poorly to propellant-driven metered-dose inhaler delivery of aerosols. In recent years, there have been two overwhelming influences for the move towards DPIs. The 1987 Montreal Protocol (53) initially limiting the use of chloro-fluorocarbon propellants and ultimately banning them in the United States by 2009 (54) because of their contribution to atmospheric ozone depletion made alternatives a key to the future success of pulmonary drug delivery (55). The need to deliver the products of biotechnology was an additional influence. Therapeutic proteins, peptides, antigens, and nucleic acids are not easily delivered by conventional routes of administration and, consequently, the lungs have been evaluated for this purpose.

The deep lung, where gas exchange occurs by passive diffusion, pro-vides a very large surface area for absorption due to its highly permeable cell layer of the alveoli, thereby potentially providing "instantaneous" absorption. Additionally, pulmonary delivery of therapeutic peptides and biopolymers (e.g., polypeptides, antigens, genes, and nucleic acids) is advantageous in potentially providing a longer duration of action due to bypassing the "first-pass effect" by the hepatic clearance metabolic pathway. Hence, much research is currently being conducted in using targeted pulmonary delivery for systemic treatment of chronic diseases and acute infections and in the development of needle-free vaccines for a variety of infectious diseases having a global impact.

DIFFERENCES FROM RELATED TECHNOLOGIES

Dry powder preparation for the delivery of small molecular weight molecules has been limited predominantly to airjet milling and spray drying. Over the past several years (17,23,56–60), an increased interest in supercritical fluid (SCF) manufacture of microparticles and nanoparticles has arisen that may ultimately lead to an ability to control more precisely the form of the particles produced. New methods may employ monodisperse nanoparticle technologies for potential use in nanomedicine applications (61).

The most closely associated technologies to DPIs are pMDI and nebulizers. Solution formulations delivered from pMDIs or nebulizers are immediately available for action or absorption. Suspension pMDI formulations deliver particles associated with any added excipients to the lungs. Dry powders are most closely related to these suspensions in terms of disposition from the lungs. It has been suggested that the efficient inhaler performance potentially improves the therapeutic effect and potentially reduces adverse systemic effects, e.g., oral candidiasis associated with inhaled corticosteroids (62). Table 3 compares the performance of dry powders with other delivery systems from an aerosol dispersion perspective.

DESCRIPTION OF TECHNOLOGY

Airjet milling is achieved by opposing jets which bring large, unmilled, particles into contact with each other, fracturing them and creating smaller particles, as illustrated in Figure 2A (45,63). Cyclone separation of particles by aerodynamic size is a feature of jet mills. A fluidizing airstream continuously mills particles until they reach a specified size, which, depending on their density, is in the range ~1–10 μm. Once this size is achieved, particles are discharged on the airstream into a collection vessel. The conveyor air is discharged through a bag filter. The conditions of mass flow rate; type of gas (usually air or nitrogen) and gas pressure (input and opposing jets) can be adjusted to optimize the process of particle production.

Spray drying, an accelerated process of solidification from the liquid state, involves the introduction of solution or suspension through a nozzle at

Table 3 Major Differences Between Dry Powder Aerosols and Propellant
Driven Metered Dose Inhalers and Nebulizers; The Means of Delivery,
Energy of Dispersion (Velocity), Particle Size Delivered, and the Nature of
the Aerosol (Including Generalized Doses)

Device	Exit velocity	Particle size range (μm)	Concentration in air	Means of delivery to lungs
MDI	Fast (30 m/sec at the actuator orifice)	1–10	Bolus, variable density as plume develops (Dose 100 μg)	Active
DPI	Variable between devices	1–10	Dense bolus (Dose ~1–10 mg)	Active or passive
Nebulizer	Slow	0.5–5	Diffuse cloud (Dose ~100–200 μg/min)	Passive

high pressure into a heated container in which the solvent evaporates, as
illustrated in Figure 2B (60). The droplets dry as evaporation proceeds and
are transported to a cyclone separator and air discharge similar to the jet
mill described above. There are four stages in the spray drying process and
they include the following (64): (*i*) spray formation by feed solution atomization; (*ii*) contact of the spray with air by flow and mixing; (*iii*) solid
particle formation as the spray dries at an elevated temperature; and (*iv*)
collection of the solid particles from the gas stream. The conditions of solute
concentration, liquid feed solution type, feed flow rate, atomization pressure, drying airflow rate and inlet/outlet temperatures can be adjusted to
optimize the process of particle production and particle characteristics.
Additionally, surfactants can be added to the feed solution to affect the
surface properties of the final solid particles. Respiratory particles produced
by spray-drying are often smooth spheres with a median diameter between 1
and 5 μm, with a relatively narrow size distribution (64,65). Additionally,
spray-dried respirable particles are often partially or completely amorphous
due to the extremely rapid speed by which the solid state comes out of the
liquid state, thereby preventing thermodynamically stable crystals to
nucleate and grow. However, carefully controlling and optimizing the various operating parameters (inlet temperature, feed solution solvent type, and
the pH of the liquid feed) does allow for crystalline polymorph formation in
the absence of any amorphous phase, as detected by X-ray powder diffraction and differential scanning calorimetry, to occur in the final solid
particle. Due to the elevated drying temperatures, biomolecules may
undergo a loss of biological activity due to uncontrolled conformational
changes, denaturation, and/or chemical degradation, either of which leads

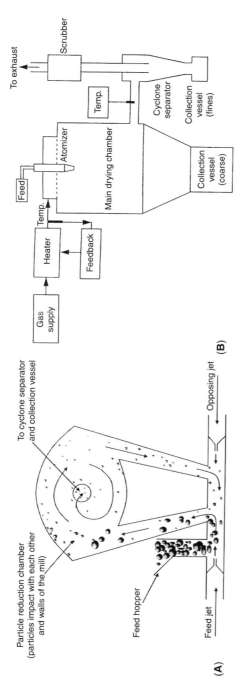

Figure 2 Schematic diagram of (**A**) airjet mill and (**B**) open system spray drier.

to therapeutic inactivity. Often, this problem can be circumvented through the incorporation of cryoprotectant sugars that maintain and stabilize the proper conformation by maintaining the intermolecular hydrogen bonds within the biomolecule as the water molecules (participating in these hydrogen bonds) are removed. If the use of cryoprotectants such as trehalose dihydrate or mannitol (e.g., insulin stabilization in Exubera) does not achieve biomolecular conformational stabilization, another type of spray drying, spray freeze drying (17), has been successfully used in engineering respirable particles; this technique will, however, not be discussed here.

SCF manufacture of particles was first investigated in the nineteenth century. In the twentieth century, SCF technology found a major application in chromatography. In the late 1980s and early 1990s, research was being conducted to further develop technologies in this area (60,66). In parallel, specific efforts were being made to utilize the principles in the manipulation of pharmaceutical solids (64,67–69), with the objective of preparing particles for inhalation (17,56–59,64,60,70,71). SCF technology is known to produce relatively monodisperse microparticles and nanoparticles. As illustrated in a typical thermodynamic phase diagram of any type of material (Fig. 3), a SCF is a single phase liquefied gas existing above its critical point, T_c.

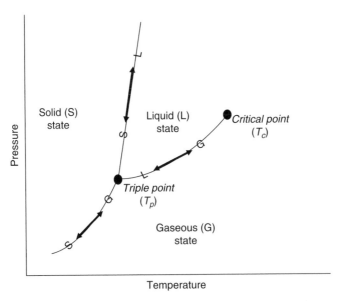

Figure 3 Phase diagram depicting the three states of matter (gaseous, liquid, and solid) and the SCF region. The gaseous, liquidus, and solidus phase boundary lines represent two-phase equilibria (coexistence). The triple point, T_p, represents the exact temperature and exact pressure where all three states of matter coexist in equilibrium. Above the critical point, T_c, the gas and liquid exist in a single phase as a liquefied gas. *Abbreviation*: SCF, supercritical fluid.

Hence, a SCF possesses advantageous properties of both its liquid (L) state and its gaseous (G) state. Some properties include the following (64): favorable solvation power; lower viscosity and higher diffusivity, which promote mass transfer and extraction of organic solvents; and near T_c, only a slight change in pressure or temperature provides careful precise control of the density and solvation power of a SCF, due to its high compressibility.

Solution-enhanced dispersion with supercritical fluids (SEDS) is a technology that always uses supercritical CO_2 (most pharmaceutical drugs are insoluble in this) as the solvent and has been successfully used in particle engineering of respirable powders (17,56,72). The particles generated are microparticles that are often crystalline. SEDS particle engineering has been successfully used in the formation of respirable albuterol sulfate/lactose (73) and budesonide/lactose blends (73), crystalline solid particles for corticosteroids, budesonide (74,75), and flunisolide (74). The SEDS drug/lactose blends exhibited reduced surface energy, improved powder homogeneity, better dose uniformity, and reduced electrostatic charges (73). Additionally, crystallization (76), polymorph control (77), polymorph separation, and pure polymorph selection can be achieved through SEDS.

A limitation of SEDS technology in multicomponent systems, such as a drug with an excipient, is that solid-state phase separation occurs. Moreover, agglomeration of the final particles has been observed, particularly when the components have surface activity or a mixture of amorphous and partially crystalline phases co-exist. Supercritical fluid extraction of emulsions (SFEE) takes advantage of relatively stable dispersed systems and using supercritical CO_2 to extract the organic phase of the emulsion or nanosuspension (17,78–80). Hence, multi-component pharmaceutical systems and drugs/excipients exhibiting amphiphilic character/surface activity are amenable to SFEE for respiratory particle generation without solid-state phase separation and/or agglomeration.

It is important to recognize that several variations of the SCF technology exist, and hence, the SCF technique is not limited to supercritical CO_2. Furthermore, these SCF technology variations greatly expand the utility of SCF technology to small molecular drugs (hydrophobic drugs, in particular), surfactant systems (e.g., emulsions and other colloidal dispersions), biopolymers, and biomacromolecules. Moreover, solid-state phase control can be achieved using other supercritical solvents, such that a range of solid-state phases in the final respirable particle can be designed, albeit, a crystal, a polymorph, a liquid crystalline, or an amorphous phase.

MECHANISM OF DRUG RELEASE

Dispersion

Small particles in the micron-size range are adhesive and cohesive. The mechanisms by which the drug particles are dispersed vary (7). Pneumatic, vibrational, or mechanical means may be employed to disperse particles (24,45,81–85). The most prominent method of dispersion is pneumatic, requiring the patient's breath to disperse the aerosol. Dispersion and delivery occurring in a single action characterize this mechanism. Active delivery devices utilizing compressed gas as a means of pneumatic dispersion do so independently of the patient's inspiratory flow and, consequently, separate the dispersion and delivery elements of inhaling aerosol particles.

Dissolution and Disposition

Dissolution occurs in the fluids within the lungs. The nature of these fluids differs depending on the region of the lung in which the aerosol deposits. Deposited particles will experience unstirred dissolution in the periphery of the lungs in the presence of lung surfactant, a monomolecular layer of a complex mixture of primarily phospholipids (90%) and surface-active proteins (10%), involved in maintaining the surface area for gaseous exchange, decreasing the work of breathing, regulating pulmonary immunity, including alveolar macrophage function and upregulation. In the conducting airways, particles will deposit in the stirred (by ciliary beat) thick mucus layers, which have a periciliary aqueous sublayer (86). Depending on the dissolution rate and surface characteristics of these particles, they will experience different dissolution phenomena in these regions of the lungs. Particles that dissolve slowly will be transported on the mucociliary escalator from the lungs and therefore have a finite period of time to release drugs in the lungs before expectoration or swallowing. Particles delivered to the periphery of the lungs may be phagocytosed by macrophages and experience the low pH and enzyme replete environment of the endosome and phago-lysosome (87). The disposition of drugs from the lungs has been discussed in detail by Byron (88) and Gonda (89,90).

Recently, the intensive effort investigating suitable and representative in vitro pulmonary cell culture models has been unveiled in a number of reviews (91–95). The A549 cell line is an in vitro cell culture model intended to represent the alveolar Type II pulmonary epithelial cell. The Calu-3 and HBE14o cell lines are in vitro models for the upper airways (bronchi). The A549 cell line (96–102), Calu-3 cell line (100,103–109), and HBE14o cultures (107,108,110,111) have been used in investigating the mechanisms of pulmonary drug absorption, transport, metabolism, and particle cell interactions. These are immortalized (continuous) cell lines possessing over expression of the P-glycoprotein (P-gp) efflux transporter, a cell membrane bound protein that actively pumps drugs out of the cell.

In an effort to use cells that are more phenotypically, morphologically, and biochemically similar to normal (noncontinuous) human pulmonary cells, a primary culture (rather than an immortalized cell line such as those mentioned previously) of human alveolar epithelial cells (99,100,107,

112–115) and pulmonary microvascular endothelial cells (101) have been used in pulmonary absorption and transport studies. Primary alveolar cell models exhibit tight junctions, and hence, are a potentially better representation of the in vivo barrier to drug absorption and transport from that of immortalized cell lines. In a recent pulmonary drug absorption and transport report (116), normal human bronchial epithelial cell monolayers at an air–liquid interface have been successfully cultured, characterized, and employed in airway drug absorption experiments.

In addition to airway epithelial cells, dendritic cells are intimately involved in pulmonary defense, immune homeostasis through cellular cross-talk, and airway inflammation for a number of pulmonary diseases (117). A novel in vitro method employs a triple co-culture model (118) of A549 cells, macrophages, and dendritic cells to decipher the biochemical mechanisms (CD14 for macrophages and CD86 for dendritic cells) of particle uptake.

Pulmonary biopharmaceutics research has also benefited from the use of ex vivo lung tissue models, namely, isolated perfused lung (IPL) from guinea pigs, rats, and rabbits. Isolated perfused rat lung (119–130) has been the IPL type most commonly used in these biopharmaceutics investigations.

RESEARCH AND DEVELOPMENT PERTAINING TO TECHNOLOGY

In Vitro Studies

In vitro studies have focused on particle size determination. The majority of DPI utilize passive dispersion of the aerosol particles. Inertial impaction is the most relevant method for the determination of particle size. The inertial, or cascade, impactor employs a defined flow rate at which it has been calibrated in terms of the aerodynamic diameter of spherical particles. This requirement renders effective evaluation of the particle size of passively dispersed dry powder aerosols difficult. A formal evaluation should be conducted over a range of selected flow rates (131,132) or over a continuously variable range of flow rates (133,134). Inertial impactors must be recalibrated for different flow rates (135). Continuously variable flow rates can be used but, since calibrations are meaningless under these conditions, the data obtained are only useful in relative terms.

Inability to deliver a complete or reproducible dose is the most significant effect of poor dispersion properties. Consequently, emitted doses must also be determined. The emitted dose will also depend upon the volumetric flow rate through the device for passive delivery systems. Both particle size determination and emitted dose are subject to compendial and regulatory specifications (136).

In Vivo Studies (Animals)

Dry powder delivery has been studied in a variety of species of animals. These studies include model compounds (137) and locally acting bronchodilators (31). Modified particles utilizing coatings (138,139) and unique aerodynamic properties (140–142) with steroid drugs have also been evaluated in animals. Tuberculosis drugs, rifampicin microspheres and para-aminosalicylic large porous particles, were administered by insufflation to guinea pigs (143) and rats (144), respectively. Albuterol sulfate large porous particles (145), and other investigational and marketed dry powder beta-2 adrenoreceptor agonists (146) have been administered to guinea pigs intratracheally. Liposomal encapsulated tobramycin DPI particles have been administered intratracheally to mice (147) following in vitro bactericidal evaluation in pseudomonas aeruginosa (148). Liposomal encapsulated non-steroidal anti-inflammatory drug DPI particles have also been given by intratracheal administration to rats (149). This range of studies demonstrates the utility of in vivo studies in evaluating a range of therapeutic agents delivered to the lungs in a range of species. However, caution should be exercised in selecting species whose lung function and biology are most relevant to the disposition and action of the drug under evaluation with respect to its ultimate use in man.

In Vivo Studies (Humans)

In recent years, many pharmacoscintigraphic (150) studies have been conducted to evaluate the site of deposition of dry powder in the human respiratory tract by combining drug substance with radiolabel [or sometimes radiolabeling the lactose carrier (151)] for the performance of gamma scintigraphy (21,152–165). In addition to using the common method of planar gamma camera scintigraphy, single photon emission computed tomography (SPECT) can be employed. SPECT generates three-dimensional imaging and has better detection sensitivity and, therefore, better analysis of regional deposition in the lung (166). Additionally, gamma scintigraphy may be potentially useful in abbreviating the clinical studies required in generic drug evaluation of DPI products. This technique has been demonstrated to help justify the dose selection used in pivotal clinical phase III trials for new DPIs with novel inhaler devices, based on those obtained for already approved DPI products with the same pulmonary drug (6). Moreover, pharmacoscintigraphic lung deposition data has functioned as a vital link between in vitro and clinical evaluations (167).

In Vitro–In Vivo Correlations

Correlations were demonstrated between dissolution properties and in vivo disposition of a model compound, disodium fluorescein, delivered as a dry powder aerosol in dogs (168). The ratio of the half-time for dissolution of coated particles to that of uncoated particles was shown to be remarkably close to similar ratios for the half-times for appearance in the plasma of dogs. On a more subtle level, it was predicted (169) that manipulation of the residence time of steroids in the lungs would lead to an improved targeting of lung receptors and this subsequently proved to be the case for a coated particulate formulation (138). Good correlation was reported with large porous particles (159).

MAJOR OBSTACLES ENCOUNTERED DURING RESEARCH AND DEVELOPMENT AND HOW THEY WERE OVERCOME

The variability in drug delivery as a function of inspiratory flow rate for passive inhalers has been seen as a potential obstacle to broad applicability of these devices. Active dispersion systems to achieve flow rate independence have been one approach to resolving this issue. However, an interesting solution has been proposed in which the formulation itself leads to device- and flow rate-independent in vitro performance. While this will inevitably vary from one drug to the next, some success has been achieved in this area by increasing the porosity of particles and thereby reducing the van der Waals forces of interaction (8,170,140). It must be remembered, however, that the deposition in the respiratory tract itself depends on inspiratory flow rate, and therefore, merely keeping the in vitro performance flow rate independent does not guarantee consistency of lung deposition, and clinical safety and efficacy. Device-independent formulations have been the subject of much research in recent years (84,85). Additionally, characterizing the aerodynamic properties of DPI systems, independent of a specific inhaler device, has been successfully attained through standardized entrainment tubes (171).

FABRICATION TECHNIQUES

It is often the case that particles cannot be manufactured easily without aggregating for a number of reasons. Aggregation may occur because of the fundamental forces of association occurring at the surfaces of particles, such as van der Waals, capillary forces, electrostatic forces or mechanical interlocking (structural cohesion) (28,35,45,52,172–176). These surface forces and interactions are significant in dry powder respiratory particles (i.e., microparticles and nanoparticles) which have large surface area-to-volume ratios. Gravitational forces become negligible in these size ranges and surface forces dominate, giving rise to strong interfacial interactions at the solid-solid interface existing between respirable particles. Additionally, pharmaceutical processing resulting in these respirable particles very often affects their surfaces by introducing "surface defects" having a higher surface free energy and often act as "active sites" for enhanced interparticulate interactions leading to aggregation. In addition, if particles have low melting points and high vapor pressures, they may deform on impact and aggregate to a larger extent on milling rather than being dispersed in small sizes.

Furthermore, particles of this nature, even when prepared as small particles, may cohere upon storage. In certain circumstances, these phenomena, as well as a tendency to be heat labile, may be overcome by low temperature milling. Any tendency to degradation by oxidation can be avoided by using inert gases rather than air as the milling fluid.

SCALE-UP PROBLEMS/MANUFACTURING ISSUES

The most serious problems in scale-up for conventional DPI are unit operations of milling, drying, blending, and filling (177,178). Pilot or large scale milling, spray drying, or blending require process optimization not unlike any other pharmaceutical unit operation being translated from the bench scale. It is important to recognize the importance of particle size distribution, crystallinity and polymorphism as output measures of the success of the process (179–181). These should be matched to products from earlier stages in the research and development process.

The filling of dry powders for aerosol products poses unique challenges. Since the total fill mass for a dry powder product may be individual milligram quantities, the dose to dose uniformity will be influenced by handling and dispensing of the powders. Most pharmaceutical manufacturers have developed individual filling systems based on their needs. Clearly, the most difficult filling process involves capsule and blister packaging. For blends which incorporate large quantities of excipient and are filled in totals of tens of milligrams, conventional capsule filling technology is sufficient. At individual milligram quantities, different solutions are required.

Since the dispersion properties of dry powder aerosols are dependent on maintaining primary particle sizes or stable aggregates, it is important that hygroscopic products are protected from water ingress. In this regard, the packaging material itself must be considered (182). It may be necessary to package capsules or blisters in aluminum to prevent moisture ingress altogether. For reservoir systems in which moisture will be expected to gain access, it may be necessary to utilize desiccant to reduce the local moisture content.

SPECIALIZED/UNIQUE REGULATORY ISSUES

Since the number of approved excipients for use in inhaled products is small, the formulation strategies are restricted. For dry powder products (183,184), the only U.S. FDA approved excipient α-lactose monohydrate. This disaccharide crystalline hydrate sugar is approved as a carrier material to help fluidize and disperse the drug and is not intended for delivery to the lungs. Consequently, to achieve controlled delivery of drugs in the lungs, other materials will be required. Some obvious choices include phospholipids, specifically lecithin, other sugars, amino acids (lysine, polylysine) and nonimmunogenic human serum albumin proteins (HSA). The use of novel materials in lung delivery will require thorough toxicological evaluation, which in turn necessitates investment of both time and money on the part of the pharmaceutical industry.

Dissolution testing is a key issue, which has yet to be addressed fully, with regard to modified-release technology. The size and surface area of particles delivered to the lungs and the environment in which they will dissolve pose a unique problem in the evaluation of their dissolution properties. Conventional dissolution studies call for the use of large volumes of dissolution media usually contained in even larger vessels and actively mixed to achieve conditions representative of those in the gastro-intestinal tract. Specific methods designed for the dissolution of particles rather than dosage forms have been adopted for aerosol products. Examples include recirculating (185) and single pass (168) small volume systems. However, these conditions remain distant from the physiological milieu to which aerosol products are exposed. Thus, novel systems must be evaluated and this will undoubtedly be an area of future development.

The bolus delivery of drug particles, dependent upon the breathing pattern of the patient, is not simply a volumetric flow event. Since the aerosol is dispersed on a single breath of the patient, the nature of the inspiratory flow cycle plays a role in powder dispersion and delivery. In this regard, the pressure drop, rate of change of linear velocity with respect to time, which is proportional to shear in the device, and total volume of air used are major contributors to the effective delivery of aerosol particles (186). Efforts have been made to harmonize the regulation of DPI products between the United States (183,184), Europe (187), and Japan.

FUTURE DEVELOPMENTS

Future developments in particle manufacture include the combination of previous techniques of manufacture with subtler drug delivery systems, such as microparticles, nanoparticles, and liposomes.

Liposomes are self-assembling structures in an aqueous environment forming colloidal dispersions having particles capable of existing in both the micron and nanometer size ranges. Their long-term physical and chemical stability in this state may not be suitable for broad applications in aerosol delivery of drugs. However, they may be prepared as freeze dried systems which can be airjet milled to produce particles that are stable on storage and can be used for a number of purposes (188–190). Spray drying of liposomes for pulmonary delivery has also been attempted and may be of interest in the future (191,192). Recently, jet-milled lyophilized liposomal powders suitable for aerosol delivery have been reported (147,193–196). Phospholipids have also been successfully incorporated into engineered particles containing pulmonary drug (18–21,197).

The advantages of coating in terms of reduced dissolution rate have been demonstrated (168,185,139). However, these studies used model coating materials with limited clinical potential. New coating technologies such as pulsed-laser ablation (138) may have more relevance to sustaining the residence time of drugs in the lungs. A laser beam impinges on a polymer surface, thereby releasing polymer molecules, which deposit on adjacent drug particles. This technique has the advantage of giving uniform coatings with small quantities of polymer, thereby maximizing the drug content.

Nanoparticle technology may also have a role to play in drug delivery to the lungs and for targeting specific immune cells, such as dendritic cells. The ability to prepare submicron dry powder particles would result in large surface areas, which would increase intrinsic solubility and dissolution rate, making the drug more readily available for action or absorption.

REFERENCES

1. Kaliner MA, Barnes PJ, Persson CGA, eds. Asthma, Its Pathology and Treatment. New York: Marcel Dekker, Inc. 1991.
2. Gringauz A. Introduction to Medicinal Chemistry: How Drugs Act and Why. New York: Wiley-VCH. 1997; 721.
3. Byron PR, Patton JS. Drug delivery via the respiratory tract. J Aerosol Med 1994; 7(1):49–75.
4. White S, Bennett DB, Cheu S, et al. EXUBERA: Pharmaceutical development of a novel product for pulmonary delivery of insulin. Diab Tech Ther 2005; 7 (6):896–906.
5. NDA 21-868/Exubera US Package Insert. ed.: Pfizer Labs. 2006; 1–24.
6. Newman SP. Drug delivery to the lungs from DPI. Curr Opin Pulmon Med 2003; 9(Suppl.):S17–20.
7. Clark AR. Pulmonary delivery technology: Recent advances and potential for the new millennium. In: Hickey AJ, ed. Pharmaceutical Inhalation Aerosol Technology, 2nd ed. New York: Marcel Dekker. 2004: 571–91.
8. Edwards DA, Caponetti G, Hrkach JS, et al. Aerodynamically light particles for pulmonary drug delivery. US Patent 5,874,064. 1999.
9. Ganderton D, Kassem NM. Aerosol Carriers. US patent 5,254,330. International, 1999.
10. Baichwal AR, Staniforth JN. Controlled Release Insufflation Carrier for Medicaments. US patent 5,738,865. 1996.
11. Clark AR, Hsu CC, Walsh AJ. Preparation of Sodium Chloride Aerosol Formulations. US Patent 5,747,002. 1998.
12. Hanes J, Edwards DA, Evora C, Langer R. Particles incorporating surfactants for pulmonary drug delivery. US Patent 5,985,309. 1999.
13. Edwards DA, Langer RS, Vanbever R, Mintzes J, Wang J, Chen D. ed. Preparation of particles for inhalation. US Patent 5,985,309.1999.
14. Boyes RN, Tice TR, Gilley RM, Pledger KL. ed. Pharmaceutical formulations comprising microcapsules. US Patent 5,384,133.1995.

15. Lechuga-Ballesteros D, Charan C, Liang Y, Stults C, Vehring R, Kuo M-C. Respiratory Drug Delivery IX, 2004; 565–8.
16. Chan H-K, Chew NYK. Novel alternative methods for the delivery of drugs for the treatment of asthma. Adv Drug Delivery Rev 2003; 55:793–805.
17. Chow AHL, Tong HHY, Chattopadhyay P, Shekunov BY; Particle engineering for pulmonary drug delivery. Pharm Res 24(3):411–37.
18. Taylor MK, Hickey AJ, VanOort MM. Manufacture, characterization, and pharmacodynamic evaluation of engineered ipratropium bromide particles. Pharm Dev Tech 2006; 11:321–36.
19. Tsapis N, Bennett D, Jackson B, Weitz DA, Edwards DA. Trojan particles: large porous carriers of nanoparticles for drug delivery. Proceedings of the National Academy of Sciences of the United States of America 2002; 99(19): 12001–05.
20. Vanbever R, J.D. Mintzes, Wang J, Nice J, Chen D, Batycky R, Langer R, Edwards DA. Formulation and physical characterization of large porous particles for inhalation. Pharm Res 1999; 16(11):1735–42.
21. Duddu SP, Sisk SA, Walter YH, Tarara TE, Trimble KR, Clark AR, Eldon MA, Improved lung delivery from a passive DPI using an engineered Pulmosphere powder. Pharm Res 2002; 19(5):689–95.
22. Edwards DA, Dunbar C. Bioengineering of therapeutic aerosols. Ann Rev Biomed Eng 2002; 4:93–107.
23. Chan H-K. Dry powder aerosol delivery systems: current and future research directions. J Aerosol Med 2006; 19(1):21–7.
24. Dalby RN, Tiano SL, Hickey AJ. Chapter 15. Medical devices for the delivery of therapeutic aerosols to the lungs. In: Hickey AJ, ed. Inhalation Aerosols: Physical and Biological Basis for Therapy, 2nd ed., New York: Informa Healthcare. 2007; 417–444.
25. Rubin LD, ed. Intal (Cromolyn Sodium) A Monograph. Bedford, MA: Fisons Corporation. 1973; 173.
26. Ganderton D, Kassem NM. Dry powder inhalers. In: Ganderton D, Jones T, eds. Advanced Pharmaceutical Science. London: Academic Press 1992; 165–91.
27. Leong KH. Theoretical Principles and Devices Used to Generate Aerosol for Research. In: Hickey AJ, ed. Pharmaceutical Inhalation Aerosol Technology, 2nd ed. New York: Marcel Dekker. 2004; 253–78.
28. Israelachvili JN. Intermolecular and Surface Forces: with applications to Colloidal and Biological Systems. 2nd ed., London, UK: Academic Press 1992; 450.
29. Pietsch W, ed. Size Enlargement by Agglomeration. New York, NY: John Wiley 1991.
30. Van Cleef J Powder Technology. The powders that lend flavor, beauty and strength to many products are created by fearsome machines that force coherent materials to fail. Am Sci 1991; 79:304–15.
31. Concessio NM, Oort MMV, Knowles M, Hickey AJ Pharmaceutical dry powder aerosols: correlation of powder properties with dose delivery and implications for pharmacodynamic effect. Pharm Res 1999; 16(6):828–34.

32. Bailey AG, Hashish AH, Williams TJ Drug delivery by inhalation of charged particles. J Electrostatics 1998; 44(1–2):3–10.

33. Peart J, Byron PR. Electrostatics. Institute of Physics Conference Series, 1999; 77–80.

34. Peart J. Powder electrostatics: theory, techniques, and applications. KONA 2001; 19:34–45.

35. Hickey AJ, Mansour HM, Telko MJ, et al. Physical characterization of component particles included in dry powder inhalers: II. Dynamic Characteristics. J Pharm Sci 2007; 96(5):1302–19.

36. Staniforth JN. Respiratory Drug Delivery: Inpterpharm, IV, Buffalo Grove, IL 1282–301. 1994; 303–12.

37. Smyth HDC, Cooney DJ, Garmise RJ, Zimmerer RO, Pipkin JD, Hickey AJ. Respiratory Drug Delivery IX, Palm Desert, CA, 2005; 805–7.

38. Peart J, Staniforth JN, Meakin BJ. Electrostatics 1995 Institute of Physics Conference Series, 1995; 271–4.

39. Byron PR, Peart J, Staniforth JN. Aerosol electrostatics I: Properties of fine powders before and after aerosolization by DPI. Pharm Res 1997; 14(6): 698–705.

40. Murtomaa M, Mellin V, Harjunen P, Lankinen T, Laine E, Leho V-P. Effect of particle morphology on the triboelectrification in DPI. Int J Pharm 2004; 282(1–2 (September 10)):107–14.

41. Murtomaa M, Strengell S, Laine E, Bailey A. Measurement of electrostatic charge of an aerosol using a grid-probe. J Electrostatics 2003; 58(3-4 (June)): 197–207.

42. Carstensen JT, ed. Pharmaceutics of Solids and Solid Dosage Forms. New York, NY: John Wiley and Sons 1989.

43. Carstensen JT, ed. Pharmaceutical Principles of Solid Dosage Forms. Lancaster, PA: Technomic 1993.

44. Mullin JW. Crystallization. 3rd ed., Oxford, UK: Butterworth-Heinemann. 1993; 527.

45. Dunbar C, Hickey AJ, Holzner P. Dispersion and characterization of pharmaceutical dry powder aerosols. KONA Powder and Particle 1998; 16:7–45.

46. Byrn SR, Pfeiffer RR, Stowell JG. Solid-State Chemistry of Drugs. 2nd ed., West Lafayette, Indiana: SSCI, Inc. 1999; 576.

47. Vippagunta SR, Brittain HG, Grant DJW. Crystalline solids. Adv Drug Delivery Rev 2001; 48:3–26.

48. Clas S-D. The importance of characterizing the crystal form of the drug substance during drug development. Current Opinion in Drug Discovery and Development 2003; 6(4):550–60.

49. Datta S, Grant DJW. Crystal structures of drugs: advances in determination, prediction and engineering. Nature Rev Drug Discovery 2004; 3(3):42–57.

50. Sheth AR, Grant DJW. Relationship between the structure and properties of pharmaceutical crystals. KONA 2005; (23):36–48.

51. Rabinowitz JD, Lloyd PM, Munzar P, Myers DJ, Cross S, Damani R, Quintana R, et al. Ultra-fast absorption of amorphous pure drug aerosols via deep lung inhalation. J Pharm Sci 2006:1–14.

52. Hickey AJ, Mansour HM, Telko MJ, Physical Characterization of Component Particles included in Dry Powder Inhalers. I. Strategy Review and Static Characteristics. J Pharm Sci 2007; 96(5):1282–301.

53. Montreal Protocol 1987. Montreal protocol on substances that deplete the ozone layers. 1987.

54. US Food and Drug Administration. Use of ozone-depleting substances; removal of essential-use designation. 2005.

55. Dunbar C, Hickey AJ. A new millenium for inhaler technology. Pharm Tech 1997; 21:116–25.

56. York P, Hanna M, Shekunov BY, Humphreys GO. Respiratory Drug Delivery VI, Hilton Head, SC, 1998; 169–76.

57. Feeley JC, Gilbert DJ, Srinivas P, Walker SE, York P. Respiratory Drug Delivery VII, Tarpon Springs, FL, 2000; 357–60.

58. York P, Hanna M. Respiratory Drug Delivery V, 1996; 231–40.

59. Clark AR, York P. Respiratory Drug Delivery 2006, Boca Raton, FL, 2006; 317–26.

60. Van Oort MM, Sacchetti M. Spray-drying and supercritical fluid particle generation techniques. In: Hickey AJ, ed. Inhalation Aerosols: Physical and Biological Basis for Therapy, 2nd ed., New York, NY: Informa Healthcare USA, Inc. 2007; 307–46.

61. Euliss LE, DuPont JA, Gratton S, DeSimone J. Imparting size, shape, and composition control of materials for nanomedicine. Chemical Society Reviews 2006; 35(11):1095–104.

62. Newman SP. Deposition and effects of inhaled corticosteroids. Clin Pharm 2003; 42(6):529–44.

63. Hickey AJ. Lung deposition and clearance of pharmaceutical aerosols: What can be learned from inhalation toxicology and industrial hygiene? Aerosol Sci Tech 1993; 18(3 (April)):290–304.

64. Tong HHY, Chow AHL. Control of Physical Forms of Drug Particles for Pulmonary Delivery by Spray Drying and Supercritical Fluid Processing. KONA Powder and Particle 2006; 24:27–40.

65. Mosen K, Backstrom K, Thalberg K, Schaefer T, Kristensen HG, Axelsson A. Particle formation and capture during spray-drying of inhalable particles. Pharm Dev Tech 2004; 9(4):409–17.

66. Tom JW, Debendetti PG. Particle formation with supercritical fluids-a review. J Aerosol Sci 1991; 22:555–84.

67. Debenedetti PG, Tom JW, Yeo S-D, Lim G-B. Application of supercritical fluids for the production of sustained delivery devices. J Controlled Release 1993; 24:27–44.

68. Kordikowski A, York P, Latham D. Resolution of ephedrine in supercritical CO_2: a novel technique for the separation of chiral drugs. J Pharm Sci 1999; 88:786–91.

69. Palakodaty S, York P. Phase behavioral effects on particle formation processes using supercritical fluids. Pharm Res 1999; 16:976–85.

70. Rehman M, Shekunov BY, York P, Lechuga-Ballesteros D, Miller DP, Tan T, Colthorpe P. Optimisation of powders for pulmonary delivery using supercritical fluid technology. Eur J Pharm Sci 2004; 22:1–17.

71. Shekunov BY. Production of powders for respiratory drug delivery. In: York P, Kompella UB, Shekunov BY, eds. Supercritical Fluid Technology for Drug Product Development, New York: Marcel Dekker. 2004; 247–82.

72. Shekunov BY, Feeley JC, Chow AHL, Tong HHY, York P. Aerosolisation behaviour of micronised and supercritically-processed powders. J Aerosol Sci 2003; 34:553–68.

73. Schiavone H, Palakodaty S, Clark A, York P, Tzannis ST. Evaluation of SCF-engineered particle-based lactose blends in passive DPI. Int J PHarm 2004; 281:55–66.

74. Velaga SP, Bergh S, Carlfors J. Stability and aerodynamic behaviour of glucocorticoid particles prepared by a supercritical fluids process. Eur J Pharm Sci 2004; 21:501–9.

75. Lobo JM, Schiavone H, Palakodaty S, York P, Clark A, Tzannis ST. SCF-engineered powders for delivery of budesonide from passive DPI devices. J Pharm Sci 2005; 94(10 (October)):2276–88.

76. Velaga SP, Berger R, Carlfors J. Supercritical fluids crystallization of budesonide and flunisolide. Pharm Res 2002a; 19:1564–71.

77. Beach S, Latham D, Sidgwick C, Hanna M, York P. Control of the physical form of salmeterol xinafoate. Org Process Res Dev 1999; 3:370–6.

78. Shekunov BY, Chattopadhaya R, Yim D, Cipolla D, Boyd B. Respiratory Drug Delivery, Boca Raton, FL, 2006; 609–12.

79. Shekunov BY, Chattopadhyay P, Seitzinger J, Huff R. Nanoparticles of poorly water-soluble drugs prepared by supercritical fluid extraction of emulsions. Pharm Res 2006; 23:196–204.

80. Chattopadhyay P, Huff R, Shekunov BY. Drug encapsulation using supercritical fluid extraction of emulsions. J Pharm Sci 2006; 95:667–79.

81. Hickey AJ, Dunbar CA. A New Millenium for Inhaler Technology. Pharm Tech 1997; 21(6):116–25.

82. Hickey AJ, Crowder TM. Dry powder inhaler devices: multidose dry powder drug packages, controlled systems, and associated methods. US697138 3B2 granted December 6, 2005.

83. Crowder TM, Louey MD, Sethuraman VV, Smyth HDC, Hickey AJ. 2001:An odyssey in inhaler formulations and design. Pharm Tech 2001; 25(7):99–113.

84. Crowder T, Hickey A. Powder specific active dispersion for generation of pharmaceutical aerosols International Journal of Pharmaceutics 2006; 327 (1–2):65–72.

85. Crowder TM. Precision powder metering utilizing fundamental powder flow characteristics Powder Technology. 2007 173(3):217–23.

86. Yeates DB, Besseris GJ, Wong LB. Physicochemical properties of mucus and its propulsion. In: Crystal RG, West JB, Weibel ER, Barnes PJ, editors. The Lung: Scientific Foundations, 2nd ed., Philadelphia, PA: Lippincott Williams & Wilken. 1997; p 487–503.

87. Bhat M, Hickey AJ. Effect of chloroquine on phagolysosomal fusion in cultured guinea pig alveolar macrophages: Implications in drug delivery. AAPS Pharm Sci 2000; 2(4):E34.

88. Byron PR. Prediction of drug residence times in regions of the human respiratory tract following aerosol inhalation. J Pharm Sci 1986; 75:433–8.

89. Gonda I. Drugs administered directly into the respiratoty tract: modeling of the duration of effective drug levels. J Pharm Sci 1988; 77(4):340–8.
90. Gonda I. Targeting by Deposition. In: Hickey AJ, ed. Pharmaceutical Inhalation Aerosol Technology, 2nd, rev. ed. New York: Marcel Dekker, 2004: 65–88.
91. Mathias NR, Yamashita F, Lee VHL. Respiratory epithelial cell culture models for evaluation of ion and drug transport. Adv Drug Delivery Rev 1996; 22(1–2):215–49.
92. Mobley C, Hochhaus G. Methods used to assess pulmonary deposition and absorption of drugs. Drug Discovery Today 2001; 6(7):367–75.
93. von Wichert P, Seifart C. The lung, an organ for absorption. Respiration 2005; 72(5):552–8.
94. Steimer A, Haltner E, Lehr C-M. Cell culture models of the respiratory tract relevant to pulmonary drug delivery. J Aerosol Med 2005; 18(2):137–82.
95. Sakagami M. In vivo, in vitro and ex vivo models to assess pulmonary absorption and disposition of inhaled therapeutics for systemic delivery. Adv Drug Delivery Rev 2006; 58:1030–60.
96. Shapiro DL, Nardone LL, Rooney SA, Motoyama EK, Munoz JL. Phospholipid Biosynthesis and Secretion by a Cell Line (A549) Which Resembles Type-II Alveolar Epithelial-Cells. Biochimica Et Biophysica Acta 1978; 530(2):197–207.
97. Foster KA, Oster CG, Mayer MM, Avery ML, Audus KL. Characterization of the A549 cell line as a Type II Pulmonary Epithelial Cell Model for Drug Metabolism. Exp Cell Res 1998; 243:359–66.
98. Forbes B, Wilson CG, Gumbleton M. Temporal dependence of ectopeptidase expression in alveolar epithelial cell culture: implications for study of peptide absorption. Int J Pharm 1999; 180(2):225–34.
99. Bruck A, Abu-Dahab R, Borchard G, Schafer UF, Lehr CM. Lectin-functionalized liposomes for pulmonary drug delivery: interaction with human alveolar epitelial cells. J Drug Targeting 2001; 9(4):241.
100. Ehrhardt C, Fiegel J, Fuchs S, Abu-Dahab R, Schaefer UF, Hanes J, Lehr CM. Drug absorption by the respiratory mucosa: cell culture models and particulate drug carriers. J Aerosol Med 2002; 15(2):131–9.
101. Hermanns MI, Unger RE, Kehe K, Peters K, Kirkpatrick CJ. Lung epithelial cell lines in coculture with human microvascular endothelial cells: development of an alveolo-capillary barrier *in vitro*. Laboratory Investigation 2004; 84:736–52.
102. Blank F, Rothen-Rutishauser BM, Schurch S, Gehr P. An optimized in vitro model of the respiratory tract wall to study particle cell interactions. Journal of Aerosol Medicine-Deposition Clearance and Effects in the Lung 2006; 19 (3):392–405.
103. Foster KA, Avery ML, Yazdanian M, Audus KL. Characterization of the Calu-3 cell line as a tool to screen pulmonary drug delivery. Int J Pharm 2000; 208:1–11.
104. Florea BI, van der Sandt ICJ, Schrier SM, Kooiman K, Deryckere K, de Boer AG, Junginger HE, Borchard G. Evidence of p-glycoprotein mediated apical to basolateral transport of flunisolide in human broncho-tracheal epithelial cells (Calu-3). Br J Pharmacol 2001; 134:1555–63.

105. Borchard G, Cassara ML, Roemele PE, Florea BI, Junginger HE. Transport and local metabolism of budesonide and fluticasone propionate in a human bronchial epithelial cell line (Calu-3). J Pharm Sci 2002; 91:1561–7.

106. Florea BI, Cassara ML, Junginger HE, Borchard G. Drug transport and metabolism characteristics of the human airway epithelial cell line Calu-3. J Controlled Release 2003; 87(1-3):131–8.

107. Forbes B, Ehrhardt C. Human respiratory epithelial cell culture for drug delivery applications. Eur J Pharm Biopharm 2005; 60(2):193–205.

108. Ehrhardt C, Kneuer C, Bies C, Lehr CM, Kim K-J, Bakowsky UU. Salbutamol is actively absorbed across human bronchial epithelial cell layers. Pulm Pharmacol & Ther 2005; 18(3):165–70.

109. Grainger CI, Greenwell LL, Lockley DJ, Martin GP, Forbes B. Culture of Calu-3 Cells at the air-water interface provides a representative model of the airway epithelial barrier. Pharm Res 2006; 23(7):1482–90.

110. Ehrhardt C, Kneuer C, Laue M, Schaefer UF, Kim K-J, Lehr CM. 16HBE14o-human bronchial epithelial cell layers express P-glyco-protein, lung resistance-related protein, and caveolin-1. Pharm Res 2003; 20 (4):545–51.

111. Manford F, Tronde A, Jeppsson AB, Patel N, Johansson F, Forbes B. Drug permeability in 16HBE14o-airway cell layers correlates with absorption from the isolated perfused rat lung. Eur J Pharm Sci 2005; 26(5):414–20.

112. Robinson PC, Voelker DR, Mason RJ. Isolation and culture of human alveolar type-II epithelial cells. Characterization of their phospholipid secretion. American Review of Respiratory Disease 1984; 130(6):1156–60.

113. Elbert KJ, Shafer UF, Shafers H-J, Kim K-J, Lee VHL, Lehr C-M. Monolayers of human alveolar epithelial cells in primary culture for pulmonary absorption and transport studies. Pharm Res 1984; 16(5):601–8.

114. Fuchs S, Hollins AJ, Laue M, Schaefer UF, Roemer K, Gumbleton M, Lehr CM. Differentiation of human alveolar epithelial cells in primary culture: morphological characterization and synthesis of caveolin-1 and surfactant protein-C. Cell and Tissue Research 2003; 311(1):31–45.

115. Bur M, Huwer H, Lehr C-M, Hagen N, Guldbrandt M, Kim K-J, Ehrhardt C. Assessment of transport rates of proteins and peptides across primary human alveolar epithelial cell monolayers. Eur J Pharm Sci 2006; 28:196–203.

116. Lin HC, Li H, Cho H-J, Bian S, Roh H-J, Lee M-K, Kim JS, Chung S-J, Shim C-K, Kim D-D. Air-liquid interface (ALI) culture of human bronchial epithelial cell monolayers as an *in vitro* model for airway drug transport studies. J Pharm Sci 2007; 96(2):341–50.

117. Upham JW, Stick SM. Interactions between airway epithelial cells and dendritic cells: implications for the regulation of airway inflammation. Current Drug Targets 2006; 7(5):541–5.

118. Rothen-Rutishauser BM, Kiama SG, Gehr P. A three-dimensional cellular model of the human respiratory tract to study the interaction with particles. Am J Respir Cell and Mol Biol 2005; 32(4):281–9.

119. Byron PR, Roberts NSR, Clark AR. An isolated perfused rat lung preparation for the study of aerosolized drug deposition and absorption. J Pharm Sci 1986; 75(2):168–71.

120. Byron PR, Niven RW. A novel dosing method for drug administration to the airways of the isolated perfused rat lung. J Pharm Sci 1986; 77(8):693–5.

121. Niven RW, Byron PR. Solute absorption from the airways of the isolated rat lung. I. The use of absorption data to quantify drug dissolution or release in the respiratory tract. Pharmaceutical Research 1988; 5(9):574–9.

122. Niven RW, Byron PR. Solute absorption from the airways of the isolated rat lung. Part 2. Effect of surfactants on absorption of fluorescein. Pharmaceutical Research 1990; 7(1):8–13.

123. Niven RW, Rypacek F, Byron PB. Solute Absorption from the Airways of the Isolated Rat Lung. III. Absorption of Several Peptidase-Resistant, Synthetic Polypeptides: Poly-(2- Hydroxyethyl)- Aspartamides. Pharm Res 1990; 7(10): 990–4.

124. Bryon PR, Sun Z, Katayama H, Rypacek F. Solute absorption from the airways of the isolated rat lung.4. Mechanisms of absorption of fluorophore-labeled poly-alpha, beta-[N(2-hydroxyethyl)-DL-aspartamide]. Pharm Res 1994; 11(2):221–5.

125. Sun JZ, Byron PR, Rypacek F. Solute absorption from the airways of the isolated rat lung. V. charge effects on the absorption of copolymers of N(2-hydroxyethyl)-DL-aspartamide with DL-aspartic acid or dimethylamino-propyl-DL-aspartamide. Pharm Res 1999; 16(7):1104–8.

126. Sakagami M, Byron PR, Venitz J, Rypacek F. Solute disposition in the rat lung in vivo and in vitro: determining regional absorption kinetics in the presence of mucociliary escalator. J Pharm Sci 2002; 91(2):594–604.

127. Sakagami M, Byron PR, Rypacek F. Biochemical evidence for transcytotic absorption of polyaspartamide from the rat lung: effects of temperature and metabolic inhibitors. J Pharm Sci 2002; 91(9):1958–68.

128. Tronde A, Norden B, Jeppsson AB, Brunmark P, Nilsson E, Lennernas H, Bengtsson UH. Drug absorption from the isolated perfused rat lung correlations with drug physicochemical properties and epithelial permeability. J Drug Targeting 2003; 11(1):61–74.

129. Pang YN, Sakagami M, Byron PR. The pharmacokinetics of pulmonary insulin in the in vitro isolated perfused rat lung: implications of metabolism and regional deposition. Eur J Pharm Sci 2005; 25(4-5):369–78.

130. Sakagami M, Omidi Y, Campbell L, Kandalaft LE, Morris CJ, Barar J, Gumbleton M. Expression and transport functionality of FcRn within rat alveolar epithelium: a study in primary cell culture and in the isolated perfused lung. Pharm Res 2006; 23(2):270–9.

131. Van Oort M. In vitro testing of DPI. Aerosol Sci and Tech 1995; 22:364–73.

132. Hindle M, Byron PR, Miller NC. Cascade impaction methods for DPI using the high flow rate Marple-Miller impactor. Int J Pharm 1996; 134(May 28): 137–46.

133. Burnell PKP, Grant AC, Haywood PA, Prime D, Sumby D, Sumby BS. Respiratory Drug Delivery VI, Hilton Head, S.C., 1998; 259–68.

134. Dunbar CA, Morgan B, VanOort M, Hickey AJ. A comparison of DPI dose delivery characteristics using power. PDA J Pharm Sci and Tec 2000; 54(6): 478–84.

135. Miller N. Respiratory Drug Delivery IV, Richmond, Virginia, 1994; 342–3.

136. Byron PR. Respiratory Drug Delivery VI, Hilton Head, South Carolina, 1998; 139–44.
137. Pillai RS, Yeates DB, Eljamal M, Miller IF, Hickey AJ . Generation of concentrated aerosols for inhalation studies. J Aerosol Sci 1994; 25(1):187–97.
138. Talton J, Fitz-Gerald J, SIngh R, Hochhaus G. Respiratory Drug Delivery VII, Tarpon Springs, Florida, 2000; 67–74.
139. Cooney DJ, Hickey AJ. Preparation of disodium fluorescein powders in association with lauric and capric acids. J Pharm Sci 2003; 92(11):2341–4.
140. Wang J, Ben-Jebria A, Edwards DA. Inhalation of estradiol for sustained systemic delivery. J Aerosol Med 1999; 12(1):27–36.
141. Ben-Jebria A, Eskew ML, Edwards DA. Inhalation system for pulmonary aerosol drug delivery in rodents using large porous particles. Aerosol Sci and Tech 2000; 32(5):421–33.
142. Codrons V VF, Verbeeck RK, Arras M, Lison D, Preat V, Vanbever R. Systemic delivery of parathyroid hormone (1-34) using inhalation dry powders in rats. J Pharm Sci 2003; 92(5):938–50.
143. Suarez S, O'Hara P, Kaazantseva M, Newcomer CE, Hopfer R, McMurray DN, Hickey AJ. Airways delivery of rifampicin microparticles for the treatment of tuberculosis. J Antimicrob Chemother 2001; 48:431–4.
144. Tsapis N, Bennett D, O'Driscoll K, Shea K, Lipp MM, Fu K, Clarke RW, Deaver D, Yamins D, Wright J, Peloquin CA, Weitz DA, Edwards DA. Direct lung delivery of para-aminosalicylic acid by aerosol particles. Tuberculosis 2003; 83(6):379–85.
145. Ben-Jebria A, Chen D, Eskew ML, Vanbever R, Edwards DA, et al. Large porous particles for sustained protection from carbachol-induced bronchoconstriction in guinea pigs. Pharm Res 2003; 16:555–61.
146. Battram C, Charlton SJ, Cuenoud B, Dowling MR, Fairhurst RA, Farr D, Fozard JR, Leighton-Davies JR, Lewis CA, McEvay L, Turner RJ, Trifilieff A. In vitro and in vivo pharmacological characterization of 5-[(R)2-(5,6-diethyl-indan-2-ylamino)-1-hydroxy-ethyl]-8-hydroxy-1H-quinolin-2-one (Indacaterol), a novel inhaled beta-2 adrenoceptor agonist with a 24-h duration of action. J Pharm and Exper Ther 2006; 317(2):762–70.
147. Beaulac C, Sachetelli S, Lagace J. Aerosolization of low phase transition temperature liposomal tobramycin as a dry powder in an animal model of chronic pulmonary infection caused by Pseudomonas aeruginosa. J Drug Targeting 1999; 7(1):33–41.
148. Beaulac C, Sachetelli S, Lagace J. In vitro bactericidal evaluation of a low phase transition temperature liposomal tobramycin formulation as a dry powder preparation against gram negative and gram positive bacteria. J Liposome Res 1999; 9(3):301–12.
149. Joshi M, Misra A 2003. Disposition kinetics of ketotifen from liposomal dry powder for inhalation in rat lung. Clinical and Experimental Pharmacology and Physiology 2003; 30:153–6.
150. Bennett WD, Brown JS, Zeman KL, Hu S-C, Scheuch G, Sommerer K. Targeting delivery of aerosols to different lung regions. J Aerosol Med 2002; 15(2):178–88.

151. Bondesson E, Asking L, Borgstrom L, Nilsson LE, Trofast E, Wollmer P. In vitro and in vivo aspects of quantifying intrapulmonary deposition of a dry powder radioaerosol. Int J Pharm 2002; 232(1–2):149–56.
152. Vidgren MT, Karkkainen A, Paronen P, Karjalainen P. Respiratory tract deposition of 99mTc-labelled drug particles administered via a DPI. Int J Pharm 1987; 39:101–5.
153. Vidgren M, Karkkainen A, Karjalainen P, Paronen P, Nuutinen J. Effect of powder inhaler design on drug deposition in the respiratory tract. Int J Pharm 1988; 42(Mar):211–6.
154. Pitcairn GR, Hooper G, Luria X, Rivero X, Newman SP. A scintigraphic study to evaluate the deposition patterns of a novel anti-asthma drug inhaled from the Cyclohaler DPI. Adv Drug Delivery Rev 1997; 26:59–67.
155. Pitcairn GR, Lim J, Hollingworth A, Newman SP. Scintigraphic Assessment of Drug Delivery from the Ultrahaler Dry Powder Inhaler. J Aerosol Med 1997 10(4):295–306.
156. Pitcairn GR, Lankinen T, Seppala OP, Newman SP. Pulmonary drug delivery from the taifun DPI is relatively independent of the patient's inspiratory effort. J Aerosol Med 2000; 13(2):97–104.
157. Newman SP, Pitcairn GR, Hirst PH, Bacon RE, O'Keefe E, Reiners M, Hermann R. Scintigraphic comparison of budesonide deposition from two DPI. Eur Respir J 2000; 16(1):178–83.
158. Hirst PH, Bacon RE, Pitcairn GR, Silvasti M, Newman SP. A comparison of the lung deposition of budesonide from Easyhaler, Turbuhaler, and pMDI plus spacer in asthmatic patients. Respir Med 2001; 95(9):720–7.
159. Dunbar C, Scheuch G, Sommerer K, DeLong M, Verma A, Batycky R. In vitro and in vivo dose delivery characteristics of large porous particles for inhalation. Int J Pharm 2002; 245(1-2):179–89.
160. Newman S, Malik S, Hirst P, Pitcairn G, Heide A, Pabst J, Dinkelaker A, Fleischer W. Lung deposition of salbutamol in healthy human subjects from the MAGhaler DPI. Respir Med 2002; 96(12):1026–32.
161. Ball DJ, Hirst PH, Newman SP, Sonet B, Streel B, Vanderbist F. Deposition and pharmacokinetics of budesonide from the Miat Monodose inhaler, a simple dry powder device. Int J Pharm 2002; 245(1-2):123–32.
162. Newman SP, Pitcairn GR, Hirst PH, Rankin L. Radionuclide imaging technologies and their use in evaluating asthma drug deposition in the lungs. Adv Drug Delivery Rev 2003; 55(7):851–67.
163. Meyer T, Brand P, Ehlich H, Kobrich R, Meyer G, Riedinger F, Sommerer K, Weuthen T, Scheuch G. Deposition of Foradil P in human lungs: comparison of in vitro and in vivo data. Journal of Aerosol Medicine-Deposition Clearance And Effects In The Lung 2004; 17(1):43–9.
164. Sebti T, Pilcer G, Van Gansbeke B, Goldman S, Michilis A, Vanderbist F, Amighi K. Pharmacoscintigraphic evaluation of lipid dry powder budesonide formulations for inhalation. Eur J Pharm and Biopharm 2006; 64(1):26–32.
165. Newhouse MT, Hirst PH, Duddu SP, Walter YH, Tarara TE, Clark AR, Weers JG. Inhalation of a dry powder tobramycin pulmosphere formulation in healthy volunteers. Chest 2006; 124:360–6.

166. Eberl S, Chan HK, Daviskas E. SPECT imaging for radioaerosol deposition and clearance studies. Journal of Aerosol Medicine-Deposition Clearance And Effects In The Lung 2006; 19(1):8–20.
167. Newman S, Wilding IR, Hirst P. Human lung deposition data: the bridge between in vitro and clinical evaluations for inhaled drug products? Int J Pharm 2000; 208:49–60.
168. Pillai RS, Yeates DB, Miller IF, Hickey AJ. Controlled dissolution from wax-coated aerosol particles in canine lungs. J Appl Physiol 1998; 84(2):717–25.
169. Hochhaus G, Suarez S, Gonzalez-Rothi RJ, Schreier H. Respiratory Drug Delivery VI, Hilton Head, SC, 1998; 45–52.
170. Edwards DA, Hanes J, Caponetti G, Hrkach J, Ben-Jebria A, Eskew ML, Mintzes J, Deaver D, Lotan N, Langer R. Large porous particles for pulmonary drug delivery. Sci 1997; 276(5320):1868–71.
171. Louey MD, Van Oort M, Hickey AJ. Standardized entrainment tubes for the evaluation of pharmaceutical dry powder dispersion. Journal of Aerosol Science 2006; 37 (11):1520–31
172. Hiestand EN. Powders: particle-particle interactions. J Pharm Sci 1966; 55 (12):1325–44.
173. Visser J. van der Waals and other cohesive forces affecting powder fluidization. Powder Tech 1989; 58(1 (May)):1–10.
174. Hickey AJ, Concessio NM, Van Oort MM, Platz RM. Factors influencing the dispersion of dry powders as aerosols. Pharm Tech 1994; 18:58–64, 82.
175. Zeng XM, Martin GP, Marriott C. Particulate Interactions in Dry Powder Formulations for Inhalation. ed., New York, NY: Taylor & Francis. 2001; 255.
176. Finlay WH. The mechanics of inhaled pharmaceutical aerosols. ed., London: Academic Press 2001.
177. Hickey AJ, Ganderton D. Pharmaceutical Process Engineering. ed., New York, NY: Marcel Dekker 2001. p 268.
178. Crowder TM, Hickey AJ, Louey MD, Orr N. A guide to pharmaceutical particulate science. First ed., Boca Raton, FL: Interpharm Press/CRC 2003; 241.
179. Hickey AJ, Jones LD. Particle-size analysis of pharmaceutical aerosols. Pharm Tech 2000; 24(9):48–58.
180. Buckton G. Respiratory Drug Delivery VI, Hilton Head, SC, 1998; 145–52.
181. Carvajal MT, Staniforth JN. Respiratory Drug Delivery VI, Hilton Head, SC, 1998; 283–9.
182. Kontny MJ, Conners JJ, Graham ET. Respiratory Drug Delivery IV, Richmond, VA, 1994; 125–36.
183. U.S. FDA. Guidance for industry:metered dose inhaler (MDI) and DPI (DPI) drug products. US FDA, CDR, ed., Washington, D.C.: U.S. FDA, CDR. 1998.
184. <601> Aerosols, Nasal Sprays, Metered-Dose Inhalers, and Dry Powder Inhalers Monograph. USP 29-NF 24 The United States Pharmacopoeia and The National Formulary: The Official Compendia of Standards, ed., Rockville, MD: The United States Pharmacopeial Convention, Inc 2006; 2617–36.
185. Pillai RS, Yeates DB, Miller IF, Hickey AJ. Controlled release from condensation coated respirable aerosol particles. J Aerosol Sci 1994; 25:461–77.

186. Clark AR, AM H. The Relationship Between Powder Inhaler Resistance and Peak Inspiratory Conditions in Healthy Volunteers - Implications for In Vitro Testing. J Aerosol Med 1993; 6:99–110.
187. European Pharmacopeia. Preparations for Inhalation. European Pharmacopeia ed.: Eur Pharmacopeia 2001.
188. Schreier H, Mobley WC, Concessio NM, Hickey AJ, Niven RW. Formulation and in vitro performance of liposome powder aerosols. STP Pharma Sci 1994; 4:38–44.
189. Ho J. Generation and analysis of liposome aerosols. In: Shek PN, ed. Liposomes in biomedical applications. Amsterdam: Harwood Academic Publishers GmBH. 1995; 199–208.
190. Mobley WC. The effect of jet-milling on lyophilized liposomes. Pharm Res 1998; 15:149–52.
191. Goldbach P, Brochart H, Stamm A. Spray-Drying of Liposomes for a Pulmonary Administration. I. Chemical Stability of Phospholipids. Drug Development and Industrial Pharmacy 1993; 19(19):2611–22.
192. Goldbach P, Brochart H, Stamm A 1993. Spray-Drying of Liposomes for a Pulmonary Administration. II. Retention of Encapsulated Materials. Drug Development and Industrial Pharmacy 1993; 19(19):2623–36.
193. Joshi M, Misra A. Dry powder inhalation of liposomal ketotifen fumarate: formulation and characterization. Int J Pharm 2001; 223:15–27.
194. Desai TR, Li D, Finlay WH, Wong JP. Determination of surface free energy of interactive dry powder liposome formulations using capillary penetration technique. Colloids and SurfacesB:Biointerfaces 2001; 22:107–13.
195. Desai TR, Wong JP, Hancock REW, Finlay WH. A novel approach to the pulmonary delivery of liposomes in dry powder form to eliminate the deleterious effects of milling. J PHarm Sci 2002; 91(2):482–91.
196. Lu D, Hickey AJ. Liposomal dry powders as aerosols for pulmonary delivery of proteins. AAPS Pharm Sci Tech 2006; 6(4):Article 80:E641-E648.
197. Cook RO PR, Kellaway IW. Novel sustained release microspheres for pulmonary drug delivery. J Control Release 2005; 104(1):79–90.

44

Adaptive Aerosol Delivery (AAD®) Technology

Kurt Nikander

Respironics, Inc., Respiratory Drug Delivery, Parsippany, New Jersey, U.S.A.

John Denyer

Respironics Respiratory Drug Delivery (UK) Ltd., Chichester, U.K.

INTRODUCTION

The modern jet nebulizer has been used for almost a century for delivery of inhaled drugs for the treatment of asthma, chronic obstructive pulmonary disease, and pulmonary infections. Recognition of the shortcomings of the conventional nebulizers in terms of drug delivery has led to the development of "intelligent" nebulizers such as the Adaptive Aerosol Delivery (AAD®) System (1,2). Diseases of the airways have traditionally been logical candidates for treatment with inhaled drugs. The introduction of the AAD technology has broadened the possibilities for inhaled treatments to include drugs with a narrow therapeutic window and drugs targeted for systemic diseases (3). The AAD System is the first commercialized technology that adapts the timing of aerosol delivery to match the patient's breathing pattern. The in vitro evidence suggests that the AAD Systems can deliver precise and reproducible doses of aerosol. The clinical evidence indicates that the AAD System is superior to conventional jet nebulizers in terms of lung deposition, elimination of waste of aerosol to the environment and true adherence. The first and second generation AAD Systems—HaloLite® and Prodose™—have been successfully used in relatively large clinical studies involving patients with asthma, cystic fibrosis, and pulmonary hypertension (3). For the purpose of this review of the AAD technology, the focus will be on I-neb, the third generation AAD System.

HISTORICAL DEVELOPMENT

The amount of aerosol delivered with a conventional nebulizer is highly variable, and the device typically wastes >50% of the total aerosol output to the environment during the patient's exhalation (1,3). The main reason for the waste is the continuous drug output which makes the amount of drug inhaled dependent on the patient's breathing pattern. The patient's duty cycle is typically 40:60, i.e., time of inspiration ~40% of a single respiratory cycle and time of expiration ~60% (4). This means that at least 60% of the drug delivered from the nebulizer will be wasted to the environment and potentially inhaled by those caring for the patient. An inhalation device which is efficient, and delivers a precise amount of aerosol with minimal waste and caregiver exposure is required for delivery of drugs with a narrow therapeutic index or for delivery of very expensive drugs. Pulsed aerosol delivery during only a part of the inhalation should minimize the amount lost during exhalation, and provide the basis for delivery of precise preset doses of drug.

The AAD technology was developed with the aim to deliver precise amounts of aerosol to the patient, to reduce the waste of aerosol to the environment, and to improve the patients' adherence to their treatment and compliance with the user instructions for the device (1,2). The technology was embodied in the AAD Systems—HaloLite the 1st generation, Prodose the 2nd generation, and I-neb® the 3rd generation commercially available since 2005. The AAD System have been designed to adapt the delivery of aerosol to the patient's breathing pattern in order to eliminate the greatest source of variability in aerosol delivery associated with conventional neb-ulizers (3). It also provides the patient with feedback on how to efficiently use the AAD System during the treatment. When the preset dose is deliv-ered, the device switches off and indicates completion of treatment.

ADAPTIVE AEROSOL DELIVERY (AAD®) TECHNOLOGY

The I-neb AAD System (Fig. 1) is a small ($150 \times 65 \times 45$ mm, h, w, d), lightweight (210 g), and virtually silent drug delivery device. The main parts are the body, the medication chamber assembly including the mesh and the drug guide, and the mouthpiece. The battery charger is not shown in Figure 1. The body includes the microprocessor that runs the AAD algorithm, the electronic aerosol generation circuit, the piezo element connected to the horn, the pressure sensor, the LCD screen, the radio frequency antenna for the AAD Disc™, the patient logging system (PLS), the infrared transmitter/receiver (for I-neb Insight™), the battery, the buzzer, and the vibration device

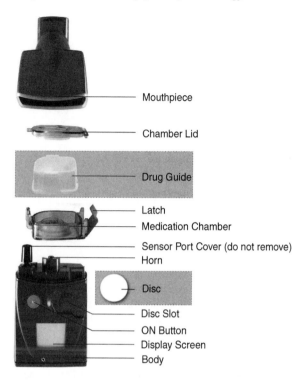

Mouthpiece

Chamber Lid

Drug Guide

Latch
Medication Chamber
Sensor Port Cover (do not remove)
Horn
Disc
Disc Slot
ON Button
Display Screen
Body

Figure 1 The I-neb AAD System without battery charges. *Abbreviation:* AAD, Adaptive Aerosol Delivery.

for tactile feedback. The piezo element connected to the horn has a variable power range (power levels 1 to 15) for the optimization of the aerosol output rate. The AAD Disc can been programmed with operational parameters such as power level, drug lot number, drug code and expiration date. The AAD Disc is usually delivered with the drug package through the pharmacy. The PLS data can be assessed through the use of I-neb Insight, which consists of a cradle and software that facilitates the download of patient usage data (5). The patient usage data downloaded from the PLS comprises device specific codes, the date and time of treatment, the drug code of the AAD Disc used, whether a full dose was delivered, and the duration of treatment.

The medication chamber assembly includes the metering chamber with optional volumes ranging from 0.25 to 1.7 mL, the platinum mesh, the latch which keeps the mesh positioned on top of the metering chamber and seals the drug in the metering chamber, and the drug guide which helps the patient fill in the drug in the metering chamber. The metering chamber volumes ranging from 0.25 to 1.7 mL might appear small, but with minimal

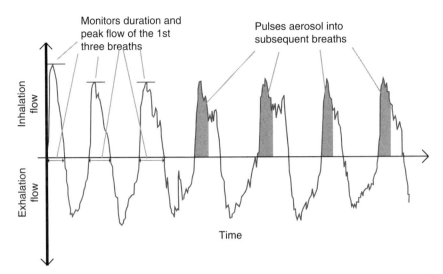

Figure 2 A schematic presentation of a patient's breathing pattern, and the way the I-neb AAD® System operating in TBM monitors the patient's breathing pattern and pulses aerosol during the inspiratory part of each breath. *Abbreviations*: AAD, adaptive aerosol delivery; TBM, tidal breathing mode.

waste during delivery and a small residual of ~0.1 mL, the 1.7 mL volume is close to the volume delivered with a conventional nebulizer filled with ~6 mL of drug.

The I-neb AAD System has been designed to deliver aerosol with two different breathing pattern algorithms, the Tidal Breathing Mode (TBM) and the Target Inhalation Mode™ (TIM, not commercially available in the United States). During TBM, the patient inhales spontaneously during tidal breathing while inspiratory flow and time are measured through the pressure sensor (Fig. 2). The aerosol is pulsed during 50–80% of the inspiration. The duration of each pulse of aerosol is determined by the breathing pattern of the patient, and varies for each subsequent breath depending on the average of the preceding three breaths. The monitoring of the preceding three breaths continues throughout the treatment, and the system continually adapts to the patient's breathing patterns. The length of the aerosol pulse is dependent on the patient's inspiratory time and tidal volume.

During TIM the patient is guided to perform slow and deep inhalations up to ~9 seconds with aerosol pulsed up to 7 seconds, leaving 2 seconds for particle deposition in the lungs (Fig. 3). To achieve the slow and deep inhalation, the flow of the patient's inhalation is limited to ~20 L/min via a high-resistance mouthpiece. The length of the inhalation is individualized to each patient, and with each breath the patient is coached to lengthen the inhalation via a vibratory feedback through the mouthpiece. As shown in

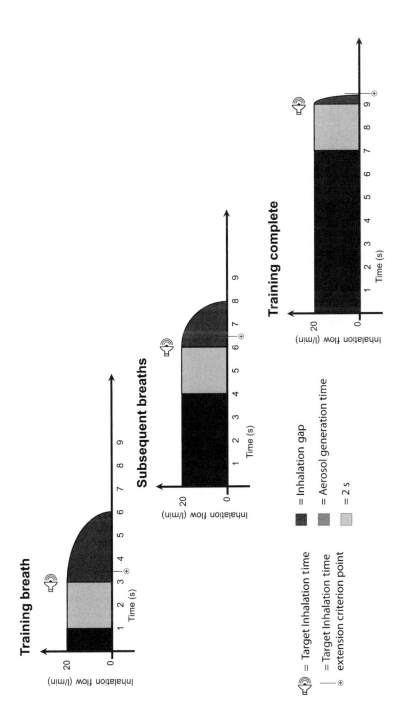

Figure 3 A schematic presentation of how the I-neb AAD System in TIM coaches a patient to gradually lengthen each inhalation through the device. *Abbreviations*: AAD, adaptive aerosol delivery; TIM, target inhalation mode.

the first panel of Figure 3, the device vibrates after 3 seconds of the patient's first inhalation, signalling for the patient to exhale. A bolus of aerosol is delivered during the first second of the 3 seconds inhalation. When inhalation exceeds the TIM extension criterion point (vertical mark on horizontal axis), as shown in the middle panel of Figure 3, the device extends the aerosol pulse in the subsequent breaths and the time of inhalation is gradually lengthened. After ~30 breaths the process is completed and the inhalation time optimized to the patient. In this case TIM is set at ~9 seconds as shown in the last panel of Figure 3 and at this point the aerosol pulse lasts for up to 7 seconds. At the end of the treatment the length of the last inhalation is stored for the next treatment. If, for some reason, the patient cannot reach the target inhalation time once the treatment time has been optimized, the I-neb AAD system gradually shortens the target inhalation time to adapt to the patient's preferred length of inhalation.

RESEARCH AND DEVELOPMENT

In Vitro Evaluation of Precise Dosage

Evaluations of the precision of drug delivery have been of special interest with I-neb in order to prove that precise preset volumes could be delivered (6,7). To determine the inter device variability of the early I-neb AAD System, 23 devices were included in an in vitro test to deliver a preset volume of 400 μL. The devices had an inspiratory filter connected to the mouthpiece and were then connected to a Harvard respirator which was used to simulate a breathing pattern with a 500-mL tidal volume, a frequency of 15 breaths/min, and a duty cycle of 0.5. An AAD Disc programmed for a medium output rate was used. The mean delivered volume on the filter was 407.1 μL with a 95% confidence interval of 401.2–412.8 μL, which was delivered during a mean nebulization time of 280.7 seconds (8).

Bridging In Vitro Data on AAD System Performance

The iloprost inhalation solution (Ventavis®, CoTherix, San Francisco, CA) has been approved by the FDA in doses of 2.5 and 5.0 μg for treatment of pulmonary arterial hypertension. Inhaled iloprost was approved for delivery with two AAD systems, Prodose and I-neb. HaloLite was the 1st generation AAD system used in the pivotal clinical documentation of inhaled iloprost, and all three AAD systems have therefore been compared in vitro in terms of mass median aerodynamic diameter (MMAD), fine particle fraction (FPF), and inhaled mass of iloprost (9). To analyze the MMAD and FPF, the AAD systems were connected to an Andersen cascade impactor which was connected to a vacuum pump and pressurized air. Air flow was regulated with flow control valves to provide inhalation and exhalation flow to the AAD System. A breathing simulator with a filter system between the simulator and the AAD System was used to measure inhaled mass of iloprost. Iloprost-specific HPLC analysis was used for quantification. The MMADs obtained with HaloLite, Prodose and I-neb were 1.4, 1.7, and 2.1 μm, respectively. The FPFs (percent <4.7 μm) were 91, 82 and 82%, respectively. The inhaled mass for the lower dose ranged from 2.8 to 2.9 μg, and for the higher dose from 4.8 to 5.2 μg. The in vitro data demonstrated that the different generations of the AAD System—despite the fact that the aerosol was created through different technologies—had comparable MMADs, FPFs and inhaled masses of iloprost.

I-neb Insight

I-neb Insight is an accessory for use with the I-neb AAD System that facilitates the download of the PLS data. In order to evaluate the I-neb Insight, an analysis of the use of I-neb for delivery of an inhaled antibiotic for three months in 29 patients with cystic fibrosis was conducted (5). The aim was to evaluate whether the PLS data downloaded using the I-neb Insight could be formatted to allow identification and interpretation of changes in patient use of the I-neb AAD System. The results indicated that I-neb Insight allowed in-depth analyses of patient usage data that could be used to give detailed feedback to the healthcare provider about both adherence to treatment and compliance with the use of the device. This could be of use in clinical studies, to ensure easy identification of non-adherent non-responders. This data could also be of use to healthcare providers when attempting to identify the reasons for lack of efficacy in patients not responding to therapy.

Lung Deposition when Using I-neb in TBM and TIM

The lung deposition of 0.5 mL of ^{99m}Tc-DTPA from I-neb in TBM and TIM (power level 10) has been evaluated in twelve healthy subjects who were enrolled in a randomized, open-label, crossover study (10). The subjects were trained in each inhalation technique prior to dosing, which was performed within 1 hour of completion of training. The training for tidal breathing during TBM and slow and deep breathing during TIM was performed using the I-neb Insight software. The radioactivity (loaded dose) dispensed into the I-neb metering chamber (0.5 mL of normal saline containing ^{99m}Tc-DTPA) was quantified with a gamma camera. Each subject underwent an ^{81m}Kr ventilation scan to define the ventilated regions of the lung. A transmission scan was also performed prior to administration of the radiolabel in order to determine regional tissue attenuation correction factors. All subjects inhaled aerosol in the seated position wearing a nose clip. Exhaled aerosol was trapped on a filter attached to the exhalation port of the I-neb device. In addition to subject imaging, radiolabel deposition on exhalation filters, and in mouthpieces was quantified. There was a washout of 24 hours between I-neb TBM and TIM sessions. The mass balance expressed as percent of loaded dose was 110% for both TBM and TIM treatments. The mean whole lung deposition was 62.8% in TBM and 73.3% in TIM, calculated as a percent of the emitted dose ex-mouthpiece. The mean exhaled fractions were 1.0% in TBM and 0.2% in TIM, and the mean mouthpiece depositions were 5.3% in TBM and 5.0% in TIM. The treatment times were 4.8 minutes in TBM and 3.0 minutes in TIM. The lung deposition achieved with I-neb in TBM was in accordance with previous lung deposition results achieved with HaloLite in healthy subjects (11). In that study nine healthy subjects inhaled ^{99m}Tc-DTPA during tidal breathing with a mean lung deposition of 60% calculated as a percent of the emitted dose ex-mouthpiece. The mean exhaled fraction in that study was less than 3%, in comparison with the I-neb results of 1% in TBM and 0.2% in TIM. The rather small amounts of aerosol that were exhaled when using I-neb in either TBM or TIM should make I-neb an ideal delivery system for drugs that healthcare providers and family members should not inhale.

REGULATORY ISSUES

In Europe, the I-neb AAD System has been approved as a medical device and classified as a small volume nebulizer for administration of medicines in spontaneously breathing patients. It is, however, only used in specific applications where it has been included on the drug licence.

In the United States, different regulatory pathways are used by FDA to approve new inhaled drugs and devices. New drug applications are handed by the Center for Drug Evaluation and Research (CDER), or Center for Biologics Evaluation and Research (CBER), and new devices by the Center for Devices and Radiological Health (CDRH). The FDA will nominate one center to take the lead for the review of an application, with other centers providing support. A review of a combination product, in which the drug is integral to the device, would most likely be lead by CDER in coordination with CDRH (for example, a Pressurized Matered Dose Inhaler (pMDI)). A drug seeking approval for delivery with a generic device would likely go to CDER (for example, dornase alpha inhalation solution for use with a nebulizer). A generic device seeking approval to deliver a range of drugs would fall to CDRH (for example, a conventional nebulizer). None of these three options seemed ideally suited for the approval of a new inhaled drug with a narrow therapeutic window that would require the use of a new drug delivery technology for precise dose delivery, but is not manufactured as a combination product (i.e., pMDI or Dry Powder Inhaler (DPI)).

The approval of iloprost inhalation solution with the I-neb AAD System in 2005 was achieved using a route different from any of the three outlined above. In this approval, the existing New Drug Application (NDA) drug process and the 510(k) device process were run in parallel, and the 510 (k) was only issued after the NDA. The I-neb device was specifically approved for administration of drugs which are approved for use with the I-neb device. This allowed the I-neb AAD System and any improvements not related to drug delivery to be controlled under the 510(k) process. The use of the 510(k) route was possible as many of the technical features of I-neb could be found in predicates, and drug specific performance data was only included in the NDA, not in the 510(k). By using this route, the device is not classified as a generic nebulizer, which means that each new drug application could attract a new reimbursement code. This would help support the cost of supplying technically advanced drug delivery systems for the delivery of new drugs. Now that the first new drug has been approved with the I-neb AAD System, the 510(k) may be referenced in future new drug developments, potentially reducing the regulatory burden on both the regulator and companies seeking approval (12).

TECHNOLOGY POSITION/COMPETITIVE ADVANTAGE

The AAD System is the first commercialized technology that adapts the timing of aerosol delivery to match the patient's breathing pattern, and delivers a precise dose of drug. The in vitro evidence confirms the ability of the I-neb AAD System to deliver precise and reproducible doses of aerosol. This has made it possible to use in vitro data in both the United States and European Union regulatory submissions to support the drug licence variation from the Prodose AAD System to the I-neb AAD System. This has significantly reduced the regulatory burden in introducing a new drug delivery system. I-neb has been approved by the FDA for the delivery of iloprost (Ventavis, CoTherix) and in the European Union for both iloprost (Ventavis, Schering AG, Delaware) and colistimethate sodium (Promixin®, Profile Pharma Ltd, Chichester, U.K.). The unique classification of the I-neb AAD System in the United States has resulted in a new reimbursement code. Furthermore, the variable dosing volume and the AAD Disc allows the I-neb AAD System to be customised to a specific pharmaceutical partner's requirements.

FUTURE DIRECTIONS

The forces driving the pharmaceutical industry to consider pulmonary drug delivery of new molecules include ever increasing competition, pricing pressures, drug patent life, life cycle management, and patient demands. The main customers for pulmonary drug delivery are the patients, the healthcare payers, and the investors. This means that new pulmonary drug delivery systems–such as the AAD System–must provide a sustainable competitive advantage by creating a technical solution that meets the patient's demands, is cost effective to meet the payer's demands, and generates a new market or extends the commercial life of the drug to meet the investor's demands. To meet these market requirements, the capabilities of the AAD Systems continue to be expanded. The novel I-neb TIM mode enhances lung deposition and reduces treatment times. I-neb Insight provides detailed information on patient adherence and compliance; this has been used in United Kingdom to pilot a direct to patient prescription service, and the monitoring of clinical outcomes. We continue to develop the AAD technology and apply its benefits in new areas such as delivery to ventilated patients.

REFERENCES

1. Nikander K. Adaptive aerosol delivery: The principles. Eur Respir Rev 1997; 7:385–7.
2. Denyer J. Adaptive aerosol delivery in practise. Eur Respir Rev 1997; 7:388–9.
3. Denyer J, Nikander K, Smith NJ. Adaptive Aerosol Delivery (AAD) technology. Expert Opin Drug Deliv 2004; 1(1):165–76.
4. Nikander K, Denyer J. Breathing patterns. Eur Respir Rev 2000; 10(76):576–9.
5. Prince I, Denyer J, Nikander K. I-neb Insight: A new tool for monitoring inhaled medication use. In: Dalby RN, Byron PR, Farr SJ, Peart J, Suman JD, eds. Respiratory Drug Delivery X. Boca Raton, FL. Davis Healthcare International Publishing, River Grove, IL, 2006: 769–72.
6. Denyer J, Prince I, Hardaker L, et al. In vitro performance of the Prodose handheld: A new portable aerosol delivery system. In: Dalby RN, Byron PR, Farr SJ, Peart J, Suman JD, eds. Respiratory Drug Delivery IX. Palm Desert, CA: Davis Healthcare International Publishing, River Grove, IL, 2004: 645–8.
7. Potter RW, Hatley RHM. Delivery of colistimethate sodium, dornase alpha and salbutamol sulphate using the I-neb AAD System. Ped Pulmonol 2006; suppl 29:341.
8. Prince I, Potts CJ, Ibanez E, et al. Uniformity of dose delivery from 23 prototype I-neb AAD System devices. Proceedings of the American Thoracic Society. San Diego, CA, 2005: 374.
9. Van Dyke R, Nikander K. Delivery of iloprost inhalation solution with HaloLite, Prodose, and I-neb Adaptive Aerosol Delivery (AAD) systems—an in vitro study. Respir Care 200: 52(2):184–90.
10. Nikander K, Prince IR, Coughlin SR, et al. Mode of breathing—tidal or slow and deep - through the I-neb Adaptive Aerosol Delivery (AAD) system affects lung deposition of 99mTc-DTPA. Proceedings of Drug Delivery to the Lungs 17. Edinburgh, Scotland, 2006: 206–9.
11. Denyer J, Dyche T, Nikander K, et al. Halolite a novel liquid drug aerosol delivery system. Thorax 1997; 52:A83.
12. Denyer J, Nikander K. Does the approval of Ventavis with the I-neb AAD System present a new approach to the regulatory approval of nebulized drugs with novel delivery devices? In: Dalby RN, Byron PR, Farr SJ, Peart J, Suman JD, eds. Respiratory Drug Delivery X. Boca Raton, FL:. Davis Healthcare International Publishing, River Grove, IL, 2006: 765–7.

45

Nebulizer Technologies

Martin Knoch

PARI Pharma GmbH, Starnberg, Germany

Warren Finlay

*Department of Mechanical Engineering, University of Alberta,
Edmonton, Alberta, Canada*

INTRODUCTION

Nebulizers today fill a niche in the delivery of high doses of drug to the respiratory tract with major applications in the treatment of asthma, COPD, and cystic fibrosis. A further advantage of nebulizers is their requirement of only minimal coordination and effort in comparison with pressurized metered-dose (pMDI) or dry powder inhalers (DPI). The earliest patents on nebulizers (1,2) indicate an amazingly long life-cycle for nebulizer technology. Although nebulizer products are suffering from price erosion and a shrinking market share in relation to MDIs and DPIs, ongoing evolutionary innovations serve to strengthen their position as niche products. The market is currently dominated by a diversity of jet nebulizers with a minor proportion of ultrasonic nebulizers. However, recent progress in manufacturing of miniaturized mechanical, electromechanical, and piezoelectric systems promises to revitalize and redefine the nebulizer market. Indeed, new piezoelectric liquid dispersion systems have the potential to form a new generation of small portable nebulizers with improved dosing capabilities, delivery efficiency, user friendliness, and safety.

In the forthcoming decade we foresee that liquid aerosol devices will split into single breath administration for lower doses, and multiple breath treatments over 1 to 3 minutes to administer larger drug volumes during spontaneous breathing. Table 1 lists some typical characteristics of these

Table 1   Classification of New Liquid Inhalers and Nebulizers

Type	Administration	Treatment duration	Aerosol inhaled per breath (μl)	Aerosol inhaled per treatment (μl)	Delivery efficiency (%)
Jet nebulizer	Consecutive spontaneous breathing	3–15 min	6–10	500–2000	20–40
Electronic nebulizer	Consecutive guided breathing	1–5 min	15–40	200–3000	60–80
Inhaler	Discrete single/ multiple breaths	<10 breaths	20–50	<500	60–80

different aerosol delivery systems. Whereas drug release with inhalers is controlled by discrete breathing maneuvers, the new generation of nebulizers may feature an incremental release of drug aerosol during guided spontaneous breathing with integrated electronic and software controlled functions. This allows improved monitoring and feedback functions that will assist the patient in receiving the most efficient treatment, enabling the clinician and practitioner to survey and optimize pulmonary treatment.

LIQUID DISPERSION PRINCIPLES

Jet Nebulizers

Jet nebulizers are driven by either a portable compressor or from a central air supply. Detailed consideration of the mechanics of jet nebulizers is given in Finlay (3). Essentially, a high speed air flow through a nozzle entrains and disperses the liquid into droplets (primary generation) via a viscosity-induced instability (3). As shown in Figure 1, droplet dispersion is improved by impaction on a baffle structure (air flow controller) adjacent to the nozzle orifice transferring kinetic energy further into increased droplet surface area (secondary generation). The resulting droplet size distribution still contains only a small fraction of respirable aerosol (droplets below 5–6 μm in size) and the large droplets are recirculated within the nebulizer by means of secondary impaction structures. This process is associated with evaporation effects that cause the gas phase to be nearly saturated with water vapor, as well as a temperature decrease within the nebulizer. A considerable part of the vapor arises from the larger recirculating droplets, thus increasing drug concentration in the remaining liquid. Therefore, assessment of nebulizer

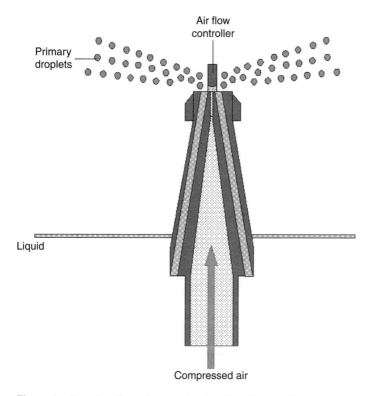

Figure 1 Droplet dispersion mechanism in a jet nebulizer.

systems cannot be done with a simple gravimetric measurement alone (4), but also requires chemical assay.

For nebulization of suspensions, preferential containment of suspension particles in larger droplets can occur if the suspended particles are of similar size to the nebulized droplets (5), so that chemical assay may be necessary for proper particle sizing of some nebulized suspensions. For liposomal formulations, disruption of liposomes can occur due to mechanical stresses during nebulization, possibly during primary generation (6) and secondary generation (3), although such disruption is device specific (7) and is most pronounced for large liposomes (8).

There are three common types of jet nebulizers: constant output (or unvented), breath enhanced (or vented), and breath activated nebulizers. Constant output nebulizers produce aerosol at a constant rate and the aerosol is diluted during inspiration by air entrainment via a T-piece or mask (9). These nebulizers require high compressed air flows (above 6 L/min) in order to achieve acceptable output characteristics and treatment times. Typically at least 50% of the aerosol is wasted to the environment during exhalation. The breath enhanced nebulizer entrains inhalation air in the droplet production region and produces aerosol at a higher rate during inspiration, but at a lower rate during expiration using a valve system. Due to this effect, approximately 70% of the aerosol will be delivered to the patient during continuous nebulization. These nebulizers may be operated by low flow compressors (3–6 L/min) and a reduced treatment time can be achieved. Breath activated nebulizers release mechanically or electronically controlled doses of aerosol only during inspiration, or a portion thereof, and theoretically may improve delivery to 100% of the generated aerosol. However, beyond dose control and reduced contamination of room air, the benefit of such systems are currently relatively low due to long treatment times and the high residual drug losses inherent with jet nebulizers.

Examples of breath enhanced nebulizers are the Ventstream® (Medic Aid) and the PARI LC PLUS® and LC STAR® nebulizers (PARI Respiratory Equipment). The concept of breath activated nebulizers has been used previously in diagnostic provocation test devices and is now entering the therapeutic arena. Examples are the Optineb® (Air Liquide), AeroEclipse® (Trudell Medical) and the HaloLite® or ProDose® systems (Profile Therapeutics).

Hygrosopic effects, whereby droplets evaporate or grow during transit through the respiratory tract, have long been thought to be an important aspect of nebulizer behavior, but probably play only a small role in high output rate nebulizers due to so-called two-way coupled effects (10). However, hygroscopic effects play an important role in proper measurement of nebulizer particle sizes, resulting in incorrect particle sizing, particularly if the nebulized aerosol is entrained with ambient air prior to size measurement, but also if the aerosol is heated in its transit through a cascade impactor (11).

Ultrasonic Nebulizers

Ultrasonic nebulizers use a piezoelectric transducer in order to create droplets from an open liquid reservoir. Pressure waves emitted from the piezo-vibrator in the bottom of the reservoir progress towards the surface forming a fountain within the wave focus. Droplets are formed by highly energetic surface instabilities in the lower part of the fountain as shown in Figure 2 (12). This process does not effectively aerosolize drug in suspensions, since the majority of the suspension particles are retained in the reservoir (13). Since the energy is transferred through the liquid container it becomes evident that formulation viscosity has a strong effect on aerosol particle size and output rate, and failure may occur with high viscosity liquids (12,14). In most ultrasonic nebulizers the heat produced by the piezo-element can result in denaturation of proteins and other thermally sensitive compounds (15). In some devices the drug formulation is in direct

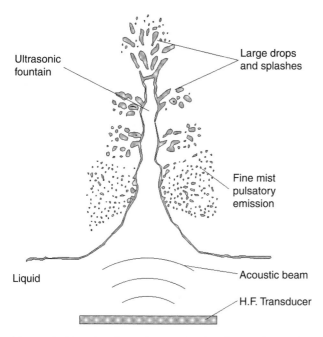

Figure 2 Droplet dispersion mechanism in an ultrasonic nebulizer. *Source*: From Ref. 12.

contact with the piezo-vibrator causing concerns regarding cleaning and microbial contamination. Later devices avoid this problem by using decalcified or distilled water as a transfer medium in which a separate, easy-to-clean or disposable drug container is inserted. The high density of the generated aerosol makes ultrasonic nebulizers ideal for airway humidification; however, the above mentioned constraints and high costs have limited their therapeutic use.

Passive Mesh-Type Piezoelectric Nebulizer

The OMRON U1 nebulizer uses an ultrasonic transducer to create a longitudinal vibration of a capillary tube. This motion pumps the liquid in contact with the lower end of the tube and ejects the liquid through a ceramic mesh adjacent to the other end. The mesh is perforated with micro-holes in the range of 5 μm in diameter. The advantage compared to jet and traditional ultrasonic nebulizers is the minimized residual volume in the drug reservoir. Drawbacks with respect to clogging of the holes and fragility of the ceramic mesh led to the development of the OMRON U14. This system feeds controlled doses of liquid into a gap between a piezo-vibrator and a mesh from where droplets are ejected. This principle is known from printer technologies. Both passive mesh-type nebulizers have a limited ability to generate sufficiently small droplets in the size range below 5 μm. The size distribution yields an MMD of approximately 7 μm and does not meet the requirements for lower respiratory tract applications. Further improvements to the technology have now been implemented in the i-Neb® nebulizer (Respironics) by combining the passive mesh technology and an intelligent breath trigger algorithm called Adaptive Aerosol Delivery (AAD®) technology (16). The iNeb has been approved for administration of Ventavis® (iloprost) inhalation solution (Actelion, formerly CoTherix) for the treatment of pulmonary arterial hypertension.

Vibrating Membrane-Type Piezoelectric Systems

With this technology, a thin perforated membrane is actuated by an annular piezo-element to vibrate in a resonant mode (17). The holes have a tapered shape with larger cross section on the liquid supply side and narrower cross section on the opposite side from where the droplets emerge. The membrane vibration in conjunction with the shape of the holes create pressure fluctuations and regular ejection of uniformly sized droplets. Depending on the therapeutic application, the hole sizes can be adjusted from 2 μm upwards, with several hundred to several thousand holes in each membrane. Figure 3 illustrates the dispersion principle, which currently is in development for a number of new aerosol delivery devices. These may cover a wide range of requirements from low dose single breath applications to treatments over several minutes for the delivery of large volumes and high doses of drug solutions or suspensions. The AeroNeb® Go and AeroNeb® Pro nebulizers (Nektar Therapeutics, formerly AeroGen) are open systems incorporating this technology for chronic treatments at home (asthma, COPD) and for hospital use in intensive care (ventilator setting), respectively. Another

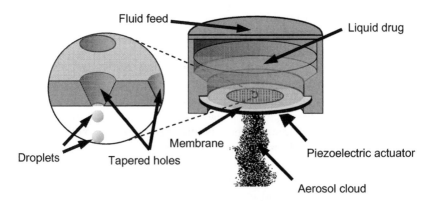

Figure 3 Droplet dispersion by a perforated vibrating membrane.

system for use with medications generally approved for administration via a nebulizer is the eFlow® rapid (PARI Pharma GmbH), marketed in the indication of cystic fibrosis (CF) in Europe. The eFlow electronic nebulizer, as a platform product, can be customized for advanced aerosol delivery of reformulated and novel drug formulations to the lungs (18) and has already entered numerous clinical studies to date, including phase III clinical trials of aztreonam lysine for inhalation, a monobactam antibiotic for the treatment of pseudomonas aeruginosa in CF (Gilead Sciences, formerly Corus Pharma). The driver for the development of this platform is to improve the delivery efficiency as compared to jet and traditional ultrasonic nebulizers.

Electrohydrodynamic Systems

Atomization by means of electrostatic charge is an old principle which has been discussed earlier for use in respiratory therapy (19). Two electrodes are charged with a high voltage of up to 30 kV. One electrode consisting of a metal shaft contains a central capillary tube for liquid supply. On the tip of the electrode, electrostatic forces shape a liquid cone with a fine mist of droplets emerging from the tip of this cone (20,21). Early stage prototypes based on this principle have demonstrated feasibility to generate aerosols suitable for inhalation (22). However, application requires drug formulations with distinct physical properties. In particular, liquids with certain conductivities and low surface tension, such as ethanol, are preferred (19). The Mystic® inhaler (formerly Battelle Pharma) was based on this principle, however, none of these systems has reached a commercial stage at this time.

REGULATORY ISSUES

In the past, a wide variety of nebulizers were accepted by regulatory bodies for use in clinical trials. Only rarely were specific requirements defined for nebulizer characteristics, and in many cases a distinct system was chosen as representative of nebulizer treatment as a whole. While pMDIs and multidose DPIs require approval as a drug product, refillable nebulizers were regarded as mechanical devices and are approved in the United States via a 510(k) marketing authorization procedure. This generic approach to nebulizers contributed to poor regulation and affected the reputation of nebulized aerosol therapy due to quality deficiencies of some nebulizer products (indeed, for a given drug the dose reaching the lungs may vary by a factor of ten among different nebulizer brands). Recognition of drug and nebulizer interactions and severe inter-device differences in lung deposition resulted in the specific selection of nebulizers for regulatory approval of new drug formulations. Examples are the FDA approval of Pulmozyme® (Genentech) for use with three distinct nebulizers in the United States and its worldwide registration for a number of nebulizers selected according to a standardized test protocol. Further examples are the FDA approval and registration in Europe of TOBI®(Novartis, formerly Chiron, formerly PathoGenesis) and the FDA approval of Pulmicort® suspension (AstraZeneca) both with the LC PLUS® nebulizer (PARI Respiratory Equipment) being selected for the final phase III clinical trials.

Better controlled clinical trials and tightened product specifications now build a link between drug and device with improved safety and efficacy in nebulizer therapy. Although use of a drug with devices other than those approved or registered cannot completely be prevented, device interfaces may be designed to prevent or discourage use with unauthorized medications. New devices and drug formulations will be conjointly developed to optimize specific therapeutic applications and be associated as unique drug/device combinations throughout the development and registration process, including the appropriate labelling. In the future, device specific liquid container systems may further support the drug/device combination concept in order to optimize safety and efficacy of inhaled therapies.

REFERENCES

1. Giffard P. Improvement in vaporizers. Patent No. 211, 234, United States Patent Office, 1878.
2. Palmer AJ, Palmer GH, Zerstaeuber P. Patent No. 47181, Kaiserliches Patentamt, 1888.
3. Finlay WH. An Introduction to the Mechanics of Inhaled Pharmaceutical Aerosols. London: Academic Press, 2001.
4. Dennis JH, Stenton SC, Beach JR, Avery AJ, Walters EH, Hendrick DJ. Jet and ultrasonic nebulizer output: Use of a new method for direct measurement of aerosol output. Thorax 1990; 45:728–32.
5. Finlay WH, Stapleton KW. Zuberbuhler P. Predicting lung dosages of a nebulized suspension: Pulmicort® (Budesonide). Particulate Sci Tech 1997; 15:243–51.
6. Taylor KMG, Farr SJ. Preparation of liposomes for pulmonary drug delivery. In: Gregoriadis G. ed. Liposome Preparations and Related Techniques. 2nd ed. Vol. 1. Boca Raton: CRC Press, 1993.
7. Finlay WH, Wong JP. Regional lung deposition of nebulized liposome-encapsulated ciprofloxacin. Int J Pharm 1998; 167:121.
8. Niven RW, Speer M, Schreier H. Nebulization of liposomes II. The effects of size and modelling of solute release profiles. Pharm Res 1991; 8:217–21.
9. Knoch M, Sommer E. Jet nebulizer design and function. Eur Respir Rev 2000; 10:183–6.
10. Finlay WH. Estimating the type of hygroscopic behaviour exhibited by aqueous droplets. J Aerosol Med 1998; 11:221–9.
11. Finlay WH, Stapleton KW. Undersizing of droplets from a vented nebulizer caused by aerosol heating during transit through an Anderson impactor. J Aerosol Sci 1999; 30:105–9.

12. Boucher RMG, Kreuter J. The fundamentals of the ultrasonic atomization of medicated solutions. Ann Allergy 1968; 26:591–600.

13. Nikander K, Turpeinen M, Wollmer P. The conventional ultrasonic nebulizer proved inefficient in nebulizing a suspension. J Aerosol Med 1999; 12:47–53.

14. Finlay WH, Lange CF, King M, Speert D. Lung delivery of aerosolized dextran. Am J Resp Crit Care Med 2000; 161:91–7.

15. Cipolla DC, Clark AR, Chan H-K, Gonda I, Shire SJ. Assessment of aerosol delivery systems for recombinant human deoxyribonuclease. STP Pharma Sci 1994; 4:50–62.

16. Denyer J, Nikander K, Smith NJ. Adaptive Aerosol Delivery (AAD®) technology. Expert Opin Drug Deliv 2004; 1(1):165–76.

17. Maehara N, Uhea S, Mori E. Influence of the vibrating system of a multi-pinhole-plate ultrasonic nebulizer on its performance. Rev Sci Instrum 1986; 57:2870–6.

18. Knoch M, Keller M. The customized electronic nebulizer: A new category of liquid aerosol drug delivery systems. Expert Opin Drug Deliv 2005; 2(2):377–90.

19. Greenspan BJ. Ultrasonic and electrohydrodynamic methods for aerosol generation. In: Hickey AJ, ed. Inhalation Aerosols. New York: Marcel Dekker, 1996: 313–35

20. Meesters GMH, Vercoulen PHW, Marijnissen JCM, Scarlett B. Generation of micron-sized droplets from the Taylor cone. J Aerosol Sci 1992; 23:37–49.

21. Jaworek A, Krupa A. Generation and characteristics of the precession mode of EHD spraying. J Aerosol Sci 1996; 27:75–82.

22. Zimlich WC, Ding JY, Busick DR, et al. The development of a novel electrohydrodynamic pulmonary drug delivery device. In: Dalby RN, Byron PR, Farr SJ, Peart J, eds. Respiratory Drug Delivery VII, Raleigh NC: Serentec Press, 2000: 241–6.

46

Formulation Challenges: Protein Powders for Inhalation

Hak-Kim Chan

Faculty of Pharmacy, University of Sydney, Australia

INTRODUCTION

Formulating protein powders for aerosol delivery is a challenge as it requires not only flowability and dispersibility of the powders but also biochemical stability of the protein molecules. To satisfy the latter requirement, proteins are usually formulated in amorphous glasses which are, however, physically unstable and tend to crystallize with inter-particulate bond formation and loss of powder dispersibility. In addition, the biochemical stability requirement limits the manufacturing processes that can be used for protein powder production. These challenges and possible ways to tackle them will be addressed in this chapter.

BIOCHEMICAL STABILITY

Proteins have secondary and higher order structures that must be maintained in order to be bioactive. During powder production, removal of water from the proteins can cause significant molecular conformational damage which can lead to further protein degradation such as aggregation, deamidation, and oxidation during storage. Amorphous glassy excipients, mainly carbohydrates, have been widely employed to stabilize proteins for inhalation: e.g., lactose for recombinant human deoxyribonuclease (rhDNase) (1,2), trehalose, lactose and mannitol for recombinant humanized anti-IgE monoclonal antibody (rhuMAbE25) (3), mannitol and raffinose for insulin (4). Other suitable excipients may include polymers (e.g., polyvinylpyrrolidone), proteins (e.g., human serum albumin), peptides (e.g., aspartame), amino acids (e.g., glycine), and organic salts (e.g., citrates). More recently, polyethylene glycol (PEG) and a diketopipirazine molecule capable of self-assembly have been used to produce insulin microspheres, ProMaxx™ (5,6) and Technosphere™ (7), respectively. Although lactose has widely been used for inhalation products for small molecule drugs, it may not be suitable for proteins. Being a reducing sugar, lactose is reactive toward the lysine residue and protein glycation has indeed been observed in both rhDNase and rhuMAbE25 (3,8). The exact mechanism for protein stabilization in the dry state is debatable. Contributing factors include (*i*) formation of a glassy state of the protein-excipient system, (*ii*) hydrogen bonding between the excipient and protein molecules, (*iii*) crystallinity of the excipients, and (*iv*) residual water content. In the glassy state, the diffusion rate and mobility of the protein molecules are much less than those in the rubbery state. Thus, any physico-chemical reactions leading to protein degradation will be diminished (9). In contrast to the amorphous excipients, crystalline excipients such as mannitol are known to reduce the stability of proteins (10). However, mannitol can be used in the amorphous form (e.g., in the presence of glycine) (11). Evidence for protein stabilization by hydrogen bonding has mainly come from the FTIR spectroscopy (12) which provides information on the protein secondary structures. The amide I absorption band ($\sim$1600–1700 cm^{-1}) of freeze-dried proteins with excipients was found to bear more similarities than the freeze-dried proteins alone to the native proteins in aqueous environment. Water affects the stability of proteins by enhancing the mobility of the protein molecules (13), as shown by solid state NMR spectroscopy (14). The crystalline or amorphous nature of the excipients is important because it controls the distribution of water between the protein and the excipient in a powder (15).

PHYSICAL STABILITY

While glassy materials are desirable for the protein stability, an immediate drawback is their physical instability. Water uptake by fine particles of hydrophilic amorphous materials can be very rapid, due to the significant specific surface area and high energy state. As exemplified by rhDNase co-spray dried with lactose (1,2), water uptake will induce crystallization which adversely affects powder dispersibility (Fig. 1).

Lactose at >34 wt% required for the biochemical stability of rhDNase was found recrystallized at moderate storage humidities of 38–57% RH (2). The probability for a glassy material to crystallize is critically determined by the storage temperature and relative humidity. In the crystallization process, water plays an essential role as a plasticiser to lower the T_g ($\sim$ 10°C decrease per 1% water in sugar-containing formulations), which, when close to the storage temperature, will enhance the molecular mobility required for

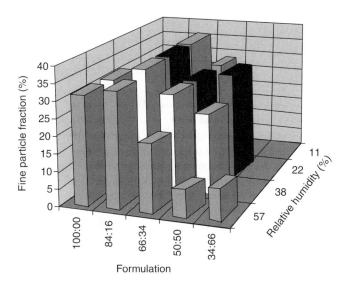

Figure 1 FPF of rhDNase:lactose formulations as a function of protein/sugar content and storage relative humidity after 4 weeks at 25°C. *Abbreviation*: FPF, fine particle fraction. *Source*: From Ref. 2.

nucleation (16). It is thus crucial to keep the powder dry in order to maintain the high T_g, or to use excipients with a high T_g, or to store the powders at a low temperature. It has been proposed to keep fragile glasses 50°C below the T_g to minimize crystallization (17), and this approach would be practical for room temperature storage for materials with a T_g of >70°C. Inhaler devices using gelatin capsules are likely to be problematic since gelatin capsules require a storage humidity of about 50% RH which may be too high for the glass materials. It is thus no coincidence that aluminum foil blisters have been chosen to store insulin powders for inhalation (18). It is also important to note that the effect of moisture on powder dispersion can be instantaneous (19). A possible way to reduce the hygroscopic effect is to use hydrophobic excipients. For example, spray dried particles of L-isoleucine, a hydrophobic amino acid, were shown to have superior physical stability at 40°C/75% RH for 6 months (20).

DISPERSIBILITY

Powder dispersibility is strongly determined by cohesion which, in turn, is related to size distribution, bulk density, surface area, surface energy, and surface morphology of the particles. The amorphous form of a given material has higher surface energy and more hygroscopic and hence, is more cohesive than the crystalline one. Dispersibility is thus strongly dependent on the physical state of the powder. Most protein drugs are prepared in the presence of one or more excipients for improved biochemical stability and/or device filling. However, the distribution of protein and excipient(s) in a particle is unlikely to be uniform. When a protein-excipient solution droplet undergoes drying to form a particle, the outer surface tends to be enriched with proteins or macromolecules that are surface active, as compared to small molecule excipients which can diffuse rapidly to the particle core. In special incidences, small excipient molecules can crystallize on the particle surface and modify the powder dispersibility (21). Various formulation approaches can be used to control the dispersibility of proteins powders.

Use of an Optimal Particle Size

Small particles are cohesive and difficult to disperse while large particles are easier to disperse but are not suitable for inhalation. Small particles can be better dispersed if a high air shear or a high efficiency inhaler is used. Thus, for a given inhaler at a given air flow, there exists an optimal particle size which will give the maximal fine particle fraction (FPF) in the aerosols. The optimal size is expected to be larger for cohesive powders and smaller for less cohesive ones. This was shown for the protein rhDNase (Fig. 2) (21), disodium cromoglycate (22), and mannitol (23) which is not only a pharmaceutical excipient, but also a diagnostic agent for asthma (24) and therapeutic agent for mucociliary clearance (25,26) when inhaled.

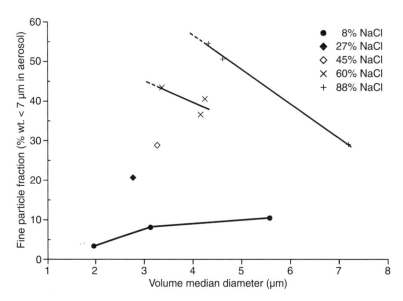

Figure 2 Dispersion properties (as FPF) versus particle size for powders of co-spray dried rhDNase and NaCl. *Abbreviation*: FPF, fine particle fraction. *Source*: From Ref. 21.

Co-Spray Drying with a Suitable Excipient

Sugars were used in co-spray dried anti-IgE antibody dry powder formulations. While lactose had no effect, both trehalose and mannitol were found to reduce the dispersibility of the antibody when the excipient:protein molar ratio was above 200:1. The deleterious effect was attributed to crystallization of the excipients. The choice of excipient is thus critical. Sodium chloride was co-spray dried with rhDNase to increase the dispersibility. In this particular case, the FPF of rhDNase increased linearly with the NaCl content and powder crystallinity (Fig. 3). Scanning electron microscopy revealed the presence of NaCl crystals on the surface of the protein particles (21). The dispersibility enhancement can be attributed to decreased cohesion as a result of changes in surface energy and morphology of the crystalline particles when the protein-salt composition changed.

Blending with a Suitable Carrier

Blending of the drug with an inert carrier to form a powder mix is generally used to give sufficient quantities for filling of low dose, potent protein drugs, and to enhance the powder flowability. However, it can also be explored to manipulate the dispersibility. Blending of spray dried pure rhDNase

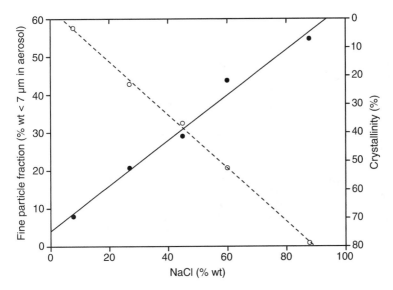

Figure 3 Relationship between NaCl content, the corresponding crystallinity (- - - -) and the dispersibility or FPF (——) of rhDNase powder aerosols. [All powders had similar primary particle size distribution before aerosolization, with median diameters of 2.7–3.3 μm (span 1.04–1.63)]. *Abbreviation*: FPF, fine particle fraction. *Source*: From Ref. 21.

with lactose was found to enhance the FPF in the aerosol by a factor of 2 and reduce the device retention 1.5–2 times, leading to a dramatic overall increase of FPF per dose loaded in the inhaler by three- to four fold (Fig. 4).

In this particular study, the improvement was found to be relatively insensitive to the carrier types, the protein/carrier blend ratio and the protein particle size (21). It is interesting to note that although monolayer-like adhesion of the protein particles on the carriers was observed, it did not appear to be a prerequisite for the FPF enhancement. Sometimes blending can reduce the dispersibility as in the case of recombinant human granulocyte-colony stimulating factor blended with PEG 8000 (27). More recently, fine carrier particles (<5 μm) have been used to enhance dispersibility (28) but the carrier deposition in the lung may raise clinical and regulatory concerns. Surface-treated carrier lactose (e.g., coating by magnesium stearate and sucrose tristearate), which has been found to enhance the aerosol performance of small molecules by reducing adhesion (29,30) is also likely to be useful for proteins drugs.

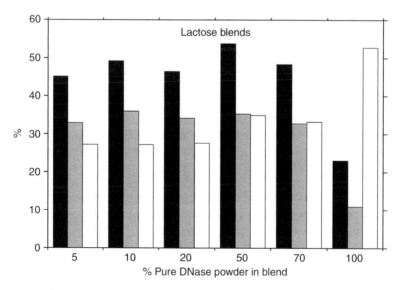

Figure 4 Dispersion properties of lactose blends containing different proportions of pure rhDNase particles (■FPF,▨dispersing efficiency, ☐device retention) [FPF is the wt% drug <7 μm in the aerosol, dispersing efficiency is the wt% drug <7 μm in the aerosol divided by the drug loaded in the inhaler device, device retention is the wt% drug retained in the inhaler (and capsules) after dispersion]. *Abbreviation*: FPF, fine particle fraction. *Source*: From Ref. 21.

USE OF LARGE POROUS PARTICLES

Large, porous particles (mean diameter 5–20 μm, specific surface area ~50–100 m^2/g) with a high degree of voids (particle mass density < 0.4 g/cc) have been found to improve FPF, as observed in particles containing insulin (20 wt%) and PLGA (80 wt%) (31). Despite the large physical size, the low particle density gave rise to a small aerodynamic size suitable for inhalation. The presence of the polymer also made these particles suitable for controlled release of the protein. The superior aerosol performance of large porous particles was also observed in anti-IgE powders (32) and was attributed to decreased cohesiveness of the porous particles.

PULMOSPHERES

These are hollow and porous particles but smaller in size (3–5 μm), also with low particle density and excellent dispersibility suitable for dry powder inhalers. These particles have been used to deliver immunoglobulin to the respiratory tract (33).

Use of Wrinkled Particles

Surface morphology can be modified to improve dispersibility. *Nonporous solid* protein particles with wrinkled surface have been reported to give a significant improvement in FPF over nonwrinkled spherical particles of bovine serum albumin (Fig. 5) (34). Surface corrugation of these particles was subsequently quantified using fractal dimension analysis which showed that a small degree of corrugation is sufficient for the FPF improvement (35). A distinct advantage of these particles, like the porous ones, is that they are less dependent on the inhaler device and air flow.

METHODS FOR PROTEIN POWDER PRODUCTION

Spray Drying

Spray drying is the most commonly used method to prepare protein powders for inhalation, e.g., rhDNase (20) rhGH, tPA (36,73), anti-IgE antibody (3,83), antibodies IgA and IgG (39), insulin (4), alpha 1-antitrypsin (40).

It involves spraying the protein solution into a concurrent stream of warm air which evaporates the spray to yield a dry powder which is collected in a cyclone. Depending on the spraying nozzle, powder nature, particle size, and the cyclone collection efficiency, the process yield varies, but can be low (< 50%), which is a major disadvantage of spray drying.

Spraying exposes the protein to mechanical shear and air-liquid interfacial denaturation while hot air drying subjects the protein to thermal stress and dry state denaturation. Thus, the major challenge during spray

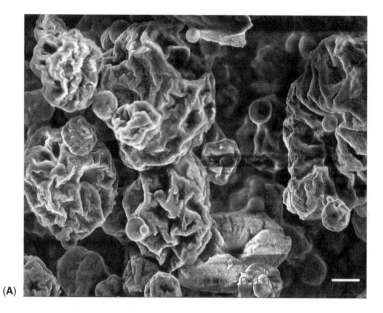

(A)

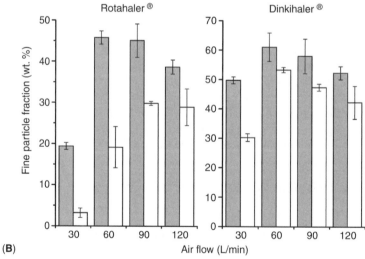

(B)

Figure 5 (**A**) Scanning electron micrograph of the spray-dried BSA wrinkled particles (scale bar 1 µm). (**B**) Dispersion properties of ■ wrinkled versus □ smooth spherical particles of BSA at various air flows. *Abbreviation*: BSA, bovine serum albumin. *Source*: From Ref. 34.

drying is to maintain the protein stability. For rhGH, interfacial denaturation has been shown to cause both soluble and insoluble aggregations which, in turn, can be suppressed by Zn^{2+} ions and surfactant polysorbate 20, respectively (36,37). A combination of polysorbate 20 and Zn^{2+}

effectively reduced the total aggregation down to 1.5% (37). While the stabilizing action of Zn^{2+} is specific to rhGH, by forming a $(rhGH-Zn^{2+})_2$ dimer, the use of surfactants should generally be applicable to other proteins which are vulnerable to air-liquid interfacial denaturation.

Spray drying is not limited to aqueous solutions and non-aqueous systems have been used. Ethanolic solutions (87%) of insulin containing human serum albumin and dipalmitoyl phosphatidylcholine as excipients were spray dried to prepare large porous particles for sustained release (41). Mixtures comprising a hIgG solution and a fluorocarbon-in-water emulsion were spray dried to obtain lipid-based hollow porous microspheres (Pulmospheres™) of human IgG. The spray dried powders were collected in perflubron and lyophilized to produce free flowing particles (33).

Spray Freeze Drying

Spray freeze drying involves spraying the protein solution into a freezing medium (usually liquid nitrogen) followed by lyophilization. The method has recently been applied to prepare rhDNase and anti-IgE antibody particles for inhalation (32). Compared with spray drying, this process produces light and porous particles with superior aerosol performance, and the production yield is almost 100%. However, this process is more costly and time consuming as it requires the additional use of liquid nitrogen and freeze drying.

Double-Emulsification Solvent Evaporation

This method was used to produce large porous particles of PLGA particles loaded with 20 wt% insulin (31). Aqueous insulin solution was sonicated with a methylene chloride solution of PLGA to form the first emulsion, which was then poured into 1% aqueous polyvinyl alcohol solution and homogenized to form the double emulsion. The major disadvantage of this method is exposing the proteins to shear or sonic stress and organic solvents during emulsification. It is also a more complicated procedure than spray drying.

Lyophilization/Milling

This is a two-step process involving protein lyophilization followed by milling. Gas-jet milling has been employed to micronize lyophilized powders of human growth hormone, interferon-beta, and granulocyte colony stimulating factor (42). However, milling produced insoluble contaminants and protein inactivation. Thus, abrasive-resistant mills utilizing high-purity nitrogen and the use of milling stabilizers such as human serum albumin and sorbitol were required. Protein degradation as well as high energy and time demands limit the general usefulness of this process.

Solvent Precipitation

Inhalable protein particles can be obtained by precipitation from aqueous solutions using non-solvents. In recent years, supercritical fluids (SCFs) are increasingly used for this application. Carbon dioxide is particularly attractive as it has a low critical temperature of 31.1°C for operation. It is also non-toxic, cheap and readily available. However, being non-polar and immiscible with water, SC CO_2 cannot be readily used as an anti-solvent to precipitate proteins from aqueous solutions. Insulin precipitated from DMSO solutions has been shown to be structurally stable for 2-year storage (43). However, DMSO is toxic and residue solvent can be a major concern. To overcome this limitation, water-based protein solutions can be used. York and co-workers have used a special coaxial nozzle to enhance mixing of water-based protein solution with SC CO_2 (44). Alternatively, fine powders can be obtained by expanding an emulsion of the aqueous protein solution and SC CO_2 through a nozzle (45). Foster and co-worker developed another approach by using high pressure CO_2 modified with ethanol, which has successfully been employed as an anti-solvent to precipitate rhDNase and insulin from aqueous solutions (46,47). A potential problem of using CO_2 is its acidic nature but solution pH can be adjusted to minimize protein degradation. Although still believed to be a promising technology to produce powdered drugs, a major SCF operation (48) has very recently been closed. This may be related to the cost, scale-up and reproducibility of the technology.

Other precipitation technologies include the use of excipients to form microparticles. Insulin is formulated into ProMaxx microspheres by mixing an aqueous insulin suspension with PEG at controlled pH and ionic strength, followed by cooling which produces the microspheres with sizes of 1–2 μm (5). In another method, insulin is encapsulated inside 2 μm agglomerates of pH-induced self-assembling small organic molecules of 3,6-bis(N-fumaryl-N-(n-Butyl)amino-2,5-diketopiperazine (7,49). This molecule, having two carboxylic acid groups, is soluble in alkaline pH and will precipitate out as the pH is lowered. During precipitation, hydrogen bonding and other molecular interactions enable formation of the self-assembled agglomerates entrapping the protein.

Mostly recently, high-gravity controlled precipitation (HGCP), coupled withspray drying, has been used to produce powers of small molecule drugs with superior aerosol performance (50,51). This technology is simple, easy to scale up and is potentialy applicable for generation of protein particles for inhalation delivery.

CONCLUSIONS

Formulation of proteins as powders for aerosol delivery is a dual challenge as it requires both powder dispersibility and protein biochemical stability.

However, a balance between these two requirements can be found and a number of proteins have successfully been formulated. Selection of appropriate excipients and minimization of powder exposure to moisture are critical as they affect both physical and biochemical stabilities. Currently, protein powders are mainly produced by spray drying but other technologies such as SCF and HGCP precipitation may prove to be useful alternatives in the future.

REFERENCES

1. Chan H-K, Gonda I. Solid state characterization of spray-dried powders of recombinant human deoxyribonuclease (rhDNase). J Pharm Sci 1998; 87: 647–54.
2. Clark AR, Dasovich N, Gonda I, et al. The balance between biochemical and physical stability for inhalation protein powders: rhDNase as an example. In: RN Dalby, PR Bryon, SJ Farr, eds. Respiratory Drug Delivery V, Buffalo Grove, IL: Interpharm Press, 1996; 167–74.
3. Andya JD, Maa Y-F, Costantino HR, et al. The effect of formulation excipients on protein stability and aerosol performance of spray-dried powders of a recombinant humanized anti-IgE monoclonal antibody. Pharm Res 1999; 16: 350–8.
4. Patton JS, Foster L, Platz RM. Methods and compositions for pulmonary delivery of insulin. US Patent 5,997,848; 1999.
5. Brown LR, Rashba-Step J, Scott T, et al. Pulmonary delivery of novel insulin microspheres. In: RN Dalby, PR Byron, J Peart, JD Suman, SJ Farr, eds. Respiratory Drug Delivery IX, Raleigh, NC: Davis Horwood International Publishing, 2004; 431–3.
6. Scott T, Sullivan A, Proos R, et al. Novel technology for fabrication of therapeutic microspheres for pulmonary delivery. In: RN Dalby, PR Byron, J Peart, JD Suman, SJ Farr, eds. Respiratory Drug Delivery IX, Raleigh, NC: Davis Horwood International Publishing, 2004; 431–33.
7. Steiner S, Pfützner A, Wilson BR, et al. Technosphere™/Insulin–proof of concept study with a new insulin formulation for pulmonary delivery. Exp Clin Endocrinol Diabetes 2002; 110:17–21.
8. Quan CP, Dasovich N, Hsu CC, et al. Susceptibility of rhDNase I to glycation in the dry-powder state. Anal Chem 1999; 71:4445–54.
9. Frank F. Long-term stabilization of biologicals. Biotech 1994; 12:253–6.
10. Izutsu K, Yoshioka S, Terao T. Decreased protein-stabilizing effects of cryoprotectants due to crystallization. Pharm Res 1993; 10:1232–37.
11. Pikal MJ, Dellerman KM, Roy ML, et al. The effects of formulation variables on the stability of freeze-dried human growth hormone. Pharm Res 1991; 8: 427–36.
12. Carpenter JF, Prestrelski SJ, Dong A. Application of infrared spectroscopy to development of stable lyophilized protein formulations. Eur J Pharm Biopharm 1998; 45:231–8.

13. Hageman MJ. Water Sorption and Solid-State Stability of Proteins. In: Stability of Protein pharmaceuticals. Part A. In: TJ Ahern, MC Manning, eds, Plenum Press, 1992; 273–309.

14. Separovic F, Lam YH, Ke X, et al. A solid-state NMR study of protein hydration and stability. Pharm Res 1998; 15:1816–21.

15. Chan H-K, Au-Yeung JK-L, Gonda I. Development of a mathematical model for the water distribution in freeze-dried solids. Pharm Res 1999; 16:660–5.

16. Roos Y, Karel M. Plasticizing effect of water on thermal behavior and crystallization of amorphous food models. J Food Sci 1991; 56:38–43.

17. Hancock B, Shamblin S, Zografi G. Molecular mobility of amorphous pharmaceutical solids below their glass transition temperatures. Pharm Res 1995; 12:799–806.

18. Patton JS. Deep-lung delivery of therapeutic proteins. Chemtech December 1997; 34–8.

19. Chew NYK, Chan H-K. Effect of humidity on the dispersion of dry powders. In: RN Dalby, PR Byron, SJ Farr, eds. Respiratory Drug Delivery VII, Raleigh, North Carolina: Serentec Press, 2000; 615–7.

20. Yamashita C, Nishibayashi T, Akashi S, et al. A novel formulation of dry powder for inhalation of peptides and proteins. In: RN Dalby, PR Byron, SJ Farr, eds. Respiratory Drug Delivery V, Buffalo Grove, IL: Interpharm Press, 1996; 483–5.

21. Chan H-K, Clark AR, Gonda I, et al. Spray dried powders and powder blends of recombinant human deoxyribonuclease (rhDNase) for aerosol delivery. Pharm Res 1997; 14:431–7.

22. Chew NYK, Bagster DF, Chan H-K. Effect of particle size, air flow and inhaler device on the aerosolisation of disodium cromoglycate powders. Int J Pharm 2000; 206:75–83.

23. Chew NYK, Chan H-K. Dispersion of mannitol powders as aerosols: influence of particle size, air flow and inhaler device. Pharm Res 1999; 16:1098–103.

24. Anderson SD, Brannan JD, Chan H-K. Use of aerosols for bronchial provocation testing in the laboratory: where we have been and where we are going. Journal of Aerosol Medicine 2002; 15:313–24.

25. Daviskas E, Anderson SD, Brannan JD, et al. Inhalation of dry-powder mannitol increases mucociliary clearance. European Respiratory Journal 1997; 10:2449–54.

26. Daviskas E, Anderson SD. Hyperosmolar Agents and Clearance of Mucus in the Diseased Airway. Journal of Aerosol Medicine 2006; 19:100–9.

27. French DL, Edwards DA, Niven RW. The influence of formulation on emission, deaggregation and deposition of dry powders for inhalation. J Aerosol Sci 1996; 27:769–83.

28. Lucas P, Anderson K, Staniforth JN. Protein deposition from dry powder inhalers: fine particle multiplets as performance modifiers. Pharm Res 1998; 15:562–9.

29. Iida K, Hayakawa Y, Okamoto H, et al. Effect of surface layering time of lactose carrier particles on dry powder inhalation properties of salbutamol sulfate. Chemical & Pharmaceutical Bulletin 2004; 52:350–3.

30. Iida K, Hayakawa Y, Okamoto H, et al. Effect of surface covering of lactose carrier particles on dry powder inhalation properties of salbutamol sulfate. Chemical & Pharmaceutical Bulletin 2003; 51:1455–7.
31. Edwards DA, Hanes J, Caponetti G, et al. Large porous particles for pulmonary drug delivery. Science 1997; 276:1868–71.
32. Maa Y-F, Nguyen P-A, Sweeney T, et al. Protein inhalation powders: spray drying vs spray freeze drying. Pharm Res 1999; 16:249–54.
33. Bot AI, Tarara TE, Smith DJ, et al. Novel lipid-based hollow-porous microparticles as a platform for immunoglobulin delivery to the respiratory tract. Pharm Res 2000; 17:275–83.
34. Chew N, Chan H-K. Use of solid corrugated particles to enhance powder aerosol performance. Pharmaceutical Research 2001; 18:1570–7.
35. Chew NYK, Tang P, Chan H-K, et al. How Much Particle Surface Corrugation is Sufficient to Improve Aerosol Performance of Powders? Pharm Res 2005; 22:147–51.
36. Mumenthaler M, Hsu CC, Pearlman R. Feasibility study on spray-drying protein pharmaceuticals: recombinant human growth hormone and tissueplasminogen activator. Pharm Res 1994; 11:12–20.
37. Maa Y-F, Nguyen P-A, Hsu SW. Spray-drying of air-liquid interface sensitive recombinant human growth hormone. J Pharm Sci 1998; 87:152–9.
38. Costantino HR, Andya JD, Nguyen P-A, et al. Effect of mannitol crystallization on the stability and aerosol performance of a spray-dried pharmaceutical protein, recombinant humanized anti-IgE monoclonal antibody. J Pharm Sci 1998; 87:1406–11.
39. Platz RM, Patton JS, Foster L, et al. Dispersible antibody compositions and methods for their preparation and use. US Patent 6,019,968. 2000.
40. Eljamal M, Patton JS. Methods and apparatus for pulmonary administration of dry powder α1-antitrypsin. US Patent 5,993,783. 1999.
41. Vanbever R, Mintzes JD, Wang J, et al. Formulation and physical characterization of large porous particles for inhalation. Pharm Res 1999; 16:1735–41.
42. Platz RM, Ip A, Whitham CL. Process for preparing micronized polypeptide drugs. US Patent 5,354,562. 1994.
43. Winters MA, Debenedetti PG, Carey J, et al. Long-term and high-temperature storage of supercritically-processed microparticulate protein powders. Pharm Res 1997; 14:1370–8.
44. Sloan R, Hollowood HE, Hupreys GO, et al. Supercritical fluid processing: preparation of stable protein particles. Proceedings of the 5th meeting of supercritical fluids, Nice, France, 1998.
45. Sievers RE, Sellers SP, Kusek KD, et al. Fine-particle formation using supercritical carbon dioxide-assisted aerosolization and bubble drying. Proceedings of 218th ACS National Meeting, New Orleans, 1999.
46. Bustami R, Chan H-K, Foster NR. Aerosol delivery of protein powders processed by supercritical fluid technology. In: RN Dalby, PR Bryon, SJ Farr, eds. Respiratory Drug Delivery VII, Raleigh, North Carolina: Serentec Press, 2000; 611–3.

47. Bustami R, Chan H-K, Dehaghani F, et al. Generation of micro-particles of proteins for aerosol delivery using high pressure modified carbon dioxide. Pharm Res 2000; 17:1360–6.
48. Nektar Therapeutics Press Releases. 26 Jul. 2006.
49. Lian H, Steiner SS, Sofia RD, et al. A self-complementary, self-assembling microsphere system: application for intravenous delivery of the antiepileptic and neuroprotectant compound felbamate. J Pharm Sci 2000; 89:867–75.
50. Chiou H, Li L, Hu T, et al. Production of salbutarmol sulfate for inhalation by high-gravity controlled antisolvent precipitation. Int J Pharm 2007; 331:93–8.
51. Hu T, Chiou H, Chan H-K, et al. Preparation of inhalable salbutamol sulphate using reactive high gravity controlled precipitation. J Pharm Sci 2008; 97:932–7.

47

The Respimat®, a New Soft Mist™ Inhaler for Delivering Drugs to the Lungs

Herbert Wachtel

Boehringer Ingelheim Pharma GmbH & Co. KG, Ingelheim, Germany

Achim Moser

Boehringer Ingelheim MicroParts GmbH, Dortmund, Germany

INTRODUCTION

The inhalation of drugs provides the most direct noninvasive route either for treating respiratory disorders topically or for administering drugs systemically. The Respimat® Soft Mist™ Inhaler (SMI) has been designed to produce a slowly moving cloud of droplets ("soft mist") with more than 60 wt% smaller than 5 µm. This "soft mist" is easy to inhale within one breath. Correspondingly, even the lung deposition of aqueous formulations is high, for example, 63% (rel. to emitted dose) of radio-labeled Berodual® was detected in the lungs of COPD patients inhaling slowly and deeply (1).

HISTORICAL DEVELOPMENT

In the past, pressurized metered-dose inhalers (pMDIs) were popular pocket-sized devices for generating inhalable aerosols. Early pMDIs containing chlorofluorocarbon (CFC) propellants are currently being phased out, and there are also concerns about the global warming potential of alternative propellants such as hydrofluoroalkanes, developed to replace CFCs. Efforts to develop alternative devices include various dry powder inhalers but these have their own shortcomings, as described by Ganderton (2). There is, therefore, an urgent need for a convenient, propellant-free inhaler device to deliver aerosols from solutions. The challenge for any solution-based system consists in the choice of a suitable atomization mechanism. In the early 1990s, the Respimat concept was demonstrated in a laboratory model, consisting of a metal body with a syringe as a solution reservoir, and it was shown to function correctly (3). The device was operated by means of a lever arm, which simultaneously tightened the mainspring and withdrew a metered volume of drug solution (about 13.5 μL) from the reservoir. Pressing a button released the spring, forcing the metered dose through the nozzle. In this first model, the nozzle openings were tiny holes pierced into a stainless steel disk. However, a nozzle design better suited for mass production was needed. This was achieved by developing a miniature "sand-wich" concept, the uniblock, consisting of a rectangle (2 ×2.5 mm) cut from a glass plate bonded to a silicon wafer. Having tested several different principles, the impinging-jet nozzle design was selected because of reproducible production of the nozzle assembly. Its striking advantages are, for example, the creation of a Soft Mist the suitable duration of the spray, and the opportunity to use a robust mechanical pump that can be easily operated by the patient (4).

DESCRIPTION OF THE TECHNOLOGY

The generation of an inhalable aerosol from a drug solution requires that the bulk liquid be dosed and then converted into appropriately sized droplets. There are several technically feasible methods for achieving the aerosolization of a drug solution in a pocket-sized device. These methods (e.g., piezoelectric effect, extrusion through micron-sized holes, electro-hydrodynamic effect) require either electric energy from a battery or mechanical energy to produce the aerosol. In any case, the energy has to be focused for the aerosolization process. This often results in acceleration of the aerosol. After atomization, it is desirable to slow down the aerosol cloud in order to minimize throat deposition.

In the case of Respimat, the technical breakthrough is based on the approach of forcing drug solution through a two-channel nozzle (5). During this process the solution is accelerated and split into two converging jets. The impinging jets, which converge at a designed angle, disintegrate into inhalable droplets. These small droplets quickly slow down and, finally, the droplets adopt the velocity of the surrounding air.

The principal parts of Respimat are shown in a schematic diagram (Fig. 1A). To use the device, the patient removes the transparent base, inserts the cartridge containing the drug solution, and mounts the transparent base again. The cartridge is now connected to the uniblock by a capillary tube (containing a nonreturn valve). When a cartridge is inserted for the first time, the device has to be primed to expel air from its inner parts. The device is then ready for use.

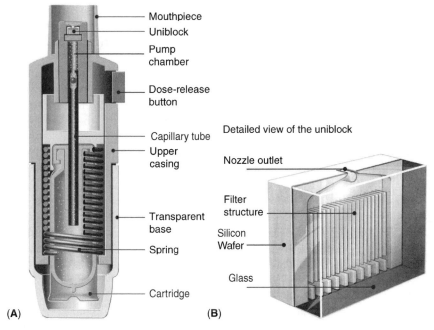

Figure 1 Schematic cross section of Respimat® Softmist™ Inhaler (**A**) and three-dimensional representation of the uniblock nozzle assembly (**B**).

To load a dose, the patient simply turns the transparent base by 180°. The helical can transforms the rotation into a linear movement, which tightens the spring and moves the capillary with the nonreturn valve to a defined lower position. During this movement, the drug solution is drawn through the capillary into a pump chamber as shown in Figure 1A. When the patient presses the dose release button, the mechanical power of the spring pushes the capillary with the now closed nonreturn valve to the upper position. This operation drives the metered volume of drug solution through the nozzle in the uniblock. At the nozzle outlets of the uniblock, two fine jets of liquid are produced. The resulting impact of the two jets of liquid generates a slow moving aerosol cloud, or Soft Mist. It is then the task of the patient to inhale slowly and deeply in order to achieve optimum delivery to the lungs.

RESEARCH AND DEVELOPMENT OF RESPIMAT®

Scale-Up Issues

The first viable prototype was obtained when a uniblock with two channels was constructed. Its liquid jets impacted at a distance of 25 µm from the nozzle outlet to produce the aerosol. A feasibility study using an aqueous drug solution of a β_2-agonist showed that the droplet size distribution in the aerosol was in the range suitable for inhalation: the majority of the particle mass was in the size range 1–5 µm.

The rise of photolithographic techniques adapted from the microelectronics industry, multiple copies of the uniblock, each comprising filter structures as well as inlet and outlet channels (Fig. 1B), are etched into the silicon wafer with high precision and accuracy. Currently, the accuracy of the photolithographic exposure process is better than 0.1 µm over a single uniblock bearing the etched nozzle microstructure. The mechanical strength of the uniblock has been optimized using finite-element simulation techniques (6). Further development of this first model included exchanging all metal parts for components made from polymers whenever possible and adapting all parts of the device for mass production. In addition, the torque required for loading the dose was minimized (approximately 40 cNm) so that the energy needed to generate the aerosol could be easily produced by hand. After initial stability and technical performance tests, the device was successfully used in the first lung deposition study, in comparison with a pMDI containing CFCs, carried out on healthy volunteers.

The experience accumulated with the various prototypes (I–IV, not shown) and the need to make a functionally practical device with a smaller number of individual components was combined with the results of device-handling studies, in which patients evaluated the four different design concepts. The resultant device, prototype IV, incorporated a radical change in design. Compared to the prototype I design, which released the dose at an angle of 90° relative to the axis of the pump chamber (i.e., the mouthpiece was at right angles to the drug cartridge), the final design releases the dose in a direction parallel to the axis. The device has been equipped with a dose-indicator. In fulfilment of regulatory requirements, life-span-blocking has been incorporated. A discussion of regulatory issues concerning the marketing authorization applications in Europe and the United States is given by Böck (7). In spring 2004, Berodual® Respimat® was launched on the German Market: a drug product using Respimat® SMI for the application of Berodual®, an aqueous formulation of fenoterol and ipratropium bromide. The latest version of Respimat (Fig. 1A) is currently being tested in clinical phase II and phase III studies with innovative formulations.

In Vitro Studies

Respimat SMI is an active system, which means that the aerosol is generated by a constantly available and consistent energy source. Its output quality ex-mouthpiece, in terms of dose and particle size distribution, is independent of both the patient's inspiratory flow and ambient conditions.

Water, ethanol, or a mixture of both, can be used as a solvent for formulating the drug solution. Aqueous drug solutions also contain the two excipients benzalkonium chloride and EDTA, as preservatives which are well tolerated (8). The optional choice of solvents and tuneable spray parameters of its nozzle make Respimat a readily available device platform for developing new inhalative therapies. Once the aerosol has left the Respimat SMI, the individual droplets interact with their environment and experimental conditions (in vitro) or the patient's morphometry or constitution (in vivo) can influence the performance, as governed by aerosol physics. The fine particle fraction, defined as the mass percentage of the aerosol consisting of particles smaller than 5 μm, is higher for an ethanolic formulation than for an aqueous formulation generated by the Respimat® SMI. Figure 2 shows typical examples of the particle size distribution of aqueous and ethanolic solutions measured in an Andersen Cascade Impactor (ACI, Andersen Instruments, Inc., Smyrna, GA), as already quoted in the previous edition for formulation A and B (5). Checking the particle size distribution also at high relative humidity (RH > 95%) shows that the droplets of formulations C and D remain small enough in order to reach their targets in the lungs (Fig. 2B and Table 1).

The fine particle fraction (Table 1) generated by Respimat SMI is higher than those of aerosol clouds from conventional portable inhaler devices, such as pMDIs and dry powder inhalers (6). The soft mist generated has relatively long spray duration. In case of Berodual, the spray duration was set to 1.5±0.2 seconds (6). The spray duration is selected in order to facilitate maximal inhalation of the dose, allowing the patient time to inhale after pressing the dose release button, in contrast to the critical need to coordinate actuation and inspiration that is required during the use of pMDIs. In addition, the soft mist produces a perceptible taste or sensation, providing appropriate feedback to indicate that the dose has been released in contrast to findings with some powder inhalers.

In Vivo Studies

The in vitro performance data of the aerosol produced by Respimat SMI led to the hypothesis that the delivery of drugs to the lungs is improved compared to the existing treatment with pMDIs. This hypothesis was tested in several scintigraphic deposition studies carried out in volunteers and patients. In these studies the radionuclide [99mTc] is added to the formulation so that it forms a physical association with the micronized drug particles in a suspension formulation (e.g., of a pMDI) or is incorporated into the droplets of a solution formulation. The topographical deposition of the aerosol in the lungs is visualized using a gamma camera and quantified in terms of the percentage of lung or oropharyngeal deposition with reference

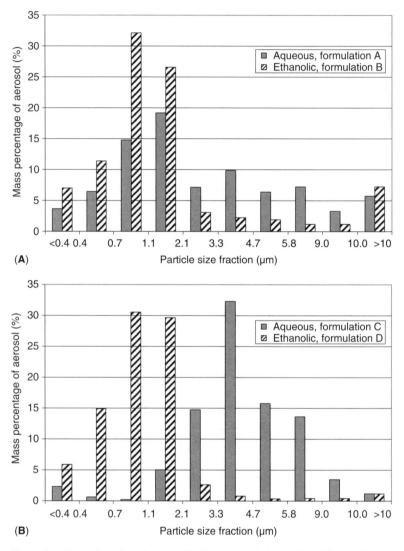

Figure 2 Examples of particle size distributions relative to the delivered dose using the Andersen Cascade Impactor: (**A**) aqueous drug solution and ethanolic drug solution measured at 22°C ± 2°C and RH = 50 ± 10%; (**B**) effect of experimental condition: aqueous and ethanolic drug solutions at 22°C ± 2°C and RH >95%.

to the metered dose. A survey of the numerical results obtained for pMDIs, dry powder inhalers, and Respimat SMI with this type of investigation is reported by Newman (9). In summary, the deposition data show that the soft mist generated by Respimat SMI, both from an aqueous solution, with

Table 1 Parameters of Typical Formulations as Determined by ACI Measurements. Drug Substance Quantified by HPLC

Formulation	Solvent	Rel. humidity (%)	FPF ($< 5 \mu m$) (%)	MMAD (μm)	GSD
A	H2O	50	63	2.0	2.6
B	EtOH	50	83	1.1	2.2
C	H2O	>95	60	4.2	2.0
D	EtOH	>95	85	1.0	1.9

Abbreviation: ACI, Andersen Cascade Impactor; HPLC, high performance liquid chromatography.

the drug fenoterol, and from an ethanolic solution, with the drug flunisolide, results in a twofold to threefold increase in lung deposition compared to the corresponding pMDI. In parallel, the oropharyngeal deposition is significantly reduced for the aerosol administered by Respimat SMI.

Finally, the ratio of deposition in peripheral regions to deposition in the central lung zone is similar for Respimat SMI and a pMDI. The increased drug delivery to the lungs from Respimat SMI measured with the gamma scintigraphy technique suggests that clinically comparable therapeutic responses should be achievable with lower doses administered to patients from Respimat SMI compared to a pMDI. In two clinical studies for aqueous drug solutions with fenoterol (Berotec®) and the combination of fenoterol/ipratropium bromide (Berodual®), this expected result was confirmed. For Berotec, 12.5 and 25 µg administered by Respimat SMI were therapeutically equivalent to either 100 or 200 µg administered via pMDI (10). For Berodual, the bronchodilatory effects of 25/10 or 50/20 µg (fenoterol/ipratropium bromide) doses administered via Respimat SMI were equal or slightly superior to the recommended dose of 100/40 µg given via pMDI (11). These results suggest that the improved lung deposition observed with Respimat SMI allows lower absolute doses to be administered for a similar clinical effect in the local treatment of lung diseases. Additionally, Respimat's high performance may result in a more efficient systemic delivery of drugs via the lungs.

TECHNOLOGY POSITION/COMPETITIVE ADVANTAGE

Demonstrating a new approach to inhalation therapy, Respimat SMI, a propellant-free, pocket-sized inhaler with a novel patented mechanism of generating a soft mist from a dosed volume of a drug solution, shows distinct advantages over contemporary inhaler devices. Like many other inhalers, Respimat SMI delivers multiple doses of an aerosol; however, Respimat SMI does this actively without the use of propellants. Respimat

SMI simply uses mechanical energy that is easily produced by the patient before each administration. The soft mist demonstrates improved particle characteristics compared to existing inhalers, especially chlorofluorocarbon pMDIs, thereby increasing the targeting of drugs to the lungs. The particle size distribution of the aerosol generated by Respimat SMI is practically influenced only by the surface tension and the viscosity of the drug solution. At ambient conditions these parameters do not change much; therefore, Respimat SMI produces the soft mist in a repeatable and consistent manner.

FUTURE DIRECTIONS

The mechanical operation principle makes Respimat SMI a versatile respiratory delivery system, which may be called a "platform" device. Besides the local treatment of lung diseases, the systemic administration of drugs with the lungs as the point of entry will become more important. This is mainly driven by the upcoming development of drugs with a protein structure. For this type of drug, the inhalative route could be a convenient and safe method of delivery into the body.

REFERENCES

1. Brand P, Hederer B, Lowe L, Herpich C, Häussermann S, Sommerer K. Flow dependence of lung deposition of an HFA pMDI and the Respimat® Soft Mist™ Inhaler in COPD Patients. Pneumologie 2007; 61(2): A1.
2. Ganderton D. Targeted delivery of inhaled drugs: current challenges and future goals. J Aerosol Med 1999; 12(Suppl. 1):S3–S8.
3. Weston TE, King A, Dunne S. Patent application WO 91/14468.
4. Spallek M, Hochrainer D, Wachtel H. Optimizing nozzles for soft mist inhalers. Respir Drug Delivery VIII 2002; 2:375–8.
5. Zierenberg B. Optimizing the in vitro performance of Respimat®. J Aerosol Med 1999; 12(Suppl. 1):S19–S24.
6. Dalby R, Spallek M, Voshaar T. A review of the development of Respimat® Soft Mist™ Inhaler. Int J Pharm 2004; 283(1–2):1–9.
7. Böck G. Comparison of the marketing authorization applications of Respimat® Soft Mist™ Inhaler in Europe and United States. In: Scheuch G. ed. Aerosole in der Inhalationstherapie VIII, Dustri-Verlag Dr. Karl Feistle, Munich-Orlando 2004; 133–44.
8. Koehler D, Pavia D, Dewberry D, Hodder R. Low incidence of paradoxical bronchoconstriction with bronchodilator drugs administered by Respimat® Soft Mist™ Inhaler: Results of phase II single-dose crossover studies. Respiration 2004; 71(5):469–76.
9. Newman SP. Use of gamma scintigraphy to evaluate the performance of new inhalers. J Aerosol Med 1999; 12(Suppl. 1):S25–S31.

10. Measen FV, van Noord JA, Streets JJ, Greefhorst APM. Dose range finding study comparing a new soft mist inhaler with a conventional metered dose inhaler (MDI) to deliver fenoterol in patients with asthma. Eur Respir J 1997; 10:128L.
11. Goldberg J, Freund E, Beckers B, Hinzmann R. Improved delivery of fenoterol plus ipratropium bromide using Respimat® compared with a conventional metered dose inhaler. Eur Respir J 2001; 17:225–32.

48

Pressurized Metered Dose Inhalation Technology

Ian C. Ashurst

GlaxoSmithKline Research and Development, Ware, Hertfordshire, U.K.

INTRODUCTION

The metered dose inhaler (MDI) has been used for over 50 years as the primary method of delivering therapeutic agents to treat lung diseases such as asthma. This chapter updates that written for the first edition of this book and specifically focuses on literature published since 2000. The major challenges over this period have been in phasing out of chlorofluorocarbon (CFC)-based MDIs and replacing them with robust hydrofluoroalkane (HFA)-based MDIs. In addition to the replacement of the propellants, there has been a focus on developing once-daily formulations either by using new chemical entities that have a longer pharmacological life or by manipulation of formulations through the use of surfactants or other long-chain additives (1). In addition, other developments have focused on a more rapid inhaled delivery of agents normally delivered via other routes, e.g., oral (2). This can also be achieved by manipulation of formulations, again typically using surfactants. Hence, this chapter primarily focuses on the approach of modifying the release of therapeutic agents by using surfactants or other long-chain molecules in the formulation of MDIs. The chapter also covers improvements in the MDI device and briefly looks at recent developments in actuator design and the addition of dose counters.

HISTORICAL DEVELOPMENT

The first HFA-based MDI was launched into the market in 1995 and consisted of an albuterol sulfate/HFA 134a formulation where oleic acid and ethanol were also used as formulation additives (3). The first combination product was launched into the market in 2001 and contained salmeterol xinafoate and fluticasone propionate in HFA134a (4). Currently, there are no sustained-release HFA-based MDIs in the market that allow once-daily dosing, except for those where the dosage level is determined by the half-life of the drug, e.g., formoterol. One of the major challenges in the CFC to HFA transition has been the replacement of surfactants readily soluble in CFC propellant but with limited solubility in HFA propellant with surfactants (e.g., oleic acid, lecithin, sorbitan trioleate) that would withstand robust preclinical testing. In recent years, there has been a significant increase in the literature of references to alternate surfactants for HFA MDIs.

A typical anatomy of the MDI is given in Figure 1, where there is a liquid phase that contains the formulation, typically a drug suspension or

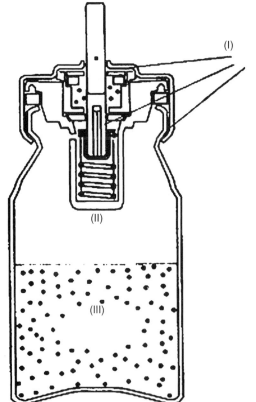

I.   Sealing mechanism of metered valve
II. Vapor phase in the MDI-propellant vapor
III. Condensed phase-drug, surfactant,
     solvent and propellant

Figure 1   Anatomy of the pressurized metered-dose inhaler: (*i*) sealing mechanism of metered valve; (*ii*) vapor phase consisting of propellant vapor and other volatile components; (*iii*) condensed phase consisting of drug, surfactant, solvent, and propellant. *Source*: From Ref. 5.

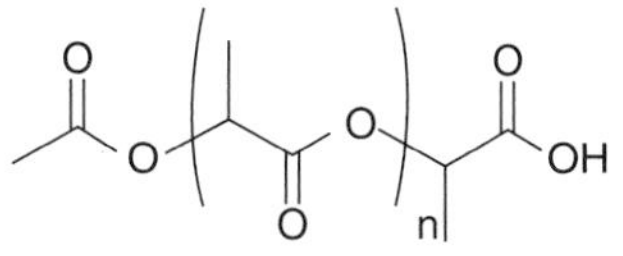

Figure 2 Oligolactic acid, *Source*: From Ref. 8.

solution, and a vapor phase that contains propellant and any other volatile components of the formulation (5). The sealing mechanism of the metered valve is also highlighted where the seals are typically constructed from elastomeric, plastic, and stainless steel or aluminum components.

MODIFIED-RELEASE SYSTEMS

Oligolactic Acid Based Surfactants

When formulating suspensions with propellant based systems, surfactant design typically consists of two key areas, a "head" group, which interacts with the drug, and a "tail," which interacts with the propellant. The head group is likely to be hydrophilic whereas the tail group would be hydrophobic. The high dielectric constant and dipole moment of the HFAs along with their hydrogen bonding capability mean that electron donors will favorably interact with the HFAs (6).

A novel excipient, oligolactic acid (OLA) has been developed specifically for use with HFA based MDIs, is biodegradable and biocompatible, and has the potential to be used either as a suspension aid, solubilizer or for sustained release (7). The OLA molecule is illustrated in Figure 2 where *n* may be varied to obtain OLAs of different solubilities and other properties (6).

An example of the use of OLAs to potentially make a formulation sustained release has been given by Li and Stefely (8). Albuterol sulfate MDI suspensions were formulated over a range of concentrations using three different OLAs with differing molecular weights or tail groups, referred to as OLA A, B, or C. As shown in Figure 3, OLAs can be used to modify the release profile of albuterol.

SURFACTANTS AS ABSORPTION ENHANCERS

Lecithin has been used to coat furosemide in the dry state, which was subsequently incorporated into an HFA 227 based MDI (2). Dissolution studies of lecithin-coated furosemide and uncoated drug demonstrated that the dissolution of furosemide was rapid and the lecithin coating had no impact on the dissolution rate or solubility. The lecithin-coated furosemide MDI and uncoated furosemide MDI were administered to rats and plasma

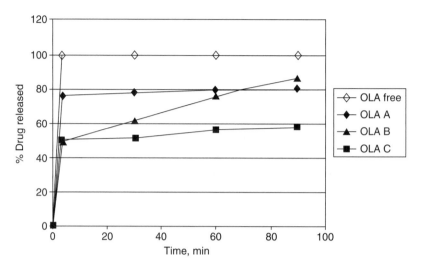

Figure 3 Effect of OLA concentration on the release profile of albuterol sulfate MDI suspensions. *Abbreviations*: OLA, oligolactic acid; MDI, metered dose inhaler. *Source*: From Ref. 8.

concentrations measured. As can be observed in Figure 4, the lecithin-coated formulation gave a significantly higher maximum plasma concentration and AUC. This is a potential way of enhancing absorption for poorly soluble drugs or of formulating a rapid-release product.

USE OF SURFACTANTS IN SOLUTION-BASED MDIs

Solution-based MDIs offer a further way to modify the release of therapeutic agents. This is mainly achieved by manipulating the fine particle fraction (FPF) of the aerosol plume, which can then target specific airway sites within the bronchial system. Lewis et al. (9) have described how an ethanol-based solution MDI can be used to modify the FPF. They derived equations which relate nonvolatile content, actuator orifice diameter, and valve-metering volume to the ex valve FPF. The higher FPF levels can be obtained by minimizing the orifice diameter and metering volume, while maximizing the HFA content. This technology offers the possibility of designing delivery of new therapeutic agents depending upon the mode of action of the agent.

A further example of solution aerosols targeting specific parts of the airway is in the beclomethasone dipropionate solution formulation (QVAR), where the drug substance is fully dissolved in ethanolic propellant. This formulation produces an extremely high FPF, which targets the alveoli with

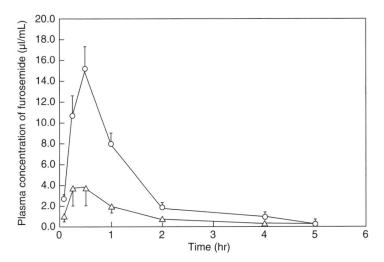

Figure 4 Plasma concentration of furosemide after intratracheal administration of furosemide or lecithin-coated furosemide using MDIs in rats: Dose was 1.25 mg furosemide/body; △ Furosemide; ○ lecithin-coated furosemide. Each data set is the mean ± SD (*n* = 5). *Abbreviation*: MDI, metered dose inhaler. *Source*: From Ref. 2.

a high degree of systemic absorption (10). This technology offers a rapid absorption route for systemic agents.

Delivery of High Molecular Weight Therapeutic Agents

There has been a renewed interest in the delivery of high molecular weight therapeutic agents to treat diseases other than asthma or COPD. One such area is the delivery of insulin by the inhaled route. While commercial inhaled insulin is now available via a dry powder device (11), no MDI is available that delivers insulin. Pritchard and Genova (12) have described an MDI development which utilizes a novel actuator called the vortex nozzle actuator (VNA) to slow down the aerosol plume and hence slow down the inhalation of the plume by the patient and subsequently maximize peripheral lung deposition. This device was used with a micronised insulin suspension in HFA 134a. The safety and efficacy of this MDI was compared to an SC Lantus™ injection in a 28-day study of type 2 diabetic patients. The results are summarized in Table 1. The key endpoint parameters are comparable for both formulations, illustrating the potential use of MDIs in the delivery of insulin. By use of surfactants, it may be possible to modify the release of insulin to match other commercial insulin products and hence offer the diabetic an alternative way to control their disease.

Table 1   Mean ± SD Data for Inhaler Insulin vs. Once-nightly SC
Injection of Lantus™

	Patient group	
Measure	pMDI Insulin	Reference - Lantus
BG reduction	51 mg/dL	43.1 mg/dL
HbA$_{1c}$	1.33 ± 0.42 %	1.05 ± 0.51 %
Mean post-prandial BG	65.6 ± 43.3 mg/dL	43.5 ± 33.8 mg/dL
BG variability (MAGE)	12.3 ± 19 mg/dL	0.4 ± 20 mg/dL
Pulmonary AE's	4	4

Abbreviation: MDI, metered dose inhaler.
Source: From Ref. 12.

RATIONAL SURFACTANT DESIGN

A more fundamental approach to rational design of surfactants for HFA-based MDIs has recently been described by Selvam et al. (13). Nonbonded pair interaction (binding) energies were calculated for the complexes between HFA134a and candidate surfactant tails; these were used as a measure of the HFA-philicity of selected moieties. A high-pressure tensiometer was used to measure the interfacial tension at the HFA134a/water interface for selected moieties. Ether-based moieties were shown to be very interfacially active compared to methyl-based moieties, which did not exhibit high activity. These results were in direct agreement with the binding energy calculations. These tools offer the potential for a more systematic and fundamental design of surfactants, especially if the work can be extended to analysis of the surfactant head group.

INNOVATIONS IN MDI DEVICES

Actuator Improvements

There have been a significant number of differently designed actuators, which have been described in the literature, both in terms of their visual appearance and in what the rationale for the design is. The VNA described earlier was designed to slow down the aerosol plume and, hence, slow down the inhalation of the plume by the patient, subsequently maximizing peripheral lung deposition for an insulin formulation (12). Example schematics of the VNA from the U.S. Patent for this device are given in Figure 5 (14). This nozzle employs a tangential inlet which imparts a swirl onto the gas-liquid internally and through the exit. By doing so, a low-pressure region is manifested in the center of the vortex. This low-pressure region eventually consists entirely of air. This "air core" is continuous from the internal rear wall of the nozzle through the exit orifice. This essentially reduces the diameter of

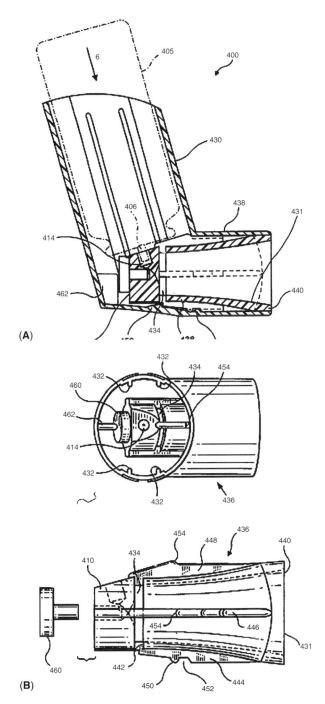

(A)

(B)

Figure 5 Example schematics of the Kos Vortex nozzle actuator from the United States Patent. *Source*: From Ref. 14.

the exit orifice and increases shear dramatically in this region, which is an effective means of deagglomerating. This process also dissipates a considerable amount of energy, which is manifested in slower exit velocities. Further, it is important to note that there is a synergistic effect when the nozzle and diffuser mouthpiece are combined.

Aerosol plumes can also be slowed down by simply reducing the size of the exit orifice diameter as with the Proventil™ HFA MDI, which contains an albuterol sulfate/HFA 134a formulation with oleic acid and ethanol as formulation additives (3). Figure 6 demonstrates the plume force of Proventil™ HFA MDI when used with a CFC actuator, the Proventil™ HFA actuator, and the Kos VNA. The plume duration is significantly longer with the VNA and the plume force much lower. It is likely that the reduction in force will make this a much more patient-friendly device, as it will avoid the well-documented Freon shock. Additionally, the ballistic component of the emerging aerosol is reduced, thereby reducing throat deposition which can hover around 55% of the dose for a standard MDI nozzle.

Lewis et al. (15) have described a series of standard actuators customized by laser drilling the exit orifices and have examined the performance of a solution BDP MDI through the different devices. The customizations ranged from single and multiple circular holes in different alignments plus a cross and slot shape orifice. The results are given in Table 2. The data show clearly that reducing the diameter of the orifice by 40% can increase the FPF below 5 μm by 2 and increase the plume duration by more than 4. The cross and slot formations can give some improvement but not to the same level as reducing the orifice diameter.

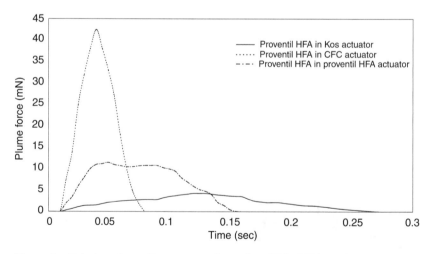

Figure 6 Relative plume force comparisons for CFC, HFA and Kos VNs tested using Proventil™ HFA MDI. *Abbreviations*: HFA, hydrofluoroalkane; CFC, chlorofluorocarbon; MDI, metered dose inhaler. *Source*: From Ref. 12.

Table 2 Performance Data for BDP HFA Formulation Delivered through Multiple Circular Laser-Drilled and Noncircular Laser-Drilled Orifices

Orifice description	Plume duration (ms)	Ex-valve FPF (% ≤ 5 μm)
Single circular 0.12 mm diameter	1421	77
Single circular 0.18 mm diameter	683	66
Single circular 0.22 mm diameter	469	48
Single circular 0.30 mm diameter	321	33
Dual circular 0.08 mm with 0.5 mm spacing	2477	68
Cross with height 0.55 mm and width 0.54 mm	606	65
Slot with height 2.0 mm and width 0.04 mm	452	54

Abbreviations: HFA, hydrofluoroalkane; FPF, fine particle fraction.
Source: From Ref. 15.

Dose Counters

The FDA has now issued a guidance document (16) that clearly recommends that manufacturers with metered-dose inhalers under development for oral inhalation integrate a dose-counting device into the development of their MDI products. It is therefore expected that many of the future MDI products to be introduced into the United States will have some form of counting device. One of the first such devices to be launched in the United States and also in Europe is the GlaxoSmithKline device illustrated in Figure 7.

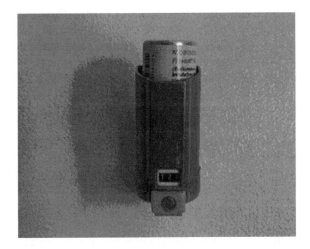

Figure 7 The GlaxoSmithKline Dose Counting Device incorporated into Flovent™ HFA. *Source*: Courtesy of GlaxoSmithKline PLC.

The whole landscape of developing dose counters has recently been reviewed by Bradshaw (17), where both count method and display method are analyzed in detail.

For the design of count method, two key failure modes need to be reviewed; undercounting through firing and not counting and overcounting through counting and not firing. Undercounting is deemed to be a more serious failure mode as it can result in the container indicating there are doses remaining where in fact there are none. There are two main types of design that are being developed, those that work on the applied force to the valve or the valve depression (displacement), the latter is the more common approach to dose counter developments. Bradshaw concludes that the more serious failure mode of undercounting is better addressed by displacement driven counters as the likely variability from force driven counters will be higher.

The types of display method used can vary significantly from a full numeric display, which increments downwards in units of one after every actuation (FDA guidance stipulates that numeric displays should count down), to a color-coded approach where the color changes as you approach the end of the inhaler.

CONCLUSIONS

This chapter update has attempted to evaluate recent developments in modifying the release of therapeutic agents from metered-dose inhalers. The focus over the past 6 years has been on transitioning CFC to HFA based MDIs, and there have been a number of developments described which indicate the potential for future modified-release formulations. Some of these developments relate to slowing down the release of therapeutic agents, while others relate to a more rapid release. As MDIs start to be used to treat diseases other than asthma and COPD, a wider range of formulation options is being developed and in some cases has been proven clinically. Additionally, new design actuators have enabled a more flexible approach to delivering an appropriate dose to specific parts of the lung and the addition of counters are further positive steps in the evolution of the MDI.

REFERENCES

1. Pritchard JN. Controlled delivery—Can you really convert a good drug into a great one? In: RN Dalby, PR Byron, J Peart, SJ Farr, eds. Respiratory Drug Delivery VIII. Raleigh, NC: Davis Horwood International Publishing, 2002; 249–56.
2. Saso Y, Seki T, Fukuchi R, et al. Effect of lecithin coating on the pulmonary absorption of furosemide in rats. Biol Pharm Bull 2006; 29(7):1445–8.
3. June DS, Schultz RK, Miller NC. A conceptual model for the development of pressurised metered-dose hydrofluoroalkane-based inhalation aerosols. Pharm Tech 1994; (October):40–52.

4. Ashurst IC, Gordon P. Consistent dose delivery from a new metered dose inhaler containing a combination of salmeterol and fluticasone propionate in HFA134a. J Aerosol Med 1999; 12(2):120.

5. Adjei AL. The Pressurized Metered-Dose Inhaler. In: Rathbone MJ, Hadgraft J, oberts MS, eds. Modified-Release Drug Delivery Technology. New York: Marcel Dekker Inc., 2003; 857–66.

6. Stefely JS, Duan DC, Myrdal PB, et al. Design and utility of a novel class of biocompatible excipient for HFA-based MDIs. In: Dalby RN, Byron PR, Farr SJ, Peart J, eds. Respiratory Drug Delivery VII. Raleigh, NC: Serentec Press, 2000; 83–90.

7. Leach CL, Hameister WM, Tomai MA, et al. Oligolactic acid (OLA) bio-matrices for sustained release of asthma therapeutics. In: Dalby RN, Byron PR, Farr SJ, Peart J, eds. Respiratory Drug Delivery VII. Raleigh, NC: Serentec Press, 2000; 75–81.

8. Li Z, Stefely J. Aerosol sustained release formulations with Oligolactic acid (OLA). In: Dalby RN, Byron PR, Farr SJ, Peart J, eds. Respiratory Drug Delivery IX. River Grove, IL: Davis Healthcare International Publishing, 2004; 321–23.

9. Lewis DA, Ganderton D, Meakin BJ, Bramhilla G. Theory and practice with solution systems. In: Dalby RN, Byron PR, Farr SJ, Peart J, eds. Respiratory Drug Delivery IX. River Grove, IL: Davis Healthcare International Publishing, 2004; 109–15.

10. Leach CL. Improved delivery of inhaled steroids to the large and small airways. Respirat Med 1998; 92(Suppl. A):3–8.

11. Smith AE. Nektar's pulmonary delivery system (PDS): Designed for usability, safety and reliability in the real world. In: Dalby RN, Byron PR, Farr SJ, Peart J, eds. Respiratory Drug Delivery X. River Grove, IL: Davis Healthcare International Publishing, 2006; 37–9.

12. Pritchard JN, Genova P. Adapting the pMDI to deliver novel drugs: Insulin and beyond. In: Dalby RN, Byron PR, Farr SJ, Peart J, eds.. Respiratory Drug Delivery X. River Grove, IL: Davis Healthcare International Publishing, 2006; 133–41.

13. Selvam P, Peguin RPS, Chokshi U, da Rocha SRP. Surfactant design for the 1,1,1,2-tetrafluoroethane—water interface: ab initio calculations and in situ high-pressure tensiometry. Langmuir 2006; (22):8675–83.

14. Genova PA, Williams III RC, Jewett W. Low spray force, low retention atomisation system. US Patent 6,418,925.

15. Lewis DA, Meakin BJ, Bramhilla G. New actuators versus old: Reasons and results for actuator modifications for HFA solution MDIs. In: Dalby RN, Byron PR, Farr SJ, Peart J, eds. Respiratory Drug Delivery X. River Grove, IL: Davis Healthcare International Publishing, 2006; 101–10.

16. U.S. FDA Guidance for Industry, "Integration of Dose-Counting Mechanisms into MDI Drug Products," March 2003

17. Bradshaw DRS. Developing Dose Counters: An appraisal based on Regulator, Pharma and user needs. In: Dalby RN, Byron PR, Farr SJ, Peart J, eds. Respiratory Drug Delivery X. River Grove, IL: Davis Healthcare International Publishing, 2006; 121–31.

49

Dry Powder Inhalation Systems from Nektar Therapeutics

Andrew R. Clark and Jeffry G. Weers

Nektar Therapeutics, San Carlos, California, U.S.A.

INTRODUCTION

In addition to offering the opportunity for topical therapy of the lung, the inhaled route also offers access to the systemic circulation. In topical therapy inhalation can enable high doses of drug to be delivered to the lungs, while avoiding high systemic concentrations. This improved targeting decreases the required therapeutic dose, while reducing systemic side effects. Topical delivery of small molecules for the treatment of asthma and lung disease has been accepted for many years. The large surface area ($\sim$100 m^2) of the peripheral (deep) lung (1) also offers the potential for systemic absorption of drugs in a generally benign metabolic environment. Inhalation can be used for systemic therapy where needle-free delivery and/or rapid onset of action may be desired. The systemic delivery of macromolecules via inhalation has recently been validated with the approval of Exubera® [insulin human (rDNA origin) inhalation powder] (2). Exubera was developed using technologies developed at Nektar Therapeutics.

UNIQUE REQUIREMENTS

Successful delivery to the lungs requires fine aerosol particles, 2–3 µm in diameter, to avoid impaction in the oropharyngeal cavity and ensure adequate deposition in the lungs (3). Therefore, medical inhalers have to maximize the generation of "fine" particles. In addition, an ideal medical inhaler should be reproducible, reliable, accurate, simple to use, durable, resistant to microbial contamination, and affordable. One must also ensure that the chemical stability of the drug and physical stability of the drug product are maintained during storage and aerosolization (4).

About a decade ago, noted aerosol scientist Richard Dalby made the following observation about inhalation of dry powders: "The forces governing dispersion are well documented and consist mainly of electrostatic, van der Waals, and capillary forces. Knowing these forces exist has not facilitated aerosol generation to any extent" (5). At the time, dry powders for inhalation were comprised of fine micronized drug crystals ($d_{geo} = 1$–5 µm). The particles were either blended with large lactose carrier particles, or spheronized to facilitate metering and fluidization. Lung deposition from passive dry powder inhalers was typically on the order of 10–30% and dependent on the patient's peak inspiratory flow rate (6). Since the Dalby quote, advances in particle engineering have led to reductions in interparticle cohesive forces, resulting in dramatic improvements in aerosol performance. Nektar has developed two technologies designed to improve powder fluidization, dispersion, and delivery.

COMPARISON TO RELATED TECHNOLOGIES

The last 50 years have seen the evolution of three main types of inhalers: The nebulizer, which atomizes aqueous solutions; the pressurized metered dose inhaler, which uses highly volatile propellant liquids; and the dry powder inhaler (DPI), which delivers powdered drug formulations. In contrast to nebulizers and solution metered dose inhalers, the formulation and physical properties of dry powders are crucial to the performance of a DPI system (7).

DPIs were introduced in the late 1960s as alternatives to pressurized metered dose inhalers. The early devices (e.g., Rotahaler®, Glaxo; Spinhaler®, Fisons) contained micronized drug packaged in hard gelatin capsules. The typical density of the particles was between 1.0 and 1.5 g/cm³, necessitating that the geometric diameter of the particles be less than about 5 µm, for effective delivery to the lungs. (Aerodynamic behavior is controlled by a particle's aerodynamic diameter, which is approximately equal to the product of the geometric diameter and the square root of the particle density.) Unfortunately, micronized particles of this size exhibit strong interparticle cohesion, resulting in poor powder flow and dispersibility. To overcome these issues the fine particles were blended with large lactose carrier particles (7). The need for a large percentage of carrier particles in the formulation, and the relatively poor efficiency of lung delivery, limits the maximum dose that can be delivered with this technology to a few milligrams. This in turn limits therapeutics that can be delivered to those which are reasonably potent (e.g., asthma therapeutics). Powder dispersion in these first generation products is achieved using the patient's inspiratory effort. A marked dependence of lung deposition with peak inspiratory flow rate

(PIF) was noted, as the degree of powder dispersion increases with increases in PIF. The resulting large degree of interpatient variability limits the technology to therapeutics with a large therapeutic index. Another disadvantage of the early DPIs is their dependence on hard gelatin capsules as a drug closure. Gelatin capsules have to be maintained within a specific relative humidity range to be successfully opened (opening is usually achieved by piercing).

Second generation DPI development focused on solving these problems through device engineering. To improve the ease of use, two different types of multidose DPIs were developed: reservoir devices in which bulk powder was metered by the device (e.g., Turbuhaler®, Astra-Zeneca), and pseudo-unit dose devices in which the dose was packaged in moisture-proof foil–foil blisters on tapes or disks (e.g., Accuhaler®, GSK). The Turbuhaler dealt with the poor powder flow properties noted with micronized drug particles by spheronization. These second generation devices were well accepted by patients, but because they still used micronized drug, their poor delivery efficiency remained. To improve powder dispersion, many of the second generation devices had increased pressure drops or tortuous paths leading to greater device resistance. This results in modest decreases in the observed flow rate dependence. Other groups developed "active" DPI devices in which powder dispersion is decoupled from patient inhalation. For example, the Exubera pulmonary delivery device (Nektar Therapeutics) utilizes a jet of compressed air to accomplish powder dispersion (8). However, although more robust in terms of reproducibility of delivery, these active devices can exhibit some degree of "reverse" flow rate dependence. Eventhough powder dispersion is consistent, variations in inspiratory flow rate lead to differences in inertial impaction in the upper airways (9).

The third generation of dry powder development is characterized by the development of "engineered" powders, and a return to the use of "simple" devices. Particle engineering is characterized by advances in formulation and/or process technology. The goal is to design desirable attributes into the particles such as: improved stability of biopolymers (10), improved powder dispersibility (11), sustained release (12), or increased drug permeability and bioavailability (13). These attributes are introduced through the use of novel excipients, or alternatively, by insightful control of particle characteristics such as particle density, morphology, microviscosity, or surface energy. In order to achieve these features new process technologies including spray-drying (11), foam-drying, and supercritical fluid technologies (14) have been investigated.

NEKTAR'S PROPRIETARY TECHNOLOGIES

In order to fulfill the requirements for pulmonary delivery, scientists at Nektar Therapeutics have developed two dry powder formulation technologies. An amorphous glass-based technology, mainly suited to the delivery of proteins and peptides, and a lipid-based technology mainly, but not exclusively, focused on the delivery of small molecules. To complement these powder technologies Nektar has developed two device technologies; an active inhaler, currently used in Exubera, and a passive inhaler, currently being used to deliver high dose anti-infectives to the lung for topical therapy. The protein dry powder formulation technology (PulmoSol™) is based on proprietary glass stabilization techniques, which dry proteins into a glassy state dramatically slowing molecular interactions and hence inhibiting peptide denaturation and promoting stability. The lipid-based PulmoSphere® technology generates hollow porous particles to reduce interparticulate forces and enhance dispersion and aerosol performance. PulmoSphere powders have also been applied to metered dose inhaler formulations where they enhance suspension stability and delivery efficiency.

PulmoSol™

Nektar's PulmoSol technology produces room temperature stable dispersible powders of soluble and insoluble peptides and proteins without the need for coarse carrier lactose. The formulations are designed with a high glass transition temperature, so as to immobilize the biomolecule in a high viscosity glassy matrix. The molecular gridlock in the glass stabilizes the biomolecule against chemical degradation. The particles have high rugosity surfaces, which facilitate dispersion. These powders coupled to a novel active inhaler device can deliver high drug doses per puff, and as with all dry powder formulations, have low microbial control requirements during manufacture (i.e., bioburden versus sterility for liquid products).

The amorphous glass powder may be delivered from an active DPI (Fig. 1). The patient slides a foil–foil blister pack into a slot on the side of the inhaler. A component called the release unit opens the blister and then utilizes a small compressed air bolus to entrain and aerosolize the powder. The device suspends and captures the fine aerosol powder in a small chamber. The aerosol is then inhaled by the patient. The chamber holds about 200 mL of air containing the medication, which an average person can easily inhale. Considering that a normal adult's tidal breath is about 700 mL and an average person's deep inhalation is from 2 to 4 L, even patients with limited lung capacities should obtain consistent results (Fig. 2). Unlike passive DPIs, Nektar's active device delivers an aerosol cloud with characteristics that are independent of the force of the patient's inhalation. The simple, durable device uses no batteries, electronics, or microchips, making it inexpensive to manufacture and extremely easy to maintain. The device has undergone a number of revisions during development. The original "proof of concept" prototype device was fairly large, but successive planned

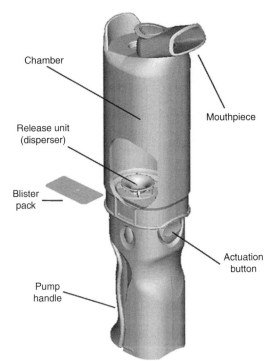

Chamber

Mouthpiece

Release unit
(disperser)

Blister
pack

Actuation
button

Pump
handle

Figure 1   The Nektar pulmonary delivery system.

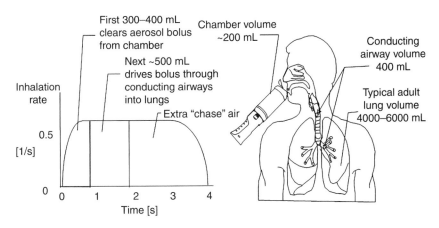

First 300–400 mL
clears aerosol bolus
from chamber

Chamber volume
~200 mL

Conducting
airway volume
400 mL

Next ~500 mL
drives bolus through
conducting airways
into lungs

Typical adult
lung volume
4000–6000 mL

Extra "chase" air

Inhalation
rate

0.5

[1/s]

0

Time [s]

Figure 2   Theory of "standing cloud" peripheral aerosol delivery using the Nektar pulmonary delivery system.

modifications during development have condensed it to commercial size (Fig. 3).

PulmoSphere®: Small Porous Particles for Inhalation

The PulmoSphere technology utilizes spray-drying from an emulsion-based feedstock to create hollow, porous particles (Fig. 4), comprised of phospholipids and the drug of interest (11). Drug is incorporated in the feedstock by dissolution in the continuous phase of the emulsion, or by dispersion of insoluble crystals in the continuous phase (15). Just like micronized drug formulations, the geometric size of PulmoSphere particles are in the range from 1 to 5 μm. However, in contrast to micronized drug, the particles need not be blended in order to achieve good powder flow characteristics.

PulmoSphere particles may be delivered using a small patient-driven inhaler, which utilizes HPMC capsules as the primary package (Fig. 5). Patients insert the capsule in the inhaler and then pierce the capsule by depressing the end of the inhaler device. Drug is only delivered from the device when the patient inhales. Emitted doses are typically >90% with RSD values less than 5% (15,16). Pharmacoscintigraphy studies have demonstrated that these small porous particles can achieve lung doses of 60% following inhalation with a simple, capsule-based DPI (16). The decreases in oropharyngeal deposition noted also leads to reductions in interpatient variability relative to micronized drug formulations (ca. 10–12% for PulmoSphere formulations) (16,17). Moreover, the lung deposition is generally independent of inspiratory flow rate, as the increases in powder

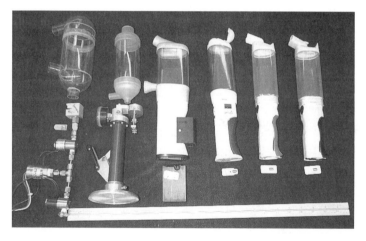

Figure 3 Prototype development sequence of the Nektar pulmonary delivery system from "proof of concept" to phase II device.

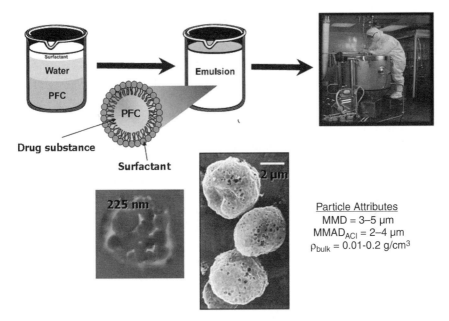

Figure 4   The PulmoSphere® manufacturing process.

dispersion and lung deposition that would occur with increasing PIF are balanced by decreases in lung deposition resulting from increased oropharyngeal impaction at the higher PIF (3)].

The fact that PulmoSphere particles need not be blended to achieve good powder fluidization and dispersion also facilitates the delivery of less

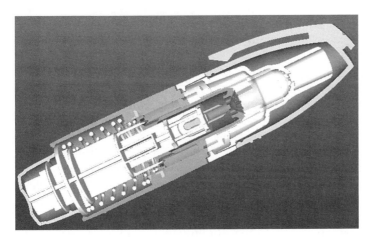

Figure 5   The Nektar passive pulmonary inhaler.

potent therapeutics (11,16,18). Newhouse et al. (17) demonstrated that a therapeutic dose of tobramycin (ca. 30 mg) could be delivered to the lungs in a few puffs from a simple DPI. This enables convenient delivery for cystic fibrosis patients who spend much of their day inhaling medication and undergoing time intensive chest percussion and physiotherapy (17,19). Tobramycin inhalation powder is currently in phase III development in a collaboration between Novartis and Nektar Therapeutics.

The PulmoSphere manufacturing process has also been applied to insoluble therapeutics (e.g., Amphotericin B, budesonide) (15,16,20). In this embodiment, microcrystals of drug are coated with a porous layer of phospholipid. The aerosol performance achieved is equivalent to that achieved with water soluble therapeutics, such as tobramycin.

The dry powder PulmoSphere particles have also shown utility in immune modulation following pulmonary administration (21,22).

The improvements in fluidization afforded with small porous PulmoSphere particles is driven by a number of factors and include the porous particle morphology (10) and the hydrophobic surface comprised of surface-active phospholipids. Note that large size (i.e., large porous particles) is not a prerequisite for achieving improvements in these properties as has been claimed by others (18).

Metered Dose Inhaler Formulations Comprising Pulmosphere Particles

The small porous PulmoSphere particles have also shown utility in reducing interparticle attractive forces in metered dose inhaler suspensions (23). Creaming times on the order of hours are observed (24). The improved suspension stability drives improved dose content uniformity. Significant improvements in delivery efficiency may also be achieved. In a comparison with the Ventolin Evohaler™, twofold increases in lung deposition were noted (25). Once again the technology works equally well when the therapeutic is either soluble in water or insoluble in water.

RESEARCH AND DEVELOPMENT

As early as 1925, it was demonstrated that insulin could be absorbed from the lung following aerosol delivery (26), although the bioavailability was only 3% and delivery was cumbersome (27,28). More recently, numerous studies in humans and animal species have shown that many proteins and peptides, including leuprolide acetate, human growth hormone, parathyroid hormone, calcitonin, and interferon, are absorbed from the deep lung (29–34). In general, biomolecules with lower molecule weights achieve higher absorption than high molecular weight biomolecules (27). Absorption ranges from 20% to 50% for proteins for molecular weights less than 30 kDa (34), and many therapeutic biomolecules fall in this size range.

For human insulin, absorption is faster following inhalation than by sub-cutaneous injection (30).

For small molecules the picture goes even further back, with references to pulmonary delivery going as far back as the Egyptians (35). However, modern treatment of asthma and COPD has evolved over the last 4 to 5 decades. Steroids and bronchodilators are the mainstay of these treatments, but inhaled antibiotics and long acting anticholinergics have been added to the arsenal. PulmoSphere technology has been applied to most of these classes of molecules, many of which have been investigated clinically.

SAFETY

The lung is a remarkably robust organ. Presumably its exposure to a variety of environmental challenges over the millennia has lead to an organ capable of tolerating a variety of inhaled materials. For example, the lungs are exposed to about 4 to 5 mg of foreign material in a smoky bar, and about 50 mg per day of low-toxicity nuisance dust in most occupational settings (36). To date, inhalation exposure to a variety of pharmacological molecules has been well tolerated (37). The mainstay of asthma treatment is the inha-lation of bronchodilators ad steroids and despite millions of years of cumu-lative patient exposure no serious toxicological issues have been noted. In the case of inhaled peptides and proteins numerous clinical studies, some lasting many years, have been conducted and there have been no observa-tions of serious adverse lung reactions, anaphylaxis, or clinically significant immune reactions (38). Measurements of insulin antibodies after exposure to inhaled insulin indicate a rise in antibodies but with no clinical implica-tions (38). In some instances measurements have also found lower levels of antibodies, for example human growth hormone following inhalation compared to subcutaneous injection in rats (38). The lungs appear to be robust and capable of exposure to milligram quantities of various classes of inhaled therapeutics.

CLINICAL TRIALS

Pulmonary delivery has, in general, demonstrated its usefulness in many clinical trials ranging from asthma through migrane to diabetes. As noted earlier, inhaled insulin was approved in 2006 based on over 50 clinical trials. The product was developed using Nektar Therapeutics' PulmoSol tech-nologies (8,39). Other early clinical investigations using this technology have involved the delivery of alpha 1 antitrypsin proteinase inhibitor, interferon-β and parathyroid hormone amongst many.

The PulmoSphere technology has undergone clinical testing with various molecules. Phase I trials have been conducted with tobramycin, budesonide, LHRH, albuterol, amphotericin B, and ciprofloxacin, while phase III trials are currently in progress with tobramycin.

SCALE UP

Both of Nektar's powder technologies utilize spray drying. To produce these powders, highly customized powder processing equipment has been developed. Proprietary atomizers and collection techniques have been developed to maintain high manufacturing efficiency and hence commercial viability. (The PulmoSphere technology also requires emulsion manufacture prior to spray drying.) The amorphous fine particles produced can be sensitive to moisture. To prevent environmental exposure, individual doses of dry powder may be packaged in foil–foil blister packs. With unit packaging, different drug strengths can also be formulated. Reproducible filling of low doses (5 mg or less) of fine powder into blister packs required development of proprietary filling methods. The SVE filling technology (39) has demonstrated the capability of filling doses as low as 1.5 mg with relative standard deviations of approximately 2–3% (Fig. 6). Although blister-filling technology is common throughout the pharmaceutical industry, no commercial technology is available to meet these special needs.

The quantity of dry powder and inhaler devices required increases as clinical programs progress. Whereas research and development and phase I trials require milligram amounts of a drug, phase III clinical trials and commercialization may call for hundreds of kilograms of drug. In 1993, PulmoSol dry powder formulations were produced in batches of 10 to 100 mg in a benchtop spray dryer, equivalent to approximately 10 g a year. By 1995, demand for batches rose and batch size was increased to 250 g manufactured in a Pilot Scale reactor. Today's phase III clinical trial materials and future large-scale commercial production is at the >5 kg per batch level. The large scale reactor capable of manufacture at this scale stands three stories tall and has required advances in both atomizer and collection technologies in order to maintain consistent high performance powder. Continued improvements in nozzle and collector design have pushed pilot scale powder production to more than a kilogram per batch. As such, pilot scale production may provide commercial capability for most other products in development.

Device manufacture over this period has also scaled accordingly. The prototype II insulin inhaler, the device designed specifically for phase II clinical trials, was manufactured in soft tools and hand assembled at Nektar, whereas commercial inhalers are being manufactured by two OEM suppliers, one in Europe and one in the United States. The patient-driven inhaler is being manufactured in Asia.

REGULATORY ISSUES

The U.S. FDA considers powder therapeutics to be "combination products." Receiving regulatory approval involves an interplay of expertise in

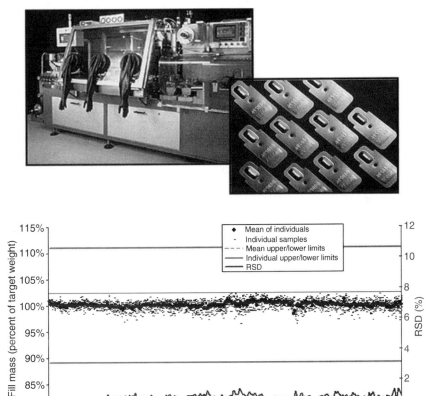

Figure 6 The PulmoSol™ blister filling equipment and dose reproducibility.

biologics, human drugs, and medical devices. The FDA's Division of Pulmonary Drug Products requires one year safety data on 200 patients, or one year in 100 patients and six months in 300 patients. Safety issues concern patient experiences with cleaning, durability, and failures of the DPI devices. The devices tested must be the same as the intended commercial devices and robust enough to withstand regular use by patients for the recommended time of use. In Europe, powder inhalation products are regulated as either a drug and device, or as a combination product. Obtaining a CE designation, which certifies that the product conforms to the relevant European Union directives relating to safety, will help the product move freely within the European Union without further national controls. All of Nektar's devices have been CE marked.

FUTURE DEVELOPMENTS

The low densities and surface energies exhibited by PulmoSphere powders can also be achieved with amorphous glass (PulmoSol) technology when hydrophobic amino acids (e.g., leucine, trileucine) are incorporated within the formulation (40,41). As observed with PulmoSphere particles, the second generation PulmoSol particles exhibit significant improvements in powder fluidization and dispersibility. Continued advances in particle engineering of amorphous glass formulations have resulted in core/shell particles in which the core of the particle contains the therapeutic and a water soluble glass forming agent with a high Tg (e.g., sodium citrate), and the shell comprises a hydrophobic amino acid. The citrate provides a high Tg and reduced molecular mobility for the peptide/protein, while the hydrophobic shell controls the excellent powder flow and dispersibility characteristics of the formulation (40). Nektar continues to develop these and other pulmonary powder technologies.

REFERENCES

1. Thurlock WM. The internal surface area of nonemphysematous lungs. Amer Rev Respir Dis 1967; 95:765–70.
2. White S, Bennett D, Stevenson C, Harper N. Exubera®: development of a novel technology solution for pulmonary delivery of insulin. In: Dalby RN, Byron PR, Peart J, Suman JD, eds. RDD Europe 2005. River Grove, IL: Davis Healthcare International Publishing, 2005; 225–7.
3. Stahlhofen W, Gebhart J, Heyder J. Experimental determination of the regional deposition of aerosol particles in the respiratory tract. Amer Ind Hyg Assoc J 1980; 41:385–98.
4. Wolff RK, Niven RW. Generation of aerosol drugs. J Aerosol Med 1994; 7:89–106.
5. Dalby RN, Tiano SH, Hickey AJ. Medical devices for the delivery of therapeutic aerosols to the lungs. In: Hickey AJ ed. Inhalation Aerosols: Physical and Biological Basis for TherapyNew York: Dekker, 1996; 441.
6. Borgstrom L, Bissgard H, O'Callaghan C, Pedersen S. Dry powder inhalers. In: Bissgard H, O'Callaghan C, Samldone GC, eds. Drug Delivery to the Lung. New York: Mauel Dekker, 2002; 421.
7. Kassem NM. Generation of deeply inspirable clouds from dry powder mixtures. Ph.D. Thesis, King's College, University of London, London, UK. 1990.
8. Burr JD, Anthony JM, Axford GS, Etter JW, Smith AE. Apparatus and methods for dispensing dry powder medicaments. US patent 6,089,228, 2000.
9. Hill M, Vaughan L, Dolovich M. Dose targeting for dry powder inhalers. In: Dalby RN, Byron PR, Farr SJ, eds. Respiratory Drug Delivery V. Buffalo Grove, IL: Interpharm Press, 1996; 197–208.
10. Blair JA, Hatley RHM. Stabilization and delivery of labile materials by amorphous carbohydrates and their derivatives. J Mol Catalysis B: Enzymatic 1999; 7:11–9.

11. Dunbar C. Porous particles for inhalation: The science behind their improved dispersibility. In: Dalby RN, Byron PR, Peart J, Suman JD, Farr SJ, eds. Respiratory Drug Delivery X. River Grove, IL: Amy Davis Biggs, 2006: 307–15.

12. Louey MD, Garcia-Contreras L. Controlled release products for respiratory drug delivery. Am Pharm Rev 2004; 7:82–7.

13. Okamoto H, Todo H, Iida K, Danjo K. Dry powders for pulmonary delivery of peptides and proteins. KONA 2002; 20:71–83.

14. Shekunov BY, Feeley JC, Chow AHL, Tong HHY, York Y. Physical properties of supercritically-processed and micronized powders for respiratory drug delivery. KONA 2002; 20:178–87.

15. Tarara T, Malcolmson R, Leung D, Weers J. Embedded crystals in low density particles: formulation, manufacture, and properties. In: Dalby RN, Byron PR, Peart J, Suman JD, Farr SJ, eds. Respiratory Drug Delivery X. River Grove, IL: Amy Davis Biggs 2006; 297–304.

16. Duddu SP, Sisk SA, Walter YH, et al. Improved lung delivery from a passive dry powder inhaler using an engineered PulmoSphere powder. Pharm Res 2002; 19:689–95.

17. Newhouse MT, Hirst PH, Duddu SP, et al. Inhalation of a dry powder tobramycin PulmoSphere formulation in healthy volunteers. Chest 2003; 124:360–6.

18. Weers J, Clark A, Challoner P. High dose inhaled powder delivery: challenges and techniques. In: Dalby RN, Byron PR, Peart J, Suman JD, Farr SJ, eds. Respiratory Drug Delivery IX. River Grove, IL: Amy Davis Biggs 2004; 281–8.

19. Geller DE, Howenstine M, Conrad C, Smith J, Mulye S, Shewsbury SB. A phase 1 study to assess the tolerability of a novel tobramycin powder for inhalation formulation in cystic fibrosis subjects. Presented at the North American Cystic Fibrosis Conference. St. Louis, MO, U.S.A 2004.

20. Weers JG, Tarara TE, Eldon MA, Narasimhan R. Aerosolizable pharmaceutical formulation for fungal infection therapy. US Patent Appl No US20040176391A1, 2004.

21. Smith DJ, Bot S, Dellamary L, Bot A. Evaluation of novel aerosol formulations designed for mucosal vaccination against influenza virus. Vaccine 2003; 21:2805–12.

22. Bot AI, Tarara TE, Smith DJ, et al. Pharm Res 2000; 17:275–83.

23. Weers JG, Tarara TE, Gill H, EnglishBS, Dellamary LA. omodispersion technology for HFA suspensions: Particle engineering to reduce dosing variance. In: Dalby RN, Byron PR, Farr SJ, eds. Respiratory Drug Delivery VII Buffalo Grove, IL: Interpharm Press Inc, 2000:91–7.

24. Dellamary LA, Tarara TE, Smith DJ, et al. Hollow porous particles in metered dose inhalers. Pharm Res 2000; 17:168–74.

25. Hirst PH, Elton RC, Pitcairn GR, et al. In vivo lung deposition of hollow porous particles from a pressurized metered dose inhaler. Pharm Res 2002; 19:258–64.

26. Gansslen M. Uber inhalation von insulin. Wien Klin Wochenschr 1925; 4:71–81.

27. Patton JS. Deep-lung delivery of therapeutic proteins. Chemtech 1997; 27:34–8.
28. Patton JS, Platz RM. Pulmonary delivery of peptides and proteins for systemic action. Adv Drug Del Rev 1992; 8:179–96.
29. Adjei A, Garren J. Pulmonary delivery of peptide drugs: Effect of particle size on bioavailability of leuprolide acetate in healthy male volunteers. Pharmacol Res 1990; 7:565–9.
30. Elliott RB, Edgar BW, Pilcher CC, Quested C, McMaster J. Parenteral absorption of insulin from the lung in diabetic children. Aust Paediatr J 1987; 23:293–7.
31. Deftos LJ, Seely BL, Clopton PC. Intrapulmonary delivery of bone-active peptides: Bioactivity of inhaled salmon calcitonin approximates that of injected calcitonin. Proc Amer Soc Bone Min Res Annual Meeting, Seattle, 1996.
32. Pillari RS, Hughes BL, Wolff RK, Heisserman JA. The effect of pulmonary delivered insulin on blood glucose levels using two nebulizer systems. J. Aerosol Med. 1996; 9:227–39.
33. Colthorpe P, Farri SJ, Smith IJ, Wyatt D, Taylor G. The influence of regional deposition on the pharmacokinetics of pulmonary delivered growth hormone in rabbits. Pharm Res 1995; 12:356–9.
34. Hastings RH, Grady M, Sakuma T, Matthay MA. Clearance of different sized proteins from the alveolar space in humans and rabbits. J Appl Physiol 1992; 73:1310–6.
35. O'Callaghan C, Nerbrink O, Vidgren MT. The history of inhaled drug therapy. In: Bissgard H, O'Callaghan C, Samldone GC, eds. Drug Delivery to the Lung. New York: Marcel Dekker, 2002: 1.
36. American Conference of Governmental Industrial Hygienists. Threshold Limit Values for chemical substances and physical agents and biological exposure indices. ACGIH, Cincinnati. 1995; 2:33.
37. Wolff RK. Safety of inhaled proteins for therapeutic use. J Aerosol Med 1998; 11:197–219.
38. Clark AR, Eldon MA, Dwivedi SK. The application of pulmonary inhalation technology to drug discovery. Annual Reports in Medicinal Chemistry, 2006:in press.
39. Rocchio MJ, Wightmam DE, Naydo K, Parks DJ, Smith AE. Powder filling systems, apparatus and methods. US patent 5,826,633, 1998.
40. Lechuga-Ballesteros D, Charan C, Liang Y, et al. Designing stable and high performance respirable particles of pharmaceuticals. In: Dalby RN, Byron PR, Peart J, Suman JD, Farr SJ, eds. Respiratory Drug Delivery IX. River Grove, IL: Amy Davis Biggs, 2004; 565–8.
41. Kuo MC, Lechuga-Ballesteros D. Dry powder compositions having improved dispersivity. US Patent 6,518,239, 2003.

50

Technosphere®/Insulin: Mimicking Endogenous Insulin Release

Andrea Leone-Bay

*Pharmaceutical Development, MannKind Corporation,
Danbury, Connecticut, U.S.A.*

Marshall Grant

*Formulation Development, MannKind Corporation,
Danbury, Connecticut, U.S.A.*

EXOGENOUS DELIVERY OF INSULIN

The effect of any medication depends heavily on the rate at which the active component is absorbed and eliminated following administration. For some therapies, such as analgesics, rapid absorption and slow elimination are desired so that the patient obtains a quick medication effect that lasts for many hours. For other therapies, both rapid drug absorption and elimination is preferred, such as the case with parathyroid hormone-mediated bone rebuilding in osteoporosis, wherein prolonged exposure can actually promote bone loss (1,2).

Analgesics and parathyroid hormone therapy are just two cases out of hundreds that demonstrate the connection between the pharmacokinetic (PK) profile of a therapeutic agent and the specific pharmacodynamic response it elicits. These PK profiles are critical to the desired safety and efficacy of drugs. For this reason, pharmaceutical researchers expend considerable time and effort developing drug formulations that provide PK profiles appropriate for both a particular drug and the specific disease state for which it is utilized.

Developing drug therapies that provide exogenous delivery of endogenous substances with PK profiles that mimic natural release is challenging. In the case of insulin, an endogenous hormone secreted by the pancreas to maintain normal blood glucose levels, healthy individuals exhibit an early insulin response, characterized by a rapid rise in circulating insulin almost immediately after the start of a meal (3,4). An exogenous insulin product with a PK profile similar to this response would be more desirable than an insulin product that does not mimic endogenous insulin secretion. Unfortunately, none of the prandial insulin products currently approved for treating diabetic patients exactly reproduces the normal pattern of endogenous insulin secretion. In particular, while endogenous insulin peaks at about 5 minutes in healthy individuals, available insulins and almost all inhaled insulins, approved and in development, reach maximum circulating concentrations 30–90 minutes after administration (5,6). Technosphere®/Insulin (MannKind Corporation, Valencia, CA) provides a more rapid rise in insulin (5) that approximates the body's natural early insulin response to a meal with peak insulin concentration occurring in about 12–14 minutes (Fig. 1).

PROPERTIES OF TECHNOSPHERE®/INSULIN

Technosphere/Insulin was developed utilizing the Technosphere technology, a novel and versatile drug delivery platform that allows pulmonary administration of therapeutics typically administered by injection. This technology is anchored in an unusual physicochemical property of a diketopiperazine

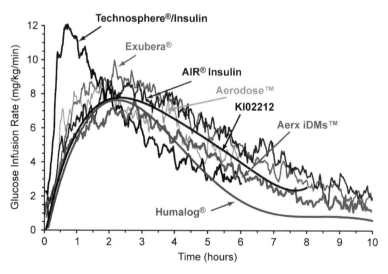

Figure 1   Composite figure with the time-action profiles obtained from a variety of inhaled insulin products in different studies. Subcutaneous injection of lispro (Humalog®) 15U is also shown for comparison. *Source*: From Ref. 5.

molecule called fumaryl diketopiperazine (FDKP). As with many small organic molecules, FDKP can be crystallized to form microcrystalline plates. Unlike other molecules that crystallize in this fashion, FDKP microcrystal plates undergo self-assembly into microparticles called Technosphere particles. Scanning electron microscopy and X-ray powder diffraction confirm that these particles comprise an array of FDKP microcrystals (Fig. 2).

The self-assembly of diketopiperazine molecules has been previously reported (7,8); however, the resultant particles are either smooth, hollow microcapsules or smooth, solid microspheres. Figure 2 shows that Technosphere particles are not characterized by a smooth exterior surface. One can visualize the architecture of a Technosphere particle by envisioning a three-dimensional sphere created from a deck of cards. Each individual card represents one FDKP microcrystal, and the sphere of cards represents a Technosphere particle. The sphere has a large surface area, composed of the face and back of each card, and the spaces between the cards provide the sphere with a high internal porosity. These features of the particles make them ideal for the adsorption of peptide and protein drug cargos.

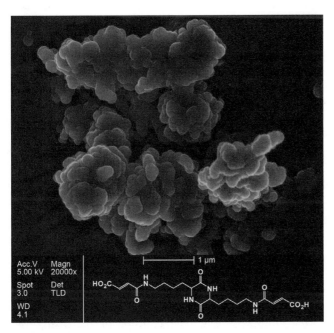

Figure 2   Scanning electron micrograph of a Technosphere® particle and the chemical structure of FDKP, the raw material from which the particles are formed. *Abbreviation*: FDKP, fumaryl diketopiperazine.

To prepare Technosphere/Insulin from Technosphere particles, insulin is precipitated onto the preformed particles. Under precipitation conditions, the insulin molecules are slightly positively charged. The FDKP molecules that make up the Technosphere particles generate a slightly negative charge on the particle surfaces. This charge difference, along with the high surface area of the Technosphere particles, promotes insulin adsorption onto the particles, forming Technosphere/Insulin. Insulin is monomeric under the conditions of the precipitation process, and it is the monomeric insulin that is deposited onto the particles. The Technosphere/Insulin particles that result have a uniform size distribution. More than 90% of the particles are in the respirable range (between 0.5 and 5.8 microns) and the typical particle diameter is 2.5 microns. Technosphere/Insulin particle morphology is essentially identical to that of Technosphere particles. The Technosphere technology is not a prodrug technology because no chemical reaction takes place between insulin and FDKP. Insulin is not covalently linked to FDKP; it is electrostatically associated with the particle surface.

Sized appropriately for inhalation into the deep lung, Technosphere/Insulin particles are inhaled using the MedTone™ inhaler, a passive, high-resistance, low-flow, dry powder device (Fig. 3). Technosphere/Insulin powder is dosed in single-use cartridges loaded into the inhaler. By inhaling on the device mouthpiece, powder is discharged and delivered to the deep lung. The inhaler does not require manual activation. Since it is activated by the patient's inhalation, it is not necessary for the patient to coordinate the timing of device activation and inhalation. Additionally, the MedTone inhaler is a compact, pocket-sized device that is easy to carry and use.

Once Technosphere/Insulin powder is inhaled, the particles are evenly distributed throughout the deep lung. Here, they dissolve rapidly due to the high surface area of the particles and to the high solubility of FDKP at the near neutral pH of the lung. Once the particles dissolve, the insulin, is quickly absorbed because it is present as monomer. The monomeric state of insulin and the rapid particle dissolution combine to give insulin, administered as Technosphere/Insulin, its unique PK profile.

MONOMER INSULIN

Although the monomer is the pharmacologically active form of insulin, most pharmaceutical dosage forms contain the zinc-complexed hexamer, which is significantly more stable and exhibits a longer shelf life than the monomer. The hexamer must dissociate into monomers to be active, and the rate of hexamer dissociation into monomer controls the rate of insulin absorption after administration. The concept of increasing the insulin absorption rate by administering monomer insulin is the basis for the design of rapid-acting insulin analogs (RAAs), such as aspart insulin (rDNA origin) (NovoLog®; Novo Nordisk Inc., Princeton, NJ) and lispro insulin

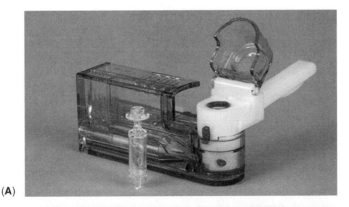

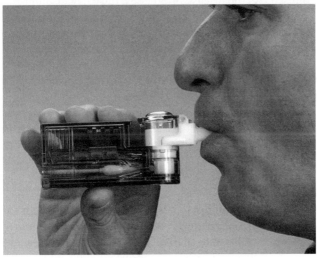

Figure 3 MedTone™ inhaler shown (**A**) with single-use cartridge, and (**B**) in use.

(rDNA origin) (Humalog®, Eli Lilly and Company, Indianapolis, IN) (9,10). The primary amino acid chain structures of these molecules have been altered for the specific purpose of destabilizing the hexamer upon administration. Following injection, both of these insulin analogs dissociate into monomer faster and are absorbed more quickly than regular human insulin. The rapid PK profiles of both aspart and lispro insulin demonstrate that monomeric insulin is absorbed faster than hexameric insulin. However, neither of these RAAs delivers insulin as rapidly as Technosphere/Insulin because, while aspart and lispro insulin favor dissociation into monomer after injection, they are not truly monomeric in the formulated product (11).

Using analytical ultracentrifugation, the monomeric state of insulin in Technosphere/Insulin has been confirmed. In analytical ultracentrifugation studies, insulin dimers and monomers are the primary species observed both in the solutions used to prepare Technosphere/Insulin and in the insulin released upon dissolution of Technosphere/Insulin particles. Further, Technosphere/Insulin formulations tend to stabilize monomer insulin without compromising shelf life.

The potential advantage of monomer insulin therapy can be best exemplified by the endogenous insulin secretion that occurs in healthy individuals (Fig. 1). When a non diabetic person begins to eat, the pancreas produces a rapid insulin rise (early insulin response) that is independent of the size of the meal. Subsequent insulin release by the pancreas is more gradual and geared to the caloric content of the meal. In patients with type 2 diabetes, however, the ability of the pancreas to release the mealtime insulin rapidly is compromised. As the disease progresses, the early insulin response is lost completely (12). Technosphere/Insulin, with its ability to deliver monomeric insulin to the bloodstream rapidly, mimics normal physiology and may compensate for an inadequate prandial insulin release.

In addition to inhaled insulin therapy, Technosphere technology has been used to deliver salmon calcitonin and parathyroid hormone by inhalation. Both drugs are approved for the treatment of osteoporosis and, with one exception, require administration by injection. The ability to administer these drugs by inhalation would facilitate compliance in patients with this chronic condition.

SUMMARY

The Technosphere technology platform is a novel inhalation system for the noninvasive administration of peptide therapeutics that are currently injected. The rapid PK profile that characterizes this delivery system may also be beneficial in the delivery of other metabolic proteins and hormones. However, this technology platform is not limited to large molecules. Formulations of small molecule drugs may find application in delivering rapid relief from pain and nausea. Ongoing studies have also demonstrated that proteins (including insulin) can be stabilized against degradation by association with Technosphere particles. This property may prove invaluable in the development of fragile protein and vaccine therapeutics. Taken together, these properties of Technosphere technology have the potential to provide drug delivery solutions across a wide variety of therapeutic areas encompassing numerous disease states.

REFERENCES

1. Hock JM, Gera I. Effects of continuous and intermittent administration and inhibition of resorption on the anabolic response of bone to parathyroid hormone. J Bone Miner Res 1992; 7:65–72.

2. Neer RM, Arnaud CD, Zanchetta JR, et al. Effect of parathyroid hormone (1–34) on fractures and bone mineral density in postmenopausal women with osteoporosis. N Engl J Med 2001; 344:1434–41.
3. Calles-Escandon J, Robbins D. Loss of early phase of insulin release in humans impairs glucose tolerance and blunts thermic effect of glucose. Diabetes 1987; 36:1167–72.
4. Polonsky KS, Given BD, Hirsch LJ, et al. Abnormal patterns of insulin secretion in non-insulin-dependent diabetes mellitus. N Engl J Med 1988; 318:1231–9.
5. Heinemann L, Heise T. Current status of the development of inhaled insulin. Br J Diab Vasc Dis 2004; 4:295–301.
6. Hirsh I. Insulin analogues. N Engl J Med 2005; 352:174–83.
7. Bergeron RJ, Phanstiel O, Yao GW, et al. Macromolecular self-assembly of diketopiperazine tetrapeptides. J Am Chem Soc 1994; 116:8479–84.
8. Bergeron RJ, Yao GW, Erdos GW, et al.An investigation of the impact of molecular geometry upon microcapsule self-assembly. J Am Chem Soc 1995; 117:6658–65.
9. Brange J, Owens DR, Kang S, et al. Monomeric insulins and their experimental and clinical implications. Diabetes Care 1990; 13:923–54.
10. White JR Jr, Campbell RK, Hirsch IB. Novel insulins and strict glycemic control: Analogues approximate normal insulin secretory response. Postgrad Med 2003; 113:30–6.
11. Richards JP, Stickelmeyer MP, Flora DB, et al. Self-association properties of monomeric insulin analogs under formulation conditions. Pharm Res 1998; 15(9):1434–41.
12. Brunzell JD, Robertson RP, Lerner RL, et al. Relationships between fasting plasma glucose levels and insulin secretion during intravenous glucose tolerance tests. J Clin Endocrinol Metabol 1976; 42:222–9.

Index

---

t = location of tables.
f = location of figures.